VETERINARY ANATOMY

VETERINARY ANATOMY
BASIC, COMPARATIVE, AND CLINICAL

By M. J. SHIVELY, D.V.M., M.S., Ph.D.

Drawings by SHARON ASHBY

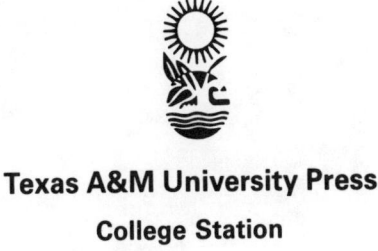

Texas A&M University Press

College Station

Copyright © 1984 by Michael J. Shively
All rights reserved

Library of Congress Cataloging in Publication Data

Shively, Michael J., 1946–
   Veterinary anatomy.

   Includes bibliographies and index.
   1. Veterinary anatomy and index.
SF761.S56   1985   636.089'1   84-40132
ISBN 0-89096-202-2

Second printing, 1987

Manufactured in the United States of America

Dedicated to . . .
 Doriann Sheri, for her warmth,
  Lorilynn Meri, for her spirit,
   James Merrill, for his strength,
    James Jefferson, for his innocence,
And especially to Annie, who made them all possible.

CONTENTS

Preface... ix
Acknowledgments... xi
Introduction.. 1
1. Thoracic Limb Osteology... 11
2. Thoracic Limb Myology... 39
3. Thoracic Limb Arthrology.. 67
4. Thoracic Limb Angiology... 87
5. Thoracic Limb Neurology.. 101
6. Plevic Limb Osteology.. 125
7. Pelvic Limb Myology.. 149
8. Pelvic Limb Arthrology... 167
9. Pelvic Limb Angiology.. 199
10. Pelvic Limb Neurology.. 209
11. Abdomen.. 231
12. Thorax... 267
13. Central Angiology and Lymphatic System..................................... 293
14. Urinary System... 325
15. Male Reproductive System... 339
16. Female Reproductive System... 363
17. Odontology... 379
18. Rachiology... 403
19. Head... 429
20. Avian Anatomy.. 469
21. Anatomy of the Pig... 489
22. Biology of Laboratory Animals.. 507
23. Integumentary System... 537
Index.. 563

PREFACE

"Anatomical study has one application for the man of science who loves knowledge for its own sake, another for him who values it only to demonstrate that nature does nought in vain, a third for the one who provides himself from anatomy with data for investigating a function, physical or mental, and yet another for the practitioner who has to remove splinters and missiles efficiently."

Galen

Veterinary Anatomy: Basic, Comparative, and Clinical is a revised version of the author's earlier work, Fundamentals of Veterinary Anatomy. Every subject area has been significantly modified, and many new illustrations have been added. The majority of the text treats the major domestic species (horse, ox, pig, dog, cat) in a comparative manner. Special sections on avian anatomy and laboratory animals are included because these species are often ignored or only superficially covered in popular texts. A section on porcine anatomy is included (even though the pig is also covered comparatively in other sections) to accommodate those who may want a quick reference on that species.

This material was assembled to serve as an accurate, readable summary of the essentials of veterinary anatomy. It was written in particular for veterinary students, who are frequently bewildered by anatomic texts in which essential facts are camouflaged by trivial details. Clinical applications of anatomy were emphasized in order to incorporate the long-range goal of contributing to the education of a practitioner.

A combination of systemic and regional approaches to anatomy have been used. Within a given area, basic and comparative features are addressed first, followed by clinical application of the involved anatomy. The anatomic nomenclature conforms to the Nomina Anatomica Veterinaria (3rd ed., 1983). Anatomic terms placed in quotes are slang, obsolete, or otherwise unofficial. Carnivore refers to the domestic dog and cat (Canis familiaris and Felis catus). Ruminant refers to the ox (Bos taurus and Bos indicus), sheep (Ovis aries) and goat (Capra hircus). Ungulate indicates the domestic species with hooves including the ruminants, pig (Sus scrofa domestica), and horse (Equus caballus). Domestic mammals refers to all of the above.

One is always concerned about what to include and what to omit in assembling a text of this type. "Detail" to one individual may be basic information to another. The author invites criticism of this work, and hopes that it will fulfill a useful position in the literature of veterinary anatomy.

M. J. Shively

College Station, Texas
July, 1984

ACKNOWLEDGEMENTS

Publication of this work represents the collective and cooperative efforts of numerous individuals. The author is indebted to his colleagues in the Department of Veterinary Anatomy, and especially to the veterinary students at Texas A&M University (particularly the classes of 1982, 1983, and 1984) for serving as critical resources. In his humble opinion, the role of students in the realization of a text of this type cannot be over-emphasized. Their motivation and curiosity cause them to question most everything; the intensity of their curriculum gives them an inherent right to offer constructive criticism; and their intelligence and resilience allow them to succeed in spite of their adversity.

Grateful appreciation is due Ms. Sharon Ashby for the illustrations. Appreciation is also extended to Dr. R. E. Habel, Dr. J. E. Smallwood, Dr. P. Popesko, and to the Paul Parey Publishing Company for permission to modify and use some of their illustrations. Similar thanks go to the Academic Press, Harvard University Press, Saunders Publishing Company, Sudz Publishing Company, and Waverly Press. Special appreciation is extended to Dr. F. J. Stein for his assistance with the chapter on anatomy of laboratory animals and, in particular, for authoring the parts on gerbils and on non-human primates. Thanks are also extended to other outstanding veterinary anatomists, like Dr. R. E. Habel, whose published knowledge in applied anatomy serves as a model of accuracy and excellence. Other members of the anatomic elite, like Dr. J. E. Stump and Dr. D. C. Van Sickle, deserve thanks for the important roles they played in the author's professional development.

Technical assistance was drawn from several sources. A number of excellent typists worked on various phases of the rough draft including Ms. Annette Gause, Ms. Lynn Dudek, and Ms. Joan Clark. The efforts of several other typists at A B Dick, Inc. is also appreciated. Ms. Pat Stroud proofread every draft to the point that she probably deserves an honorary degree in Anatomy. Ms. Dori Pye also made a number of editorial improvements.

Finally, the author expresses gratitude to his gracious wife, Ann, for the dedication, love, and children that bring such joy to his life. She so fulfills his life that he always has a smile in his heart.

INTRODUCTION

Anatomic Nomenclature

The study of anatomy involves three basic facets of information: name, location, and function. The names of anatomic structures are very important because of their use throughout the scientific community. Some individuals argue that names of structures do not matter as long as their locations and functions are understood. However, this position is only valid for isolated individuals who lack access to scientific literature, presentations, and/or colleagues.

Historically, the efficiency of anatomic nomenclature has been compromised by the use of multiple names for anatomic structures. To combat the confusion resulting from this practice, a nomenclature committee was formed to select and assemble a list of proper (official) anatomic names. The resulting list was published in 1968, as the Nomina Anatomic Veterinaria (NAV), and then revised in 1973 and again in 1983 [1]. Although the committee which formulated the NAV has often been accused of fabricating new names for structures, most of the names selected were already widely used by the scientific community. Seven guidelines were followed by the committee in compiling the official nomenclature [1]:

1. Aside from a very limited number of exceptions, each anatomic concept should be designated by a single term.

2. Each term should be in Latin in the official list, but the anatomists of each country are free to translate the official Latin terms into the language of instruction.

3. Each term should be as short and simple as possible.

4. The terms should be easy to remember and should have, above all, both instructive and descriptive value.

5. Structures that are closely related topographically should have similar names: for example, arteria femoralis, vena femoralis, nervus femoralis.

6. Differentiating adjectives should generally be opposites, as major and minor, superficialis and profundus.

7. Terms derived from proper names (eponyms) should not be used.

Obviously, not every term listed by the NAV [1] can properly reflect all 7 of these principles. "Fetlock" joint, for example, is a shorter and simpler term than the recommended metacarpophalangeal joint (or metatarsophalangeal joint). However, "fetlock" has little instructive or descriptive value and it can refer to either thoracic or pelvic limbs; therefore, it does not conform to principles 1 or 4 [2].

Body Planes and Directional Terms

The study of vertebrate anatomy involves continual references to body planes and directional terms. Because of the postural differences between man and the quadrupeds, many of the descriptive directional terms from human anatomy (anterior, posterior, superior, inferior) have different meanings when applied to quadrupeds [3]. Consequently, these terms are used in veterinary anatomy only in reference to some organs in the head (especially the eye and ear).

Plane--a surface, real or imaginary, along which any two points can be connected by a straight line.

Median plane--a plane which longitudinally divides the head, neck, or trunk into equal right and left halves. The concept is also used in dividing a limb along its axis (although the resulting halves are not equal).

Sagittal plane--a plane parallel to the median plane. A "mid-sagittal" plane is a median plane.

Transverse plane--a plane which intercepts the long axis of a body part perpendicularly.

Dorsal plane--a plane perpendicular to the median plane and simultaneously perpendicular to a transverse plane through a given body part.

Cranial--toward or relatively closer to the head. This term is used in reference to the neck, the trunk, and on the limbs proximal to the carpus and tarsus. On the head, the term rostral is used (in reference to the nose) for the same directional concept (Figure I-1).

Caudal--toward or relatively closer to the tail. This term is used on the head, neck, trunk, and on the limbs proximal to the carpus and tarsus.

Dorsal--toward or relatively closer to the back (top) of the head, neck, trunk, or tail. On the limbs, dorsal is used instead of cranial on the manus and pes.

Ventral--toward or relatively closer to the underside of the head, neck, trunk, or tail.

Palmar--the aspect of the manus on which the supporting surface is located. It is used instead of caudal or volar from the carpus distally.

Plantar--the aspect of the pes on which the supporting surface is located. It is used instead of caudal or volar from the tarsus distally.

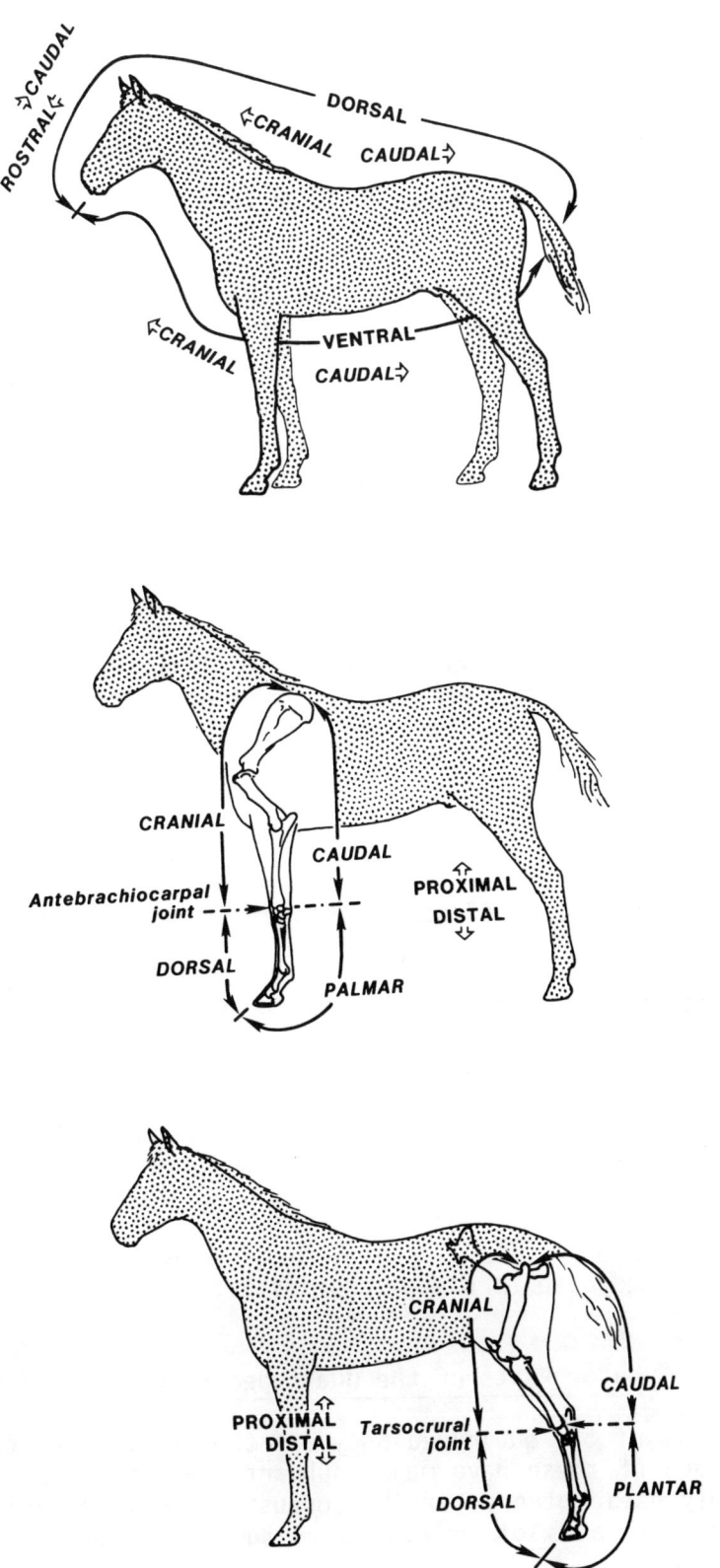

Figure I-1

Application of Directional Terms to Various Parts of the Body

From Shively, 1983 [4]

Medial--toward or relatively closer to the median plane.

Lateral--away from or relatively further from the median plane.

Axial, abaxial--terms which indicate a position relatively closer (axial) or further (abaxial) from the longitudinal axis of the limb. Use of these terms is generally restricted to the digits of multidigited species where the functional axis of the limb is considered to course between the third and fourth digits.

Proximal--commonly used in reference to the limbs where it implies a position near or relatively closer to the trunk. In other usages, it may refer to an obvious point of reference. When applied to vessels, it implies a position closer to the heart; within the kidney, it refers to the portions of the uriniferous tubule closer to the glomerulus, etc.

Distal--commonly used in reference to the limbs where it implies a position away from or relatively further from the trunk. In other usages, it may refer to another obvious point of reference (see proximal).

Superficial--near or relatively closer to the outer aspect of the body or part.

Deep--near or relatively closer to the central aspect of the body or part.

External--near or relatively closer to the outer surface.*

Internal--near or relatively closer to the center of a structure.*

Intermediate--a position between medial and lateral aspects (intermediate tubercle of the equine humerus).

Middle--the position between any paired directional terms except medial and lateral (i.e., cranial and caudal, dorsal and ventral, superficial and deep, proximal and distal, etc.).

Major Parts of the Quadruped Body

The major parts of the quadruped body are the head, neck, trunk, tail, and the limbs. Each of these have major subparts, as listed below. Some of these are commonly used, others rarely. Confusion sometimes arises because of similarity in the names of related structures (carpus, carpal bones, carpal joint).

---

*More restrictive definitions of internal and external limit their use to hollow organs or body cavities.

Head
    Cranium
        vertex--the crown of the head (uppermost part)
        sinciput--the dorsal half of the cranium
            frons--forehead (brow)
        occiput--the caudal aspect of the head
        tempora--the left and right lateral aspects of the head
            dorsal to the zygomatic arch
        horn (cornu)
        ear (auris)
        auricle--external ear, pinna

    Face
        eye
            superior and inferior palpebrae (eyelids)
            palpebral rim (margin)
            eyeball
            infrapalpebral sulcus (groove)
        nose
            dorsum of the nose
            apex (tip of the nose) ⎫
            wing of the nose   ⎪ Individuality of the nose and
            naris (nostril)   ⎬ superior lip as well as their
            nasal plane   ⎪ morphological interactions
            nasolabial plane   ⎪ vary among domestic animals.
            rostrum   ⎭ (See Chapter 23.)
            rostral
        mouth
            superior and inferior lips
            oral rim (margin)
            oral cavity
            tongue
            fauces--the junction of the oral cavity and the pharynx
            bucca (cheeks)

        mentum (chin)

        mentolabial groove

Neck
    nucha--the dorsum (nape) of the neck
    juba (mane)
    palear (dewlap)
    larynx
        laryngeal prominence
    pharynx
    trachea
    esophagus

Trunk
    dorsum (back)
        vertebral column
        vertebral canal

thorax
- thoracic cavity
- pectus (chest)--the ventral aspect of the thorax
    - thoracic mammae
        - mammary papillae

abdomen
- abdominal cavity
- epigastric fossa--the area just caudal to the xiphoid process
- umbilicus
- latus--flank
    - plica lateralis--fold of the flank or lateral fold
- lumbus--the lumbar portion of the back (loin)
- inguen--the caudolateral aspect of the ventral abdomen
- abdominal mammae
    - mammary papillae
- intermammary groove
- uber (udder)
- prepuce
- scrotum

Pelvis
- pelvic cavity
- coxa (hip)
- nates (clunes, buttocks)--the area caudal to the hips
- perineum
- anus
- crena ani--the notch (groove) between the nates
- pudendum femininum (vulva)

Tail
- root
- cirrus caudae (the "switch" or tail tuft of oxen)

Thoracic limb
- axilla
    - axillary fold
- brachium
    - cranial, caudal, medial, and lateral surfaces and lateral and medial bicipital grooves
- cubitus
- antebrachium
    - cranial, caudal, medial, and lateral surfaces
- manus
    - dorsum of manus
    - palm of manus
    - carpus
        - carpal pad
    - metacarpus
        - dorsal, palmar, medial, and lateral surfaces
        - metacarpal pad
        - ergot (equine homologue of metacarpal pad)

        digits of manus
            digit I (pollux)
            digits II-V
                dorsal, palmar, medial, and lateral surfaces
                solar surface
                axial and abaxial surfaces (in multidigited species)
            paradigit--a reduced digit ("dewclaw")
            paraungula (ungulates), paraunguicula (carnivores)--a paradigit which lacks skeletal components (formed of soft tissue only)
            ungula (hoof)
            unguicula (nail, claw)

    Pelvic limb
        femur--the thigh. It is supported by the os femoris.
            cranial, caudal, medial, and lateral surfaces
        genu (stifle)
            poples--the caudal aspect of the genu
            patella
        crus--leg
            cranial, caudal, medial, and lateral surfaces
            sura--the calf of the leg
            medial and lateral malleoli
        pes
            dorsum of the pes
            plantum of the pes
            tarsus
            calx--heel
            torus tarseus (horse only; see Chapter 23)
            metatarsus
            dorsal, plantar, medial, and lateral surfaces
            metatarsal pad
            ergot (equine homologue of metatarsal pad)
            digits of the pes
                digit I (hallux)
                digits II-V
            remaining parts of digits are homologous to their counterparts in the manus

Major Regions of the Body

Considerable inventive nomenclature pervades the professional literature in regard to the regions of the body. Most official regional names correspond to major bones or other organs located in the area.

    Regions of the Head
        cranial regions
            occipital region
            parietal region
            temporal region
            supraorbital region
            frontal region
            cornual region

       regions of the face
           nasal region
               dorsal and lateral nasal regions
               region of the naris
           oral region
               region of the maxillary lip
               region of the mandibular lip
           mental region (region of the chin)
           orbital region
               region of the superior eyelid (palpebra)
               region of the inferior eyelid
           zygomatic region
           infraorbital region
           region of the temporomandibular joint
           masseteric region
           buccal region
           maxillary region
           mandibular region
           subhyoid region

Regions of the Neck
    dorsal border of the neck
    dorsal and lateral regions of the neck
    parotid region
        retromandibular fossa
    retroauricular region
    pharyngeal region
    brachiocephalic region
    jugular groove
    sternocephalic region
    prescapular region
    ventral regions of the neck
        region of the larynx
        region of the trachea

Pectoral Regions
    presternal region
    median and lateral pectoral grooves
    sternal region
    region of the thoracic mammae
    scapular region
        region of the scapular cartilage
        supraspinous region
        infraspinous region
        acromial region
    costal region
    cardiac region
    costal arch

Abdominal Regions (see Chapter 11)
    cranial abdominal region
        hypochondriac region (left and right)
        xiphoid region

    middle abdominal region
      lateral abdominal region (left and right)
        paralumbar fossa
        region of the lateral fold
      umbilical region
    caudal abdominal region
      inguinal region (left and right)
      pubic region
      preputial region
    region of the abdominal mammae
    region of the inguinal mammae
    region of the udder

Regions of the Back
    region of the thoracic vertebrae
      interscapular region (includes the withers in large domestic
        mammals)
    lumbar region

Regions of the Pelvis
    sacral region
    gluteal region
    region of the tuber coxae
    clunial region
    region of the ischiatic tuberosity
    region of the tail
    perineal region
      anal region
      urogenital region
    scrotal region
    supramammary region

Regions of the Thoracic Limb
    region of the humeral joint
    axillary region
    brachial region
    tricipital region
    tricipital border
    cubital region
    olecranon region
    antebrachial regions (cranial, caudal, medial, and lateral)
    carpal regions (dorsal, palmar, medial, and lateral)
    metacarpal regions (dorsal, palmar, medial, and lateral)
    metacarpophalangeal region
    region of the proximal phalanx (compedal region in ungulates =
      pastern region)
    region of the middle phalanx (coronal region in ungulates)
    interdigital space (absent in horse)
    unguicular region (region of the nail)
    ungular region (region of the hoof)

Regions of the Pelvic Limb
    region of the coxal joint
        trochanteric region
    femoral regions (cranial, caudal, medial, and lateral)
    genual regions (cranial, caudal, medial, and lateral)
        patellar region
    popliteal region
    crural regions (cranial, caudal, medial, and lateral)
        region of the common calcanean tendon
    tarsal regions (dorsal, plantar, medial, and lateral)
        region of the calcaneus
    metatarsal regions (dorsal, plantar, medial, and lateral)
    metatarsophalangeal region
    (other digital regions same as thoracic limb)

References

1. International Committee on Veterinary Gross Anatomical Nomenclature. 1983. Nomina Anatomica Veterinaria, third ed. Published by the Committee, Ithaca, New York.

2. Shively, M. J. 1977. Anatomic nomenclature: past, present, and future. JAVMA 170(1):69-72.

3. Habel, R. E. 1982. Applied Veterinary Anatomy, second ed. Published by the author, Ithaca, New York.

4. Shively, M. J. 1983. Anatomic nomenclature used in equine practice. Equine Prac. 5(6):6-16.

THORACIC LIMB OSTEOLOGY

The bones of the thoracic limb include the scapula, humerus, radius and ulna, carpal bones, metacarpal bones, phalanges, and a number of sesamoid bones. For each of these, a list of the significant anatomic features which are present in most domestic mammals is given. This is followed by comparative, clinical, and developmental information. Minor anatomic features with no obvious clinical significance have been intentionally omitted.

I. SCAPULA (a triangle with 2 surfaces, 3 angles, 3 borders)

   A. Major features:

   costal surface--the whole medial side of the bone
      serrated surface--the dorsal aspect of the costal surface (where the serratus ventralis m. attaches)
      subscapular fossa--the ventral aspect of the costal surface (where the subscapularis m. attaches)
   lateral surface
      spine--the ridge on which the trapezius and deltoideus mm. attach
      supraspinous fossa--the depression craniodorsal to the spine
      infraspinous fossa--the depression caudoventral to the spine
   cranial, caudal, and ventral angles--the 3 corners of the triangular shape
   cranial, caudal, and dorsal borders--the 3 sides of the triangular shape
   acromion--the distal extremity of the spine
   neck--the constriction near the ventral angle
   infraglenoid tubercle--the roughened area near the caudal aspect of the neck where the teres minor m. attaches
   supraglenoid tubercle--the projection near the ventral aspect of the cranial border for the attachment of the biceps brachii m.
   coracoid process--the projection at the cranial aspect of the ventral angle for the attachment of the coracobrachialis m.
   glenoid cavity--the articular surface at the ventral angle
   scapular cartilage--a cartilaginous extension of the dorsal border

   B. Selected comparative, clinical, and developmental features:

   1. A bony enlargement called the spinal tuber is present near the middle of the lateral border of the spine in the pig and horse [1]. Some authors consider the ox [2] and cat [3] to have one also, but it is poorly developed in these species (Fig. 1-1A).

   2. The horse lacks an acromion [4].

   3. The acromion of the cat has a caudal projection termed the suprahamate process [3]. Other domesticated mammals do not have a suprahamate process, but it is present in many laboratory species. This feature of the feline scapula should be recognized as normal radiographically. The distal portion of the acromion in cats is termed the hamate process (Fig. 1-1B).

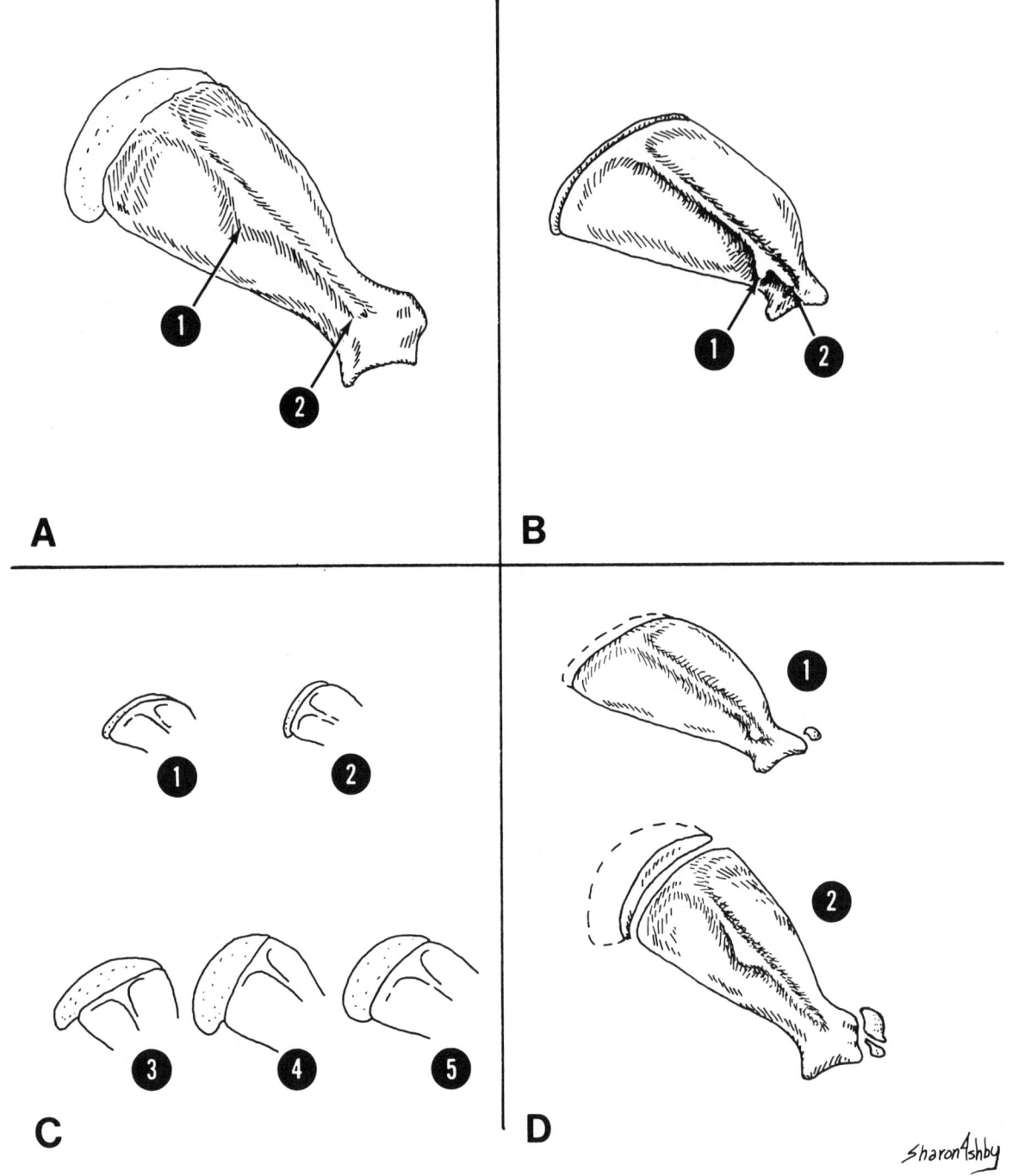

Figure 1-1

Selected Comparative, Clinical, and Developmental Features of the Scapula

- A. Equine scapula: spinal tuber (1) and lack of acromion (2).
- B. Feline scapula: suprahamate (1) and hamate (2) processes.
- C. Scapular cartilages: cat (1), dog (2), pig (3), ox (4), and horse (5).
- D. Centers of ossification: dog (1) and horse (2)--dotted lines indicate scapular cartilage.

4. The scapular cartilage is well developed in the ungulates and poorly developed in the carnivores [2]. It serves as an additional area of attachment of the rhomboideus m. (Fig. 1-1C).

5. In carnivores, a secondary center of ossification for the supraglenoid tubercle appears at about 6 weeks of age and is usually fused to the parent bone by 6 to 8 months of age [5] (Fig. 1-1D1).*

6. In the horse there are 4 centers of ossification [4] (Fig. 1-1D2). The centers for the main part of the bone, supraglenoid tubercle, and cranial part of the glenoid cavity are primary centers which fuse to each other at about a year of age. The dorsal border of the scapula is a secondary center which unites some time after the third year.

7. Fractures of the scapula are usually limited to its neck in carnivores, but in the horse, where the neck is comparatively thicker, they have been reported in several parts of the bone [6].

II. CLAVICLE

In man and many other vertebrates, the clavicle articulates with the sternum and scapula. Pigs, ruminants, and horses do not have a clavicle, and it is vestigial in the carnivores. In both dogs and cats, the clavicle is embedded in soft tissue on the deep surface of the brachiocephalicus muscle, and it does not articulate with the rest of the skeleton. The feline clavicle is consistently osseous and is obvious radiographically. In the dog, it is usually so small and mineralized so poorly (if at all) that it is often difficult to find (either grossly or radiographically).

III. HUMERUS

A. Major features:

head--the rounded, proximal end which articulates with the glenoid cavity
neck
greater (major) tubercle--on the proximal, craniolateral aspect
    crest of major tubercle--cranial ridge from greater tubercle
lesser (minor) tubercle--on the proximal, medial aspect
intertubercular groove--transmits the tendon of biceps brachii m.
tricipital line--attachment for lateral head of triceps brachii m.
body
    deltoid tuberosity--where the deltoideus m. attaches (craniolateral)
    brachial groove--where the brachialis m. lies
    teres major tuberosity--the subtle roughened area on the medial side,
        where the teres major and latissimus dorsi mm. attach
condyle--the whole distal end of the humerus
    capitulum--the lateral part of the articular surface
    trochlea--the medial part of the articular surface

---

*A primary center of ossification in a bone is an area which mineralizes before birth. A given bone may have one, more than one, or none. A secondary center of ossification is an area which begins mineralizing after birth. In bones which have no primary centers (carpal bones of carnivores) the areas of mineralization that subsequently develop are usually just termed "centers of ossification" rather than secondary centers. Some authors definte "primary center" as the first area to ossify. Using this definition, every bone has one and only one.

Figure 1-2

Selected Comparative, Clinical, and Developmental Features of the Humerus

    A.   Craniolateral aspect of left equine humerus (proximal end):
          1.   lesser tubercle
          2.   intermediate tubercle
          3.   cranial part of greater tubercle
          4.   caudal part of greater tubercle

    B.   One method of repair of a T or Y fracture of the humeral condyle in a dog showing the relation of the condylar screw, intramedullary pin, and supratrochlear foramen (a) from cranial (1) and medial (2) perspectives. An intramedullary pin will seat distally inside the medial epicondyle rather than the lateral one because the medial epicondyle is directly in line with the diaphysis.

    C.   Cranial aspect of the right humeral condyle of a cat:
          1.   supracondylar foramen
          2.   coronoid fossa
          3.   radial fossa

    D.   Lateral aspect of the humeral condyle. In all species the caudal aspect of the medial epicondyle (1) has a square profile and that of the lateral epicondyle (2) has a rounded outline.

    E.   Centers of ossification in the humeri of the dog (1) and horse (2). Primary centers (areas mineralized at birth) are stippled. The main part of the equine condyle develops from a single center. The additional center in the distal epiphysis of the equine humerus is in the caudal aspect of the medial epicondyle. The dog has a single center of ossification for the proximal epiphysis and three for the distal epiphysis. The horse has two proximally and two distally. Both species have a single center of ossification for the humeral diaphysis (body).

    F.   A lateral perspective of a canine humerus to illustrate how the curvature of the bone allows a retrograded intramedullary pin to miss the humeral head and emerge from the bone by penetrating the craniolateral cortex.

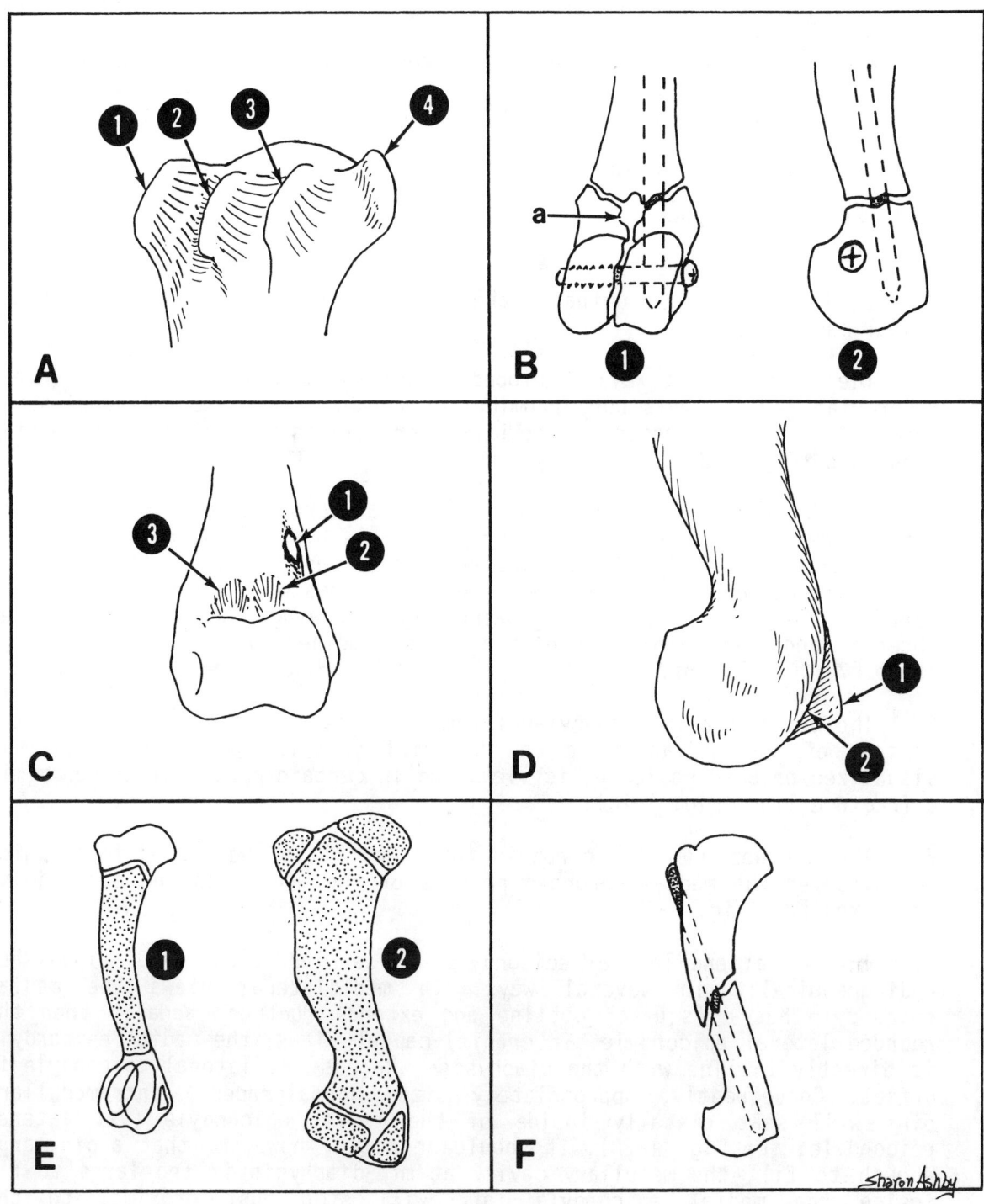

Figure 1-2

olecranon fossa--receives the ulnar anconeal process during extension of the cubital joint (located caudally)
    radial fossa--receives the radial head during marked cubital flexion
medial epicondyle--attachment for caudomedial antebrachial muscles
lateral epicondyle--attachment for craniolateral antebrachial muscles
    crest of lateral epicondyle--origin of extensor carpi radialis m.

B. Selected comparative, clinical, and developmental features:

1. The greater tubercle has cranial and caudal parts in the ungulates. In the carnivores, a division is not obvious [2].

2. In the horse and ruminants the lesser tubercle also has cranial and caudal parts [2].

3. The horse has a well-developed intermediate tubercle in the intertubercular groove. This bony prominence may act as a brake shoe against an indentation in the tendon of the biceps brachii as part of the equine stay apparatus (Fig. 1-2A).

4. The dog (and occasionally the pig) has a supratrochlear foramen in the distal humerus through which nothing passes [1]. This foramen forms because of the close proximity of the olecranon fossa and the radial fossa. "T" or "Y" fractures of the distal humerus of carnivores often fracture into this foramen. They are commonly repaired by screwing the two epicondyles together and then pinning or plating this combined distal fragment to the shaft [7] (Fig. 1-2B).

5. The cat has a supracondylar foramen in the medial epicondyle for the passage of the median nerve and brachial vessels [3]. This foramen is visualized on some radiographic views and in certain perspectives can mimic a fracture line (Fig. 1-2C).

6. The cat has a subtle coronoid fossa medial to the radial fossa which accommodates the medial coronoid process of the ulna when the elbow joint is flexed [3] (Fig. 1-2C).

7. The medial and lateral epicondyles of carnivores can be distinguished radiographically in several ways. In mediolateral views the medial epicondyle has a "square" outline and extends further caudally than the rounded lateral epicondyle. In cranial-caudal views, the medial epicondyle is directly in line with the diaphysis* whereas the lateral epicondyle is offset. Consequently, appropriately sized normalgraded** intramedullary pins will seat distally inside of the medial epicondyle (vs. lateral epicondyle; see Fig. 1-2D). It should be noted, however, that a pin large enough to fill the medullary cavity at mid-diaphysis is too large to fit inside the medial epicondyle, and will stop just proximal to the supratrochlear foramen.

---

*The diaphysis is the shaft of any long bone. Either end of a long bone is an epiphysis. In growing long bones, the term metaphysis refers to the portion of the diaphysis immediately adjacent to either epiphysis.

**The term normalgrade as used in intramedullary pinning refers herein to driving a pin distally in a bone or bone fragment. The term retrograde refers to driving a pin proximally.

8. Retrograded intramedullary pins will emerge on the craniolateral aspect of the humerus, and will miss the humeral head because of the curvature of the bone (Fig. 1-2F).

9. Carnivores typically have 5 centers of ossification for the humerus: a primary center for the diaphysis and 4 secondary centers (Fig. 1-2E):
    a. proximal epiphysis (head and greater tubercle)
    b. medial part of condyle
    c. lateral part of condyle
    d. caudal part of medial epicondyle

10. The equine humerus has 5 centers of ossification. All five centers are present at birth (Fig. 1-2E). In contrast to the pattern in carnivores, a separate center is present for the greater tubercle (resulting in two centers proximally), and the main part of the condyle develops from only a single center (resulting in only two centers distally).

11. The humeral shaft may be approached craniolaterally between the brachiocephalicus and brachialis mm. and medially between the biceps brachii and triceps brachii mm. The distal end (condyle) may be approached by a "transolecranon" procedure in which the tuber olecrani of the ulna is temporarily removed (see Chapter 3) [9].

IV. RADIUS

  A. Major features:

    head--the proximal epiphysis
        fovea capitis--articulates with humeral condyle
    neck--part adjacent to the head
    body
    trochlea--the distal epiphysis
        carpal articular surface
        (radial) styloid process--on the medial side

  B. Selected comparative, clinical, and developmental features:

    1. The radius and ulna remain separate and distinct in the pig and carnivores, but they fuse in the ruminants and horse (Fig. 1-3A). In the ruminants, the two bones can be easily differentiated even though they are fused, but in the horse, they blend indistinguishably.

    2. The radial tuberosity (for the attachment of the biceps brachii m.) is a general feature present in all species, but it is small and difficult to distinguish (especially in carnivores).

    3. The radius develops from a primary center (body) separated from two secondary centers (head and trochlea) by proximal and distal physes [5] (Fig. 1-3B). In carnivores, about 40% of the increase in length of the radius during growth occurs proximally and about 60% occurs distally (some workers have reported 30% and 70%; the exact percentage is academic). This is important in growth related deformities of the limb (see ulna) [10].

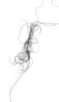

4. Some foals require correction of uneven growth at the distal radial physis (Fig. 1-3C). Large metal staples across the physis have been used to slow growth on the longer (faster growing) side. By bridging the physis on the "long" side, growth is slowed and the "short" side catches up. For this treatment to be effective, the animal must be young enough so that sufficient corrective growth remains, and the staples must be removed at the proper time to prevent over-correction [11]. A more recent surgical correction of this problem is periosteal stripping on the short side to release theoretical tension and allow it to "catch up" in growth [12].

5. On the cranial aspect of the junction of the radial body and trochlea, there are grooves which accommodate tendons (Fig. 1-3D). From medial to lateral directions these grooves are occupied by the tendons of the abductor digit I (pollicis) longus, extensor carpi radialis, and common digital extensor muscles. Surgical approaches to this area to remove fracture chips in dogs and horses are made between these tendons [9,13].

Figure 1-3

Selected Comparative, Clinical, and Developmental Features of the Radius

- A. Radius and ulna of the pig (1), ox (2), and horse (3) showing the progressive fusion of the two bones. In the pig (and carnivores) they remain unfused. In the ruminants they are fused but easily distinguishable, and in the horse they are visually separable only at their proximal aspects.

- B. Cranial view of the radius of a dog showing the approximate positions of the proximal (1) and distal (2) physes. The head (3) and trochlea (4) develop as secondary centers of ossification and their physes contribute about 40% and 60%, respectively, of the total radial elongation during growth.

- C. Correction of uneven growth at the distal radial physis of a foal by use of a metal staple to bridge the "long" side of the physis:

    1. appearance just after insertion of the staple.

        a. distal epiphysis of radius
        b. proximal row of carpal bones
        c. distal row of carpal bones

    2. appearance after growth on the "long" side has been slowed sufficiently to allow the "short" side to catch up.

- D. Cranial aspect of the right radial trochlea of a horse to illustrate the grooves occupied by the tendons of the:

    1. common digital extensor--most lateral.
    2. extensor carpi radialis.
    3. abductor pollicis longus [abductor digit I longus]--most medial.

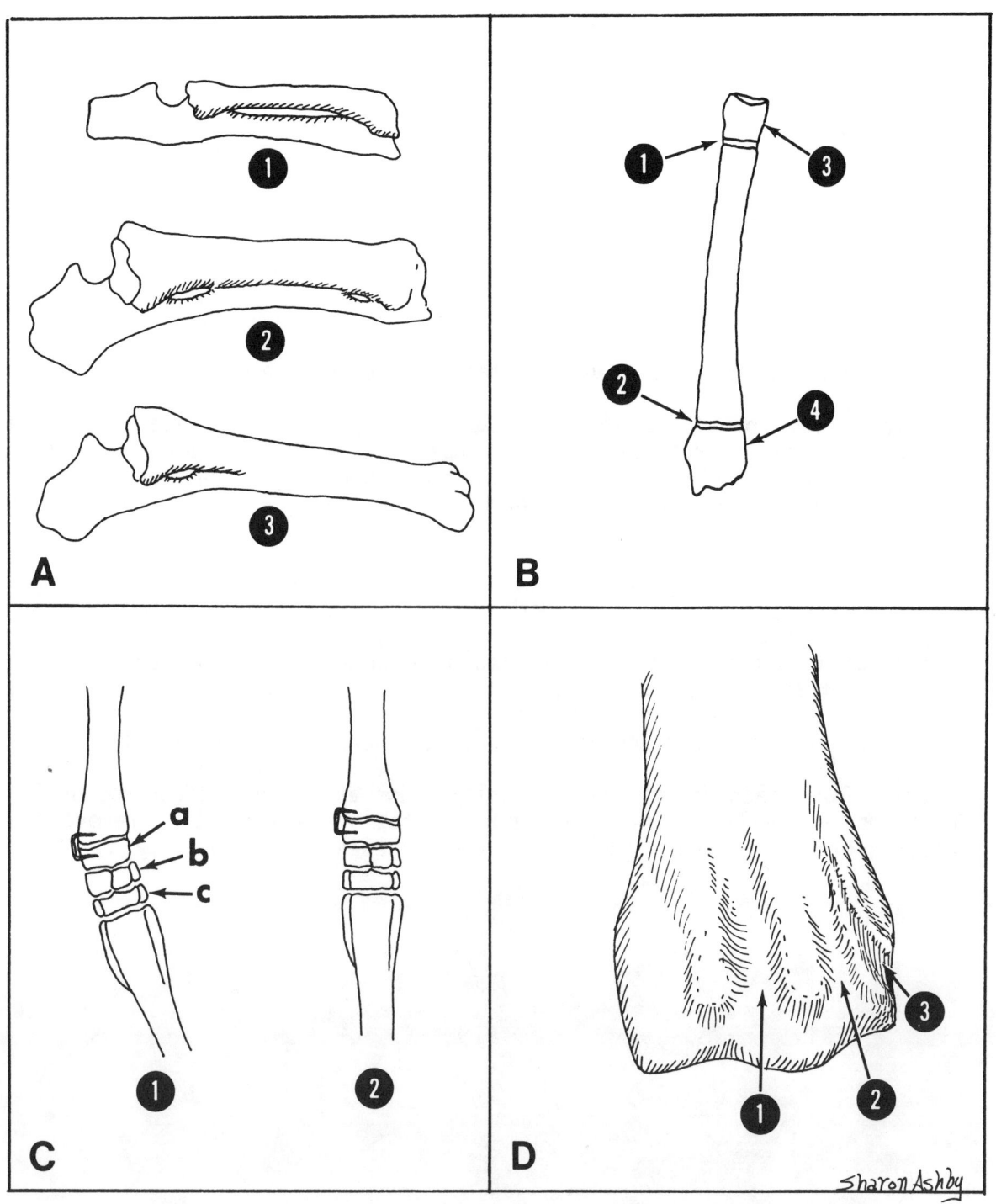

Figure 1-3

Figure 1-4

Selected Comparative, Clinical, and Developmental Features of the Ulna

    A.   Cranial aspect of the distal left radius of a horse. The lateral styloid process (1) forms from the ulna and fuses to the radius during the first few months of age. Complete fusion may not occur for several years and the remaining epiphyseal line should be recognized radiographically as a normal feature.

    B.   Ulna of a carnivore showing the secondary centers of ossification for the ulnar styloid process (1), the anconeal process (2), and the tuber olecrani (3). Only the distal physis (the one associated with the head of the ulna) contributes to the length of the ulna between the elbow and carpus. If it does not keep correct growth pace with bone physes of the radius (Fig. 1-3B), subluxations of the cubital joint, curvature of the antebrachial skeleton, and/or deviations of the manus at (near) the carpus will result.

    C.   Method of reattachment of the anconeal process as a surgical correction for ununited anconeal process (UAP) in dogs. Most surgeons opt to remove the process except in larger dogs where it is necessary for stability.

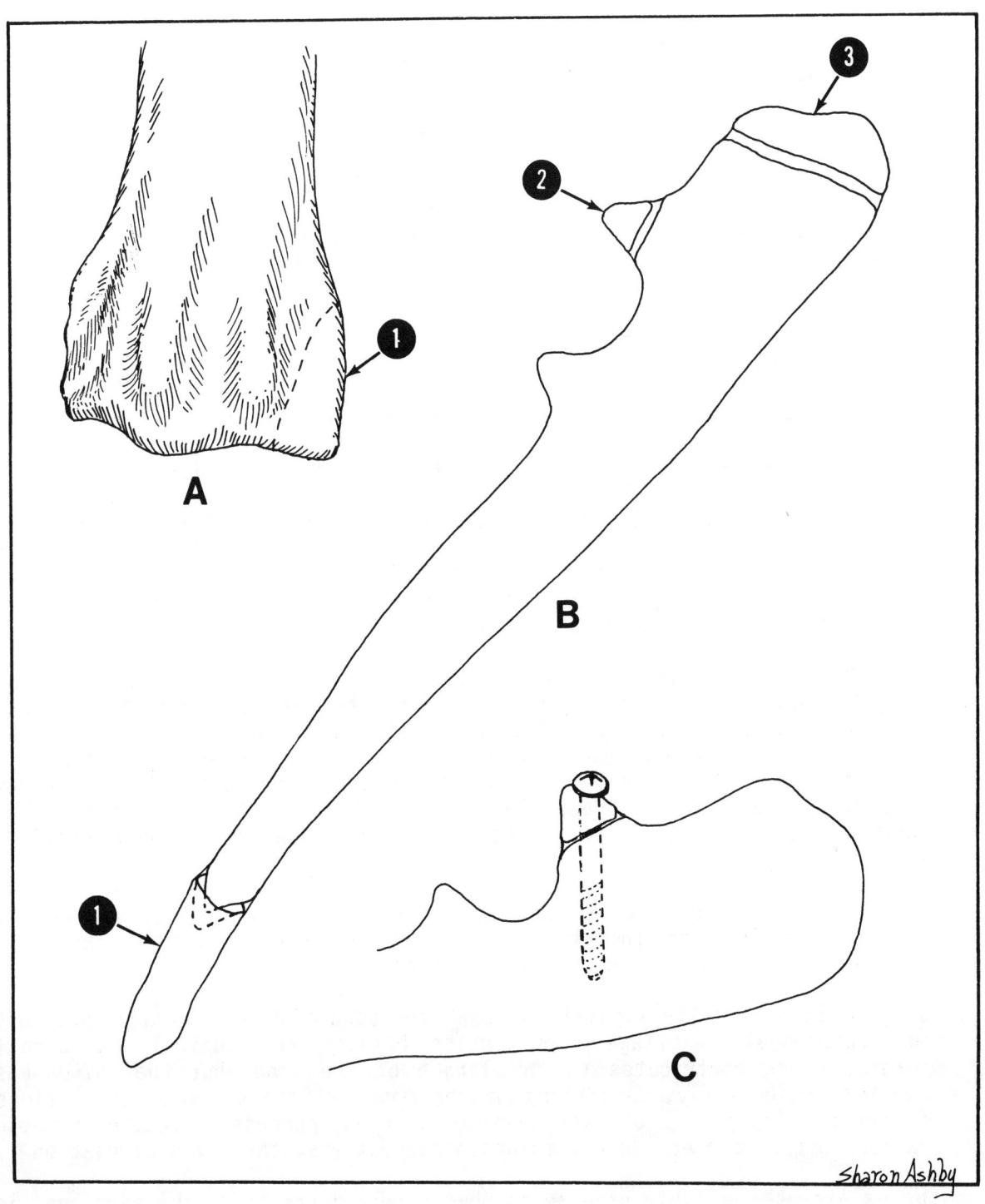

Figure 1-4

V. ULNA

    A. Major features:

        olecranon--the part proximal to the trochlear notch
            tuber olecrani
            anconeal process
        trochlear notch--articulates with the humerus
        medial coronoid process--distal to the trochlear notch
        lateral coronoid process--distal to the trochlear notch
        body
        head--the distal end*
            (ulnar) styloid process
            carpal articular surface

    B. Selected comparative, clinical, and developmental features:

        1. In the horse and ruminants, the ulna fuses to the radius.

        2. In the horse, the ulnar styloid process becomes indistinguishable from the radius after the two bones fuse (Fig. 1-4A). For this reason, the equine radius is considered to have medial and lateral styloid processes. In other words, the equine ulnar and radial styloid processes are termed lateral and medial styloid processes of the radius, respectively [1].

        3. The ulna of carnivores develops from a primary center (in the body) and at least two secondary centers; one in the head and one in the tuber olecrani. Most large dogs have an additional secondary center in the anconeal process which fuses to the parent bone at 4 to 5 months of age [5]. Failure to fuse results in ununited anconeal process (UAP) which may have to be removed [7] (resulting in some loss of cubital stability) or screwed into place [14] (often resulting in osteoarthritic changes)(Fig. 1-4C).

        4. The medial coronoid process may develop from a separate center of ossification in some individuals. Fragmented coronoid process (ununited coronoid process) has been reported in carnivores [16].

        5. It is clinically significant that the ulna of the carnivores has only one epiphyseal cartilage ("physis")** between the cubital and carpal joints, which contributes to the length of the bone, but the radius has two.*** Consequently, deviations of the manus at the carpus, dislocations of the cubital joint, or even ununited anconeal process may occur if these various growth centers do not maintain correctly synchronized elongation

---

*All long bones except the tibia have an epiphysis termed the head. The term head is based on the shape of the corresponding skeletal element in man, and bears no relationship with the orientation of the bone. The heads of the humerus, radius, femur, and fibula are located proximally, but in the metacarpal and metatarsal bones, proximal and middle phalanges, and also in the ulna, the heads are located distally.
**Epiphyseal cartilages are located between centers of ossification. Epiphyseal cartilage is the proper name among a host of unofficial synonyms, including "physis," "growth plate," "growth cartilage," and "epiphyseal plate."
***A proximal physis of the ulna is present, but it does not contribute to ulnar length between the cubital and carpal joints.

("premature closure"). Because the radius elongates in two places between the elbow and carpus, but the ulna does so in only one, the radius must slide distally along the ulna during growth. Consequently, cross-pinning the radius and ulna to stabilize a fracture in a young animal is contraindicated since the same abnormalities may result as noted above for asynchronous premature closures [10].

6. In young growing carnivores, both the radius and ulna are considerably enlarged at the locus of their distal epiphyseal cartilages (physes). The distal epiphyseal cartilage of the ulna is normally shaped like a hollow cone which causes a V-shaped radiolucency (Fig. 1-4B).

7. Hypertrophic osteodystrophy is a disease of young, rapidly growing dogs. It usually affects the larger breeds and is characterized by inflammation at the distal ends of the long bones, especially the radius and ulna. Radiographically, a radiolucent band appears in the metaphysis adjacent to the physis, and an irregular collar of bone forms around the metaphysis within a few days. Hypertrophic osteodystrophy may be differentiated from scurvy by the fact that the physes usually remain normal in width (in scurvy they widen) and by the collar of new bone. It may be differentiated from hypertrophic osteoarthropathy because the latter characteristically involves palisade periosteal new bone formation in the long bones and phalanges [15].

8. Olecranon bursitis (capped elbow, bursitis of the point of the elbow)* is an inflammation over the tuber olecrani in which a subcutaneous bursa forms. (The bursa under the triceps brachii tendon is usually not involved.) In large dogs, the complaint may be precipitated by lying on a hard surface. In horses, it may be caused by elbow hitting (striking the tuber olecrani with the hoof of the same leg) and is also known as "shoe boil" [11].

VI. CARPAL BONES

  A. Major features:

Name	Commonly used abbreviations**	Official Synonyms
radial carpal bone	Cr	os scaphoideum
intermediate carpal bone	Ci	os lunatum
ulnar carpal bone	Cu	os triquetrum
accessory carpal bone	Ca	os pisiforme
first carpal bone	C1	os trapezium
second carpal bone	C2	os trapezoideum
third carpal bone	C3	os capitatum
fourth carpal bone	C4	os hamatum

*There is no Nomina Clinica. Consequently, one cannot designate an "official" name for a given diagnosis or procedure. Those which contain official anatomic terms, however, are often more descriptive than those which do not (i.e., olecranon bursitis vs. shoe boil).

**When using abbreviations, the context of their usage becomes very important. For example, C1 may be used for either the first carpal bone or the first cervical vertebra. Likewise, T1 may refer to the first tarsal bone or to the first thoracic vertebra.

B. Selected comparative, clinical, and developmental features (Fig. 1-5):

1. The differences in the carpal bone patterns of domestic mammals result from fusions of some of the bones to one another and from the absence of certain bones in some species. The generalized carpal bone pattern consists of eight units in two rows with named bones forming the proximal row and numbered bones forming the distal row (Fig. 1-5). In the proximal row, the radial carpal bone is medial, the ulnar carpal bone is lateral, and the intermediate carpal bone lies between them. The accessory carpal bone is lateral and palmar. The distal carpal bones are numbered from medial to lateral.

   a. The pig has the generalized pattern of 8 separate bones (Fig. 1-5A).
   b. The carnivores have fusion of the radial and intermediate carpal bones to form the intermedioradial carpal bone and therefore have only 7 separate carpal bones. This fused bone has been commonly called the "radial" carpal bone (Fig. 1-5B). The tiny bone radiographically visualized on the medial side of the carpus is the sesamoid of the abductor digiti I (pollicis) longus muscle (see below, Part IX, B1c).
   c. In ruminants, the first carpal bone is absent. The second and third carpal bones are fused so that a total of 6 carpal bones are present. The fused entity is usually referred to as the fused second and third carpal bone (C2 and C3) rather than by its official synonym, os trapezoideocapitatum [1] (Fig. 1-5C).
   d. The horse may have 7 or 8 carpal bones on each side because the first carpal bone is often absent (unilaterally or bilaterally). Rare individuals have a fifth carpal bone on the palmarolateral aspect of the distal row, resulting in a total of 8 bones (if C1 is absent) or 9 bones (if C1 is present) [11]. The origin of the diminutive fifth carpal bone remains undocumented (Fig. 1-5D).

2. In carnivores, except for the intermedioradial carpal bone (3 centers) and the accessory carpal bone (2 centers), each carpal bone develops from a single center of ossification [5].

3. The third ossification center for the intermedioradial carpal bone in dogs may be radiographically identified only in very young individuals. It is the central carpal bone which is present developmentally in all of the domestic mammals. The central carpal bone fuses to one or more of the other carpal bones and does not become a definitive bone in any domestic species [5].

4. The accessory carpal bone is the only carpal bone which serves as a point of attachment for muscles (extensor carpi ulnaris and flexor carpi ulnaris). It is occasionally fractured in horses and treatment is complicated by the pull of the muscles [11].

VII. METACARPAL BONES

A. Major features:

   metacarpal bones (first through fifth, often abbreviated Mc1-5)
      base--the proximal epiphysis
      body--the diaphysis
      head--the distal epiphysis

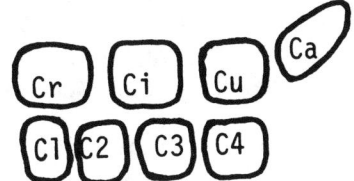

A

Generalized carpal pattern (pig).

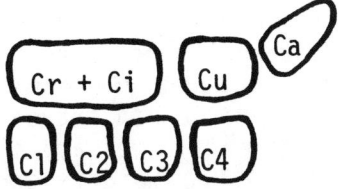

B

Fusion of the radial and intermediate carpal bones to form the intermedioradial carpal bone (carnivores).

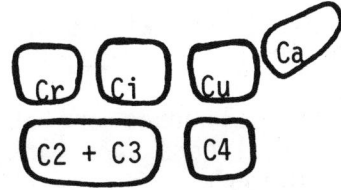

C

Absence of first carpal bone and fusion of second and third carpal bones (ruminants).

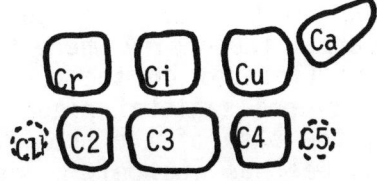

D

Frequent absence of first carpal bone. Rare presence of fifth carpal bone (horse).

Figure 1-5

Schematic Comparison of the Carpal Bones in the Domestic Mammals

    Cr = radial carpal bone
    Ci = intermediate carpal bone
    Cu = ulnar carpal bone
    Ca = accessory carpal bone
    C1, C2, C3, C4, & C5 = first, second, third, fourth, and
      fifth carpal bones

B. Selected comparative, clinical, and developmental features (Fig. 1-6).

1. Species differences in the metacarpal bones result from reduction in the number present and from osseous fusion. Five bones are present in the generalized mammalian metacarpus, and they are numbered 1-5 from medial to lateral. Each metacarpal bone normally bears a digit.
    a. The carnivores have the generalized pattern of five metacarpal bones (Fig. 1-6B). The first metacarpal bone is markedly reduced and supports a correspondingly reduced digit. Digits 2-5 bear weight.
    b. The pig has no first metacarpal bone (Fig. 1-6C). The abaxial metacarpal bones (Mc2 and Mc5) are notably smaller than the axial metacarpal bones (Mc3 and Mc4). All four of the metacarpal bones support digits, but only the axial digits normally bear weight.
    c. In the ruminants the first and second metacarpal bones are absent (Fig. 1-6D). The third and fourth metacarpal bones are fused to form a single bony mass known as the third and fourth metacarpal bone (Mc3+4). "Cannon bone" and "large metacarpal bone" are slang terms used for this structure. It supports the weight-bearing third and fourth digits and has the following specific features (Fig. 1-7A):
      (1) dorsal and palmar longitudinal grooves
      (2) proximal and distal metacarpal canals
      (3) intertrochlear notch
The fifth metacarpal bone is markedly reduced ("small metacarpal bone") and does not support a digit. It should be recognized as normal radiographically.
    d. In the horse, the first and fifth metacarpal bones are absent (Fig. 1-6E). The second and fourth metacarpal bones are markedly reduced and are commonly called "splint bones" as are their pelvic limb counterparts. This name should not be conceptually confused with a "fractured splint" or with pathological inflammation of the interosseous ligaments* between the metacarpal bones (known clinically as the disease "splints"). The third metacarpal bone is notably larger than the second and fourth metacarpal bones and it is the only one which supports a digit. Major features of Mc3 include the metacarpal tuberosity where the extensor carpi radialis muscle attaches (located on the dorsal aspect near the base) and the well-developed sagittal ridge on the head which fits into a groove on the base of the proximal phalanx. The third metacarpal bone, as well as its pelvic limb counterpart, is loosely called "cannon bone." The second and fourth metacarpal bones are not only medial and lateral (respectively) to Mc3, but they are also slightly palmar (Fig. 1-7B).

2. Metacarpal bones typically develop from three centers of ossification (one each for the base, body, and head) separated by two epiphyseal cartilages. Fusion of the base and body usually occurs in utero so that after birth only the distal epiphyseal cartilage typically remains

---

*The metacarpal (or metatarsal) interosseous ligaments should not be confused with the interosseous muscle. In horses, the interosseous muscle is commonly called the "suspensory ligament."

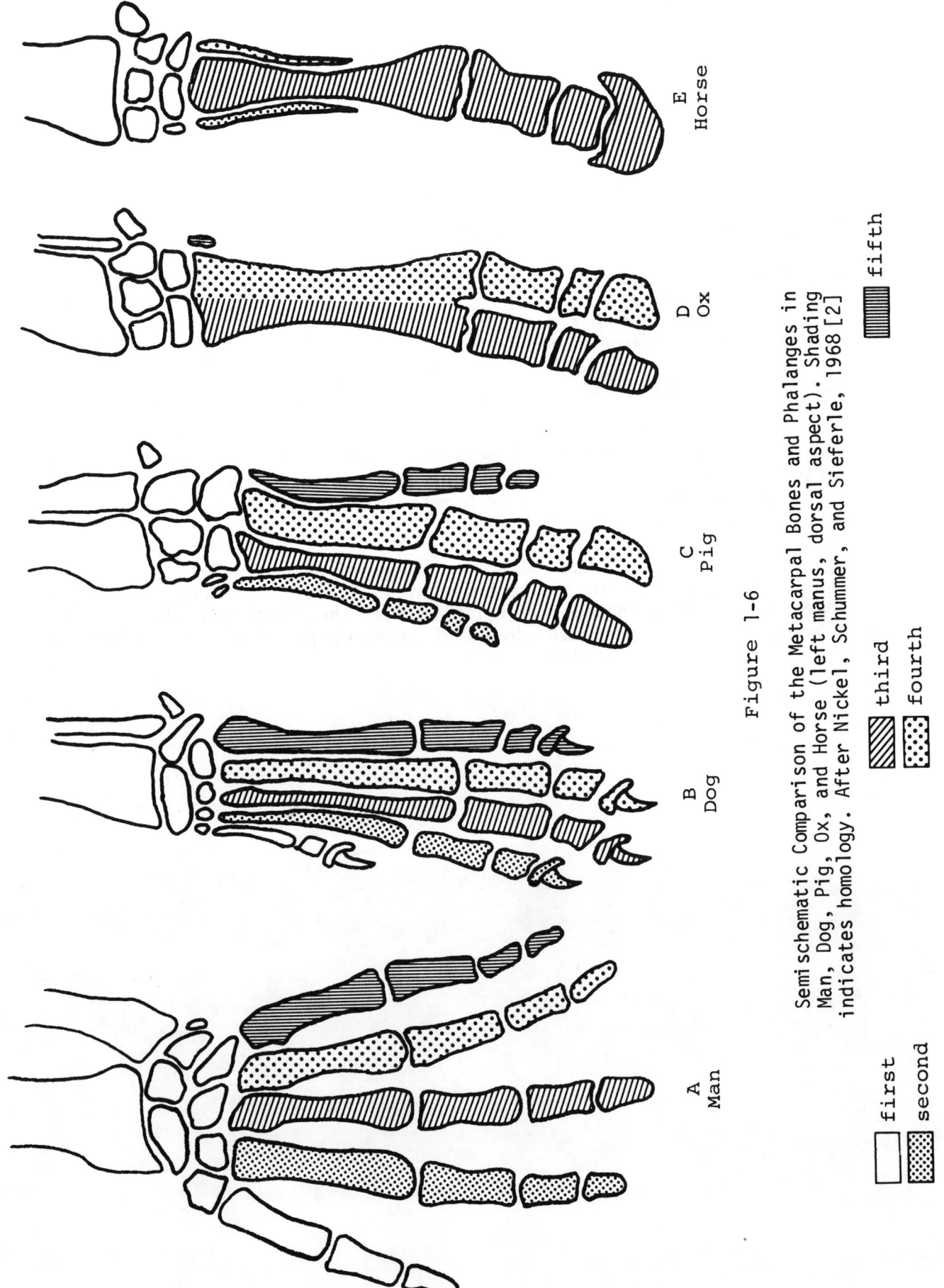

Figure 1-6

Semischematic Comparison of the Metacarpal Bones and Phalanges in Man, Dog, Pig, Ox, and Horse (left manus, dorsal aspect). Shading indicates homology. After Nickel, Schummer, and Sieferle, 1968 [2]

Figure 1-7

Selected Comparative, Clinical, and Developmental Features of the Metacarpal Bones

A. Dorsal aspect of the left metacarpal bones of an ox:

1. fused third and fourth metacarpal bones
2. fifth metacarpal bone
3. dorsal longitudinal groove
4. proximal metacarpal canal
5. distal metacarpal canal
6. intertrochlear notch

B. Transverse section through the metacarpal bones of a horse showing their relative sizes and positions. Oblique views are necessary to radiographically isolate the second and fourth metacarpal bones (1) because they are not truly medial and lateral to Mc3.

C. Dorsal aspect of the skeleton of a manus of a four-week-old dog. The unmineralized physes of the second, third, fourth, and fifth metacarpal bones are distally located (1) while that of the first metacarpal bone is proximal (2). Unmineralized physes of proximal phalanges (3) and middle phalanges (4) are proximally located.

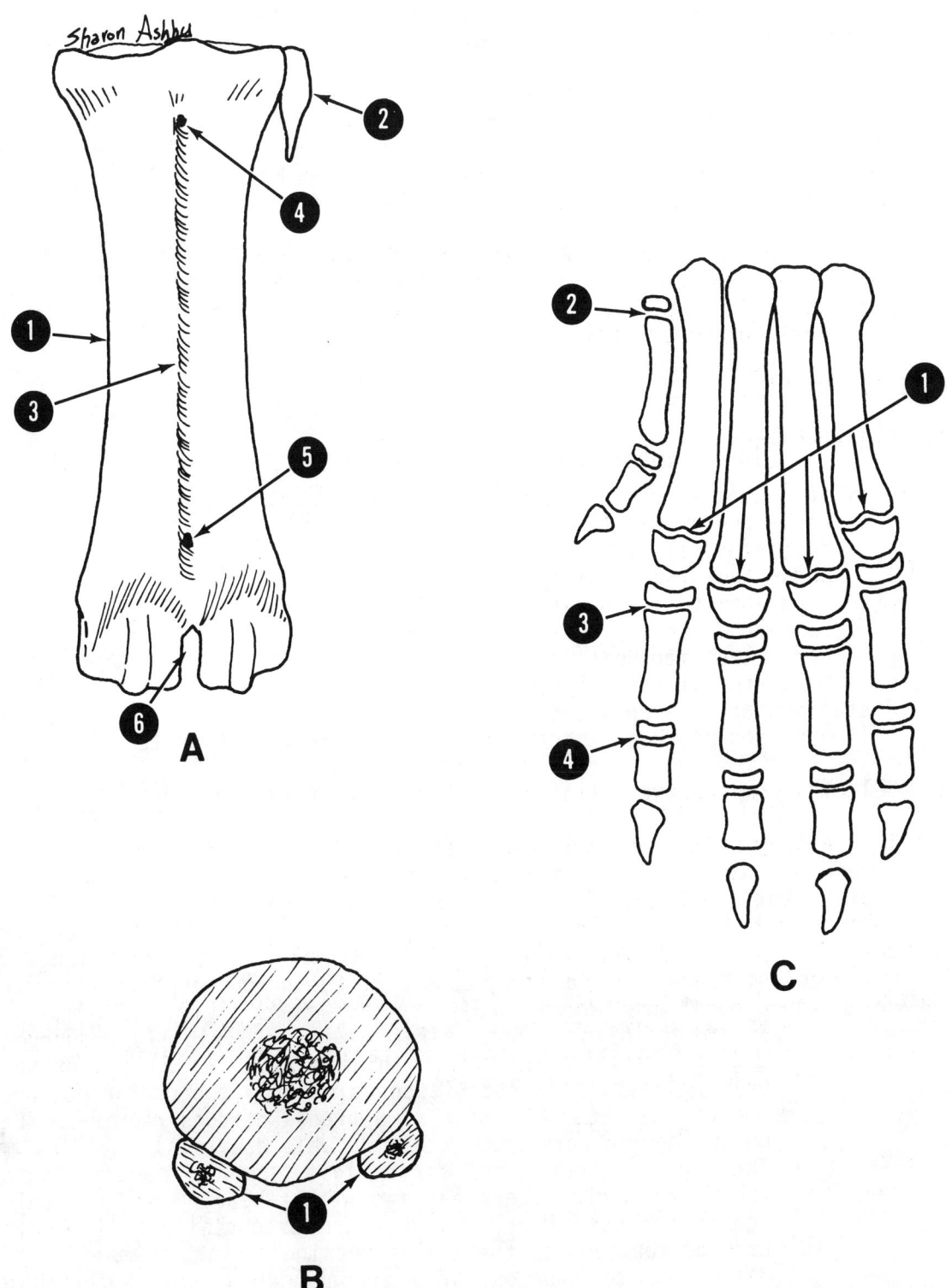

Figure 1-7

unmineralized. These structures should be recognized as normal radiographic radiolucencies. It is a curious fact that in the vestigial first metacarpal bone of carnivores, however, the proximal epiphyseal cartilage remains unmineralized after birth instead of the distal one. This should not be mistaken for a fracture line when viewed radiographically (Fig. 1-7C) [17].

3. The axis of the limb courses distally between the third and fourth metacarpal bones and digits, except in the horse where it passes through the longitudinal midline of the third metacarpal bone and the third digit. The axis is the basis for the terms axial (relatively closer to the axis) and abaxial (relatively further from the axis) [1].

4. In young horses, periostitis of the dorsal surface of the third metacarpal (or metatarsal) bone is termed bucked shins. It is usually manifested by swelling and pain on palpation. Horses over 3 years of age are rarely affected [11].

VIII. BONES OF THE DIGITS

A. Major features:

proximal phalanx (os compedale)
    base--the proximal epiphysis
    body--the diaphysis
    head--the distal epiphysis
middle phalanx (os coronale)
    base--the proximal epiphysis
    body--the diaphysis
    head--the distal epiphysis
distal phalanx (os ungulare)
    extensor process--where the extensor tendons terminate

B. Selected comparative, clinical, and developmental features:

1. A digit is the segmental part of a limb corresponding to a human finger or toe. The phalanges are the main skeletal components of the digits, but the proximal and distal sesamoid bones are also included (see below, Part IX). Species differences in the digital skeleton are related primarily to which digits are present and which ones bear weight. Digits which do not reach the plane of support of their counterparts (i.e., do not reach the ground) are termed paradigits ("dewclaws") [1].
    a. In the carnivores, the first digit is typically reduced (para-digit), but the other four (digits 2, 3, 4, 5) are present and bear weight. The paradigit contains only two phalanges, proximal and distal. Standards for some breeds of dogs require a specific morphology in this area (e.g., "double dewclaws).
    b. The pig is missing the first digit, has two paradigits (second and fifth digits), and has two weight-bearing digits (third and fourth digits). The paradigits are essentially fully formed but reduced versions of the weight-bearing digits. However, they lack distal sesamoid bones. They probably lend some support in soft ground.
    c. The ox has a pattern similar to the pig with two paradigits (2 and 5), two weight-bearing digits (3 and 4), and no first digit.

The paradigits, however, have no metacarpal support, and they contain only misshapen, vestigial remnants of phalanges which typically do not articulate with each other or with the rest of the skeleton.
    d. The modern horse has only one digit on each limb (digit 3), but evolutionary predecessors of the horse had multiple digits. The reduced second and fourth metacarpal bones provide morphological evidence of other digits which can be observed on fossilized skeletal remains of equine ancestors.

2. Proximal and middle phalanges normally develop from three centers of ossification (one each for the base, body, and head) separated by two epiphyseal cartilages. By the time of birth, the bodies and heads typically fuse and only the proximal epiphyseal cartilages remain unmineralized. (Contrast this pattern with that of the metacarpal bones, where only the distal epiphyseal cartilage typically remains unmineralized after birth; Fig. 1-7C).

3. Each distal phalanx usually develops from a single center of ossification, but a small separate one for the extensor process has been identified in horses. Distal phalanges of the various species have the following distinctive features [1]:
    a. carnivores (Fig. 1-8A)
        (1) ungual crest
        (2) ungual process--the osseous support of the claw
    b. ungulates (Fig 1-8B, C)
        (1) parietal surface--adjacent to the hoof wall
        (2) surface of the sole--adjacent to the sole (ground)
        (3) coronary border--proximal edge of the parietal surface. The extensor process of ungulates is located along this border.
        (4) border of the sole--junction of (1) and (2)
    c. horse only (Fig. 1-8B, C)
        (1) marginal notch of the sole--this osseous defect is variable in its development and may be mistaken radiographically for a lytic area.
        (2) medial and lateral foramina of the sole--the distal ends of the medial and lateral digital arteries enter these.
        (3) canal of the sole--this vascular channel and several of the larger ones which arborize from it form distinctive radiographic shadows which mimic fracture lines.
        (4) medial and lateral palmar processes ("angles," "wings")--the cartilages of the hoof attach to their coronary borders.
        (5) medial and lateral parietal grooves--vascular channels in the parietal surface which are parallel to the border of the sole. They are most pronounced near the palmar processes.
        (6) medial and lateral cartilages of the hoof (ungual cartilages)--inflammation of these is termed quittor (either limb) and is characterized by draining tracts in the coronary region. Ossification of the cartilages is termed sidebone [11].

4. Unofficial terms frequently used for the proximal, middle, and distal phalanges of the horse and occasionally of the ox are the "long pastern bone," "short pastern bone," and "coffin bone," respectively.

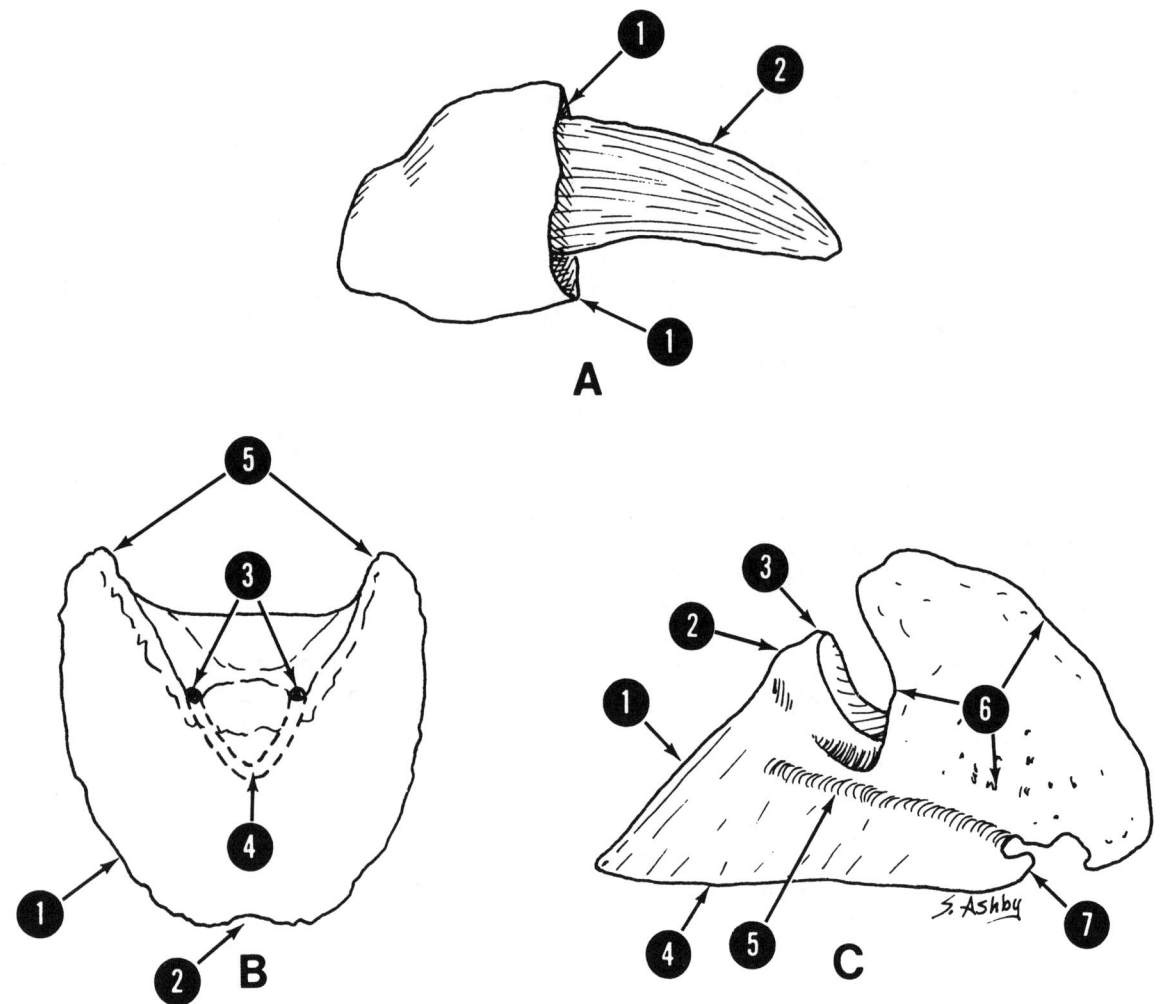

Figure 1-8

Selected Comparative, Clinical, and Developmental Features of the Distal Phalanx

A. Lateral aspect of a distal phalanx of a dog:
   1. ungual crest
   2. ungual process

B. Solar surface of a distal phalanx of a horse:
   1. border of the sole
   2. marginal notch of the sole
   3. medial and lateral solar foramina
   4. canal of the sole (dotted lines)
   5. medial and lateral palmar processes
   6. solar surface

C. Lateral aspect of an equine distal phalanx and attached cartilage of the hoof:
   1. parietal surface
   2. extensor process
   3. coronary border
   4. border of the sole (solar border)
   5. parietal groove (lateral one)
   6. cartilage of the hoof (lateral one)
   7. lateral palmar process

5. Ringbone is periosteal bone deposition on the phalanges of horses. It is classified as "high" if it occurs near the proximal interphalangeal joint (involvement of proximal and/or middle phalanges) and "low" if it occurs near the distal interphalangeal joint (involvement of middle and/or distal phalanges). The terms articular or periarticular are also used to describe ringbone depending on whether the articular surface is actually involved in the disease [11].

6. Pyramidal disease (buttress foot) is new bone deposition at the extensor process of the distal phalanx in horses. It may occur because of a fracture of the extensor process or it may be a form of low ringbone [11].

7. Pedal osteitis is a demineralization of the distal phalanx of horses resulting from inflammation [11].

8. Chronic laminitis in horses results in rotation of the distal phalanx, which is observed radiographically as non-parallelism between the dorsal aspect of the hoof wall and distal phalanx [11].

9. Hypertrophic osteoarthropathy (hypertrophic pulmonary osteopathy) is a disease of dogs characterized by periosteal new bone formation on the long bones and phalanges. It is often associated with a space-occupying lesion in the thorax or with abdominal disease, and its unknown etiology may involve circulatory disturbances. The periosteal reaction is in a characteristic "palisade" pattern (trabeculae laid down at right angles to the long axis of the bone). In time, the periosteal reaction may become smooth. Resolution of the space occupying lesion or vagotomy on the side of the lesion results in regression of the disease.

IX. SESAMOID BONES

A. Major features:

The typical sesamoid bones which are present in the thoracic limb include two proximal sesamoid bones on the palmar aspect of the metacarpophalangeal joint of each major digit. These are embedded in the tendon of the interosseous muscle and articulate primarily with the palmar aspects of the heads of the metacarpal bones. In addition, there is a single distal sesamoid bone on the palmar aspect of each distal interphalangeal joint which articulates with the middle and distal phalanges (Fig. 1-9). In contrast to the other sesamoid bones of the body, the distal sesamoid bones are not embedded in tendons. The tendon of the deep digital flexor courses superficial to the distal sesamoid bone, and the podotrochlear ("navicular") bursa occurs between the tendon and the bone (Fig. 3-6).

B. Selected comparative, clinical, and developmental features:

1. Carnivores
   a. In contrast to the situation in the ungulates, the distal sesamoid bone of each digit usually remains cartilaginous.
   b. A single dorsal sesamoid bone is embedded in the extensor tendons on the dorsal aspect of the metacarpophalangeal joints. Some individuals also have these bones at the proximal and distal interphalangeal joints.

Figure 1-9

Selected Comparative, Clinical, and Developmental Features of the Equine and Bovine Digital Skeletons

    A.   Lateral and palmar aspects of the skeleton of a left equine digit:

           1.   proximal sesamoid bones

           2.   distal sesamoid bone

           3.   third metacarpal bone

           4.   proximal phalanx

           5.   middle phalanx

           6.   distal phalanx

    B.   Lateral and palmar aspect of the skeleton of the left bovine digits:

           1.   proximal sesamoid bones of digit 4

           2.   distal sesamoid bone of digit 4

           3.   proximal phalanx of digit 4

           4.   middle phalanx of digit 4

           5.   distal phalanx of digit 4

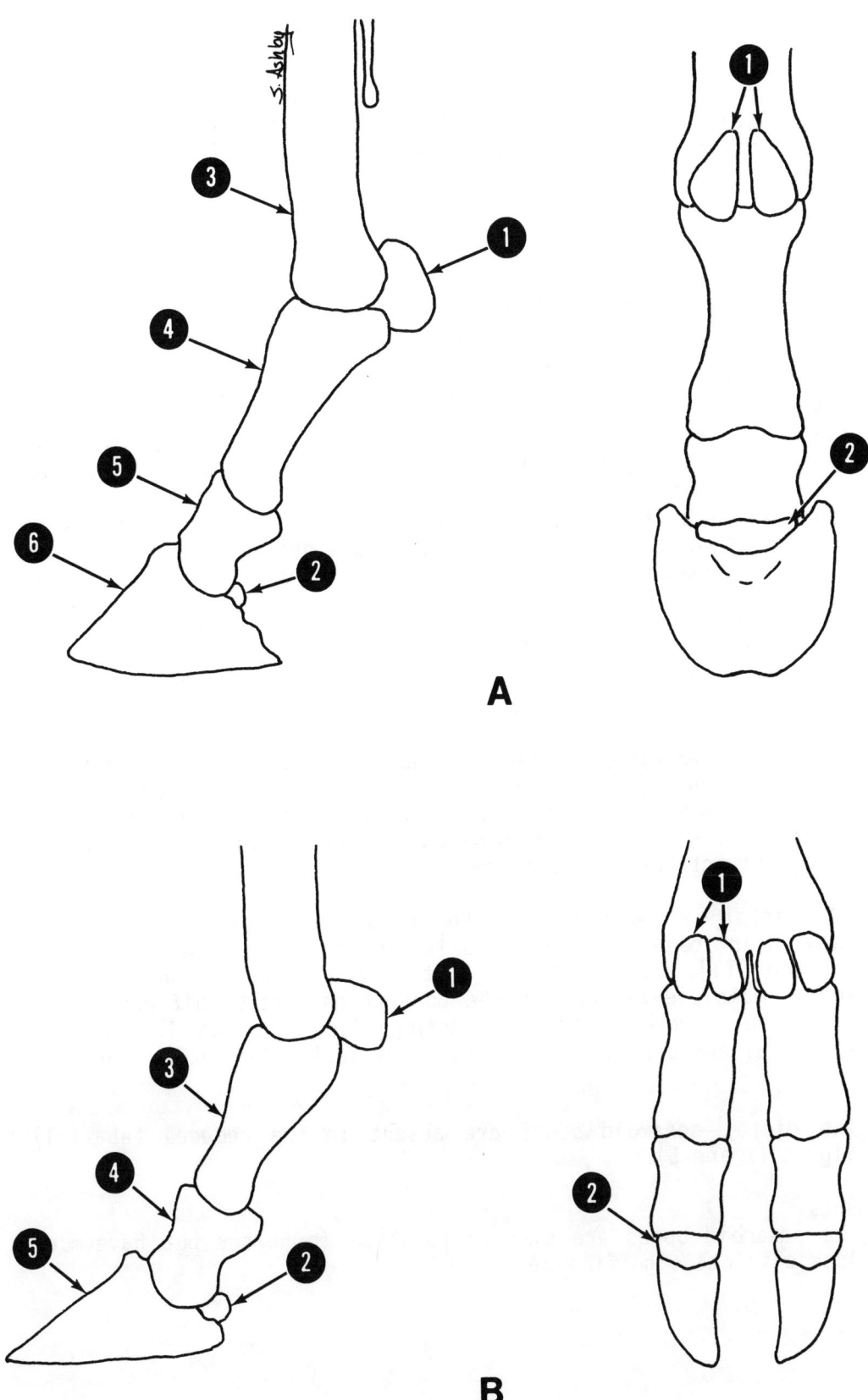

Figure 1-9

  c. A sesamoid bone is embedded in the tendon of the abductor digiti I (pollicis) longus on the medial side of the carpus. It may be confused with a chip fracture of one of the carpal bones.

 2. Horse
  a. The proximal sesamoid bones may fracture in racing animals. Trauma from contact of this region of the limb with the ground has been implicated as a cause. Another suggested etiology is improper positioning of the bones relative to the articular surface on the head of Mc3 at the moment when the deep digital flexor m. contracts [11].
  b. Each proximal sesamoid bone has three defined surfaces [1] (Fig. 1-9A, B):
   (1) articular surface--on the dorsal aspect where it articulates with Mc3 (there is also a small articular facet distally for articulation with the proximal phalanx).
   (2) flexor surface--on the palmar aspect where it is joined to its contralateral counterpart by the palmar annular ligament ("intersesamoidean ligament") to form a groove for the flexor tendons.
   (3) interosseous surface--on the abaxial aspect where the interosseous muscle ("suspensory ligament") attaches.
  The "base" as used by some clinicians is an unofficial term which refers to the distal aspect.

  c. It is of radiographic significance that the lateral proximal sesamoid bone is a little taller than its medial counterpart. This may help differentiate them in unlabeled or improperly labeled films. The lateral proximal sesamoid bone is also concave along its interosseous surface.

  d. The distal sesamoid bone of the horse is popularly termed the "navicular" bone and associated lamenesses are termed "navicular" disease [11]. Radiographically, this condition is manifested as small radiolucent areas in the bone which must be differentiated from the normal vascular foramina. The bone has two borders (proximal and distal) and two surfaces (articular and flexor).

 3. Pig
  a. The distal sesamoid bones are absent in the reduced (abaxial) digits (2 and 5).

 4. Ruminants
  a. The sesamoid bones are similar to those in horses but have much less clinical significance.

References

1. International Committee on Veterinary Gross Anatomical Nomenclature. 1983. Nomina Anatomica Veterinaria, third ed. Published by the Committee, Ithaca, New York.

2. Nickel, R., A. Schummer, and E. Seiferle. 1968. Lehrbuch der Anatomic der Haustiere. Band I. Paul Parey, Berlin.

3. McClure, R. C., M. J. Dallman, and P. G. Garrett. 1973. Cat Anatomy: An Atlas, Text and Dissection Guide. Lea and Febiger, Philadelphia.

4. Getty, R. 1975. Sisson and Grossman's The Anatomy of the Domestic Animals, fifth ed. W. B. Saunders, Philadelphia.

5. Hare, W. 1960. Radiographic anatomy of the canine pectoral limb. Part II. Developing Limb. JAVMA 135(6):305-310.

6. Hickman, J. 1964. Veterinary Orthopedics. Lippincott, Philadelphia.

7. Archibald, J., ed. 1974. Canine Surgery. American Veterinary Publications, Santa Barbara, California.

8. Wingfield, W. E., and C. A. Rawlings. 1979. Small Animal Surgery. W. B. Saunders, Philadelphia.

9. Piermattei, D. L., and R. G. Greeley. 1979. An Atlas of Surgical Approaches to the Bones of the Dog and Cat, second ed. W. B. Saunders, Philadelphia.

10. Olson, N. C., C. B. Carrig, and W. O. Brinker. 1979. Asynchronous growth of the canine radius and ulna: Effects of retardation of longitudinal growth of the radius. Am. J. Vet. Res. 40:351-355.

11. Adams, O. R. 1974. Lameness in Horses, third ed. Lea and Febiger, Philadelphia.

12. Auer, J. A., R. J. Martens, and E. H. Williams. 1982. Periosteal transection for correction of angular limb deformities in foals. JAVMA 181(5):459-466.

13. Milne, D. W., and A. S. Turner. 1979. An Atlas of Surgical Approaches to the Bones of the Horse. W. B. Saunders, Philadelphia.

14. Herron, M. R. 1971. Ununited anconeal process in the dog. Vet. Clin. N. Amer. 1:417.

15. Kealy, J. K. 1979. Diagnostic Radiology of the Dog and Cat. W. B. Saunders, Philadelphia.

16. Tirgari, M. 1980. Clinical, radiographical and pathological aspects of ununited medial coronoid process of the elbow joint in dogs. J. Small Anim. Pract. 21:595-608.

17. Shively, M. J. 1978. First metacarpal bone or proximal phalanx? J. Am. Vet. Rad. Soc. 19(2):50-52.

THORACIC LIMB MYOLOGY

A general knowledge of the muscles of the thoracic limb has obvious clinical application to many surgical procedures. Familiarity with the general actions of the muscles is also a prerequisite to the diagnosis of specific neuropathies. Although a number of references to vascularity and innervation are made in this chapter, more complete discussions are available in Chapters 4 and 5. The muscles of the thoracic limb can be divided into two major groups:

Extrinsic Muscles--those that attach the limb to the head, neck, and trunk. Some of them attach to the scapula and some to the humerus. The extrinsic muscles* are innervated by unnamed branches of the cervical and thoracic spinal nerves, as well as by the accessory nerve (cranial nerve 11) and by several named branches of the brachial plexus.

Intrinsic Muscles--those that attach to the bones within the limb itself. These are innervated by named derivatives of the brachial plexus and may be further divided into seven groups according to their position in the body:

    A. Lateral muscles of the shoulder
    B. Medial muscles of the shoulder
    C. Cranial muscles of the brachium
    D. Caudal muscles of the brachium
    E. Craniolateral muscles of the antebrachium
    F. Caudomedial muscles of the antebrachium
    G. Muscles of the manus

I. EXTRINSIC MUSCLES OF THE THORACIC LIMB (Figs. 2-1, 2-2, 2-3, 2-4)

    A. Superficial pectoral (descending pectoral and transverse pectoral mm.)

Origin: Sternum.
Termination: Crest of greater tubercle and cranial border of humerus (also fascia of antebrachium in large animals and cat).
Action: Adduct the thoracic limb.

The name descending pectoral is synonymous with the obsolete "cranial superficial pectoral" and transverse pectoral is synonymous with "caudal superficial pectoral" (Fig. 2-2). The superficial pectoral is partially transected during a cranial approach to the shoulder in carnivores [1].

---

*Extrinsic muscles of the thoracic limb do not comprise a recognized group in the N.A.V. [2]. They belong to three other groups: muscles of the neck (brachiocephalicus); muscles of the thorax (superficial pectoral, deep pectoral, subclavius, and serratus ventralis thoracis); and muscles of the back (omotransversarius, rhomboideus, latissimus dorsi, trapezius, and serratus ventralis cervicis).

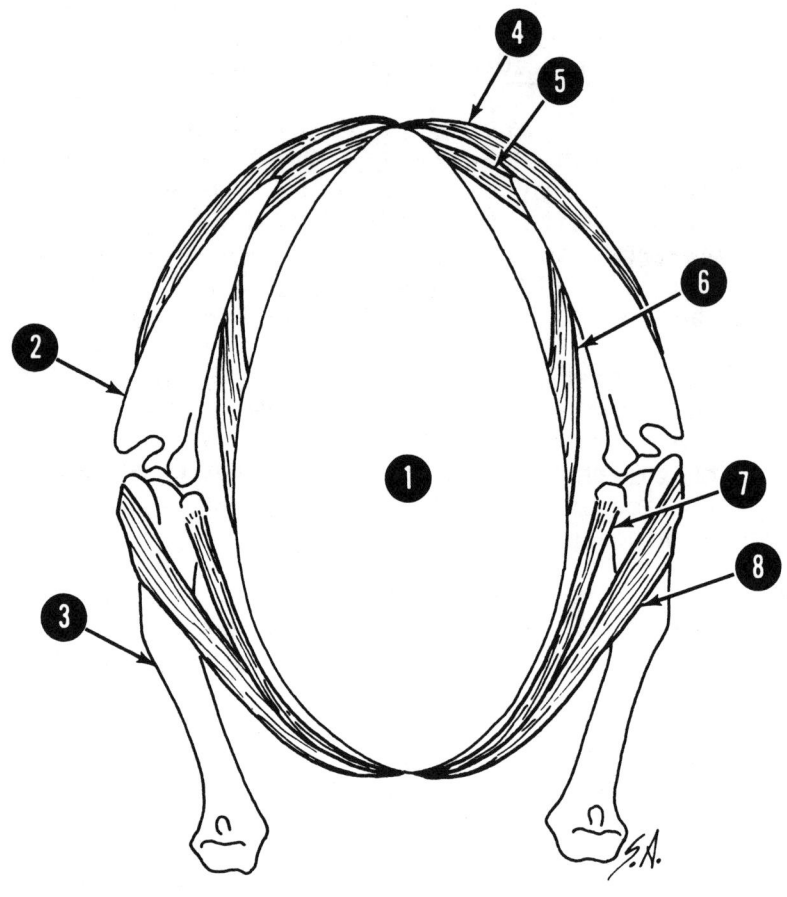

Figure 2-1

Schematic Relationship of Selected Extrinsic Muscles
to the Scapula, Humerus, and Thorax

1. Transverse section of thorax
2. Scapula (cranial aspect)
3. Humerus (cranial aspect)
4. Trapezius m.
5. Rhomboideus m.
6. Serratus ventralis m.
7. Deep pectoral m.
8. Superficial pectoral m.

The omotransversarius, brachiocephalicus, and latissimus dorsi mm. are not shown because their origins were too far cranial or caudal to the plane of this transverse section.

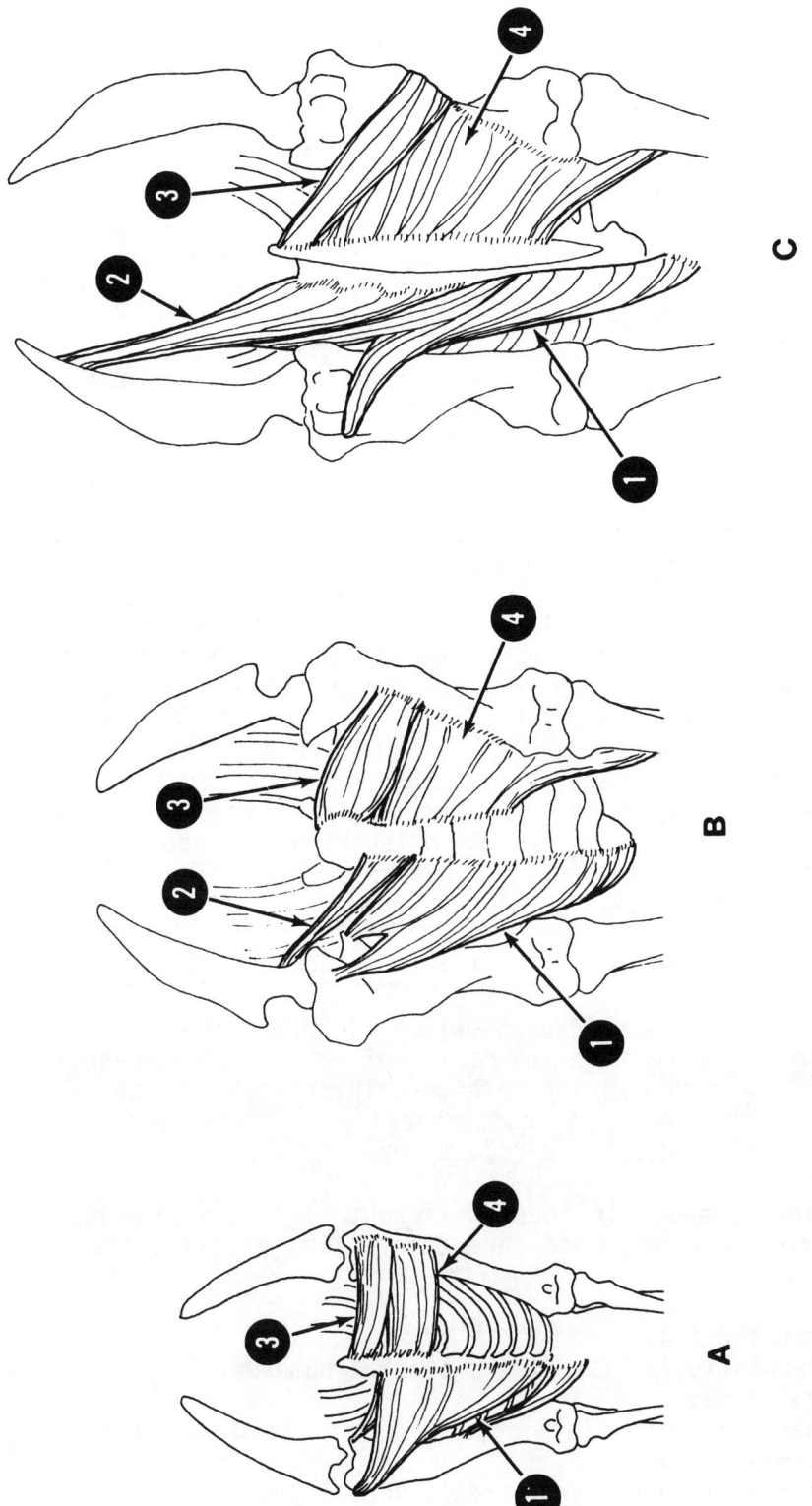

Figure 2-2

Differences in the Pectoral muscles of the Dog (A), Ox (B), and Horse (C) (Cranioventral aspect of the thorax with the right deep pectoral m. and left superficial pectoral m. illustrated.)

1. Ascending pectoral m.
2. Subclavius m.
3. Descending pectoral m.
4. Transverse pectoral m.

After Nickel, Schummer, Seiferle, 1968 [12]

B. Deep pectoral (ascending pectoral) and subclavius m.

   Origin: Sternum.
   Termination: Lesser and greater tubercles (ascending pectoral); scapular
                fascia (subclavius m.).
   Action: Adduct limb and pull it caudally.

   Ascending pectoral is synonymous with the obsolete "caudal deep pectoral" and subclavius is synonymous with "cranial deep pectoral" and "cleidoscapularis" [2]. The carnivores do not have the subclavius portion and it is vestigial in the ox, attaching to the deep surface of the brachiocephalicus muscle. In the goat and horse the subclavius is well developed and lies along the cranial border of the scapula [3]. Ascending, transverse, and descending, as applied to the various pectoral muscles, describe the general orientation of the respective muscle fibers from the sternum to the limb and are more descriptive of the bipedal (erect) posture of man. The muscles may be divided along their ventral median raphe during mid-sternal thoracotomies [4].

C. Brachiocephalicus

   The name brachiocephalicus implies that this muscle attaches to the arm and to the head. It has two major subdivisions which are separated by a tendinous intersection in all domestic mammals: cleidobrachialis (clavicle to the arm) and cleidocephalicus (clavicle to the head) (Fig. 2-3). The clavicular intersection may be difficult to identify. The cleidocephalicus is further subdivided, in all species except the horse, into two parts. One of these is the mastoid part (because it attaches to the mastoid part of the temporal bone). The other one is termed the cervical part in the carnivores (because it attaches to the neck) and the occipital part in the ruminants and pig (because it attaches to the occipital bone). For purists interested in belaboring this point, all species have a cleidobrachialis and a cleidocephalicus. The cleidocephalicus has further subdivisions as follows [2]:

Species	Named parts of the cleidocephalicus m.
horse	mastoid part only ("cleidomastoideus")
ruminants and pig	mastoid and occipital parts ("cleidomastoideus" and "cleidooccipitalis")
carnivores	mastoid and cervical parts ("cleidomastoideus" and "cleidocervicalis")

   The confusion inherent in these different names can be reduced by the realization that the names are descriptive of the sites of attachment.

   Origin: clavicular intersection.
   Termination: cleidobrachialis (all species), cranial humerus.
                cleidocephalicus
                        mastoid part (all species), mastoid process of
                        temporal bone.
                        cervical part (carnivores), dorsal neck.
                        occipital part (ruminants and pig), occipital bone.

Action: Pull the limb forward and/or depress and pull the head and neck laterally.

In the horse, the terms cleidocephalicus and mastoid part are synonymous since the equine cleidocephalicus has no subdivisions. The equine "cleidotransversarius" of older anatomy textbooks was considered at one time to be a subdivision of the cleidocephalicus. However, the cleidotransversarius is now considered to be the omotransversarius [2] (see omotransversarius). In the cat, the cleidobrachialis extends distally far enough to attach to the proximal ulna [5].

In carnivores, the brachiocephalicus muscle is reflected cranially during a craniolateral approach to the humerus (see brachialis m.) [6] and caudally (laterally) during a cranial approach to the shoulder [1].

The sternocephalicus is not an extrinsic muscle of the thoracic limb. However, because of its importance in forming the jugular groove (along with the brachiocephalicus) it is included here. The sternocephalicus attaches to the sternum and to the head. It is divided into two subparts in the carnivores, ox, and goat, and these are named according to their attachments (Fig. 2-3). In the pig and sheep, the undivided sternocephalicus is also known as the mastoid part because of its cephalic attachment; similarly, the undivided sternocephalicus of the horse is also known as the mandibular part.

To summarize the subdivisions of the sternocephalicus [2]:

Species	Named parts of the sternocephalicus
horse	mandibular part only ("sternomandibularis")
pig and sheep	mastoid part only ("sternomastoideus")
carnivores	mastoid and occipital parts ("sternomastoideus" and "sternooccipitalis")
ox and goat	mastoid and mandibular parts ("sternomastoideus" and "sternomandibularis")

Origin: Sternum.
Termination: Mastoid part (all species except horse), mastoid process of temporal bone.
    Occipital part (carnivores only), occipital bone.
    Mandibular part (horse and ruminants), mandible.
Action: Depress the head and neck and/or draw them laterally.
    (Open the mouth in the horse, ox, and goat.)

The jugular groove of horses and ruminants is located between the brachiocephalicus and sternocephalicus muscles. Its deep wall is formed by the omohyoideus muscle in the horse (a cervical muscle) and by the mastoid part of the sternocephalicus in ruminants [3].

D. Omotransversarius

Origin: Wing of the atlas.
Termination: Spine of the scapula (directly or indirectly).
Action: Depress the head and neck and/or advance the limb.

Figure 2-3

Differences in the Brachiocephalicus and Sternocephalicus Muscles

A   Dog
    Brachiocephalicus m.
        Cleidobrachialis m.
        Cleidocephalicus m.
            Mastoid part
            Cervical part
    Sternocephalicus m.
        Mastoid part
        Occipital part

B   Ox
    Brachiocephalicus m.
        Cleidobrachialis m.
        Cleidocephalicus m.
            Mastoid part
            Occipital part
    Sternocephalicus m.
        Mastoid part
        Mandibular part

C   Horse
    Brachiocephalicus m.
        Cleidobrachialis m.
        Cleidocephalicus m. (Mastoid part)
    Sternocephalicus m. (Mandibular part)
    Omotransversarius (Cleidotransversarius) m.

After Nickel, Schummer, and Seiferle, 1968 [12]

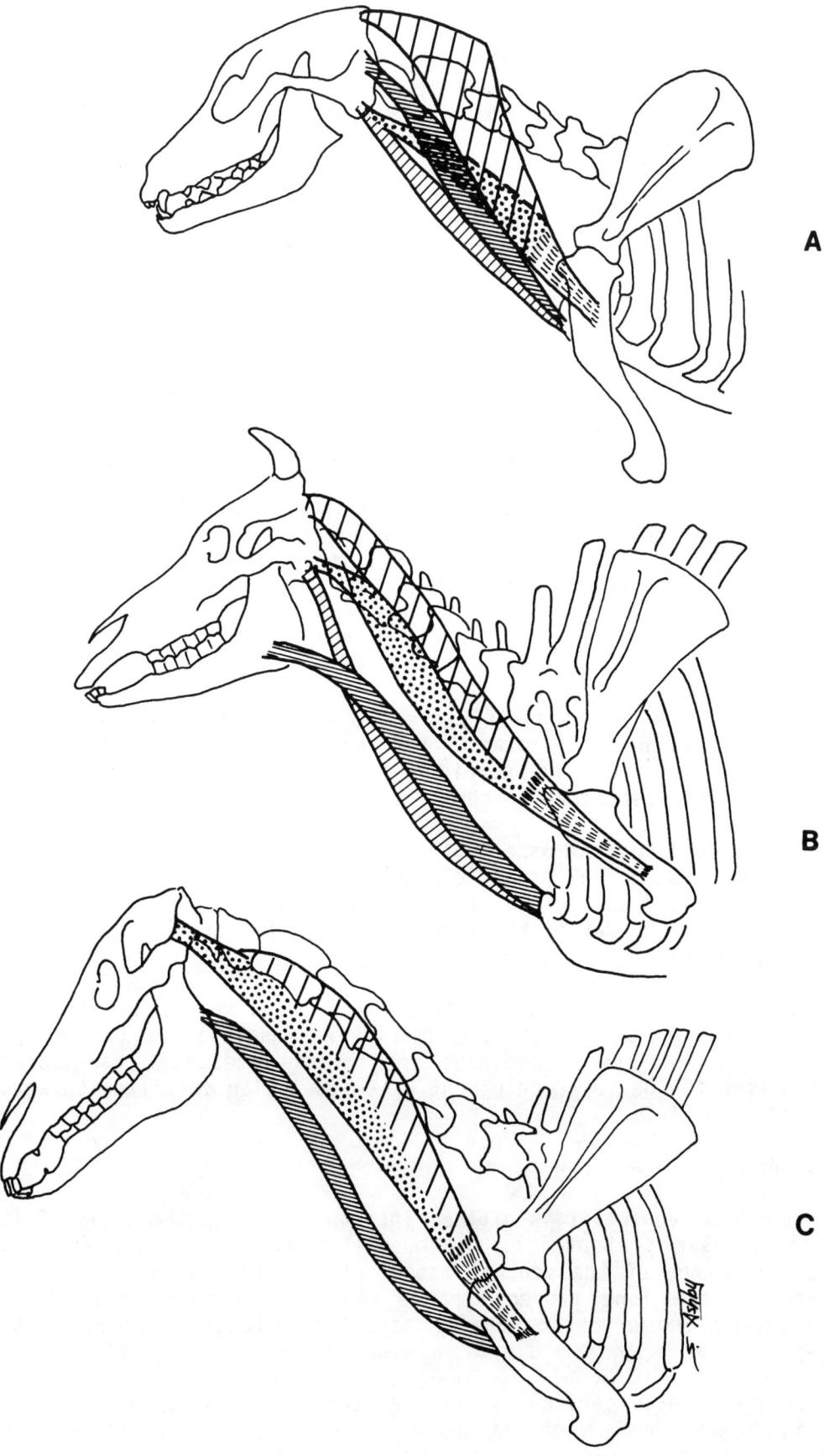

45

In the horse and ruminants, the omotransversarius ends in the lateral fascia of the shoulder and attaches to the scapular spine only indirectly. In the horse, the omotransversarius lies along the dorsal aspect of the cleidocephalicus part of the brachiocephalicus, attaches to several other cervical vertebrae as well as to the atlas, and was formerly known as the cleidotransversarius [2]. Its indirect (weak) attachment to the scapular spine in the horse may be related to the lack of an acromion in this species.

E. Trapezius

Origin: Dorsal neck and thorax.
Termination: Spine of the scapula.
Action: Elevate the limb.

The trapezius muscle is the most superficial muscle on the dorsal aspect of the cervicothoracic junction. It may be divided into cervical and thoracic parts on the basis of its origin. These are more obviously separable in the carnivores and horse than in the other species. The trapezius is innervated by the accessory (11th cranial) nerve which also partially innervates the brachiocephalicus, sternocephalicus, and omotransversarius muscles.

F. Rhomboideus

The rhomboideus is immediately deep to the trapezius and is divided into at least two parts (thoracic and cervical) on the basis of its origin in all species. The carnivores and pig have a small third (capital) part which attaches to the head.

Origin: R. thoracis, dorsal aspect of thorax.
       R. cervicis, dorsal aspect of neck.
       R. capitis, nuchal crest of occipital bone.
Termination: Dorsal border of the scapula and/or its cartilage.
Action: Elevate the limb.

In Bos indicus, the well-developed rhomboideus muscle along with a considerable deposition of fat is primarily responsible for the "hump". The larger size of the rhomboideus in the ungulates (vs. carnivores) correlates with the better development of the scapular cartilage to which it attaches (Fig. 1-1).

G. Serratus ventralis

The serratus ventralis is divided into two parts on the basis of its origin (cervical and thoracic). The muscle receives its name from the serrated appearance of the ventral aspect of the thoracic portion. It is innervated by the long thoracic nerve which is a derivative of the brachial plexus and courses caudally across the lateral aspect of the muscle.

Origin: Cervical part, cervical vertebrae; thoracic part, ribs.
Termination: Serrated face of scapula.
Action: Support and/or elevate the trunk by depressing the scapula.

Functionally, the serratus ventralis muscles serve to "sling" the body between the scapulae (Fig. 2-1/6). Rarely, the muscle is ruptured from trauma. In one such case from the medical records file at Texas A&M University, a dairy cow ruptured this muscle on one side when she slipped on the floor of a milking parlor. She did not progress satisfactorily and was ultimately euthanized.

H. Latissimus dorsi

Origin: Thoracolumbar fascia.
Termination: Teres major tuberosity.
Action: Draw the humerus caudally.

The latissimus dorsi is positioned over the dorsolateral aspect of the thorax. It is innervated by the thoracodorsal nerve. Both the latissimus dorsi and the serratus ventralis may be partially severed (preferably split along its fibers) during intercostal thoracotomies [4].

II. INTRINSIC MUSCLES OF THE THORACIC LIMB (Figs. 2-4, 2-5, 2-6)

A. Lateral muscles of the shoulder

The four muscles of this group are primarily flexors of the humeral joint. The supraspinatus, however, is a humeral joint extensor.

1. Deltoideus

Origin: Spine and acromion of scapula.
Termination: Deltoid tuberosity of humerus.
Action: Flex the humeral joint.

In the pig and horse the deltoideus appears undivided but in the other domestic species it has distinct acromial and spinous subdivisions. In carnivores different manipulations of the deltoideus m. account for the major variations in lateral approaches to the humeral joint. At least four variations are described:
   a. sever the acromial head near the acromion [6];
   b. osteotomize the acromion [6];
   c. dissect between the spinous and acromial heads [6];
   d. avulse the proximal part of the insertion on the deltoid tuberosity (leaving the distal part intact) [6,7].
Methods a and b above are the most traumatic but give the best exposure. Method c is least traumatic but gives the poorest exposure.

2. Supraspinatus

Origin: Supraspinous fossa of the scapula.
Termination: Greater tubercle of the humerus.
Action: Extend the humeral joint.

The supraspinatus of the ungulates attaches to the cranial parts of both the greater and lesser tubercles. The suprascapular nerve supplies both the supraspinatus and infraspinatus muscles and its dysfunction in horses results in classic (shoulder) sweeny [8].

Figure 2-4

Superficial Muscles of the Neck, Thorax, and Brachium
of Dog (A), Ox (B), and Horse (C)
(lateral aspect)

1. Triceps brachii m. (lateral head)

2. Ascending pectoral m.

3. Triceps brachii m. (long head)

4. Latissimus dorsi m.

5. Trapezius m.

6. Cleidocephalicus m. (the cephalic part[s] of the brachiocephalicus m.)

7. Sternocephalicus m.

8. Omotransversarius m.

9. Cleidobrachialis m.

10. Deltoideus m.

11. Serratus ventralis m. (shows on horse only)

12. Subclavius m. (shows on horse only)

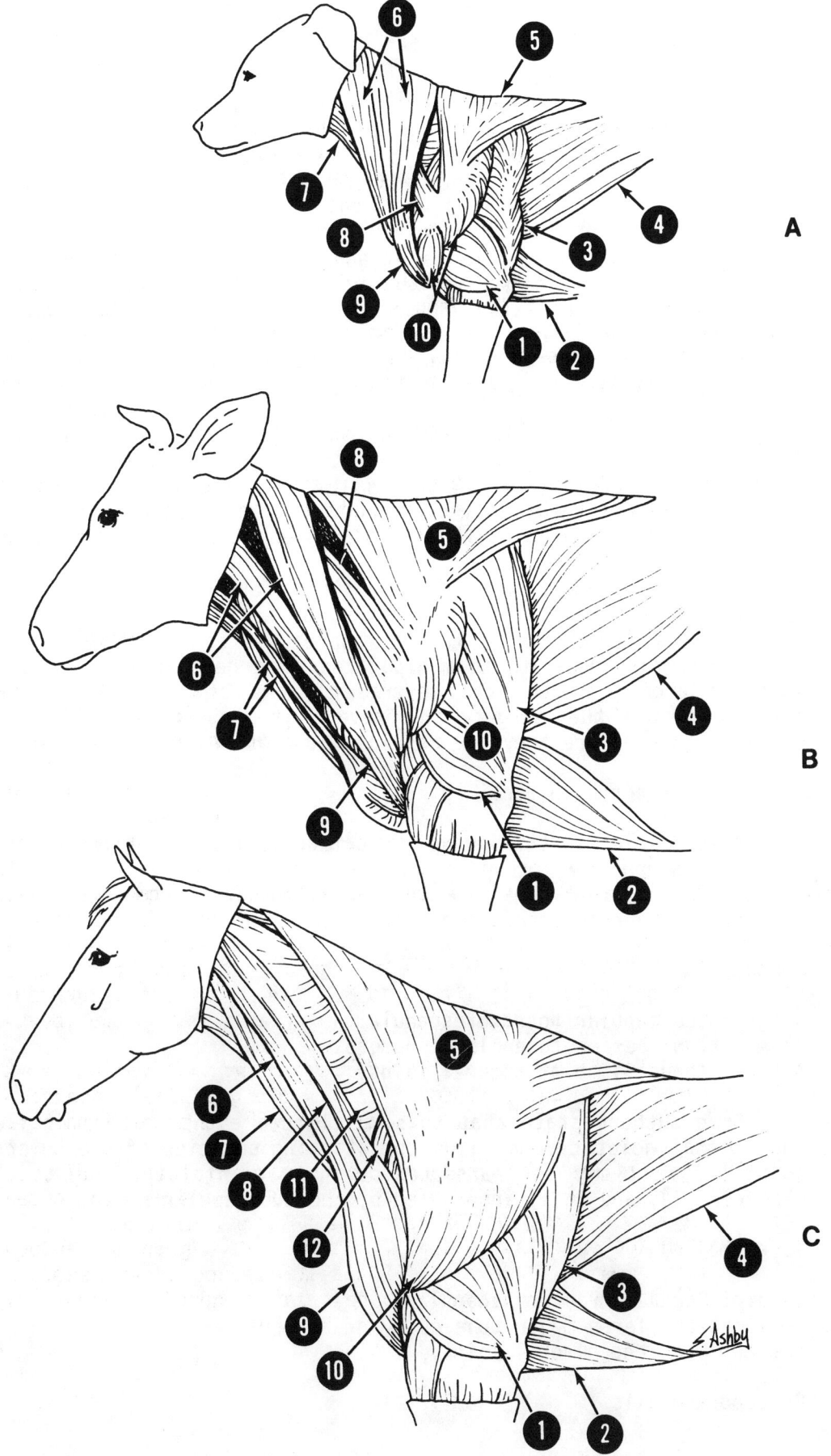

3. Infraspinatus

   Origin: Infraspinous fossa of the scapula.
   Termination: Greater tubercle of the humerus.
   Action: Flex the humeral joint; abduct limb at the humeral joint.

   The ungulates have cranial and caudal parts of the greater tubercle, and the infraspinatus attaches to both parts in the horse and ruminants. In the pig it terminates in a depression distal to the greater tubercle. In the horse, the tendon is a landmark for injection of the humeral joint. The needle is passed just cranial to the tendon, craniodorsal to the greater tubercle, and it is directed distally, medially, and caudally [9].

4. Teres minor

   Origin: Infraglenoid tubercle of scapula.
   Termination: Teres minor tuberosity.
   Action: Flex the humeral joint.

   The small teres minor is partially covered by the infraspinatus. The tendons of the teres minor and/or infraspinatus are commonly transected during lateral approaches to the humeral joint after the deltoideus m. is manipulated (see deltoideus) [6]. Some surgeons prefer to tag the severed tendons of the muscles with sutures during the surgery to prevent them from retracting and becoming lost before they are rejoined at closure.

B. Medial muscles of the shoulder (Fig. 2-5)

   The three muscles in this group are primarily flexors of the humeral joint. The subscapularis occupies much of the costal surface of the scapula. The teres major parallels the caudal border of the scapula. The coracobrachialis courses across the medial aspect of the humeral joint.

   1. Subscapularis

      Origin: Subscapular fossa of scapula.
      Termination: Lesser tubercle of humerus.
      Action: Adduct limb at humeral joint.

      Some authors state that this muscle can either extend or flex the humeral joint depending on the starting position of the humeral joint [10]. It may be transected during a cranial approach to the shoulder [1], and it is innervated by the subscapular nerve.

   2. Teres major

      Origin: Caudal border of scapula.
      Termination: Teres major tuberosity of humerus.
      Action: Flex the humeral joint.

   3. Coracobrachialis

Origin: Coracoid process of the scapula.
Termination: Proximal, medial humerus.
Action: Flex the humeral joint. (Some authors state that it extends the humeral joint in the dog [10].)

C. Cranial muscles of the brachium

The two cranial muscles of the brachium are primarily flexors of the cubital joint and are innervated by the musculocutaneous nerve. the biceps brachii is located medially and the brachialis muscle is on the lateral side, deep to the triceps brachii.

1. Biceps brachii

    Origin: Supraglenoid tubercle.
    Termination: Radial tuberosity.
    Action: Flex the cubital joint and extend the humeral joint.

    In the carnivores and the pig the biceps brachii also terminates on the proximal ulna. In the horse and to a lesser extent in the ox, a strong fibrous band, the lacertus fibrosus, joins the biceps brachii to the extensor carpi radialis. This can be palpated on the craniomedial aspect of the cubitus in the depression where the leg joins the trunk. The proximal end of the biceps brachii is bound into the intertubercular groove by the transverse humeral retinaculum which is better developed in some species than in others. In carnivores with chronic shoulder luxations, this ligament may be transected and the biceps tendon translocated to a new position (medially or laterally) to counteract the luxation [1]. In the horse the portion of the biceps tendon in the intertubercular groove is deeply indented on its caudal aspect by the intermediate tubercle of the humerus.

2. Brachialis

    Origin: Brachial groove of humerus.
    Termination: Proximal radius and/or ulna.
    Action: Flex the cubital joint.

    The humeral shaft may be approached craniolaterally in carnivores between the brachialis and brachiocephalicus muscles [6].

D. Caudal muscles of the brachium

These three muscles are primarily extensors of the cubital joint. They all insert on the tuber olecrani of the olecranon, and they are innervated by muscular branches of the radial nerve.

1. Triceps brachii (long, medial, and lateral heads)

    Origin: Caudal border of scapula (long head); proximal humerus (other heads).
    Termination: Tuber olecrani of olecranon.
    Action: Extend the cubital joint (all heads); flex the humeral joint (long head).

Figure 2-5

Intrinsic Muscles of the Thoracic Limb
(medial aspect of equine limb with most of the extrinsic muscles removed)

1. Scapular cartilage
2. Latissimus dorsi m. (transected)
3. Teres major m.
4. Long head of triceps brachii m.
5. Tensor fasciae antebrachii m. (transected)
6. Tuber olecrani
7. Subscapularis m.
8. Supraspinatus m.
9. Subclavius m. (transected)
10. Deep pectoral m. (transected)
11. Coracobrachialis m.
12. Medial head of triceps brachii m.
13. Biceps brachii m.
14. Brachialis m.
15. Lacertus fibrosus
16. Extensor carpi radialis m.
17. Medial collateral ligament of cubital joint
18. Ulnar head of deep digital flexor m.
19. Flexor carpi ulnaris m.
20. Flexor carpi radialis m.
21. Radius
22. Abductor pollicis longus m. (extensor carpi obliquus m.)
23. Third metacarpal bone
24. Tendon of common digital extensor m.
25. Second metacarpal bone ("medial splint bone")
26. Interosseous m. ("suspensory lig.")
27. Tendons of superficial and deep digital flexor mm.
28. Extensor branch of interosseous m.
29. Palmar annular lig.
30. Tendon of superficial digital flexor m.
31. Proximal digital annular lig.
32. (Medial) cartilage of hoof

After Pasquini et al, 1983 [15]

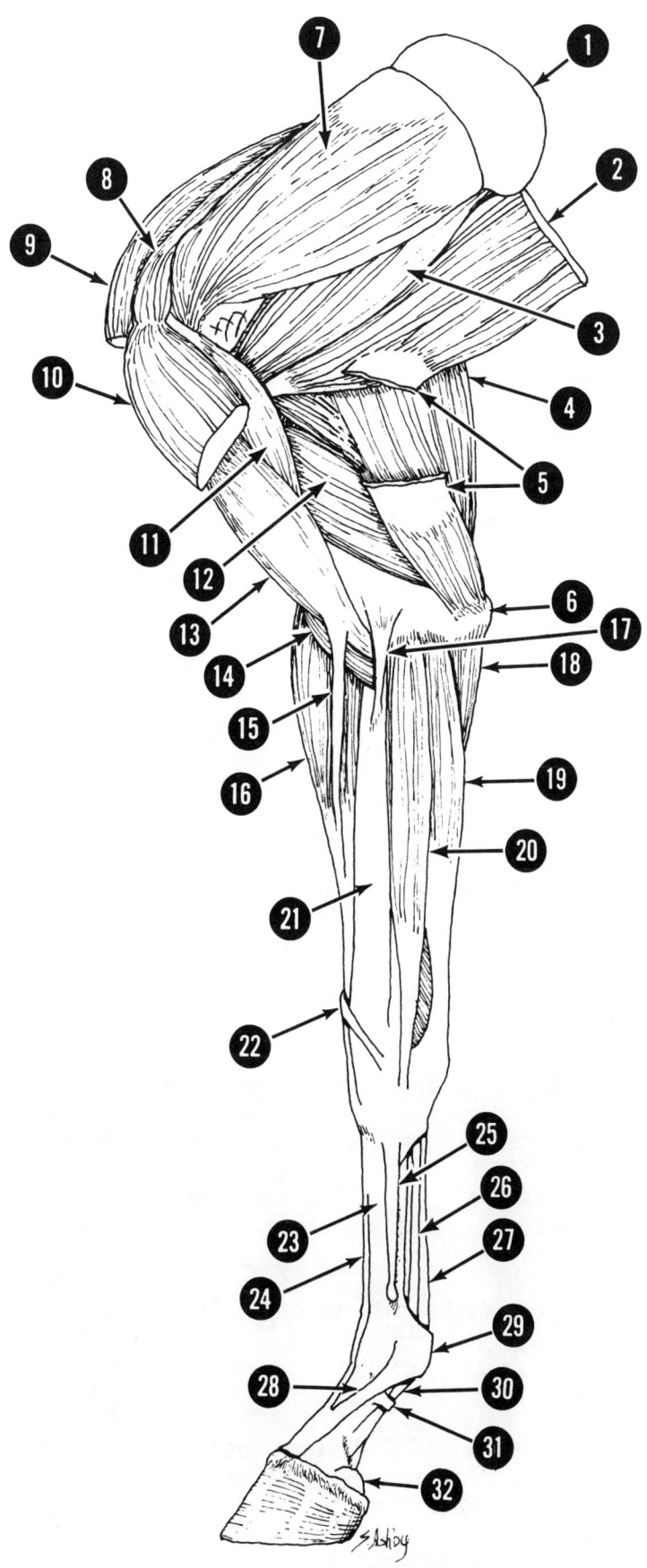

The triceps brachii of carnivores has a fourth (accessory) head. (An accessory head can also be partially separated from the medial head in some ruminants, especially in goats.) The humeral shaft may be approached medially between the triceps brachii and biceps brachii, but the three nerves and two vessels in the field should be preserved (musculocutaneus, median, and ulnar nerves; brachial a. and v.) [6].

A bursa exists between the tendon of termination of the triceps brachii and the tuber olecrani. In the bursitis which occasionally affects horses (shoe boil, capped elbow, olecranon bursitis) a "false" subcutaneous bursa forms and the bursa under the triceps tendon is not usually involved [8].

2. Tensor fasciae antebrachii

Origin: Latissimus dorsi and fascia on caudal border of scapula.
Termination: Tuber olecrani of olecranon.
Action: Extend the cubital joint (and tense the deep antebrachial fascia).

In the horse, the belly of the tensor fasciae antebrachii is divided into two parts that may appear to be two separate muscles.

3. Anconeus

Origin: Caudal aspect of the distal humerus.
Termination: Tuber olecrani of the olecranon.
Action: Extend the cubital joint.

The diminutive anconeal muscle lies primarily under the triceps brachii. It is incised during a lateral approach to the cubital joint [6].

Before reviewing the craniolateral and caudomedial antebrachial muscles, it may be helpful to recall these basic facts:

1. There are at least nine antebrachial muscles in any domestic mammal:

    2 digital extensors   (common and lateral)
    2 digital flexors   (superficial and deep)
    2 carpal extensors   (radial and ulnar)
    2 carpal flexors   (radial and ulnar)
    abductor pollicis longus

    In fact, these are the only antebrachial muscles present in a horse. Mammals progressively less specialized for running have additional minor antebrachial muscles (pronator teres, pronator quadratus, supinator, and others).

2. There is often considerable fusion between the bellies of adjacent antebrachial muscles, and they may be separated most easily by working distally to proximally from their tendons of termination. In addition, by

following the tendons distally, the carpal extensors and flexors can be easily (and always) distinguished from the digital extensors and flexors.

3. In regard to the most distal attachment of the digital flexors and extensors, the following statements are true for either limb in any domestic mammal:

   a. Superficial digital flexor muscles attach to the middle phalanges of the weight-bearing digits.
   b. Deep digital flexor muscles attach to the distal phalanges of the weight-bearing digits.
   c. Digital extensor muscles (common, long, and lateral) extend distally to the distal phalanges of the weight-bearing digits (except the lateral digital extensor of the thoracic limb of the horse which attaches to the proximal phalanx). Common and long digital extensors are distributed to all of the major digits while lateral digital extensors are distributed only to some of the lateral digits.

4. Two antebrachial muscles, the extensor carpi ulnaris (ulnaris lateralis), and flexor carpi ulnaris attach to the accessory carpal bone. No other carpal bone serves as a point of muscular attachment.

5. The tendons of the abductor pollicis longus, extensor carpi radialis, and common digital extensor muscles all lie in grooves in the distal radius (from medial to lateral, respectively). Surgical approaches to the carpus for chip and slab fractures are made between these tendons [6,11].

E. Craniolateral antebrachial muscles (Fig. 2-6)

   These muscles are primarily extensors of the carpal and digital joints. Most of them originate on or near the lateral epicondyle of the humerus. Some of them actually originate from the radius and ulna, but (with the exception of the abductor digiti I longus) these points of origin are still near the lateral epicondyle. Many of these muscles have some flexor action on the cubital joint because of their origin above it, but this is a minor action in most cases (except for the extensor carpi radialis). The craniolateral muscles are innervated by the deep branch of the radial nerve. Surgical approaches to the radius may be made between their bellies.

   1. Extensor carpi radialis

      Origin: Lateral epicondyle of the humerus (and its crest).
      Termination: Third metacarpal bone.
      Action: Extend the carpal joint and flex the cubital joint.

      The extensor carpi radialis is the largest craniolateral antebrachial muscle. Its tendon is obliquely crossed by the abductor pollicis longus. In the cat and partially in the dog, the extensor carpi radialis is divisible into a long part which inserts on metacarpal 2 and a short part which inserts on metacarpal 3. In the horse, the tendon occasionally ruptures with the presenting sign of exaggerated flexion of the carpus [8].

Figure 2-6

Craniolateral Antebrachial Muscles of the Dog (A), Pig (B), Ox (C), and Horse (D)

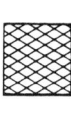 Brachioradialis m. (present in carnivores only)

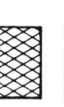 Extensor carpi radialis m.

Common digital extensor m.

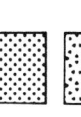 Lateral digital extensor m.

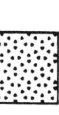 Extensor carpi ulnaris (ulnaris lateralis) m.

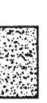 Abductor pollicis longus m.

Interosseous m.

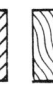 Deep digital flexor m. (ulnar head - not visible in the dog)

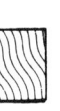 Superficial digital flexor m. (not visible in the dog)

 Flexor carpi ulnaris m. (visible in dog only)

 First and second digital extensor m. (dog), first digital extensor m. (pig)

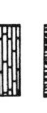

After Nickel, Schummer, and Seiferle, 1968 [12]

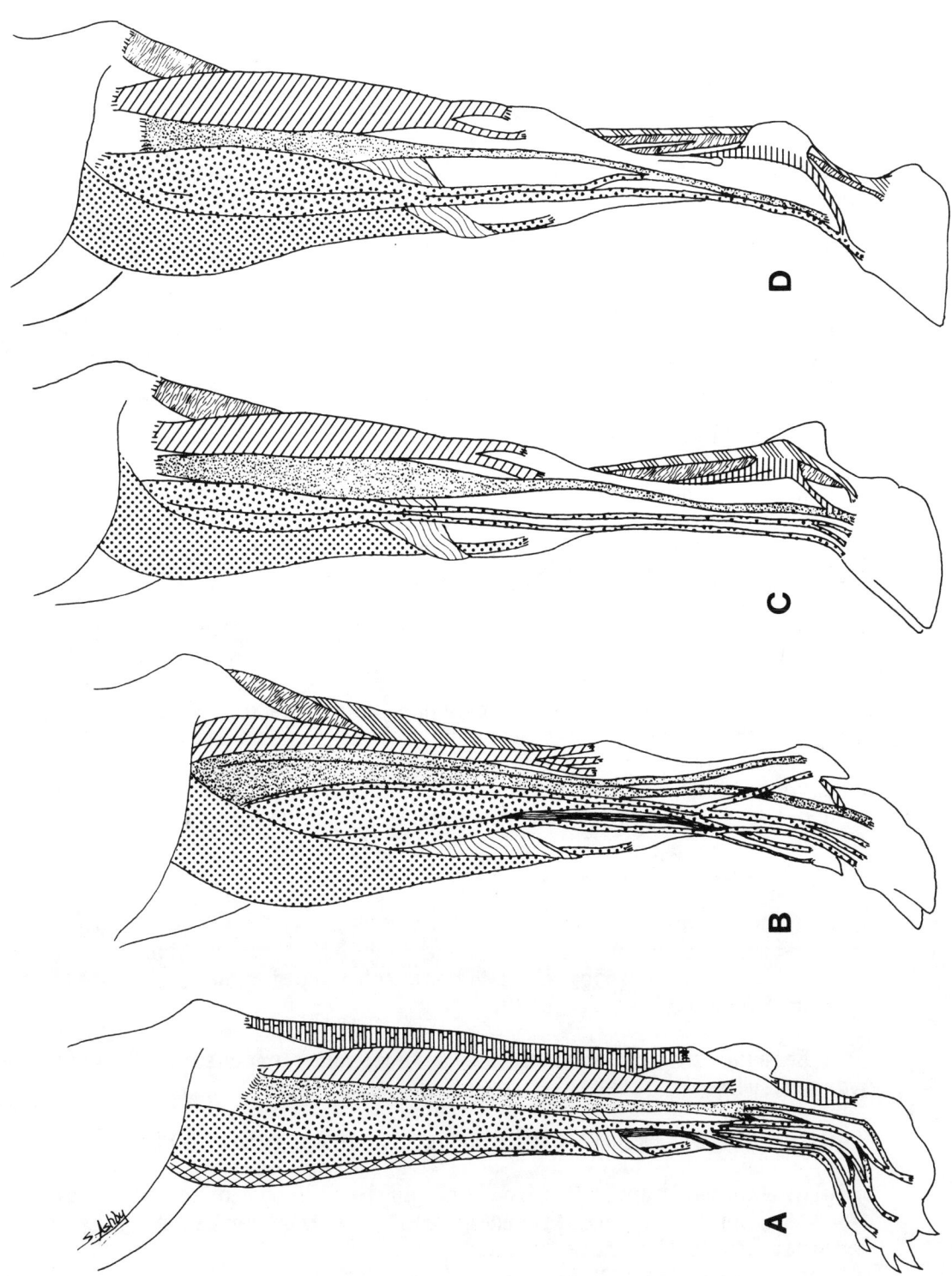

2. Common digital extensor

   Origin: On or near the lateral epicondyle.
   Termination: Extensor processes of the distal phalanges.
   Action: Extend carpal and digital joints.

   In domestic animals with more than one functional digit on each limb (i.e., all except the horse) the tendon is divided into parts which are distributed to each digit. In the artiodactyles this division separates the muscle distinctly into a medial belly, the tendon from which is distributed only to the medial digit(s), and a lateral belly, the tendon from which divides into parts for the medial and lateral digits. The medial belly has been termed "medial digital extensor" by some authors in reference to the pig and "proper extensor of digit III" in reference to the ruminants [12]. In the carnivores, dorsal sesamoid bones are embedded in the tendons at the metacarpophalangeal joints and occasionally at the interphalangeal joints. The ungulates do not have these bones.

3. Lateral digital extensor

   Origin: On or near the lateral epicondyle.
   Termination: Distal phalanges (also the proximal and/or middle phalanges) of the lateral digit(s).
   Action: Extend the digital joints.

   In the horse the lateral digital extensor attaches only as far distally as the proximal phalanx after receiving a communicating tendinous slip from the common digital extensor. This is the only exception to the general rule of thumb that the distal-most point of termination of any digital extensor (any species, either limb) is on the distal phalanges. For the purist, the actual digits which receive tendons of the lateral digital extensor are: cat--2, 3, 4, 5; dog--3, 4, 5; pig--4, 5; ruminants--4; horse--3.

4. Extensor carpi ulnaris [ulnaris lateralis]

   Origin: On or near the lateral epicondyle.
   Termination: Accessory carpal bone and the fourth (horse, ox) or fifth (pig, carnivores) metacarpal bone.
   Action: Flex the carpal joint.

   Because this muscle is not a functional extensor, the official synonym, ulnaris lateralis, is often used.

5. Abductor digiti I [pollicis] longus [extensor carpi obliquus]

   Origin: Proximal antebrachium. For purists: body of radius (horse); ulna (carnivores); radius and ulna (ruminants, pig).
   Termination: Medial metacarpus.
   Action: Extend the carpal joint (ungulates), abduct the first digit (carnivores).

   The tendon of this muscle crosses obliquely over that of the extensor carpi radialis from lateral to medial. For the purist, the termination is Mc1 in the carnivores, Mc2 in the horse and pig, and Mc3 + 4 in the ruminants. In the carnivores, there is a sesamoid bone embedded in the tendon on the medial side of the carpus.

Several other minor craniolateral antebrachial muscles are present in some species. In the cat and often in the dog, a brachioradialis muscle is present (Fig. 2-6). It lies cranial to the extensor carpi radialis, originates on the humerus, inserts on the radius, and functions in supination of the paw. It has been mistaken for the cephalic vein by the novice venipuncturist. The carnivores also have a small supinator muscle which is sometimes present in the pig. It lies under the extensor carpi radialis and common digital extensor. Other vestigial muscles in this group include the tiny extensor digiti I et II ("extensor pollicis longus et indicus proprius") which is present in carnivores and the extensor digiti I in pigs.

Clinically, the craniolateral antebrachial muscles are significant during surgical approaches to the radius and ulna and in the evaluation of radial nerve dysfunctions.

F. Caudomedial antebrachial muscles (Fig. 2-5)

The caudomedial antebrachial muscles are primarily flexors of the carpal and digital joints. They originate on or near the medial epicondyle of the humerus and are innervated by the median and ulnar nerves. Many of these muscles have some minor action on the cubital joint because of their origin proximal to it, but their major actions concern the carpal and digital joints.

Clinically, these muscles are significant in some approaches to the ulna, in tendon translocations to treat radial paralysis, and in the assessment of median and ulnar nerve damage.

1. Flexor carpi radialis

   Origin: Medial epicondyle of humerus.
   Termination: Proximal aspect of metacarpal bones.
   Action: Flex the carpal joints.

   For the purist, the termination in the horse is Mc2; carnivores, Mc2 and 3; pig, Mc3; and ruminants Mc3 + 4.

2. Flexor carpi ulnaris (2 heads: humeral and ulnar)

   Origin: Medial epicondyle and olecranon.
   Termination: Accessory carpal bone.
   Action: Flex the carpal joint.

   In the horse and ox, the ulnar head of this muscle can be confused with the similarly sized ulnar head of the deep digital flexor. Following their tendons distally allows differentiation.

3. Superficial digital flexor

Origin: On or near the medial epicondyle of the humerus.
Termination: Middle phalanges of the digits.
Action: Flex the carpal and digital joints.

In domestic animals with more than one functional digit on each limb (i.e., all except the horse) the tendon, and sometimes the muscle belly, is divided into parts which are distributed to each digit. Near the metacarpophalangeal joints, each branch of the tendon forms a loop or collar (Figs. 2-7 A/6 and 2-7 B/7). The tendon branches of the deep digital flexor pass through these collars to gain the "superficial" positions necessary to continue on to the distal phalanges. Likewise, the collars allow the superficial digital flexor tendons to gain the "deep" positions necessary for their attachments on the middle phalanges.

In the horse, the superficial digital flexor attaches to the distal end of the proximal phalanx in addition to its attachment to the middle phalanx. This may help prevent the "dorsal buckling" of the proximal interphalangeal joint which can otherwise occur. ("Dorsal buckling" is hyperflexion of the proximal interphalangeal joint with simultaneous hyperextension of the metacarpophalangeal joint). The horse also has a "radial head" of the superficial digital flexor which consists of a strong tendinous band from the radius to the main tendon just proximal to the carpus (Fig. 2-7 A/1 and 2-7 B/1). Obsolete synonyms for this structure include the popular "radial check ligament" as well as "superior check ligament" and "proximal check ligament." Its proper name is accessory ligament of the superficial digital flexor. In foals with flexor deformities (i.e., contracted tendons--see deep digital flexor) the accessory ligament is sometimes surgically severed, and in severe cases, the main superficial and deep digital flexor tendons may be transected as a corrective procedure [8].

In the ruminants, the superficial digital flexor is divided into two bellies, and the tendon of the superficial belly does not pass through the carpal canal with that of the deep belly. Instead, it passes through the heavy flexor retinaculum and joins the deep tendon in the mid-metacarpal region.

4. Deep digital flexor (3 heads: humeral, radial, ulnar)

Origin: Medial epicondyle of the humerus, radius, ulna. The radial head may be absent in the horse.
Termination: Distal phalanges.
Action: Flex the carpal and digital joints.

In animals with more than one functional digit on each limb, the tendon and/or muscle bellies are divided into parts which are distributed to each digit. In the horse, a strong tendinous band (as big as the tendon of the muscle) from the palmar carpal ligament joins the tendon distal to the carpus. Its proper name is the accessory ligament of the deep digital flexor (Fig. 2-7 B/4). Obsolete, but more popular, synonyms for this structure include "carpal check ligament", "inferior check ligament", and "distal check ligament." This ligament is surgically resected in one surgical correction for "contracted tendons" in foals [13].

Contracted tendons is a clinical syndrome of horses which involves shortening of the superficial and/or deep digital flexor muscles or their accessory ("check") ligaments. It may be congenital or acquired and may be treated surgically (resection) or conservatively [8,13].

Tendosynovitis* of the superficial and/or deep digital flexor tendons in horses is termed bowed tendon. It may occur in either thoracic or pelvic limbs and it produces a swelling on the palmar or plantar side of the metacarpus or metatarsus. The condition is classified as high, middle, or low, depending on which part of the metapodium is involved.

In the cat, the deep digital flexor is primarily responsible for the protrusion of the claws, although it has been shown that some contraction by extensor muscles must also occur (see Chapter 3, VIII, B2). Flexion of the distal interphalangeal joints causes the claws to be "extended" (protrude) [5].

5. Pronator teres

   Origin: On or near the medial epicondyle of the humerus.
   Termination: Medial body of radius.
   Action: Weak elbow flexion and weak pronation of the manus.

   The pronator teres is absent in the horse and very small in the ox. "Teres" means round, referring to a transverse section of the muscle belly.

6. Pronator quadratus

   Attachments: Opposed surfaces of the radius and the ulna.
   Action: Pronation of paw.

   The pronator quadratus is absent in the horse and ruminants (their radius and ulna are fused). "Quadratus" means four-sided and refers to the transectional shape of the muscle belly.

G. Muscles of the manus

   A number of small and generally insignificant muscles are associated with the manus. Most of them lie on the palmar aspect of the metacarpus, are best developed in the carnivores, and are even less significant or absent in the larger domestic animals. Included among them are several tiny muscles associated with the first, second, or fifth digits whose names are usually larger than the muscles themselves (abductor digiti I brevis, adductor digiti V, extensor digiti II, etc., ad nauseam). Some

---

*Tendosynovitis should be differentiated from synovitis, tendinitis, and tenosynovitis. Synovitis is a nonspecific term which indicates inflammation of the synovial lining of a joint, bursa, or tendon sheath. Tenosynovitis (tenovaginitis) is the term applied when the synovitis involves a tendon sheath. If the tendon is inflamed as well as its sheath, the term tendosynovitis (tendovaginitis) is used. If only the tendon is involved, the term tendinitis is applied [8].

Figure 2-7

Accessory Ligaments of the Superficial and Deep Digital Flexor Muscles
(thoracic limb of the horse)

A. "Radial check ligament" and related structures (medial aspect)

1. "radial check ligament" (accessory lig. of superficial digital flexor)

2. belly of deep digital flexor muscle

3. belly of superficial digital flexor muscle

4. tendon of superficial digital flexor in metacarpus

5. tendon of deep digital flexor in metacarpus

6. collar or ring formed by the tendon of the superficial digital flexor through which the tendon of the deep digital flexor courses

7. division of the superficial digital flexor tendon into 2 parts for insertion on the distal end of the proximal phalanx and the proximal end of the middle phalanx

8. distal continuation of the deep digital flexor tendon (displaced palmarly in this illustration for clarity)

B. "Radial and carpal check ligaments" and related structures (medial aspect)

1. "radial check ligament" (accessory lig. of superficial digital flexor)

2. belly of deep digital flexor muscle

3. belly of superficial digital flexor muscle

4. "carpal check ligament" (accessory lig. of deep digital flexor)

5. junction of "carpal check ligament" and deep digital flexor tendon

6. transected tendon of superficial digital flexor

7. collar or ring formed by the tendon of the superficial digital flexor to transmit the tendon of the deep digital flexor

8. points of termination of the superficial digital flexor on the proximal and middle phalanges

9. termination of the deep digital flexor on the distal phalanx

From Shively, 1983 [14]

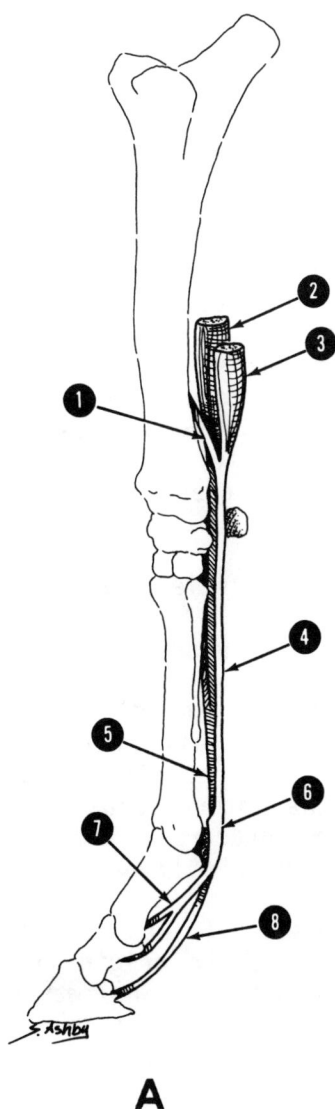
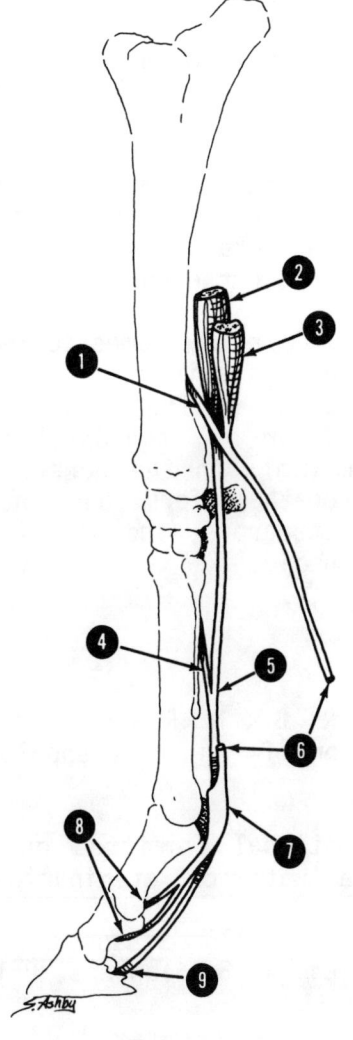

authors term these "special muscles of digits I, II and V" [10]. Another group of three weak flexor muscles includes the short digital flexor, the lumbricales, and the interflexorius mm. The one muscle of the manus which deserves special attention is the interosseous muscle--especially important in large animals.

Domestic mammals have one functional interosseous muscle for each weight-bearing digit (the two in ruminants are fused). The interossei originate near the proximal ends of the metacarpal bones and each one divides to insert on the proximal sesamoid bones. A tendinous extensor branch from each of these continues around each side of the metacarpophalangeal joints to join the digital extensor tendon (these extensor branches are palpable in the horse). The interossei are flexors of the metacarpophalangeal joints and they also support these joints. Comparative points about them include the following:

1. In the carnivores and pig, the interosseous muscles are fleshy.

2. In the horse, three interosseous muscles are present, but the medial one and lateral one are insignificant and play out in the fascia near the "fetlock." The interosseous medius (middle interosseous muscle) becomes tendinous (non-contractible) with maturity and is often called the "suspensory ligament" or "proximal sesamoidean ligament" [3]. One should not confuse the interosseous muscle with the interosseous ligaments between the metacarpal and metatarsal bones (inflammation of which results in "splints").

3. In the ruminants the two interosseous muscles (3 and 4) have fleshy and tendinous parts. They are fused near their origin and send a band to the superficial digital flexor tendon about halfway down the metacarpus. The axial extensor branches are fused during their course through the intertrochlear notch of Mc3 + 4 (Fig. 3-6/2) [3].

In any domestic mammal, the three major anatomical entities present between skin and bone on the palmar aspect of the metacarpus (or plantar aspect of the metatarsus) are the tendon(s) of the superficial digital flexor m., tendon(s) of the deep digital flexor m., and interosseous m.(mm). In the horse, the superficial and deep digital flexor tendons together form one of the two heavy palpable bands on the palmar metacarpus, and deep to them the other one is formed by the interosseous muscle.

References

1. Hohn, R. B., H. Rosen, R. H. Bohning, and S. G. Brown. 1971. Surgical stabilization of recurrent shoulder luxation. Vet. Clinics of North Am. 1(3):537-548.

2. International Committee on Veterinary Gross Anatomical Nomenclature. 1983. Nomina Anatomica Veterinaria, third ed. Published by the Committee, New York.

3. Getty, R. 1975. Sisson and Grossman's The Anatomy of the Domestic Animals, fifth ed. W. B. Saunders, Philadelphia.

4. Archibald, J., ed. 1974. Canine Surgery. American Veterinary Publications, Santa Barbara, California.

5. McClure, R. C., M. J. Dallman, and P. G. Garrett. 1973. Cat Anatomy: An Atlas, Text and Dissection Guide. Lea and Febiger, Philadelphia.

6. Piermattei, D. L., and R. G. Greeley. 1979. An Atlas of Surgical Approaches to the Bones of the Dog and Cat, second ed. W. B. Saunders, Philadelphia.

7. Hohn, R. B. 1973. Osteochondritis dissecans of the humeral head. JAVMA 163:69-70.

8. Adams, O. R. 1974. Lameness in Horses, third ed. Lea and Febiger, Philadelphia.

9. Habel, R. E. 1981. Applied Veterinary Anatomy, second ed. Published by the author. Ithaca, New York.

10. Evans, H. E., and G. C. Christensen. 1979. Miller's Anatomy of the Dog, second ed. W. B. Saunders, Philadelphia.

11. Milne, D. W., and A. S. Turner. 1979. An Atlas of Surgical Approaches to the Bones of the Horse. W. B. Saunders, Philadelphia.

12. Nickel, R., A. Schummer, and E. Seiferle. 1968. Lehrbuch der Anatomic der Haustiere. Band I. Paul Parey, Berlin.

13. McIlwraith, C. W., and J. R. Fessler. 1978. Evaluation of inferior check ligament desmotomy for treatment of acquired flexor tendon contracture in the horse. JAVMA 172(3):293-298.

14. Shively, M. J. 1983. Functional and clinical significance of the check ligaments. J. Equine Pract. 5(2):37-42.

15. Pasquini, C., V. Reddy, and M. Ratzlaff. 1978. Atlas of Equine Anatomy, second ed. Sudz Publishing Company, Eureka, California.

THORACIC LIMB ARTHROLOGY

The major joints of the thoracic limb consist of the humeral (shoulder) joint, cubital (elbow) joint, carpal joint(s), metacarpophalangeal joints, and the proximal and distal interphalangeal joints. In addition to these, there are radioulnar joints and intermetacarpal joints. In domestic mammals there is no bony connection between the thoracic limb skeleton and the axial skeleton. In man, the clavicle serves in this capacity by articulating with the scapula and the sternum.

I. HUMERAL JOINT ("SHOULDER JOINT," "SCAPULOHUMERAL JOINT")

   A. General features

   The humeral joint has no well-developed ligaments to insure its integrity. However, the heavy tendons which cross the joint serve as active ligaments: two laterally (supraspinatus and infraspinatus), one medially (subscapularis), and one cranially (biceps brachii). The glenoid cavity of the scapula is considerably smaller than the humeral head with which it articulates.*

   B. Comparative and clinical considerations

   1. Although thickenings in the joint capsule can be identified medially and laterally in the dog and cranially in the horse (glenohumeral ligg.), they are poorly developed and are not very significant clinically. A poorly developed skeletal muscle is associated with the joint capsule (articularis humeri m.) in the cat, pig, and horse.

   2. Dislocations of the humeral joint rarely occur even though "true" supporting collateral ligaments are lacking. This is because the muscles (tendons) which surround the joint (those of the supraspinatus, infraspinatus, subscapularis and biceps brachii mm.) serve as functional ligaments. However, in a relaxed, and particularly in an anesthetized animal, the articular surfaces can be subluxated to a marked degree.

   3. There is a distinct intertubercular ("bicipital") bursa associated with the tendon of the biceps brachii at the level of the intertubercular groove in the horse and ruminants. Inflammation of this area results in bicipital bursitis [1]. In the pig and carnivores, this bursa communicates with the shoulder joint cavity [2].

   4. Osteochondrosis lesions commonly affect the canine humeral head. They are found in the midcaudal aspect and are best isolated radiographically by a mediolateral view. Since little or no bony involvement may be present, contrast medium may help outline the

---

*All freely moveable joints have either a surface area size differential between their components or only a portion of their articular surfaces in contact at any instant (genual joint). Otherwise, any movement would cause subluxation.

cartilaginous lesion. In severe cases, typical radiographic lesions consist of a focal flattening of the bony contour of the midcaudal humeral head, and free osteocartilaginous bodies (joint mice) may be present. Osteochondrosis has also been reported involving the cubital, genual, and tarsal joints of dogs [3] and it has been reported in several joints in horses and cattle.

5. Injections into the shoulder joint in carnivores can be made by directing the needle medially just caudal to the end of the acromion [3]. In large animals it is done in a similar manner just cranial to the tendon of the infraspinatus m. (Table 3-1).

6. The carnivores have a well-developed transverse humeral retinaculum ("intertubercular lig.") which spans the intertubercular groove to hold the tendon of the biceps brachii in place. In large animals this retinaculum is less distinct.

7. To obtain good mediolateral radiographs of the humeral joint, the limb must be pulled cranially and ventrally to a marked degree to avoid superimposing the joint on the cranial thorax or caudal neck [4].

II. CUBITAL JOINT ("ELBOW JOINT," "HUMERORADIOULNAR JOINT")

A. General features

The cubital joint is a compound joint including the humeroulnar, humeroradial, and the proximal radioulnar joints. All of these individual components are included within the same capsule (i.e., all joint cavities communicate). Its major ligaments include:

1. Medial collateral ligament ("radial collateral lig.")--attaches to the medial epicondyle of the humerus and divides distally into two parts.

2. Lateral collateral ligament ("ulnar collateral lig.")--attaches to the lateral epicondyle of the humerus and, in the carnivores, it divides distally into two parts. In the dog, a small sesamoid bone is occasionally observed radiographically in the lateral collateral ligament just lateral to the head of the radius.

B. Comparative and clinical considerations

1. The specific points of attachments of the collateral ligaments vary considerably among the domestic species and are not noted here because the differences have no clinical significance. In general, the ligaments attach to the proximal radius and/or ulna.

2. Luxations of the cubital joint rarely occur medially because the enlarged medial epicondyle of the humerus prevents the radius and ulna from dislocating in that direction. To reduce lateral luxations, the cubital joint should first be placed in extreme flexion. This will allow the joint to be reduced with the fewest intervening bony processes. Extreme flexion of the joint is also required to obtain good radiographic visualization of the anconeal

process to evaluate suspected cases of ununited anconeal process in dogs [4].

3. Three syndromes of the canine cubital joint may have similar clinical manifestations (lameness) in the early stages: osteochondrosis of the humeral trochlea, ununited anconeal process, and ununited (fragmented) coronoid process. All may be bilateral which makes the condition difficult for an owner to detect [3,5].

4. In the carnivores, two small additional ligaments are present: a radial annular ligament (around the head of the radius) and an olecranon ligament (extending from the lateral aspect of the medial epicondyle of the humerus to the cranial border of the ulna). The oblique ligament of the dog, which has been described by some authors, may be considered to be a regional thickening in the joint capsule [6]. These have no clinical significance.

5. Although the cubital joint may be approached surgically from the lateral aspect, the best exposure of the distal humerus and anconeal process is via a transolecranon procedure [7]. In this approach, the olecranon is transected and reflected (with its attached triceps tendon) and then reattached with pin and wire or a screw after the procedure is completed. The pilot hole for reattachment pins or screws should be drilled before the olecranon is transected. In dogs, this hole should be angled laterally (about 15-20°) because of the angulation of the tuber olecrani with the ulnar diaphysis. Otherwise, the medial aspect of the olecranon will be penetrated. In the cat, the olecranon is nearly in line with the diaphysis, and angulation of the pilot hole is contraindicated. When transecting the tuber olecrani, care should be taken not to injure the ulnar nerve which courses between the olecranon and the medial epicondyle of the humerus.

6. The cubital joint of carnivores can be injected by directing a needle between the tuber olecrani and the lateral epicondyle of the humerus, or by directing a needle caudomedially at the lateral border of the proximal aspect of the extensor carpi radialis m. The cubital joint of an ox can also be injected by these techniques or by the procedure described for the horse (Table 3-1).

III. RADIOULNAR ARTICULATIONS

There are proximal and distal radioulnar joints. The proximal radioulnar joint ossifies in the horse and ruminants. In the carnivores, it occurs where the edge of the head of the radius (articular circumference) articulates with the radial notch of the ulna. In the carnivores, a heavy antebrachial interosseous ligament occupies much of the interosseous space and binds the radius and ulna together. The distal radioulnar joint also typically ossifies in the horse and ruminants, although fusion is often still incomplete in many horses over four years of age [8]. In carnivores, a radioulnar ligament connects the distal radius and ulna to lend support to the distal radioulnar joint.

IV. CARPAL JOINTS

A. General features

The carpal joint complex includes the antebrachiocarpal joint, the intercarpal joints (between individual carpal bones) and some authors also include the carpometacarpal joints under the general heading "carpal joints". The collective intercarpal joints which lie between the proximal and distal rows of carpal bones comprise the middle carpal joint. "Intercarpal joint" is popularly, but incorrectly, used to designate the middle carpal joint. Intercarpal joints between adjacent carpal bones (side to side) have no specific designations (Fig. 3-1) [6]. Horsemen commonly refer to the carpus as the "knee."

Numerous individual ligaments are involved in the joint complex and there is considerable species variation. Most of the joint movement occurs at the antebrachiocarpal joint (made up of the larger radiocarpal joint and the smaller ulnocarpal joint) and the middle carpal joint. Very little movement occurs at the carpometacarpal joint(s). In the horse (at least) the synovial cavity of the antebrachiocarpal joint is distinct from the cavities of the rest of the complex, and the middle carpal and carpometacarpal joints communicate [9,10,11]

The carpal canal serves as a passageway for the flexor tendons, as well as for nerves and vessels. It is formed by the accessory carpal bone (laterally), by several of the other carpal bones (dorsally), and by the flexor retinaculum (palmarly).

B. Comparative and clinical considerations

1. Five radiographic views are normally used for a "complete" radiographic examination of the carpus. These include [10]:

   a. dorsopalmar (DP = "AP")
   b. lateromedial or mediolateral (LM or ML)
   c. flexed lateromedial or flexed mediolateral (LMF or MLF)
   d. dorsopalmar mediolateral oblique (DPMLO = "APLO")*
   e. dorsopalmar lateromedial oblique (DPLMO = "APMO")*

   In addition to these, some specialized views are occasionally used. Some views are more useful in locating lesions than others. In horses, some studies have shown that the LMF view is of more value in this regard than any other single view [12]. In carnivores, stress views (weight-bearing or simulated weight-bearing) of the carpus are often necessary to demonstrate ligamentous injuries.

2. "Lateral view" is commonly (and incorrectly) used in reference to both lateromedial radiographic projections and mediolateral projections. In practice, "lateral views" of large animal limbs are usually exposed as lateromedial views and "lateral views" of carnivore limbs are usually exposed as mediolateral views because of the ease of positioning the animals for these perspectives.

---

*A special committee of radiologists and anatomists has recently recommended that even the oblique views should be designated from the point of entry of the x-ray beam to the point of exit. Using this reasoning, a DPMLO view is designated DM-PLO and a DPLMO view is designated DL-PMO.

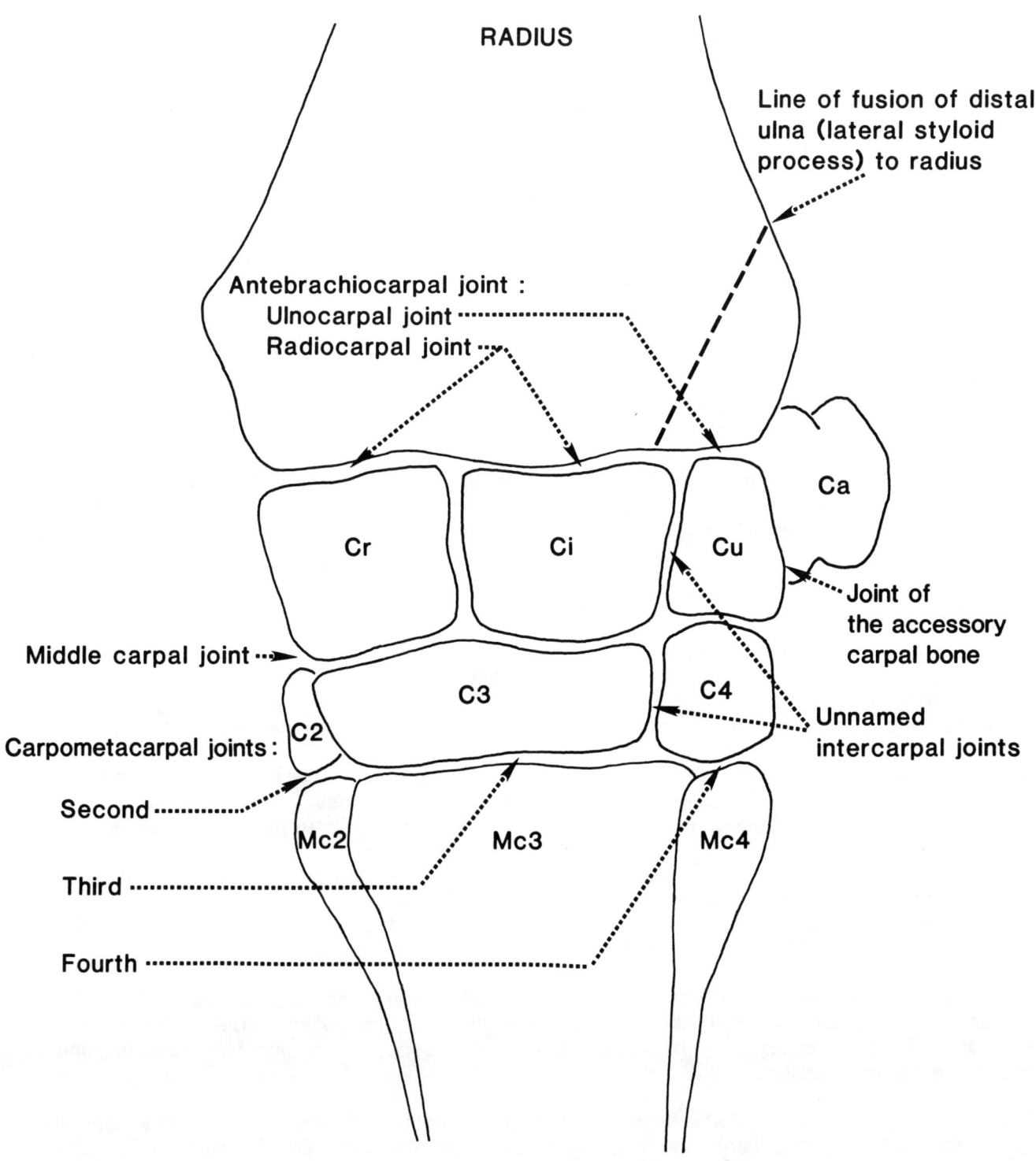

Figure 3-1

Proper Anatomic Designations of the Carpal Joint Complex
(dorsal aspect of left equine carpus)

Cr = radial carpal bone
Ci = intermediate carpal bone
Cu = ulnar carpal bone
Ca = accessory carpal bone

C2, C3, C4 = second, third, and fourth carpal bones
Mc2, Mc3, Mc4 = second, third, and fourth metacarpal bones

From Shively, 1982 [14]

Table 3-1

Synoviocentesis Techniques for the Equine Thoracic Limb

Shoulder joint--insert the needle 2 cm proximal to the greater tubercle at the cranial border of the tendon of the infraspinatus m. Direct the needle medially, distally, and caudally 5-10 cm until synovium is encountered.

Intertubercular bursa--insert the needle at the cranial border of the humerus 2 cm proximal to the deltoid tuberosity and just caudal to the lateral border of the biceps brachii tendon. Direct the needle medially until bone is encountered and then proximally under the biceps several cm (6-8) until synovium is encountered.

Cubital joint--insert the needle at the cranial border of the lateral collateral ligament of the cubital joint. Direct the needle medially to the bone and then sharply proximally until synovium is encountered.

Olecranon bursa--insert the needle over the proximal end of the olecranon to one side of the triceps brachii tendon.

Carpal joints--flex the joint and insert the needle between the radius and proximal row of carpal bones (for the antebrachiocarpal joint) or between the proximal and distal rows of carpal bones (for the middle carpal joint and carpometacarpal joints). The needle can be directed to the side of the extensor tendons.

Synovial sheath of the digital flexor tendons--insert the needle between the deep digital flexor tendon and the interosseous muscle about 5 cm proximal to the proximal sesamoid bones. Direct it horizontally until synovium is encountered.

Metacarpophalangeal joint--insert the needle into the center of an area halfway between the distal tip of Mc4 and the proximal sesamoid bone. The needle should be directed between Mc3 and the interosseous muscle, and it should be advanced distomedially. A similar technique can be used from the medial side.

Proximal interphalangeal joint--insert the needle along the lateral border of the digital extensor tendon about 2 cm proximal to the joint. Direct the needle about 4 cm distomedially between the dorsal aspect of the proximal phalanx and the extensor tendon.

Distal interphalangeal joint--insert the needle about 2 cm proximal to the dorsal border of the hoof and about 2 cm lateral (or medial) to the midline of the limb. Direct the needle distomedially along the dorsum of the middle phalanx 1-4 cm.

Podotrochlear bursa--insert the needle between the heels and direct it dorsally and slightly proximally in a line parallel to the proximal hoof border (as viewed laterally). When hard tissue is encountered the needle tip should be in the bursa.

3. Slab and chip fractures of carpal bones occur in racing horses and dogs. Most of these occur on the dorsal aspects of the bones and are believed to result from the excess forces put on the dorsal surfaces by hyperextension of the carpal joint. The bones most frequently fractured in the equine carpal region are the radial carpal bone, third carpal bone, distal radius, intermediate carpal bone, and accessory carpal bone (in that order) [12,13].

4. The second and fourth metacarpal bones of the horse ("splint bones") articulate with the distal row of carpal bones as well as with the third metacarpal bone [9]. In the ox, the fifth metacarpal bone articulates only with the fourth metacarpal bone and not with any of the carpal bones [11]. In the carpometacarpal joints of the horse, it is of value in radiographic orientation to note that, on the medial side of the carpus, the second carpal bone articulates with only one metacarpal bone (Mc2). Laterally, however, C4 articulates with both Mc3 and Mc4.

5. Particularly in reference to large animals, the entire antebrachiocarpal joint is popularly termed the "radiocarpal" joint. As noted under general considerations, however, in precise usage the latter term refers to only the medial part of the antebrachiocarpal joint [14].

6. Medial and lateral collateral carpal ligaments, joining the bones of the antebrachium and metacarpus, are present in the ungulates. These have long superficial and short deep parts and may send bands to some of the carpal bones. In the carnivores, these ligaments extend distally only to the intermedioradial and ulnar carpal bones ("short radial and ulnar collateral ligaments").

7. A number of ligaments attach the accessory carpal bone to adjacent bones and also distally to the metacarpus. This anchoring is necessary because of the proximal pull of the flexor carpi ulnaris and extensor carpi ulnaris (ulnaris lateralis) muscles. These ligaments are named according to the other bones to which they attach, but the offical names are not well known (accessory-ulnar lig., accessory-ulnocarpal lig., accessory-quartal lig., accessory-metacarpal lig.) [6].

8. The carpal joint is sometimes surgically fused (carpal arthrodesis) in cases of radial nerve paralysis.

9. Traumatic arthritis of the carpus in horses is termed carpitis (popped knees). Sometimes a subcutaneous bursa forms which produces a swelling on the dorsal aspect of the carpus (hygroma) [1].

10. Carpal canal syndrome is a condition caused by a space-occupying lesion in the carpal canal which results in pressure against the flexor retinaculum. Often this is caused by a soft tissue lesion (such as high bowed tendon in horses) and may result in pressure necrosis of the vascular and/or nervous supply to the distal limb. Surgical resection of the flexor retinaculum (usually done on the medial side) may be necessary [15]. Fracture of the accessory carpal bone has also resulted in this problem [16].

11. Various configurations of the equine carpus and adjacent regions of the limb have specific clinical designations. Some of them are pathological and some are simply conformational defects with little clinical significance (Fig. 3-2):

   a. Calf knees--palmar deviation of the carpus [1].
   b. Buck knees, knee sprung, goat knees, over at the knee--dorsal deviation of the carpus.
   c. Knock knees, knee narrow, valgus* deformity of the carpus-- medial deviation of the carpus, lateral angulation at the carpus - correction may require casting, staples across the distal epiphyseal cartilage of the radius, or periosteal stripping procedures (see Chapter 1).
   d. Bow legs, bandy-legged, varus* deformity of the carpus--lateral deviation of the carpus, medial angulation at the carpus.
   e. Cut out under the knees--a noticeable indentation when viewed laterally on the dorsal aspect of the thoracic limb just distal to the carpus.
   f. Tied in knees--a noticeable indentation when viewed laterally on the palmar aspect of the thoracic limb just distal to the carpus.
   g. Bench knees--a noticeable indentation when viewed cranially on the medial aspect of the limb just distal to the carpus. It is due to laterally offset metacarpi.
   h. Open knees--an irregular profile of the carpal joint when viewed from the lateral side due to enlargement of the distal radial epiphysis. This typically affects only young horses (1-2 years) and is attributed to the enlargement around the epiphyseal cartilages.

12. The carpal joint(s) in any domestic mammal may be easily injected from the dorsal aspect by flexing the joint to separate the carpal bones (Table 3-1) [19]. Synovial fluid may be withdrawn for analysis [20].

V. INTERMETACARPAL JOINTS

The proximal ends of the metacarpal bones in all species articulate with their adjacent counterparts to form the intermetacarpal joints. These are primarily fibrous joints formed by dense tissue (interosseous ligaments). In the dog, cat, and pig, these ligaments bind only the proximal portions of the metacarpal bones together because the metacarpal bones diverge as they course distally to form distinct intermetacarpal spaces. In the horse, the three metacarpal bones are bound together for much of their length by exceptionally well developed metacarpal interosseous ligaments which may become inflamed (interosseous desmitis or "splints") and may ossify with time. Similar

---

*The correct usages of valgus and varus are often confused by well-meaning authors. "Valgus" actually means bent outward and refers here to the lateral angulation of the distal limb which occurs at the carpus. The carpus itself is positioned or deviated medially. Similarly, "varus" refers to an inward (medial) angulation of the distal limb [18].

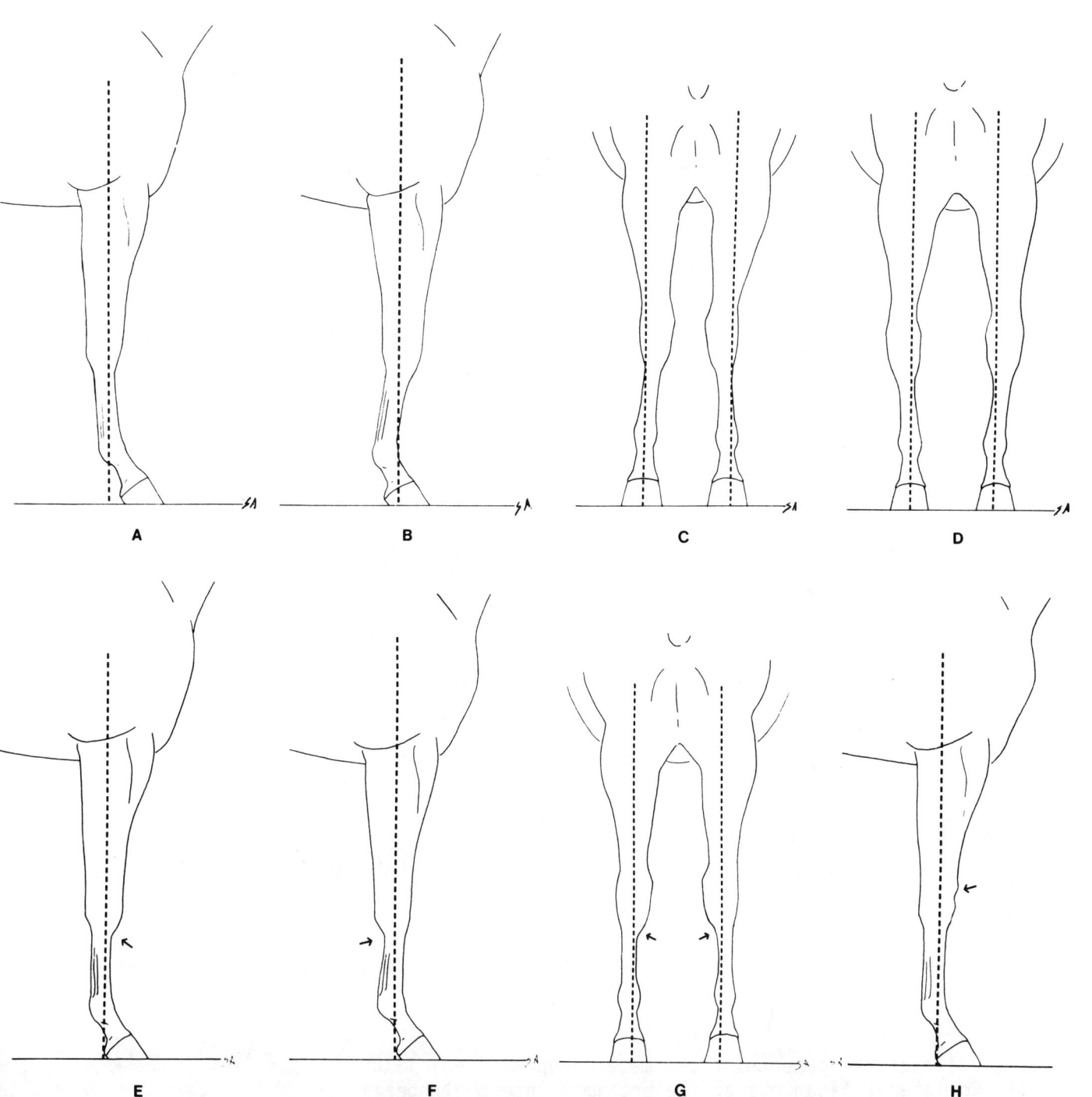

Figure 3-2

Abnormal Configurations of the Equine Carpus and Adjacent Regions

    A. Calf knees
    B. Buck knees (knee-sprung, goat knees, over at the knee)
    C. Knock knees (knee narrow, valgus deformity of the carpus)
    D. Bow legs (bandy-legged, varus deformity of the carpus)
    E. Cut out under the knees
    F. Tied in knees
    G. Bench knees
    H. Open knees

From Shively, 1982 [17]

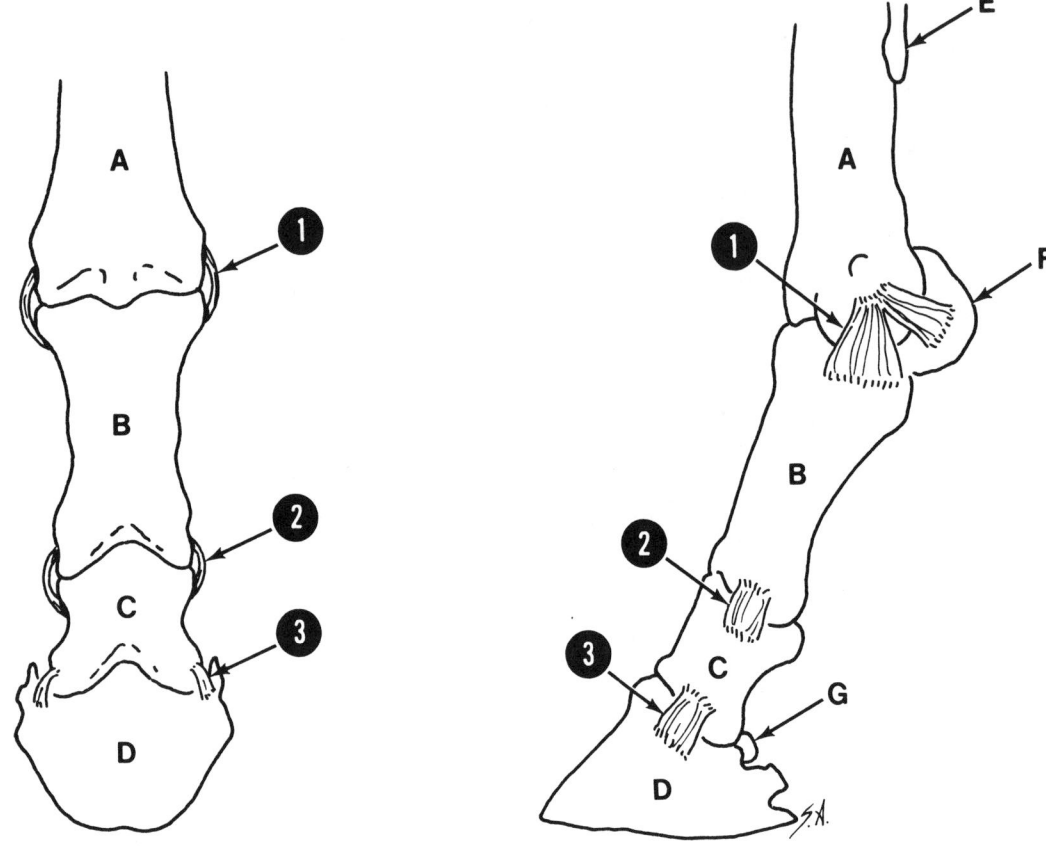

Dorsal Aspect   Lateral Aspect

Figure 3-3

Collateral Ligaments of the Digital Joints of the Horse
(ungual cartilages removed)

1. Collateral ligaments of the metacarpophalangeal joint
2. Collateral ligaments of the proximal interphalangeal joint
3. Collateral ligaments of the distal interphalangeal joint
4. Collateral sesamoidean ligament (the part to the proximal phalanx is not illustrated - see Fig. 3-5/1)

Skeletal Components:

A. Third metacarpal bone
B. Proximal phalanx
C. Middle phalanx
D. Distal phalanx
E. Fourth metacarpal bone
F. Proximal sesamoid bone (lateral)
G. Distal sesamoid bone

ligaments that suffer the same maladies are present in the pelvic limbs. In the ox, the joint between the third and fourth metacarpal bones is obliterated by the fusion which forms the single third and fourth ("large") metacarpal bone. The fifth ("small") metacarpal bone of the ox remains separate.

VI. METACARPOPHALANGEAL JOINTS

A. General features

The metacarpophalangeal joints occur between the heads of the metacarpal bones and the bases of the proximal phalanges. Medial and lateral collateral ligaments are present (Fig. 3-3/1. The articular surfaces of the proximal sesamoid bones are included within the same synovial capsule. A number of ligaments are associated with the proximal sesamoid bones, and since these sesamoids and their associated ligaments are best developed and most easily observed in the horse, the major features of the equine pattern will be used as a model (Figs. 3-4, 3-5):

1. The palmar ligament ("intersesamoidean lig.") attaches the proximal sesamoid bones together and provides a bearing surface for the flexor tendons. It contains a considerable amount of cartilage which extends proximal to the sesamoid bones (Fig. 3-5/2) [5].

2. The medial and lateral collateral sesamoidean ligaments attach to the interosseous surface of each sesamoid bone and divide into two branches. One of these attaches to the side of the head of the metacarpal bone and the other one attaches to the ipsilateral side of the base of the proximal phalanx. These ligaments blend into the collateral ligaments of the metacarpophalangeal joints and are not clearly separable from them (Fig. 3-5/1) [2].

3. The straight ("superficial") sesamoidean ligament joins the proximal sesamoid bones to a fibrocartilage on the proximal end of the palmar aspect of the middle phalanx (Fig. 3-4/3) [2].

4. The oblique ("middle") sesamoidean ligament joins the proximal sesamoid bones to the proximal phalanx attaching distally to the "V" shaped ridges on the palmar aspect of the proximal phalanx. This ligament is very thin axially and much thicker along its medial and lateral borders (Fig. 3-4/4) [2].

5. The cruciate ("deep") sesamoidean ligaments join the distal aspects of each sesamoid bone to the base of the proximal phalanx. They are very short and cross each other to join the contralateral aspect of the base of the proximal phalanx (Fig. 3-4/5).

6. The short sesamoidean ligaments join the sesamoid bones to the proximal phalanx without crossing (these are very small - Fig. 3-5/3).

The unofficial term "distal sesamoidean ligaments" refers collectively to the straight, oblique, and cruciate sesamoidean ligaments. "Proximal sesamoidean ligaments" refers to the interosseous muscle ("suspensory ligament"). "Suspensory apparatus" refers collectively to the interosseous muscle and the "distal sesamoidean ligaments".

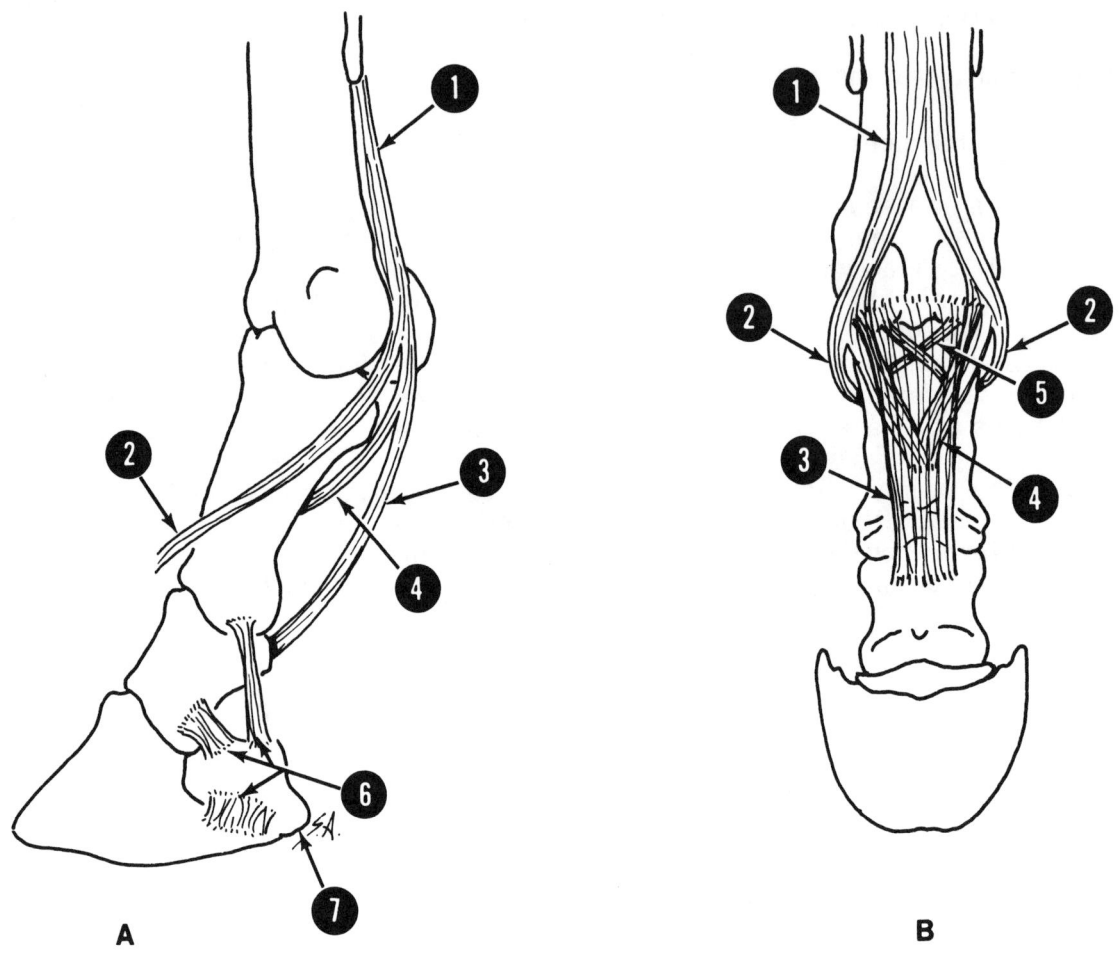

Figure 3-4

"Suspensory Ligament," Distal Sesamoidean Ligaments, and Ligaments of the Ungual Cartilages of the Horse

    A.   Lateral aspect

    B.   Palmar aspect (cartilages of distal phalanx not shown)

        1.   Interosseous m. ("suspensory lig.")
        2.   Branch of interosseous m. to extensor tendon
        3.   Straight sesamoidean ligament
        4.   Oblique sesamoidean ligament
        5.   Cruciate sesamoidean ligament
        6.   Ligaments of the ungual cartilage
        7.   (Lateral) ungual cartilage (cartilage of the hoof)

B. Comparative and clinical considerations

1. The interdigitation of the sagittal ridge on the head of each metacarpal bone with the groove in the base of each proximal phalanx imparts additional lateral stability to the metacarpophalangeal joints. The ridge is especially well developed in horses, and it divides the head of the third metacarpal bone into a slightly larger (wider) medial part and a slightly smaller (narrower) lateral part--a differentiation which is sometimes of value radiographically [21]. The ridge may be responsible for occasional longitudinal and oblique fractures of the proximal phalanx. Perhaps it acts like a screwdriver blade to produce these injuries either acutely or as the culmination of repeated stress [22].

2. The collateral ligaments of the metacarpophalangeal joints of the horse have superficial and deep layers: the deep layers are much stronger and send attachments to the abaxial surfaces of the proximal sesamoid bones as well as attachments to the proximal phalanx (Fig. 3-3/1).

3. In the ruminants, the two axial collateral ligaments result from the bifurcation of a single band which arises in the intertrochlear notch.

4. Species variations in the sesamoidean ligament pattern include the following:

   a. In the carnivores, these ligaments are not significant clinically. There are a number of differences from the equine pattern including the absence of short sesamoidean ligaments and straight sesamoidean ligaments.

   b. No good descriptions for the pig are available or necessary.

   c. In the ruminants, the straight sesamoidean ligament is absent. The oblique sesamoidean ligament is paired for each digit because the thin central portion, which is present in the horse and connects the thicker abaxial parts (see VI-A-4), is absent in the ox (Fig. 3-7). The palmar ligament, attaching the axial sesamoid bones of the third and fourth digits, is given the name interdigital intersesamoidean ligament. Ligaments occurring between one pair of proximal sesamoid bones and the proximal phalanx of the opposite digit are termed interdigital phalangosesamoidean ligaments [5].

5. Note that the metacarpophalangeal joints in domestic mammals are normally in a hyperextended position. In a galloping racehorse, this may be exaggerated during a stride so that the whole palmar surface of the proximal phalanx may be adjacent to the ground. This may be a contributing factor in compression fractures of the proximal sesamoid bones. Exaggerated metacarpophalangeal hyperextension may contribute to fractures of the dorsal aspect of the base of the proximal phalanx, since the extension may force it into the dorsal aspect of the third metacarpal bone and chip off a small piece.

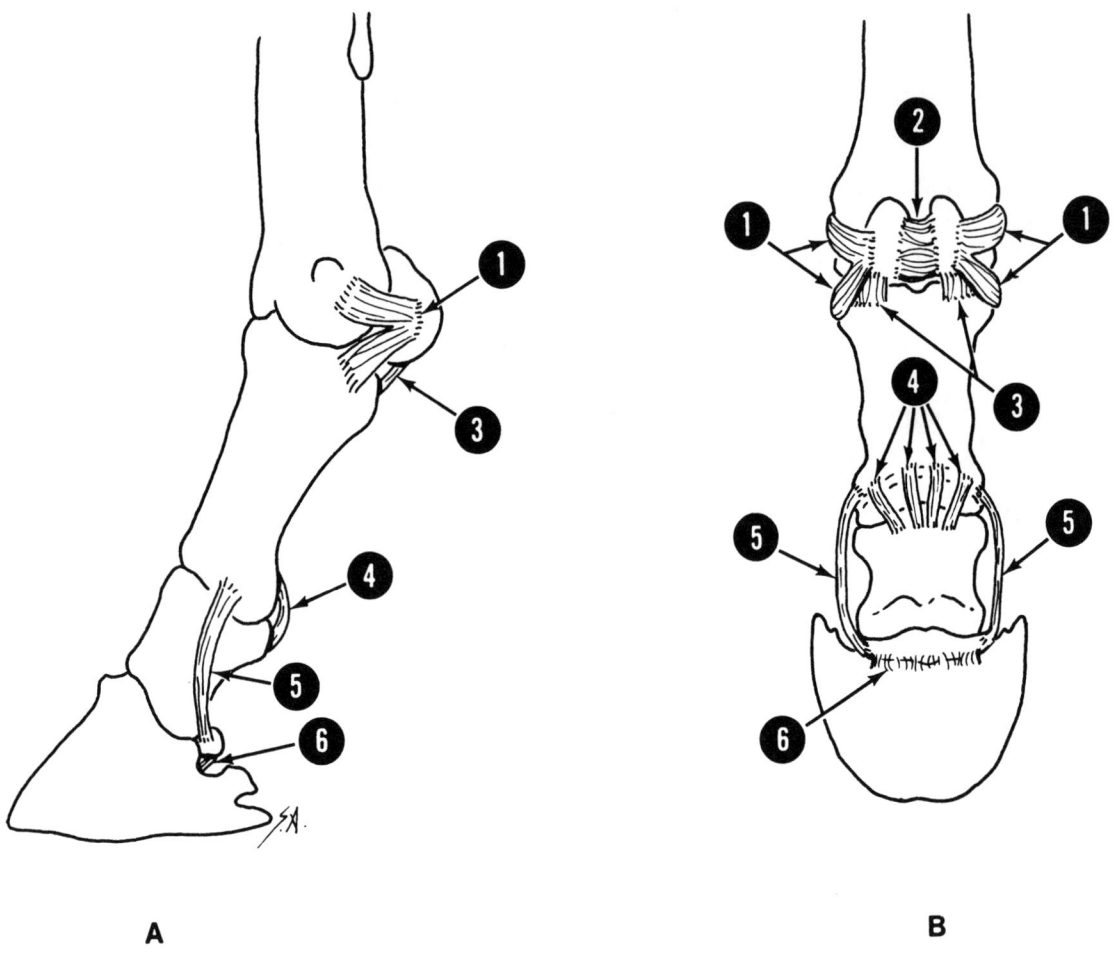

Figure 3-5

Miscellaneous Ligaments of the Manus of the Horse
(ungual cartilages removed)

A. Lateral aspect

B. Palmar aspect

1. Collateral sesamoidean ligaments
2. Palmar ("intersesamoidean") ligament
3. Short sesamoidean ligaments
4. Palmar ligaments of proximal interphalangeal joints
5. Collateral sesamoidean ligaments (of distal interphalangeal joint)*
6. Distal sesamoidean impar ligament

*These ligaments were formerly called suspensory ligaments of the distal sesamoid bone.

6. In horses, traumatic arthritis of the metacarpophalangeal joint is commonly termed osselets [1]. It is manifested by swelling and often by periosteal reactions near the joint. When no radiographic changes are present, the term green osselets is used. At necropsy, the only signs of inflammation in such cases may be villous hyperplasia of the synovial membrane.

7. The metacarpophalangeal joints (and metatarsophalangeal joints) of the horse, and occasionally of the ruminants as well, are popularly known as "fetlock joints."

8. Arthrocentesis of the metacarpophalangeal joints is rarely done in any domestic species except the horse [19,20]. In the ox, a technique similar to that described for the horse (Table 3-1) can be used.

VII. PROXIMAL INTERPHALANGEAL JOINT(S)

A. General features

A proximal interphalangeal joint occurs between the head of the proximal phalanx and the base of the middle phalanx of each weight-bearing digit. Medial and lateral collateral ligaments are present (Fig. 3-3/2).

B. Comparative and clinical considerations

1. The proximal interphalangeal joints may be surgically fused (arthrodesed) with few ill effects to relieve the pain associated with various arthropathies.

2. The proximal interphalangeal joint of a given digit is less mobile in ungulates than either the metacarpophalangeal joint or the distal interphalangeal joint.

3. In the horse, and often in ruminants, the proximal interphalangeal joints are popularly termed "pastern joints".

4. In the horse and in ruminants, some palmar ligaments are present in addition to the collateral ligaments. These consist of a central pair, bordered by medial and lateral bands, all four of which join the palmar aspects of the proximal and middle phalanges (Fig. 3-5/4). In ruminants the central pair fuse to form a single band (Fig. 3-7/5) [2].

VIII. DISTAL INTERPHALANGEAL JOINT(S)

A. General features

A distal interphalangeal joint occurs between the head of each middle phalanx and the articular surface of each distal phalanx. The articular surface of the distal sesamoid bone articulates with the palmar aspect of both phalanges. Medial and lateral collateral ligaments are present (Fig. 3-3/3).

B. Comparative and clinical considerations

1. The distal interphalangeal joints of horses, and often of ruminants, are popularly termed "coffin joints." A technique for arthrocentesis in the horse has been described (Table 3-1) [1].

2. The carnivores have a pair of dorsal ligaments for each digit which are elastic in nature and tend to keep the distal interphalangeal joints in a hyperextended position. In the dog, these ligaments are symmetrical and poorly developed. In the cat, they are heavier and one is longer than the other. Cats also have a third ligament which assists the other two. These ligaments keep the claws of cats retracted by keeping the distal interphalangeal joints (hyper-) extended. Flexion of the distal interphalangeal joint protrudes the claws. Although this action would appear to be a function of the deep digital flexor muscle only, an investigation has shown that simultaneous contraction of both flexors and extensors is necessary for the claws to protrude [23]. Declawing (onychectomy) in cats is typically done by amputation through the distal interphalangeal joint [24]. Most cats, incidentally, can still climb trees after this surgery if the claws on the pes are left intact.

3. In the horse, medial and lateral ungual cartilages (cartilages of the hoof) attach to the palmar processes of the distal phalanges and extend above the coronary region. They often mineralize with age to form "sidebone," which has little or no clinical significance [1]. These cartilages are joined to each phalanx by ligaments (Fig. 3-4/6).

4. Special ligaments of the distal sesamoid bone, best developed in the horse, include the paired collateral sesamoidean ligaments ("suspensory ligaments of the distal sesamoid bone"--Figs. 3-5/5, 3-6/6) which extend from its extremities to the distal end of the proximal phalanx. There is also a distal sesamoidean impar ligament that extends from the distal border of the distal sesamoid bone to the solar surface of the distal phalanx (Figs. 3-5/6, 3-6/10) [25].

5. In the horse, inflammation of the podotrochlear ("navicular") bursa is associated with "navicular" disease. It is more common in the thoracic limbs than in the pelvic limbs, and bony lesions occur in chronic cases. The pain may be relieved by digital neurectomies [1]. However, proprioception is reduced, and the animal may be more prone to stumbling and less safe to ride. Arthrocentesis of the podotrochlear bursa has been described (Table 3-1) [1].

6. In the ruminants, no ungual cartilages are present. The ligaments associated with the distal sesamoid bones resemble those in the horse.

IX. ADDITIONAL LIGAMENTS OF THE THORACIC LIMB

A. In ruminants (except sheep), adjacent proximal phalanges are bound by proximal interdigital ligaments (Fig. 3-7/6). Distal interdigital ligaments join the proximal, abaxial aspect of the middle phalanges to

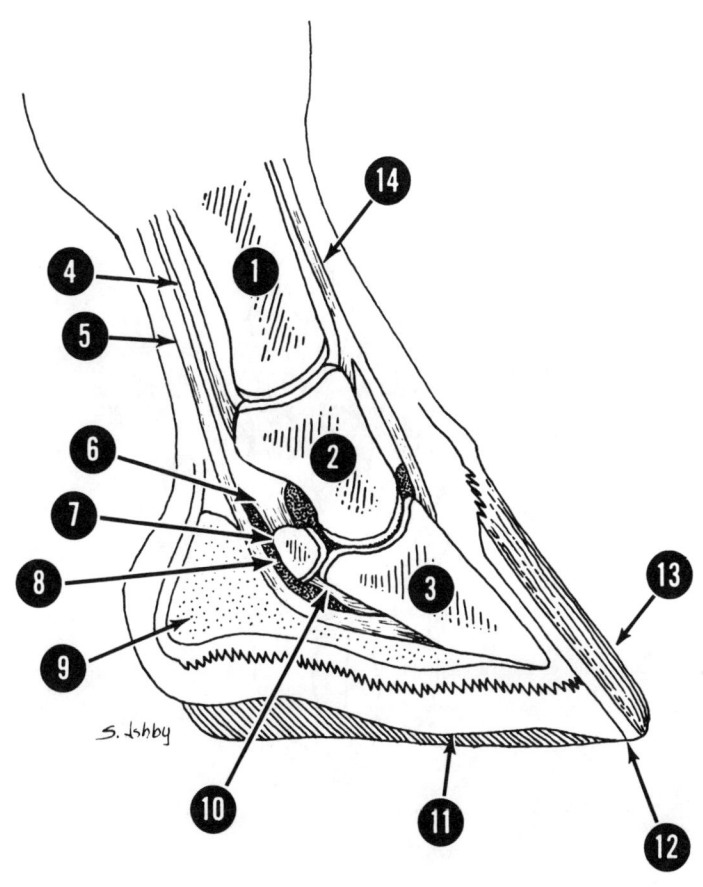

Figure 3-6

Sagittal Section of Equine Digit

1. Proximal phalanx
2. Middle phalanx
3. Distal phalanx
4. Tendon of superficial digital flexor m.
5. Tendon of deep digital flexor m.
6. Collateral sesamoidean lig.
7. Distal sesamoid bone
8. Podotrochlear ("navicular") bursa
9. Digital cushion
10. Distal sesamoidean impar lig.
11. Sole
12. White zone
13. Hoof wall
14. Tendon of common (or long) digital extensor m.

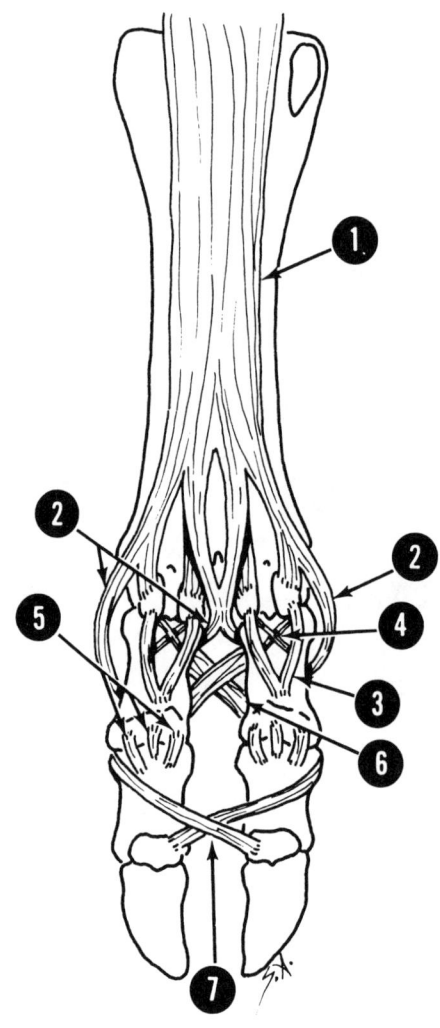

Figure 3-7

Selected Ligaments* of the Manus of the Ox (palmar aspect)

1. Interosseous muscle ("suspensory ligament")
2. Branches of interosseous m. to extensor tendons
3. Oblique sesamoidean ligaments
4. Cruciate sesamoidean ligaments
5. Palmar ligaments of proximal interphalangeal joint
6. Proximal interdigital ligaments
7. Distal interdigital ligaments (superficial parts)

*Ligaments not illustrated include the collateral ligaments of the various joints, ligaments of the distal sesamoid bones (collateral and impar), interdigital intersesamoidean ligament, palmar (intersesamoidean) ligaments of the metacarpophalangeal joints, and the interdigital phalangosesamoidean ligaments.

the opposite distal sesamoid bone and distal phalanx (Fig. 3-7/7). Finally, ruminants have interdigital phalangosesamoidean ligaments between the proximal phalanx of the digit and the proximal sesamoid bones of the other digit.

B. Note that the flexor tendons are bound in position at the metacarpophalangeal joint and to the proximal and middle phalanges by the palmar annular ligament (Fig. 2-5/29), the proximal digital annular ligament (Fig. 2-5/31), and the distal digital annular ligament respectively.

References

1. Adams, O. R. 1974. Lameness in Horses, third ed. Lea and Febiger, Philadelphia.

2. Getty, R. 1975. Sisson and Grossman's The Anatomy of the Domestic Animals, fifth ed. W. B. Saunders, Philadelphia.

3. Olsson, S. E. 1977. Osteochondrosis in the dog. In Current Veterinary Therapy VI, edited by R. Kirk. W. B. Saunders, Philadelphia.

4. Schebitz, H., and H. Wilkens. 1973. Atlas of Radiographic Anatomy of Dog and Horse. Paul Parey, Berlin.

5. Goring, R. L., and M. S. Bloomberg. 1983. Selected developmental anomalies of the canine elbow: radiographic evaluation and surgical management. Comp. Cont. Ed. 5(3):178-188.

6. International Committee on Veterinary Gross Anatomical Nomenclature. 1983. Nomina Anatomica Veterinaria, third ed. Published by the Committee, Ithaca, New York.

7. Piermattei, D. L., and R. G. Greeley. 1979. An Atlas of Surgical Approaches to the Bones of the Dog and Cat, second ed. W. B. Saunders, Philadelphia.

8. Myers, V. S. 1965. Confusing radiologic variations at the distal end of the radius of the horse. JAVMA 147(2):1310-1312.

9. Habel, R. E. 1981. Applied Veterinary Anatomy, second ed. Published by the author, Ithaca, New York.

10. Smallwood, J. E., and M. J. Shively. 1979. Radiographic and xeroradiographic anatomy of the equine carpus. J. Equine Prac. 1(1):22-38.

11. Shively, M. J., and J. E. Smallwood. 1978. Normal radiographic and xeroradiographic anatomy of the bovine manus. Swest Vet. 31(3):220-226.

12. Park, R. D., J. P. Morgan, and T. R. O'Brien. 1971. Chip fractures in the carpus of the horse: a radiographic study of their incidence and location. JAVMA 157(1):1305-1312.

13. Thrall, D. E., L. L. Jacques, and T. R. O'Brien. 1981. A five-year survey of the incidence and location of equine carpal chip fractures. JAVMA 158(8):-1366-1368.

14. Shively, M. J. 1982. Correct anatomic nomenclature for the joints of the equine carpus. J. Equine Prac. 4(6):6-10.

15. Mackay-Smith, M. P., L. S. Cushing, and J. A. Leslie. 1972. "Carpal canal" syndrome in horses. JAVMA 160(7):993-997.

16. Radue, P. 1981. Carpal tunnel syndrome due to fracture of the accessory carpal bone. J. Equine Prac. 3(5):8-18.

17. Shively, M. J. 1982. Equine English dictionary: Part I--Standing conformation. J. Equine Pract. 4(5):10-27.

18. Shively, M. J. 1983. Use of the terms varus and valgus in describing angular limb deformities of the limbs. J. Equine Prac. 5(3):15-17.

19. Van Pelt, R. W. 1962. Intra-articular injection of the equine carpus and fetlock. JAVMA 140:1181-1191.

20. Sokolowski, J. H. 1982. Methylprednisolone acetate in the treatment of equine osteoarthritis. J. Equine Prac. 4(6):15-28.

21. Shively, M. J. 1977. The normal radiographic anatomy of the equine digit. Swest. Vet. 30(2):193-199.

22. Fackelman, G. E. 1973. Sagittal fractures of the first phalanx in the horse. VM/SAC 68(6):622-636.

23. Gonyea, W., and R. Ashworth. 1975. The form and function of retractile claws in felidae and other representative carnivores. J. Morph. 145:229-238.

24. Herron, M. R. 1967. Declawing the cat. Med. Vet. Pract. 48(10):40-43.

25. Stump, J. E. 1967. Anatomy of the normal equine foot, including microscopic features of the laminar region. JAVMA 151:1588-1598.

4

THORACIC LIMB ANGIOLOGY

Knowledge of the vessels of the thoracic limb has clinical application in:

1. Venipunctures for drug administration, blood sampling, and insertion of indwelling catheters.
2. Arteriopunctures for special angiographic procedures and blood gas determinations.
3. Surgical procedures involving the thoracic limb. It is undesirable to unexpectedly sever vessels in surgery because the blood makes orientation in the surgical field difficult. In orthopedic cases, preservation of as much of the normal blood supply as possible may be essential to promote proper healing.

Vessels of the limb are also clinically significant in wire injuries in ungulates. Carelessly discarded baling wire or the thicker rims of rusty cans occasionally become embedded in the distal limb, where they may cause circulatory disturbances. However, most of the major channels in either thoracic or pelvic limbs can be ligated in a normal individual with no (or only temporary) ill effects [2,3]. Hemostasis is, nonetheless, an important surgical principle.

The main arterial channel that supplies the thoracic limb is divided into several segments from proximal to distal: the axillary a., brachial a., median a., common digital aa., and proper digital aa. To appreciate the significance of this vasculature, the landmarks for regional name changes and the primary branches should be considered because they are relatively constant regardless of species. The second and third order branches, however, are more variable and have less clinical significance. Therefore, in the following discussion, only the major arteries which constitute a general pattern applicable to all domestic mammals have described. Other vessels are present in the various species either as unnamed muscular branches or as minor named vessels. The more significant of these are cited as species-specific variations.

Arteries of the Thoracic Limb (Fig. 4-1)

I. AXILLARY ARTERY

The axillary artery is the most proximal arterial channel supplying the thoracic limb. It is the extra-thoracic continuation of the subclavian artery and begins where the latter vessel exits the thoracic cavity by coursing around the first rib. The axillary a. supplies the following branches and then continues as the brachial a. after the origin of the subscapular a.:

A. External thoracic a.--a small vessel which supplies the pectoral muscles. It may originate from a source other than the axillary a. (quite often from a branch of the superficial cervical a. in carnivores).

B. Cranial circumflex humeral a.--courses around the cranial aspect of the proximal humerus. It may arise from the brachial artery or from the subscapular artery in some species and/or individuals [3].

Figure 4-1

Schematic Pattern of the Major
Arteries of the Thoracic Limb
     (medial aspect)

A. Branches of the axillary a.

   1. external thoracic a.
      (enters pectoral mm.)

   2. cranial circumflex humeral a.
      (encircles humerus cranially)

   3. subscapular a.
      (courses between teres major
      and caudal border of scapula)
      a. caudal circumflex humeral a.
         (encircles proximal
         humerus)
      b. thoracodorsal a.
         (courses caudally on deep
         surface of l. dorsi m.)

B. Branches of the brachial a.

   4. deep brachial a.
      (enters triceps brachii m.)

   5. bicipital a.
      (enters biceps brachii m.)

   6. collateral ulnar a.
      (crosses caudomedial aspect
      of cubital joint)

   7. transverse cubital a.
      (courses laterally between
      biceps brachii m. and
      humerus)

   8. common interosseous a.
      (one branch courses laterally
      between radius and ulna)

C. Branches of the median a.

   9. deep antebrachial a.
      (enters caudomedial
      antebrachial mm.)

   10. radial a.
       (courses cranial to the major channel)

   11. continuation of median a.

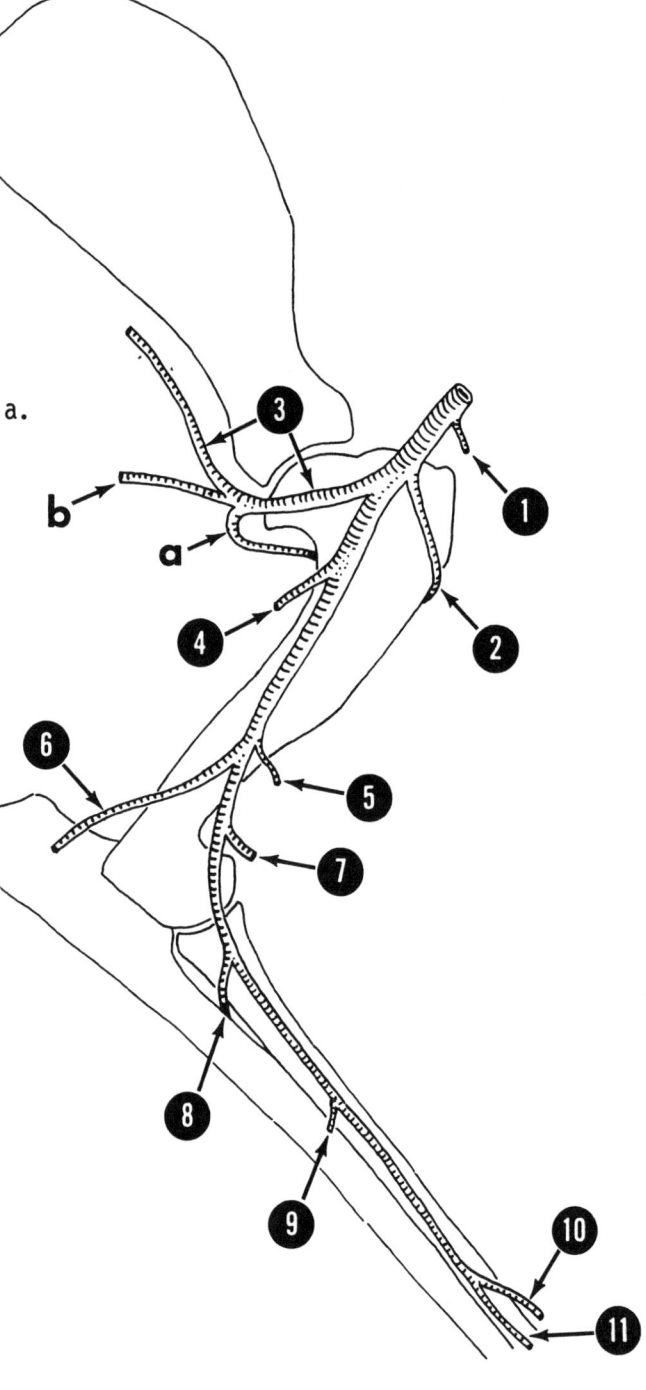

C. Subscapular a.--a large vessel which marks the termination of the axillary artery. The subscapular artery courses along the caudal border of the scapula and supplies two large named branches:

1. Caudal circumflex humeral a.--courses around the caudal aspect of the proximal humerus. This large vessel often divides near its origin.

2. Thoracodorsal a.--courses caudally on the deep surface of the latissimus dorsi m.

D. In addition to the above three branches of the axillary a., which are found in all domestic mammals, the following species variations may be of interest:

1. The carnivores have a lateral thoracic a. which accompanies the lateral thoracic n. It has a variable origin from either the axillary a., the brachial a., or the subscapular a. It courses subcutaneously and caudally along the junction of the deep pectoral and latissimus dorsi mm. and is further ventral but somewhat parallel to the thoracodorsal a. [4,5].

2. The ox and horse have a suprascapular a. which originates from the axillary a. and accompanies the suprascapular nerve. In other species (small ruminants, pig, carnivores) the suprascapular artery originates from another vessel [3].

II. BRACHIAL ARTERY

The brachial artery is the continuation of the axillary a., distal to the origin of the subscapular a. The brachial artery supplies several branches and is continued distally as the median a. after the common interosseous a. arises. In the cat, note that the brachial artery passes through the supracondylar foramen of the humerus along with the median nerve. This restricts a surgeon's ability to reflect it during medial approaches to the humerus [4]. The major branches of the brachial a. include the following:

A. Deep brachial a.--a large vessel primarily distributed to the triceps brachii. It courses into the muscles between the medial and long heads, along with the radial nerve.

B. Bicipital a.--a small branch which enters the biceps brachii. It may arise directly from the brachial a., or in the carnivores, it may arise from the superficial brachial a. (see F-2) [3].

C. Collateral ulnar a.--a small artery originating in the distal half of the brachium which sends branches to the cubital joint and antebrachium (see F-2 for a variation in carnivores).

D. Transverse cubital a. (formerly termed "distal collateral radial a.")--a large vessel near the cubital joint passing laterally between the humerus and biceps brachii to be distributed to the craniolateral antebrachial muscles.

E. Common interosseous a.--the last branch of the brachial a. It divides into the cranial interosseous a. and the caudal interosseous a. (and in the carnivores it also supplies an ulnar a.--see F-1 below). The cranial interosseous a. penetrates the interosseous space to supply the craniolateral antebrachial mm. The caudal interosseous a. remains on the caudal side of the antebrachial skeleton. In the carnivores, the caudal interosseous a. courses distally in the interosseous space between the radius and ulna where it is susceptible to injury by fractures and may cause significant hemorrhage during surgical repairs.

F. There are a number of species variations in the branches of the brachial a.

1. The common interosseous a. of the ungulates has only two branches (cranial and caudal interosseous aa.) and these may arise separately from the brachial a. [3]. The dog has a third branch (ulnar a.). The cat has no "common" interosseous a. because the cranial and caudal interosseous aa. typically originate as separate entities. Also in the cat, the ulnar a. is a branch of the caudal interosseous a. [5]. The ulnar a. of both carnivores is the vessel which accompanies the ulnar nerve in the antebrachium.

2. The carnivores have a superficial brachial a. (formerly termed "proximal collateral radial a.") the terminal branches of which are distributed superficially to the cranial antebrachium. In the cat, and sometimes in the dog, the collateral ulnar a. may originate from the superficial brachial a. [3].

3. In the horse, the nutrient a. of the humerus typically arises directly from the brachial a., but it may arise from other branches as it does in other species [7].

4. In the pig, the deep antebrachial a. typically arises from the brachial a. instead of from the median a. (i.e., it arises proximal to the origin of the common interosseous a.).

III. MEDIAN ARTERY

The median artery is the antebrachial continuation of the brachial a. after the origin of the interosseous complex. It is the largest artery that continues to the manus in all domestic mammals except the cat, in which the radial a. (a branch of the median a.) is the largest channel coursing distally. Distal to the carpus, the median artery terminates by forming the superficial palmar arch from which the palmar common digital arteries arise. In ungulates no true "arch" occurs, but its position is marked (but difficult to find) by anastomoses with other vessels coursing distally from the antebrachium. The median a. has only 2 named branches in most species.

A. Deep antebrachial a.--supplies the caudomedial antebrachial muscles. It usually originates a few centimeters distal to the interosseous vessels and is the largest of the "muscular" branches of the median a.

B. Radial a.--courses distally to contribute to the digital vascular supply.

C. The horse has 2 species-specific variations in the median a. branches:

1. The horse has a proximal radial a. as well as a radial a. which originates separately from the median a. Together they supply the field of distribution of the radial a. of other species.

2. The horse also has a palmar branch which anastomoses with the collateral ulnar a. and contributes to the palmar arch vasculature. It is also a major feeder of the small third palmar common digital a. (lateral palmar a.).

IV. DIGITAL ARTERIES

The vascular network which continues distally to supply the digits varies somewhat in its specific pattern among the various domestic mammals. However, two general principles of nomenclature hold true in any species:

A. Superficial aa. of the metacarpus are termed common digital aa. and are numbered medially to laterally to correspond to the metacarpal skeleton (i.e., a first common digital a. parallels the groove between Mc1 and Mc2, a second common digital a. is found between Mc2 and Mc3, etc.). All domesticated mammals have these vessels on the palmar side and they are termed palmar common digital arteries [3]. They originate from the superficial palmar arch and each one terminates by dividing near the bases of the digits to form the palmar proper digital arteries. The palmar proper digital arteries extend distally down the axial and abaxial sides of the digits (axial and abaxial palmar proper digital aa. of the individual digits). Carnivores have small superficial vessels on the dorsal side of the metacarpus, too. These dorsal common digital aa. are terminal branches of vessels supplied by the superficial brachial a.

B. Deep aa. of the metacarpus are termed dorsal or palmar metacarpal aa. with respect to the side of the manus on which they occur [3]. They parallel the common digital aa., are typically much smaller, and are also numbered from medial to lateral. The metacarpal aa. are derivatives of vascular networks arising primarily from branches of the radial a. They typically contribute to the formation of the proper digital arteries.

Knowledge of the details of the vascular supply to the digits of the carnivores and pig has little, if any, clinical application. However, a review of the vessels supplying the manus of the horse and ox is appropriate.

Horse

In the horse (Fig. 4-2), the single largest arterial channel coursing distal to the carpus is the second palmar common digital a. (medial palmar a.). The medial palmar a. may be considered to be the direct continuation of the median a. distal to the carpus. Technically, it does not begin until the level of the superficial palmar arch, but the latter is an anastomosis of the main channel with other branches distal to the carpus and may be absent or difficult to find [8]. Just proximal to the metacarpophalangeal joint, the second palmar common digital artery divides into the medial and lateral palmar proper digital arteries. These vessels are commonly called "medial" and "lateral digital arteries." They are the major arterial supply to the digit and supply numerous dorsal and palmar branches before their distal ends enter the solar foramina of the distal phalanx where they anastomose in the solar canal to form the terminal arch.

Figure 4-2

Major Arteries of the Equine Manus (right limb)
A. Palmar aspect
B. Transverse section through mid-metacarpus

1. Median a.
2. Proximal radial a.
3. Radial a.
4. Palmar branch of median a.
5. Second palmar common digital a. (medial palmar a.). In the transverse section, the medial palmar vein and nerve which accompany the artery are shown.
6. Third palmar common digital a. (lateral palmar a.). In the transverse section, the lateral palmar vein and nerve which accompany the artery are shown.
7. Second (medial) palmar metacarpal a.
8. Third (lateral) palmar metacarpal a.

In the transverse section, note the medial and lateral palmar metacarpal nn. which accompany the palmar metacarpal arteries and note also the single palmar metacarpal vein between them.

9. Medial palmar proper digital a. (medial digital a.)
10. Lateral palmar proper digital a. (lateral digital a.)
11. Dorsal and palmar branches to the proximal phalanx
12. Dorsal and palmar branches to the middle phalanx
13. Dorsal branch to the distal phalanx
14. Branch to the digital cushion
15. Terminal arch
16. Second (medial) dorsal metacarpal a.
17. Third (lateral) dorsal metacarpal a.
18. Second metacarpal bone
19. Third metacarpal bone
20. Fourth metacarpal bone
21. Common digital extensor tendon
22. Lateral digital extensor tendon
23. Superficial digital flexor tendon
24. Deep digital flexor tendon
25. Accessory ligament of deep digital flexor
26. Interosseous muscle

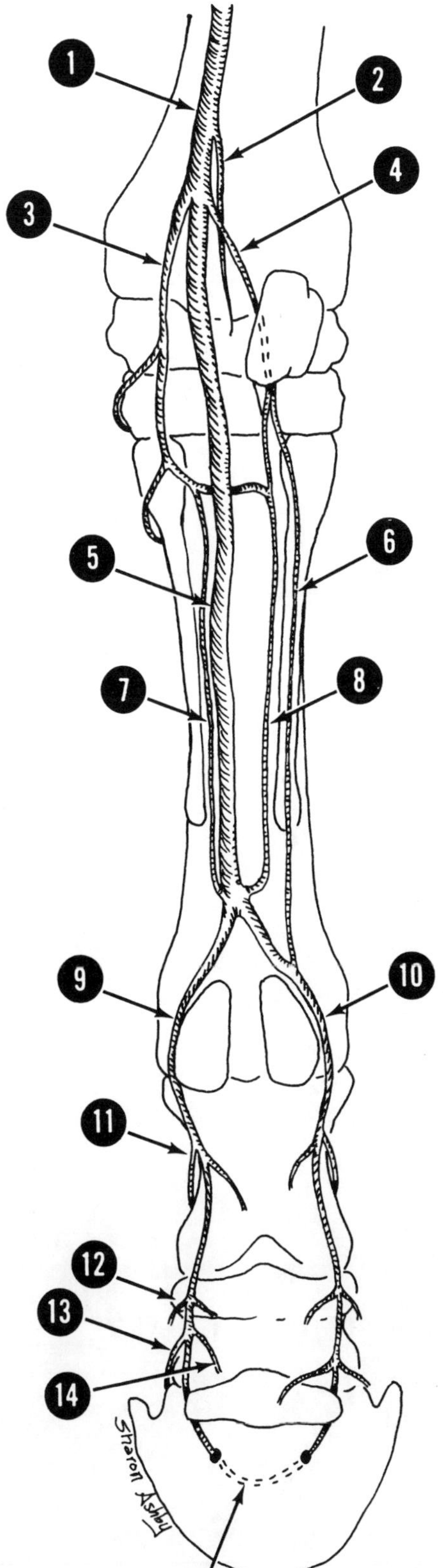

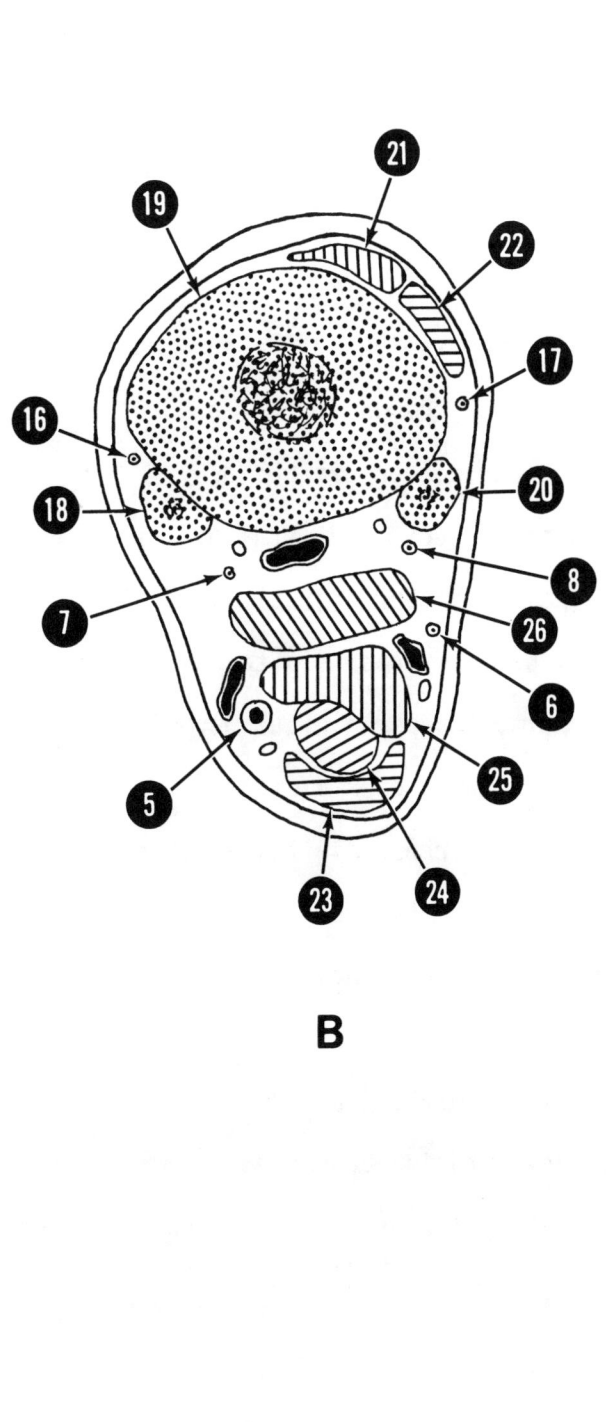

A

B

Figure 4-3

Major Arteries of the Bovine Manus

(palmar aspect of right limb)

1. Median a.
2. Radial a.
3. Cranial interosseous a. (palmar branch)
4. Second palmar common digital a.
5. Third palmar common digital a.
6. Fourth palmar common digital a.
7. Axial palmar proper digital a. of digit 2
8. Abaxial palmar proper digital a. of digit 3
9. Axial palmar proper digital aa. of digits 3 and 4
10. Abaxial palmar proper digital a. of digit 4
11. Axial palmar proper digital a. of digit 5
12. Second palmar metacarpal a.
13. Third palmar metacarpal a.
14. Fourth palmar metacarpal a.
15. Proximal perforating branch
16. Distal perforating branch
17. Vestigial phalanges in the second digit (medial paradigit, "dewclaw")

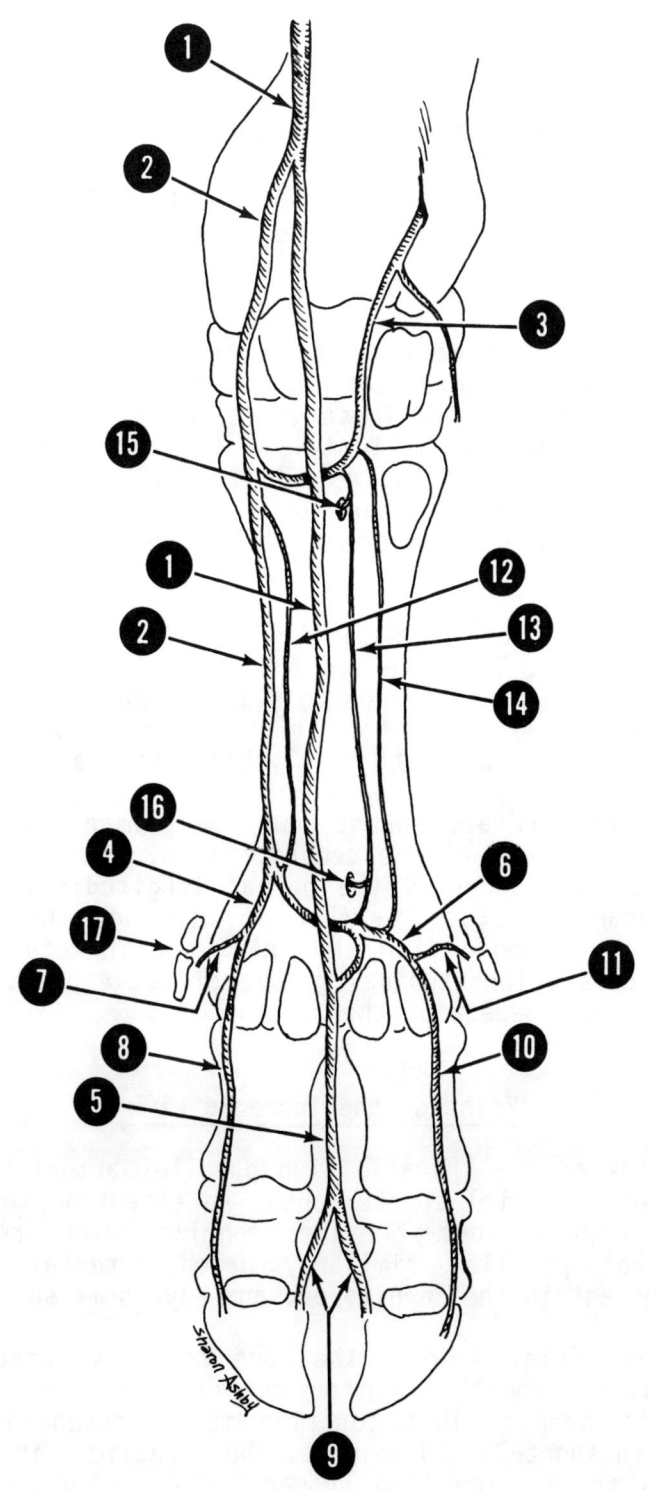

95

In addition to the medial palmar a., there are several other arterial pathways down the equine metacarpus (Fig. 4-2). The lateral palmar a. (third palmar common digital a.--Fig. 4-2/6) is the lateral counterpart to the main channel. It is much smaller than the medial palmar a. and is derived primarily from the palmar branch of the median a. The deeply located metacarpal aa. (Fig 4-2/7, 8, 16, 17) parallel the more superficial vessels. The palmar ones (Fig. 4-2/7, 8) are derived from the radial aa. and are better developed than the dorsal ones which arise from a network of small vessels on the dorsal aspect of the carpus. The exact pattern of origin and anastomoses of these vessels varies among individuals.

Ox

In the ox (Fig. 4-3), the median artery continues to the distal fourth of the metacarpus where it receives anastomotic branches from the cranial interosseous artery and the radial artery [8]. These anastomoses form the superficial palmar arch which is an arch in name only. Distal to the arch, the major channel is the third palmar common digital a. (Fig. 4-3/5) which courses distally on the medial side of the deep digital flexor tendon. It supplies some branches and ultimately divides into the axial palmar proper digital arteries of the third and fourth digits (Fig. 4-3/9).

The second and fourth palmar common digital arteries (Fig. 4-3/4, 6) are much smaller than the third one. They are fed primarily by the radial a. (Fig. 4-3/2) and supply axial palmar proper arteries to digits 2 and 5 (Fig. 4-3/7, 11) as well as abaxial palmar proper arteries to digits 3 and 4 (Fig. 4-3/8, 10). Dorsal branches from the digital aa. arise to supply the dorsal aspects of the digits.

Three deep (metacarpal) aa. course down the palmar aspect of the metacarpus (Fig. 4-3/12, 13, 14). These are the second, third, and fourth palmar metacarpal aa. The axial (third) one occupies the palmar longitudinal groove of Mc3+4, and sends perforating branches (Fig. 4-3/15, 16) through the proximal and distal metacarpal canals to anastomose with the third dorsal metacarpal a. This latter vessel occupies the dorsal longitudinal groove of Mc3+4 and is the only artery of significance of the dorsal aspect of the metacarpus.

Veins of the Thoracic Limb

Most of the veins of the thoracic limb parallel arterial channels and assume the same name as their arterial counterparts. An exception that has some clinical significance is the cephalic network. The cephalic veins are superficial venous channels that do not parallel similarly named arterial channels. They are clinically more important in the carnivores, and have some species variation.

In the carnivores (Fig. 4-4/A), the more medially located cephalic vein is joined by the accessory cephalic vein on the cranial aspect of the antebrachium just proximal to the carpus. This junction is a convenient place to direct a venipuncture needle in short-legged animals. The cephalic vein anastomoses with the brachial vein via a short connecting segment (the median cubital vein) near the flexor surface of the elbow joint (Fig. 4-4A/2, 4-5/2). A "hold-off" proximal to this anastomosis will fail to raise the cephalic vein adequately for a venipuncture. The cephalic vein courses deep to the brachiocephalicus muscle just distal to the humeral joint, and ultimately joins the external jugular vein. Just before it disappears under the caudal border of the brachiocephalicus m., the

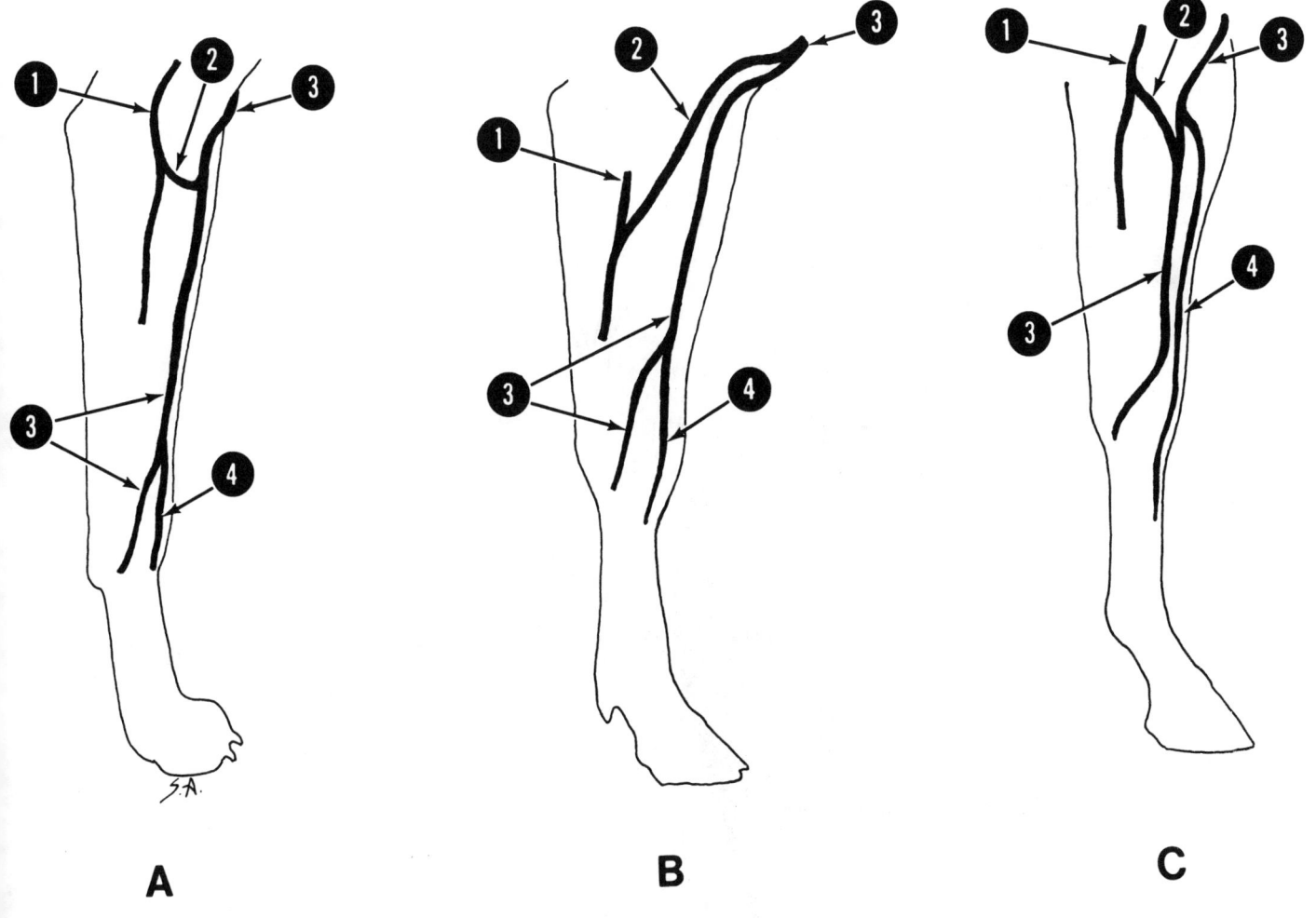

Figure 4-4
Anastomoses of Major Superficial Venous Channels in the Thoracic Limb
of the Dog (A), Ox (B), and Horse (C)
(medial aspects of the limbs)

1. Brachial vein
2. Median cubital vein
3. Cephalic vein
4. Accessory cephalic vein

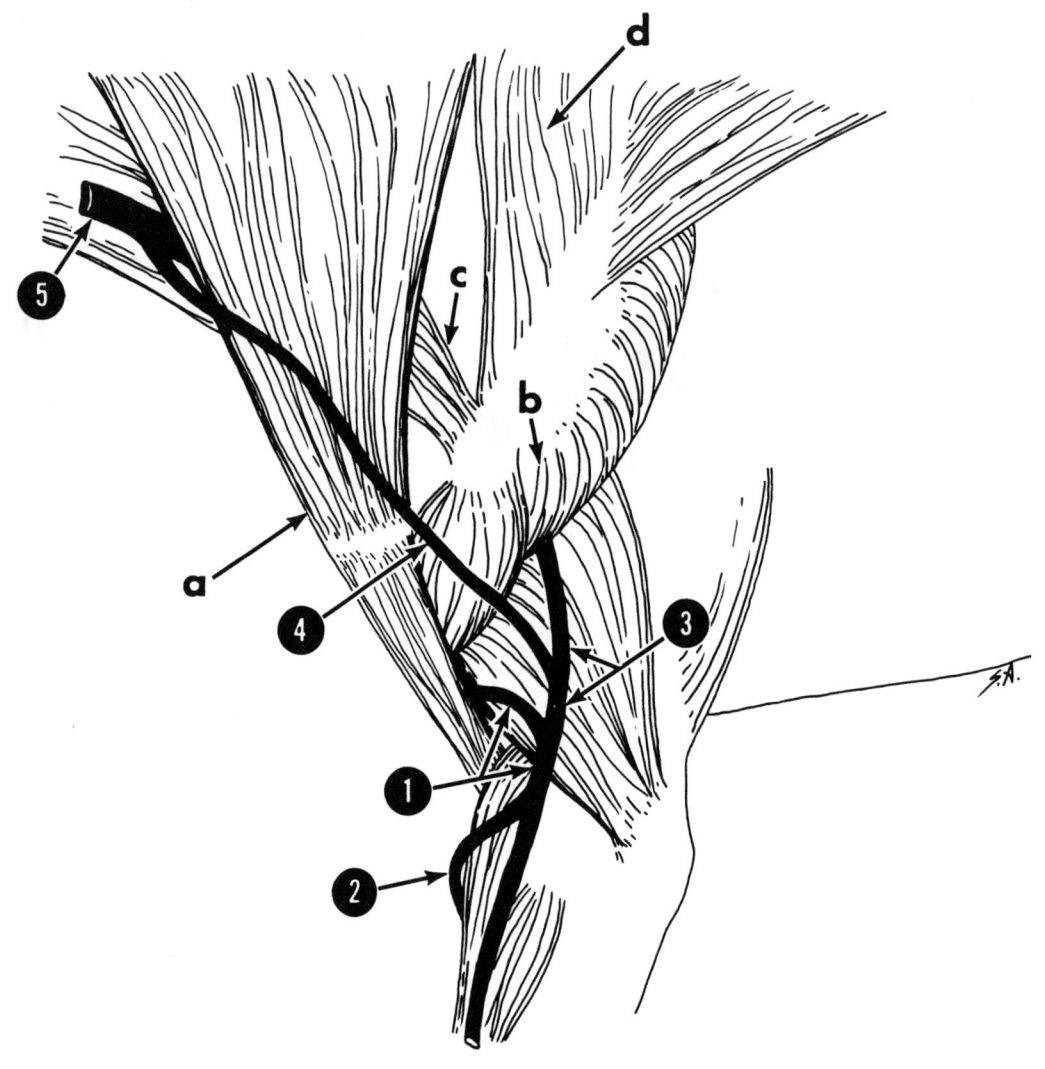

Figure 4-5

Branches of the Cephalic Vein in the Dog
(lateral aspect of the left brachial region)

1. Cephalic v.
2. Median cubital v.
3. Axillobrachial v.
4. Omobrachial v.
5. External jugular v.

a. brachiocephalicus m.
b. deltoideus m.
c. omotransversarius m.
d. trapezius m.

cephalic vein gives rise to the axillobrachial vein (Fig. 4-5/3). This vessel courses dorsocaudally across the shoulder, penetrates the musculature at the caudal border of the deltoideus m. and anastomoses with the axillary vein. In dogs, a branch of the axillobrachial vein, the omobrachial vein, passes superficially over the brachiocephalicus m. and ultimately joins the external jugular vein (Fig 4-5/4). The omobrachial vein must be ligated and/or reflected in most of the lateral approaches to the humeral joint. The omobrachial vein is absent in cats [3].

In the ox (Fig. 4-4/B), the cephalic and accessory cephalic veins join just proximal to the carpus as they do in carnivores. However, the median cubital vein is much longer [8]. It attaches to the brachial vein near the cubital joint as in other domestic animals, but then it courses proximally in the groove between the descending pectoral and brachiocephalicus muscles. It finally joins the more laterally located cephalic vein near the junction of the latter with the external jugular vein.

In the horse (Fig. 4-4/C), several superficial cutaneous veins are often visible. The cephalic vein is the large one on the craniomedial side of the antebrachium. The accessory cephalic vein is smaller and more cranially located. In contrast to the situation in the carnivores and ox, the cephalic and accessory cephalic veins of the horse do not anastomose until they reach a point near the cubital joint [8]. The large median cubital vein leaves the cephalic near the junction of the cephalic and accessory cephalic veins and crosses the medial surface of the distal aspect of the biceps brachii.

References

1. Cummings, B. C. 1962. Collateral circulation of the canine thoracic limb. Small Anim. Clin. 2:584-592.

2. Cummings, B. C. 1961. Collateral circulation of the canine pelvic limb. Small Anim. Clin. 1:260-268.

3. International Committee on Veterinary Gross Anatomical Nomenclature 1983. Nomina Anatomica Veterinaria, third ed. Published by the Committee, Ithaca, New York.

4. Evans, H. E., and G. C. Christensen. 1979. Miller's Anatomy of the Dog, second ed. W. B. Saunders, Philadelphia.

5. McClure, R. C., M. J. Dallman, and P. G. Garrett. 1973. Cat Anatomy. An Atlas, Text and Dissection Guide. Lea and Febiger, Philadelphia.

6. Habel, R. E. 1981. Applied Veterinary Anatomy, second ed. Published by the author, Ithaca, New York.

7. Getty, R. 1975. Sisson and Grossman's The Anatomy of the Domestic Animals, fifth ed. W. B. Saunders, Philadelphia.

8. Schummer, A. H., H. Wilkens, B. Vollmerkaus, and K. H. Habermehl. 1981. The Circulatory System, the Skin, and the Cutaneous Organs of the Domestic Mammals. Translated by W. Siller and A. Wight. Paul Parey, Berlin.

THORACIC LIMB NEUROLOGY

I. BRACHIAL PLEXUS

The nerves which supply the intrinsic muscles of the thoracic limb are named nerves which are derived from the brachial plexus. Brachial plexus derivatives also supply some of the extrinsic muscles of the thoracic limb. The brachial plexus is an exchange network of fibers from the ventral branches of the last few cervical spinal nerves and the first one or two thoracic spinal nerves.* The last three cervical and first two thoracic spinal nerves (C6, 7, 8, T1, 2) are typically involved in most domesticated mammals.

It has been shown experimentally for a given individual that the definitive fiber components within a particular thoracic limb nerve (radial n. for example) are derived from certain segments of the spinal cord which contribute to the brachial plexus. But attempts to equate which segments ultimately give rise to exactly which named nerves are primarily of academic interest because of species variation, individual variation, and a lack of specific clinical application. For these reasons, it seems inappropriate and generally impossible to claim that specific spinal cord segments, applicable to all species, contribute to given nerves. To illustrate this point, in the dog it is accepted for purposes of discussion that the brachial plexus is derived from the ventral branches of spinal nerves C6, 7, 8, T1, 2. In an actual study of this area, however, the following individual variation was found [1]:

% of specimens (n=58)	Brachial plexus derivation
58.6	C6, 7, 8, T1
20.7	C5, 6, 7, 8, T1
17.2	C6, 7, 8, T1, 2
3.5	C5, 6, 7, 8, T1, 2

Even with these variations, it may be of value to consider a general scheme of the spinal cord's contribution to the six nerves of greatest clinical importance in the thoracic limb (as presented by Habel after the work of Bowne) [2,3]:

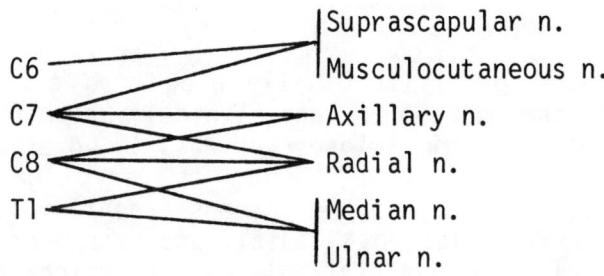

*A spinal nerve has two principal parietal branches: a dorsal one which is primarily sensory and motor to epaxial structures, and a ventral one which is primarily sensory and motor to hypaxial structures. The limbs, as a whole, are hypaxial structures and the brachial plexus is derived only from the ventral branches of the involved nerves.

II. MAJOR NERVES OF THE THORACIC LIMB

Most of the nerves which supply the thoracic limb are derivatives of the brachial plexus (Figs. 5-1, 5-2, 5-3,). They include:

- A. radial n.
- B. ulnar n.
- C. median n.
- D. musculocutaneous n.
- E. suprascapular n.
- F. axillary n.
- G. subscapular nn.
- H. thoracodorsal n.
- I. long thoracic n.
- J. lateral thoracic n.
- K. pectoral nn.
- L. muscular branches

There are relatively few species in regarding the pattern of distribution of these nerves except for those related to differences in the numbers of digits. Consequently, information regarding one species applies well to the others. At least three categories of information are useful clinically in regard to nerves:

1. the muscle groups they supply. This will aid in the diagnosis and prognosis of nerve injuries.

2. a working concept of the cutaneous sensory dermatomes. This will also aid in the diagnosis of neuropathies.

3. a general knowledge of their location and distribution. This will avoid iatrogenic damage during surgical procedures and will aid in performing and interpreting diagnostic and surgical nerve blocks.

A. Radial nerve

The radial nerve supplies the caudal brachial muscles and the craniolateral antebrachial muscles (extensors of the cubital, carpal, and digital joints). After leaving the brachial plexus, it courses between the medial and long heads of the triceps brachii with the deep brachial vessels. It then supplies numerous branches to the caudal brachial muscles, and continues laterally and cranially around the humerus. This latter part of the nerve is vulnerable to injuries from midshaft fractures of the humerus. After encircling the humerus, the radial nerve emerges at the cranial border of the lateral head of the triceps brachii. It divides near this point (usually further proximally) into a deep branch which supplies the craniolateral antebrachial muscles and a superficial branch which is cutaneously distributed. One of the named branches of the superficial branch is the lateral cutaneous antebrachial nerve which is distributed to the craniolateral antebrachium in all domestic animals and to the dorsal manus in all but the horse.

Radial (nerve) paralysis usually occurs as a result of traumatic injury and it is the most common and clinically significant paralysis of the thoracic limb. The animal loses the ability to extend the carpal and digital joints, but unless the injury is very high (proximal to the muscular branches which supply the triceps brachii m.), extension of the cubital joint is not affected.* Radial paralysis must be differentiated from avulsion of the brachial plexus in which there is greater functional loss to the limb [2,4,5]:

---

*Flexion of the cubital joint may be weakened in these cases because of loss of innervation to the extensor carpi radialis. This is probably more of academic curiosity than of clinical significance.

1. low radial paralysis--loss of extension of carpal and digital joints (i.e., deep branch is damaged). The dorsum of the manus drags the ground and/or knuckles over. All species may learn to compensate for low radial paralysis by learning to flip the carpus and digits into the normal extended position. Loss of sensation from the cutaneous dermatome and paralysis of the craniolateral antebrachial musculature are diagnostic, although one can occur without the other if the superficial or the deep branch only is damaged. Temporary low radial paralysis may occur as a post-surgical complication in large animals restrained in lateral recumbency. It has been suggested that direct compression [6] or temporary circulatory disturbance [7] may be involved. In carnivores, low radial paralysis may be surgically treated by carpal arthrodesis or by flexor tendon translocations.

2. high radial paralysis--inability to extend the cubital, carpal, and digital joints (i.e., main nerve trunk is damaged above the branches to the triceps m.). The limb cannot bear weight and is carried in a flexed position.

3. brachial plexus involvement--(i.e., the damage occurs further proximally and involves other nerve trunks)--the limb is flaccid and the manus drags on the ground.

B. Ulnar nerve

The ulnar nerve is one of the three thoracic limb nerves which course distally on the medial side of the brachium in close association with the brachial vessels. The others are the musculocutaneous nerve and the median nerve. All three of these components should be identified and preserved in a medial approach to the humerus. Near the cubital joint the ulnar nerve is the most caudal component of this triad. It courses distally between the medial epicondyle of the humerus and the tuber olecrani, and it should be identified and preserved during a trans-olecranon approach to the cubital joint. Proximal to the elbow, the ulnar nerve gives rise to a cutaneous branch, the caudal cutaneous antebrachial nerve. This nerve and other cutaneous branches of the ulnar nerve are sensory to the skin on the caudal antebrachium and palmar manus. The ulnar nerve also supplies some of the caudomedial ante-brachial muscles and the muscles of the manus.

Damage to the ulnar nerve has little clinical significance. The gait is not altered, but in carnivores, a slight spreading of the digits occurs [2].

C. Median nerve

The median nerve parallels the brachial vessels down the medial side of the brachium. In the carnivores and ruminants, it arises with the ulnar nerve and the two course distally as a common trunk for a variable distance. However, they are easily distinguished near the elbow joint, because the ulnar nerve courses caudodistally and the median nerve remains in close association with the brachial vessels. In the

Figure 5-1

Nerves of the Equine Thoracic Limb, Medial Aspect

1. Roots of the brachial plexus derived from the ventral branches of C6-C8
2. Roots of the brachial plexus derived from the ventral branches of T1-T2
3. Cranial pectoral nerve--to superficial pectoral and subclavius mm.
4. Suprascapular nerve--to supraspinatus and infraspinatus mm.
5. Musculocutaneous nerve
6. Proximal branch of 5--to coracobrachialis and biceps brachii mm.
7. Axillary artery
8. Ansa axillaris--a communication distal to the axillary artery
9. Subscapular nerve--to subscapularis m.
10. Thoracodorsal nerve--to latissimus dorsi m.
11. Lateral thoracic nerve--to cutaneous trunci and cutaneous omobrachialis mm.
12. Axillary nerve--to teres major, teres minor, and deltoideus mm.
13. Radial nerve--to extensors of the cubital joint and the joints of the manus
14. Ulnar nerve--to certain flexors of the joints of the manus
15. Combined musculocutaneous and median nerves
16. Distal branch of musculocutaneous nerve--to brachialis m.
17. Cranial cutaneous antebrachial nerve--from axillary nerve
18. Medial cutaneous antebrachial nerve--from 16
19. Median nerve--to certain flexors of the joints of the manus
20. Caudal cutaneous antebrachial nerve--from ulnar nerve
21. Dorsal branch of ulnar nerve
22. Palmar branch of ulnar nerve
23. Medial palmar nerve (p.c.d.n. 2)
24. Lateral palmar nerve (p.c.d.n. 3)
25. Superficial branch of 22, combined with 24 to form lateral palmar nerve
26. Deep branch of ulnar nerve--to interosseous m.
27. Communicating branch from medial palmar nerve to lateral palmar nerve
28. Medial palmar metacarpal n. (p.m.n. 2)--from the deep branch of the ulnar n.
29. Medial palmar digital nerve
30. Dorsal branch of medial palmar digital nerve

The long thoracic nerve to the serratus ventralis m. is not illustrated.

Used with permission of Dr. J. E. Smallwood

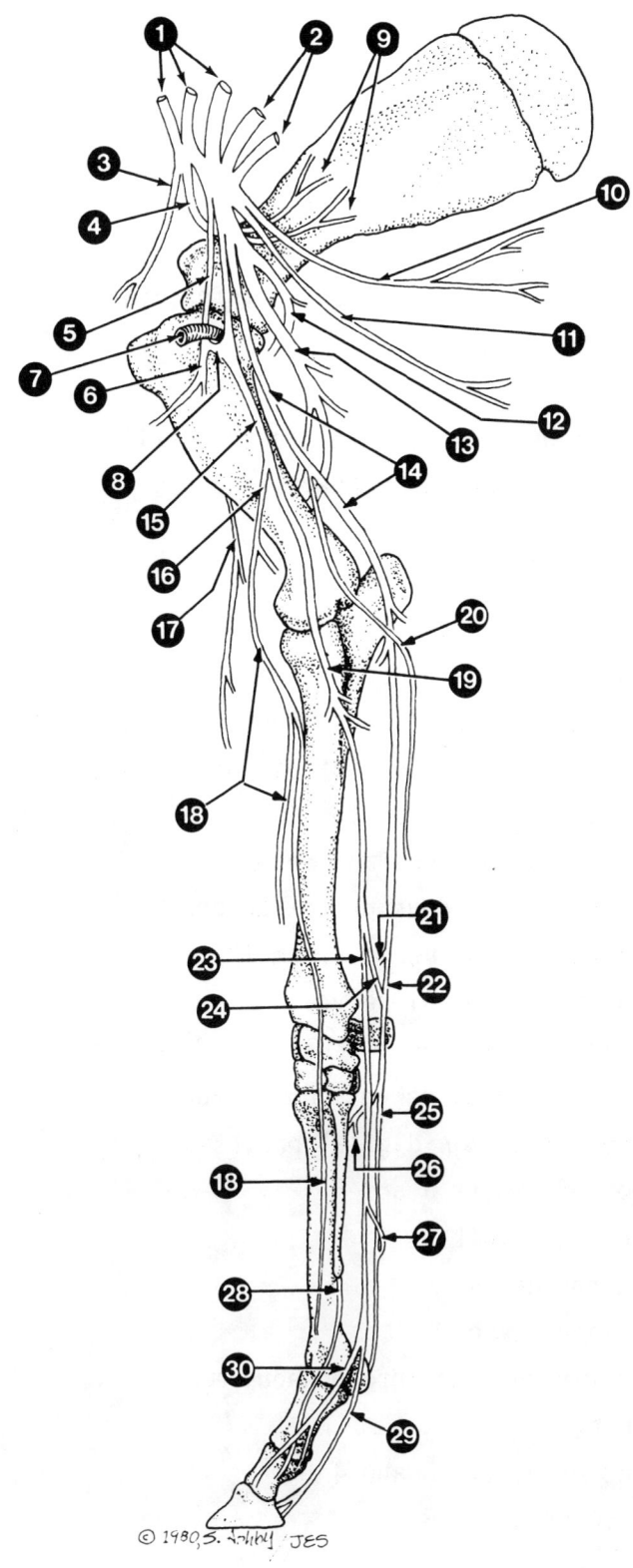

Figure 5-2

Nerves of the Bovine Thoracic Limb, Medial Aspect

1. Roots of the brachial plexus derived from the ventral branches of C6-C8
2. Roots of the brachial plexus derived from the ventral branches of T1-T2
3. Cranial pectoral nerve--to superficial pectoral mm.
4. Suprascapular nerve--to supraspinatus and infraspinatus mm.
5. Musculocutaneous nerve
6. Axillary a.
7. Ansa axillaris--a communication distal to the axillary artery.
8. Proximal branch of 5--to coracobrachialis and biceps brachii mm.
9. Subscapular nerve--to subscapular m.
10. Long thoracic nerve--to serratus ventralis m.
11. Thoracodorsal nerve--to latissimus dorsi m.
12. Lateral thoracic nerve--to cutaneous trunci and cutaneous omobrachialis mm.
13. Axillary nerve--to teres major, teres minor, and deltoideus mm.
14. Radial nerve--to extensors of the cubital joint and joints of the manus
15. Ulnar nerve--to certain flexors of the joints of the manus
16. Combined musculocutaneous and median nerves
17. Distal branch of musculocutaneous nerve--to brachialis m.
18. Medial cutaneous antebrachial nerve--from 17
19. Superficial branch of the radial nerve
20. Median nerve--to certain flexors of the joints of the manus
21. Caudal cutaneous antebrachial nerve--from ulnar nerve
22. Second and third dorsal common digital nerves
23. Axial dorsal nerves of digits 3 and 4
24. Abaxial dorsal nerve of digit 3
25. Dorsal branch of ulnar nerve
26. Palmar branch of ulnar nerve
27. Deep branch of ulnar nerve--to interosseous mm.
28. Communicating branch
29. Axial palmar nerves of digits 3 and 4
30. Abaxial palmar nerve of digit 3

Used with permission of Dr. J. E. Smallwood

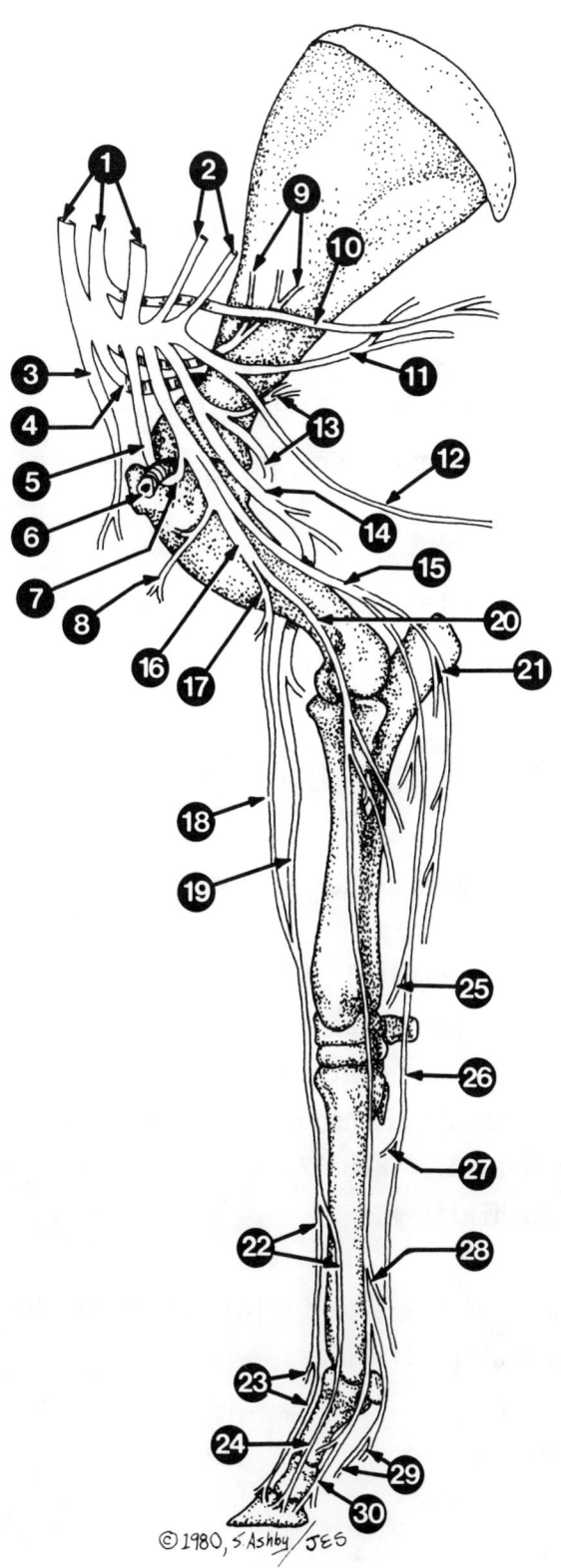

Figure 5-3

Nerves of the Canine Thoracic Limb, Medial Aspect

1. Roots of the brachial plexus derived from the ventral branches of C6-C8
2. Root of the brachial plexus derived from the ventral branch of T1
3. Subscapular n.--to subscapularis m.
4. Branch of brachial plexus to brachiocephalicus m.
5. Suprascapular nerve--to supraspinatus and infraspinatus m.
6. Axillary n.--to teres major, teres minor, and deltoideus mm.
7. Cranial pectoral n.
8. Musculocutaneous n.
9. Proximal branch of musculocutaneous n.--to coracobrachialis and biceps brachii mm.
10. Cranial cutaneous antebrachial n. (from 6)
11. Long thoracic n.--to serratus ventralis m.
12. Thoracodorsal n.--to latissimus dorsi m.
13. Combined median and ulnar nerves
14. Lateral thoracic n.--to cutaneous trunci m. and skin
15. Caudal pectoral n.
16. Radial n.--to extensors of the cubital joint and joints of the manus
17. Ulnar n.--to some flexors of the joints of the manus
18. Median n.--to some flexors of the joints of the manus
19. Communicating branch from musculocutaneous n. to median n.
20. Caudal cutaneous antebrachial n. (from 17)
21. Distal branch of 8--to brachialis m.
22. Deep branch of radial n.
23. Medial and lateral branches of the superficial branch of the radial n.
24. Medial cutaneous antebrachial n. (from 8)
25. Dorsal branch of the ulnar n.
26. Palmar branch of the ulnar n.
27. Dorsal proper digital nn.
28. Palmar proper digital nn.

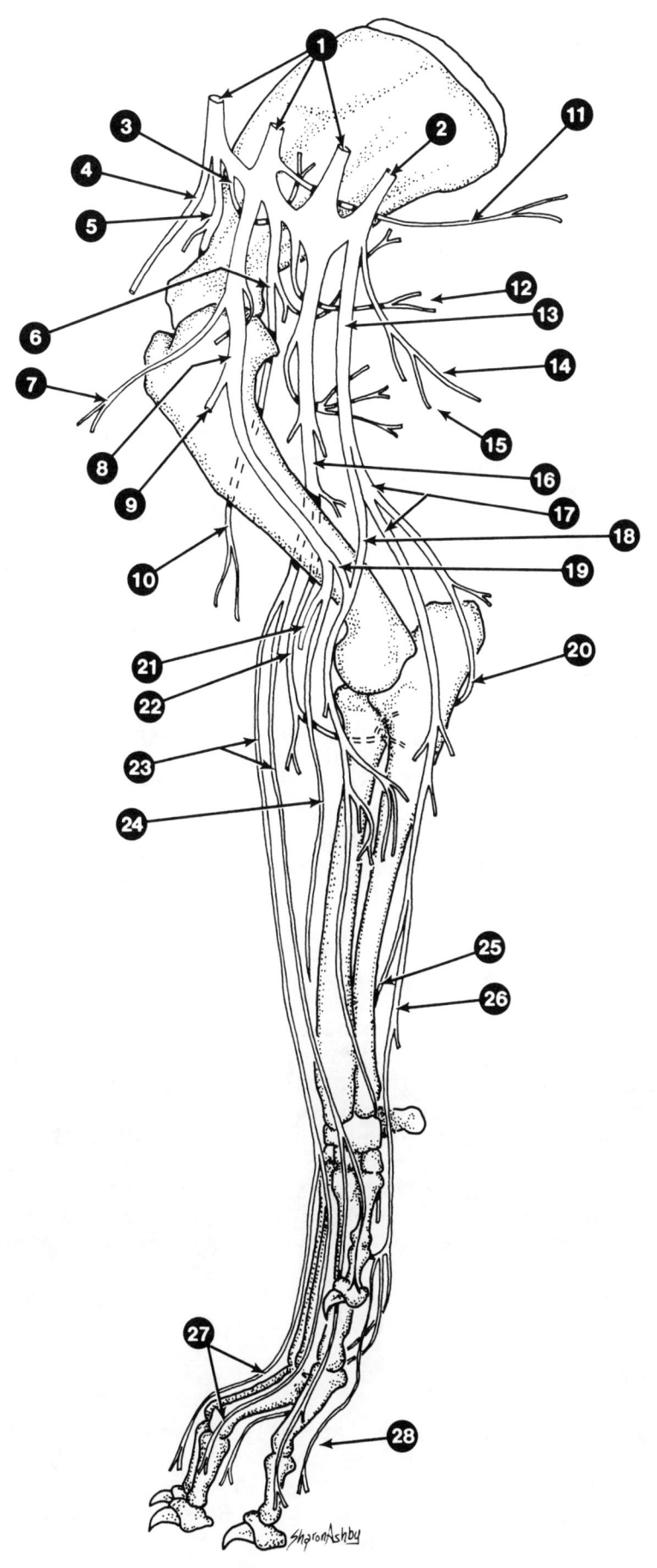

cat, the median nerve accompanies the brachial artery through the supracondylar foramen of the humerus. The median nerve supplies some of the caudomedial antebrachial muscles and is sensory to the palmar aspect of part of the manus.

In carnivores, damage to the median nerve causes little change in gait, but there is some hyperextension of the metacarpophalangeal joints (i.e., sinking of "fetlocks") and a lack of the ability to "dig in" with the claws. In addition, the claws are raised off the ground and the foot splays [2]. In cattle, when both the median and the ulnar nerves are sectioned, hyperextension of various joints occurs with a characteristic "goose-step." [5].

D. Musculocutaneous nerve

The musculocutaneous nerve supplies the cranial muscles of the brachium and the coracobrachialis muscle. Near the humeral joint, its proximal muscular branch enters the coracobrachialis and biceps brachii mm. The nerve then courses down the medial side of the brachium and supplies a distal muscular branch to the brachialis m. near the cubital joint. In ungulates, the musculocutaneous nerve is so closely associated with the median nerve that its proximal and distal muscular branches appear to arise from the latter. In the carnivores, the musculocutaneous nerve is distinctly separate from the median nerve, but it does communicate with the median near the cubital joint. The medial cutaneous antebrachial nerve is a sensory continuation of the musculocutaneous nerve which arises as a continuation of the distal muscular branch. It supplies the skin over the medial antebrachium in all species, and additionally, the dorsomedial manus as far distally as the fetlock in the horse. Damage to the musculocutaneous nerve results in very little change in the gait, but paw placing in carnivores (requiring flexion of the cubital joint) is markedly affected if the nerve is injured proximally [4].

E. Suprascapular nerve

The suprascapular nerve passes between the supraspinatus and subscapularis mm. along the cranial border of the scapula. It supplies only the supraspinatus and infraspinatus mm. and has no cutaneous distribution. Surgeons repairing scapular fractures or using an acromion osteotomy to approach the humeral joint should be cognizant that the nerve passes from the supraspinous fossa to the infraspinous fossa deep in the muscles under the acromion. Injury to the suprascapular nerve results in classic shoulder sweeny due to rapid neurogenic atrophy of the supraspinatus and infraspinatus muscles, but the gait is often unchanged [2]. In some horses, a lateral buckling of the humeral joint may occur [8]. In calves, experimental transection of the suprascapular nerve produces a curious abduction of the limb as well as the expected muscular atrophy. Some gait alteration also occurs [5].

F. Axillary nerve

The axillary nerve passes laterally between the teres major and subscapularis muscles. It supplies several flexors of the humeral joint (the teres major, teres minor, and deltoideus mm.) and part of the subscapularis. It terminates as cutaneous branches, the lateral cutaneous brachial n. and cranial cutaneous antebrachial n. These supply the skin over the craniolateral brachium and part of the antebrachium. Damage to the axillary nerve results in little change in the gait [4], evidently because other muscles (such as the triceps brachii and latissimus dorsi) can adequately flex the shoulder joint.

G. Subscapular nerve(s)

The subscapular nerve supplies the subscapularis muscle. Typically two trunks are present and they have no cutaneous distribution.

H. Thoracodorsal nerve

The thoracodorsal nerve courses caudally across the deep face of the latissimus dorsi muscle which it supplies. It has no stated cutaneous distribution.

I. Long thoracic nerve

The long thoracic nerve is distributed to the thoracic part of the serratus ventralis muscle and can be seen coursing caudally across its lateral surface. It has no cutaneous distribution.

J. Lateral thoracic nerve

The lateral thoracic nerve supplies the cutaneous trunci and is cutaneously distributed to the ventrolateral abdominal wall. It may be used to assess thoracolumbar spinal cord integrity by the panniculus reflex. In this reflex, the afferent information from a pin prick enters the cord through spinal nerves at the local level receiving the prick. If a skin twitch occurs, it is a positive sign that the cord is intact from the level of the stimulation up to the cervical area since the motor information to the cutaneous trunci (via the lateral thoracic nerve) leaves the cord at that level.

K. Pectoral nerves

The variable pectoral nerves are distributed to the pectoral muscles and may be divided into cranial ones and caudal ones.

L. Muscular branches

A number of unnamed muscular branches arise from the brachial plexus. Most of these are distributed to the extrinsic muscles. Several muscles are innervated by more than one source. (For example, the serratus ventralis m. is partly innervated by the long thoracic nerve and partly by cervical spinal nerves.) The subscapularis m. is partly innervated by the axillary n. as well as by the subscapular n.

III. NERVE SUPPLY TO THE MANUS

The nomenclature of superficial and deep nerves in the metacarpus follows the same pattern described for the vasculature (see Chapter 4, IV).* The specific

---

*Superficial nerves in the metacarpus are termed common digital nerves and deep nerves are termed metacarpal nerves. Both sets of nerves are numbered medial to lateral in the same manner as the blood vessels of the manus.

details of the nerves in the manus have little clinical application in the carnivores and pig. In the horse and ox, the patterns vary sufficiently to warrant separate descriptions.

   A.   Nerve Supply to the Digit of the Horse (Fig. 5-4)

   The major nerve supply to the digit of the horse is derived from the median and ulnar nerves. In other domestic species, the radial nerve (superficial branch) also has a significant role, but in the horse the superficial branch of the radial nerve is reduced to only the lateral cutaneous antebrachial nerve. This nerve is cutaneously distributed only as far as the carpus. Further distally, the dorsal cutaneous innervation of the metacarpus is taken over by the medial cutaneous antebrachial nerve (from the musculocutaneous nerve) on the dorsomedial side, and by the dorsal branch of the ulnar nerve on the dorsolateral side.

   The median nerve divides several centimeters proximal to the carpus to form the medial and lateral palmar nerves (palmar common digital nn. 2 and 3) which are the major nerves to the digit (Fig 5-4/8, 9). The ulnar nerve divides at about the same level into a dorsal branch which supplies the dorsolateral aspect of the metacarpus and a palmar branch. The palmar branch of the ulnar n. joins the lateral palmar n. (from the median n.) and the combined nerve continues distally as the lateral palmar n. Both the medial and the lateral palmar nerves pass through the carpal canal. Just distal to the carpus the lateral palmar nerve gives off a deep branch* which supplies the interosseous mm. and also forms the medial and lateral palmar metacarpal nn. which continue distally in a deep position adjacent to the metacarpal bones. To summarize, coursing down the palmar aspect of the metacarpus are the two large superficial nerves adjacent to the edges of the digital flexor tendons (Fig. 5-4/8, 9--medial and lateral palmar nn.) and two small deeply located nerves (Fig. 5-4/13, 14--medial and lateral palmar metacarpal nn.) [9]:

   1.   The medial palmar nerve (Fig. 5-4/8) follows the medial border of the flexor tendons down the metacarpus. About halfway down the metacarpus it sends a communicating branch** obliquely across the surface of the superficial digital flexor tendon to join the lateral palmar nerve. In blocking the medial and lateral palmar nerves, this communicating branch assumes clinical significance because if one nerve is blocked above and the other one below the communicating branch, total desensitization of both palmar nerves will not be affected. The medial palmar n. continues to the digit to become (as it crosses the metacarpophalangeal joint) the medial palmar digital n. (m.p.d.n.). Near the metacarpophalangeal joint, the m.p.d.n. gives off a dorsal branch which ramifies over the dorsal aspect of the metacarpophalangeal joint and the rest of the digit. It may be joined by a second dorsal branch. These dorsal branches innervate skin over the dorsal aspect of the

---

*The proper name for this nerve is the deep branch of the ulnar n., but studies have shown that it contains fibers from the median n. (lateral palmar n.) as well.
**Nerves have communicating branches. Vessels have anastomotic branches.

metacarpophalangeal joint as well as the dorsal parts of the interphalangeal joint capsule. (The palmar aspects are supplied by the medial palmar digital nerve itself rather than by the dorsal branches.) The medial palmar digital nerve then continues down the digit just palmar to the medial palmar artery which it accompanies. This nerve and its symmetrical lateral counterpart are often resected to relieve the pain associated with navicular disease. The ligament of the ergot, which crosses the digital artery, vein, and nerve obliquely, should not be confused with the nerve [9]. Distal to the metacarpophalangeal joint, the (palmar proper) digital artery, vein, and nerve are in a "VAN" order (vein-artery-nerve) from dorsal to palmar, and they are parallel. The ligament of the ergot crosses them obliquely from palmar to dorsal, as it courses distally [9].

2. The lateral palmar n. (Fig. 5-4/9) is distributed similarly to the medial palmar n. The distal continuation of the medial and lateral palmar nerves (i.e., medial and lateral palmar digital nerves) constitute the only innervation to the palmar aspect of the foot including the navicular bursa.

3. The medial palmar metacarpal nerve (Fig. 5-4/13--derived from the deep branch of the ulnar n.) is usually larger than its lateral counterpart. It emerges at the distal end of Mc2 (where it may be conveniently blocked) and may reach the coronary border of the hoof [10].

4. The small lateral palmar metacarpal nerve (Fig. 5-4/14-derived from the deep branch of the ulnar nerve) is distributed similarly to its medial counterpart. Together they innervate the metacarpophalangeal joint capsule (as do some branches of the medial and lateral palmar nn.).

B. Nerve Supply to the Digits of the Ox (Figs. 5-5, 5-6)

The median nerve of the ox divides distal to the carpus into the second and third palmar common digital nerves (p.c.d.n.). A communicating branch from p.c.d.n. 3 joins the palmar branch of the ulnar nerve in forming the fourth palmar common digital nerve. The major distribution of these nerves is [9]:

1. p.c.d.n. 2--the major branch courses distally as the abaxial palmar nerve of the digit 3. (p.c.d.n. 2 also supplies a palmar branch to the medial paradigit--digit 2).

2. p.c.d.n. 3--divides to form the axial palmar nerve of digit 3 and the axial palmar nerve of digit 4. (Sometimes these remain separate rather than coursing together as p.c.d.n. 3).

3. Communicating branch--continues distally to join the palmar branch of the ulnar n. in forming the fourth palmar common digital nerve (p.c.d.n. 4).

Figure 5-4

Nerves of the Equine Manus (left limb)

    A.   Dorsal aspect
    B.   Palmar aspect

1. Cranial cutaneous antebrachial nerve (from axillary n.)
2. Lateral cutaneous antebrachial nerve (from radial n.)
3. Medial cutaneous antebrachial nerve (from musculocutaneous nerve)
4. Dorsal branch of the ulnar nerve
5. Dorsal branch of the medial palmar digital nerve
6. Dorsal branch of the lateral palmar digital nerve
7. Median nerve
8. Medial palmar nerve (p.c.d.n. 2)--circle at site for palmar block
9. Lateral palmar nerve (p.c.d.n. 3)--circle at site for palmar block
10. Ulnar nerve
11. Palmar branch of the ulnar nerve
12. Deep branch of the ulnar nerve
13. Medial palmar metacarpal nerve
14. Lateral palmar metacarpal nerve
15. Communicating branch from medial to lateral palmar nerves
16. Medial palmar digital nerve (circle at site for palmar digital block)
17. Lateral palmar digital nerve (circle at site for palmar digital block)

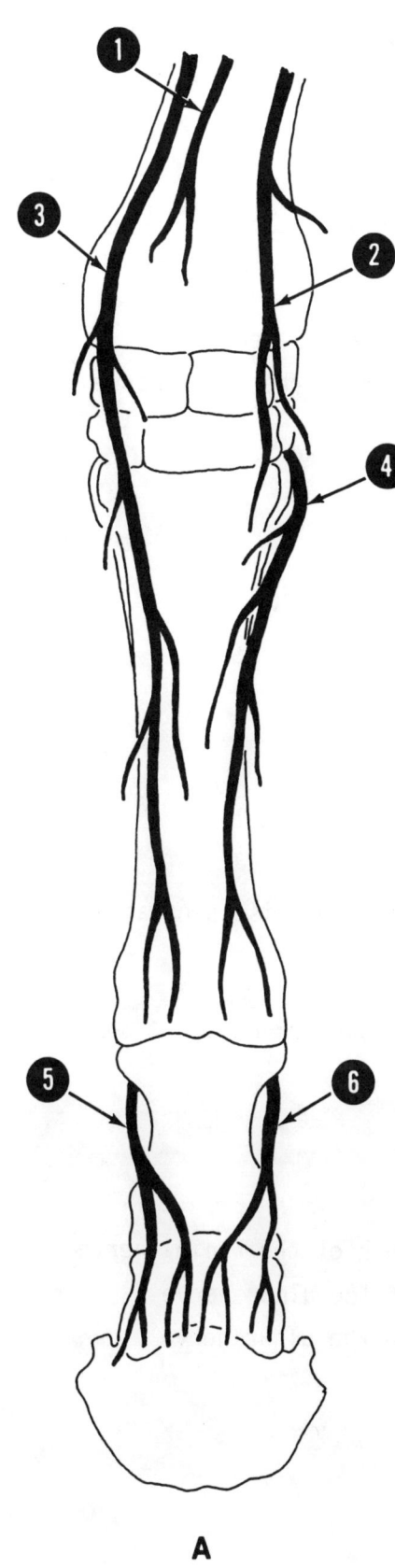
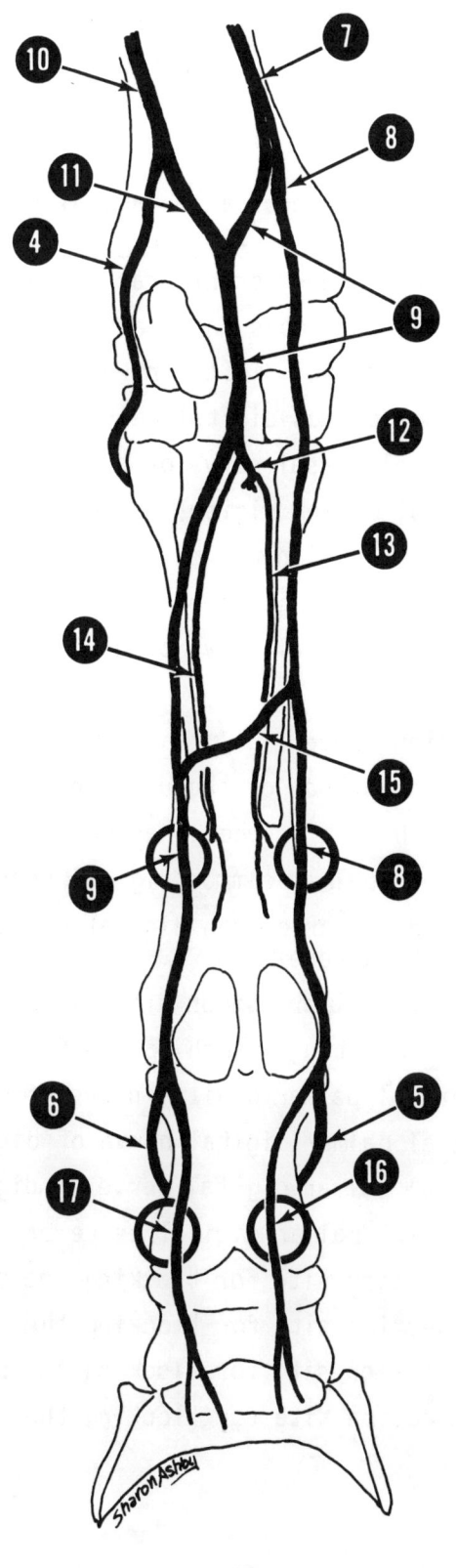

A

B

Figure 5-5

Nerves of the Bovine Manus (left limb)
  A. Dorsal aspect
  B. Palmar aspect

1. Caudal cutaneous antebrachial nerve (from ulnar n.)
2. Superficial branch of the radial nerve (exchanges some fibers with the medial cutaneous antebrachial n.)
3. Medial cutaneous antebrachial n. (from musculocutaneous nerve)
4. Dorsal common digital n. 4 (from the dorsal branch of the ulnar nerve
5. Dorsal common digital nerve 2
6. Abaxial dorsal nerve of digit 3
7. Dorsal common digital nerve 3 (very short)
8. Axial dorsal nerve of digit 3
9. Axial dorsal nerve of digit 4
10. Abaxial dorsal nerve of digit 4
11. Ulnar nerve
12. Median nerve
13. Palmar branch of the ulnar nerve
14. Deep branch of the ulnar nerve
15. Second palmar common digital nerve
16. Third palmar common digital nerve (the components may arise separately as shown here)
17. Fourth palmar common digital nerve
18. Communicating branch to the fourth palmar common digital nerve
19. Abaxial palmar digital nerve of digit 4
20. Axial palmar digital nerve of digit 4
21. Axial palmar digital nerve of digit 3
22. Abaxial palmar digital nerve of digit 3
23. Injection site for blocking the superficial branch of the radial nerve
24. Injection site for blocking the dorsal branch of the ulnar nerve
25. Injection site for blocking the palmar branch of the ulnar nerve
26. Injection site for blocking the median nerve

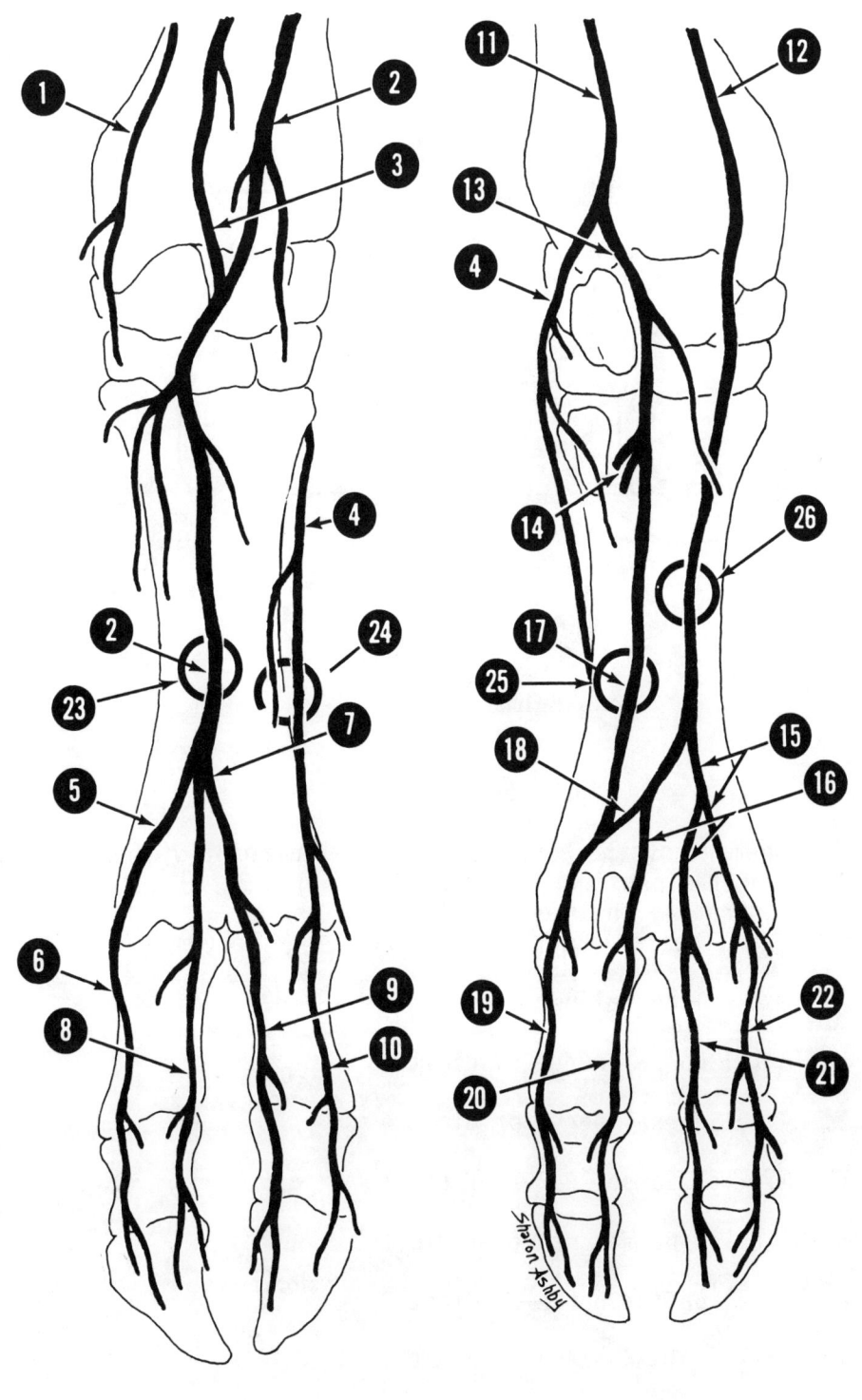

A

B

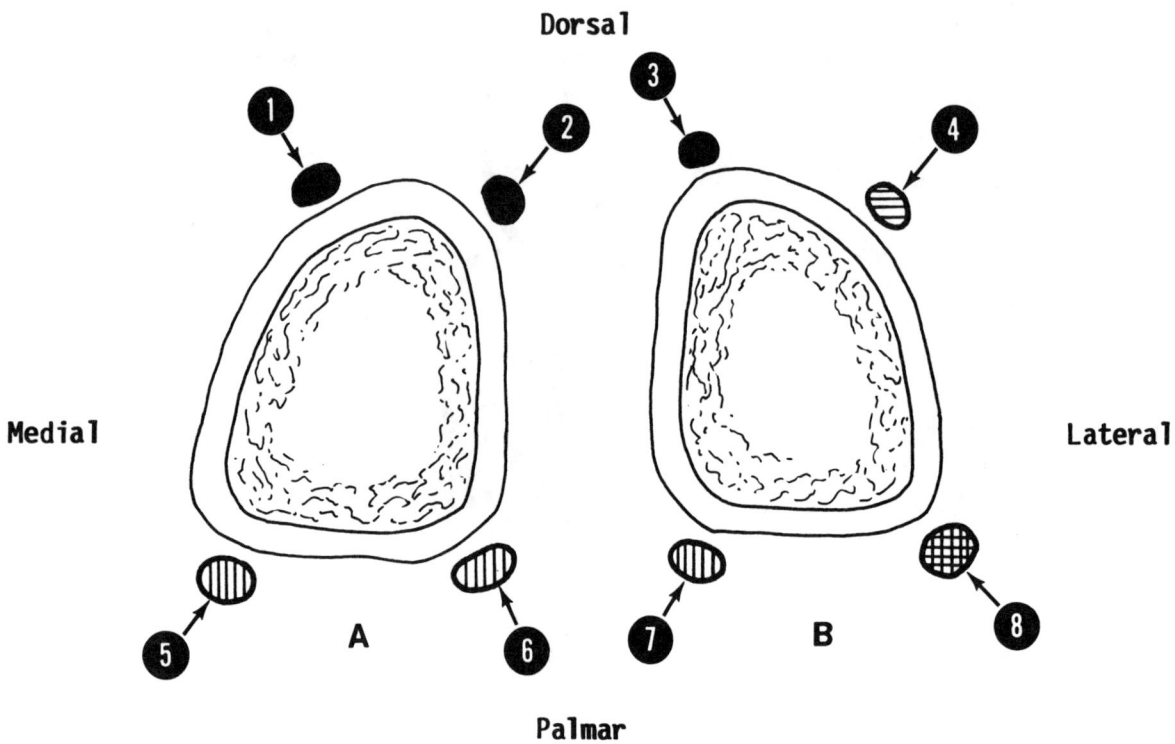

Figure 5-6

Schematic Arrangement of the Nerves around the Ruminant Digits
(transverse sections of the proximal phalanges of digits 3 [A] and 4 [B])
Illustrating their Derivation from the
Radial ● , Median 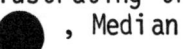 , and Ulnar 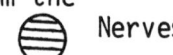 Nerves

1. Abaxial dorsal nerve of digit 3
2. Axial dorsal nerve of digit 3
3. Axial dorsal nerve of digit 4
4. Abaxial dorsal nerve of digit 4
5. Abaxial palmar nerve of digit 3
6. Axial palmar nerve of digit 3
7. Axial palmar nerve of digit 4
8. Abaxial palmar nerve of digit 4

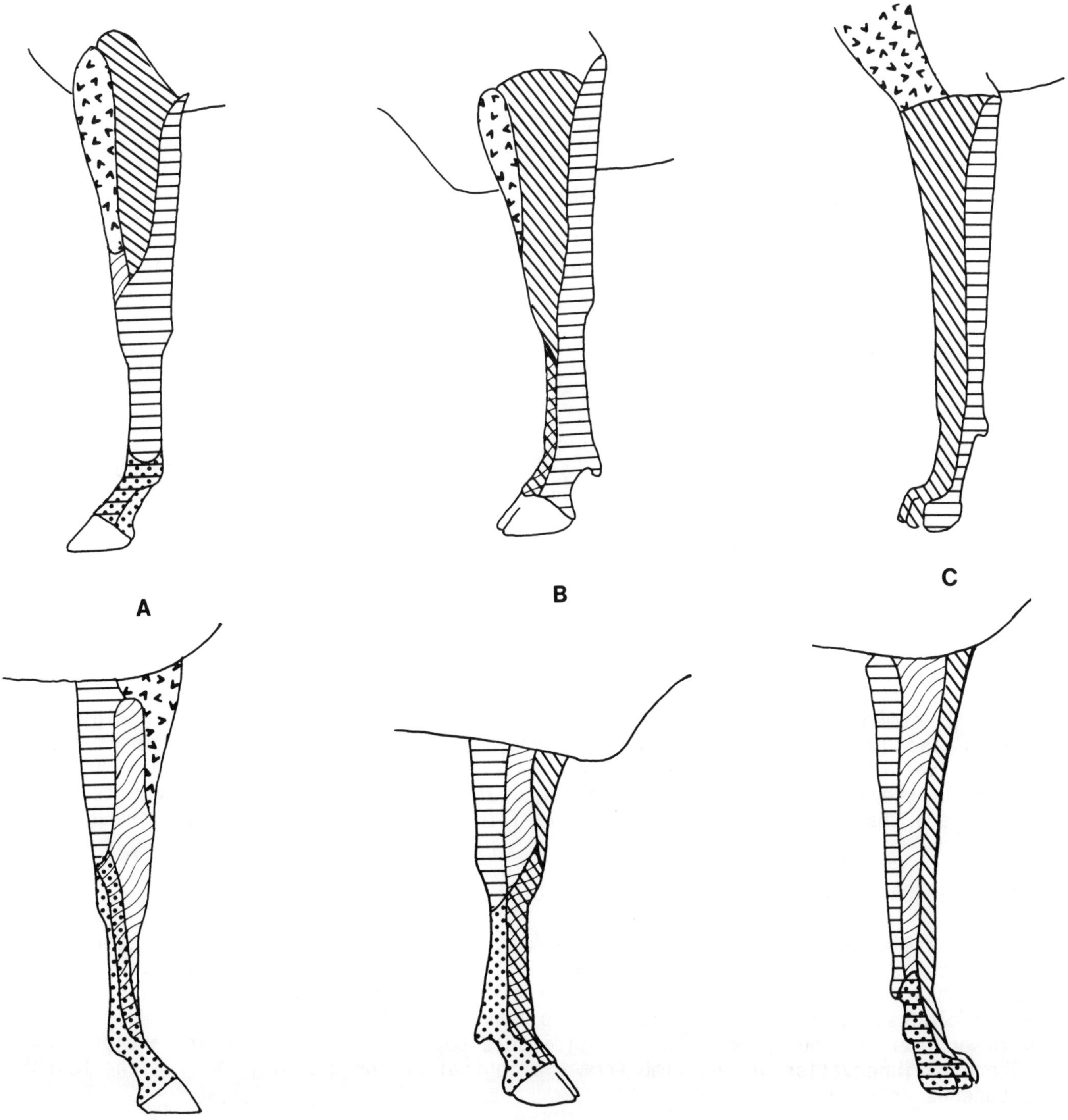

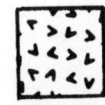

Figure 5-7

Cutaneous Dermatomes of the Thoracic Limbs of the Horse (A), Ox (B), and Dog (C)
(Lateral aspects are illustrated at the top and medial aspects are shown at the bottom.)

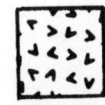 Axillary nerve (lateral cutaneous brachial and/or cranial cutaneous antebrachial nerves)

 Musculocutaneous nerve (medial cutaneous antebrachial nerve)

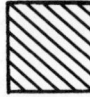 Radial nerve (superficial branch including the lateral cutaneous antebrachial nerve)

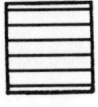 Ulnar nerve (caudal cutaneous antebrachial nerve and the cutaneous distribution of the dorsal and palmar branches of the ulnar nerve)

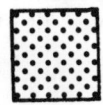 Median nerve

The ulnar nerve divides above the carpus into a dorsal branch and a palmar branch. The dorsal branch continues distally through the metacarpus as the dorsal common digital n. 4. Its main distal continuation becomes the abaxial dorsal nerve of digit 4, but it also supplies a dorsal branch to the lateral paradigit (digit 5). The palmar branch of the ulnar nerve supplies a deep branch to the interosseous muscles distal to the carpus and then continues distally as the fourth palmar common digital nerve (p.c.d.n. 4). It receives a communicating branch from p.c.d.n. 3 (or from the axial palmar nerve of digit 4). Distally the main continuation of p.c.d.n. 4 is the abaxial palmar nerve of digit 4, but it also supplies a palmar branch to the lateral paradigit (digit 5).

The radial nerve (the superficial branch which separated from the deep branch above the cubital joint) divides distal to the carpus into two dorsal common digital nerves (d.c.d.n. 2 and 3) [2]:

1. d.c.d.n. 2--the major branch continues as the abaxial dorsal nerve of digit 3 and it also supplies a dorsal branch to the medial paradigit (digit 2).

2. d.c.d.n. 3--divides to form the axial dorsal nerve of digit 3 and the axial dorsal nerve of digit 4.

To summarize the digital innervation, there are four dorsal proper digital nerves and four palmar ones. On the dorsal aspect, the three medial ones are derivatives of the radial nerve and the lateral one is from the ulnar nerve (Fig. 5-6). On the palmar aspect, the three medial nerves are derived from the median nerve, and the lateral one contains fibers from both the median nerve and the ulnar nerve.

IV. SENSORY DERMATOMES OF THE THORACIC LIMB (Fig. 5-7)

Familiarity with the sensory dermatomes can be used to help diagnose specific neuropathies by the presence or absence of a response to a pin prick test. The dermatomes can also be used to check the effectiveness of surgical and diagnostic nerve blocks. It is important to keep in mind that the junctions of one dermatome with another are not precise and considerable overlap occurs. A major part of the cutaneous innervation of the limb from the cubital region distally is from the four cutaneous antebrachial nerves:

1. The cranial cutaneous antebrachial nerve from the axillary nerve.

2. The medial cutaneous antebrachial nerve from the musculocutaneous nerve.

3. The caudal cutaneous antebrachial nerve from the ulnar nerve.

4. The lateral cutaneous antebrachial nerve from the radial nerve.

Although the exact pattern of distribution of these nerves varies somewhat among the domestic species, the general pattern is fairly constant. One significant variation involves the cutaneous distribution of the radial nerve in the horse. In the other domestic mammals, the radial nerve is distributed to the craniolateral and dorsolateral aspects of the antebrachium and manus, respectively. In the horse, however, the radial distribution plays out at the carpus and further distally its cutaneous function is taken over primarily by the cutaneous branches of the musculocutaneous and ulnar nerves.

V. DIAGNOSTIC AND SURGICAL NERVE BLOCKS

Local and regional nerve blocks in the thoracic limb are frequently and routinely performed in horses, but less often in other species. It is important to realize that diagnostic nerve blocks begin distally in a limb, and if soundness is not gained, move progressively higher until the lesion is localized [11]. They are not made proximal to motor branches of the involved nerves because the altered gait from the block cannot be differentiated from the original lameness. Surgical blocks are made far above the desired field so that collateral unblocked branches do not interfere with the desired anesthesia. A few selected blocks and their uses will be considered. The blocks themselves are "cookbook" procedures and one should always consider what nerves are affected and reason out the consequences of successful blocks (as well as failures). Understanding the nerve distribution (anatomy) allows expansion of the following selected blocks into the specific variations used by individual veterinarians:

A. Horse

1. Palmar digital block--inject at the border of the flexor tendons about halfway between the metacarpophalangeal joint and coronary border of the hoof. If done properly, and on both medial and lateral sides, this block will desensitize the distal sesamoid bone and its bursa and will imitate the results of a palmar digital neurectomy. Palmar digital neurectomies are performed on the palmar branches of the medial and lateral digital nerves. If done higher (so that the dorsal branch is also included), a number of atrophic lesions may occur including exungulation, digital flexor tendon rupture, or fractures [2].

    In interpreting palmar digital blocks relative to navicular disease versus other lameness of the distal limb, Habel offers this differential [2]:

    Pain relieved by:

Site of lesion	Palmar digital block	Injection of distal Interphalangeal joint
Navicular bursa	+	+
Distal interphalangeal jt.	-	+
Digital pad, frog, sole	+	-

    The reason that injection of the distal interphalangeal joint causes relief of pain in the navicular bursa is that anesthetic can diffuse from the joint cavity into the bursa even though they do not directly communicate. A palmar digital block will not relieve pain from a distal interphalangeal joint lesion because at least part of the joint is supplied by other nerves (dorsal branches of the digital nerves).

2. Palmar block--inject on both sides of the flexor tendons in the distal metacarpal region to block the medial and lateral palmar nerves. They can be blocked above or below the communicating branch, but care should be taken to block both sides above it or both below it. Otherwise, total desensitization of the palmar nerves will not be effected. This will desensitize most of the foot but the palmar metacarpal nerves must also be blocked for total desensitization. These nerves can be blocked by infiltrating anesthetic distal to the distal ends of Mc 2 and 4. Even this procedure will not totally desensitize the metacarpophalangeal joint because the capsule receives some unblocked, deeper branches from the palmar metacarpal nerves.

To anesthetize the metacarpus and metacarpophalangeal area, the ulnar, median, and musculocutaneous nerves must be blocked [2]. This procedure may be of value for regional analgesia in cases of traumatic injuries or for minor surgical procedures.

3. Ulnar nerve block--inject in the groove between the flexor carpi ulnaris and the extensor carpi ulnaris (ulnaris lateralis) mm. This groove can be located 10 or more centimeters proximal to the accessory carpal bone [2].

4. Median nerve block--inject at the distal edge of the transverse pectoral m. on the caudomedial aspect of the proximal radius [2]. The nerve can also be blocked in the distal half of the antebrachium between the flexor carpi radialis and flexor carpi ulnaris [8].

5. Musculocutaneous (medial cutaneous antebrachial) nerve block - inject where the nerve crosses the lacertus fibrosus or on the sides of the cephalic and accessory cephalic veins [2,8]. The carpus can be anesthetized with these last three blocks plus a block of a branch of the radial nerve (on the deep surface of the common digital extensor just proximal to the carpus) [12]. The interior of the joint, however, is blocked more simply by carpocentesis [2].

B. Dog

1. The median, ulnar, and musculocutaneous nerves can all be blocked on the medial side of the brachium where they lie adjacent to the brachial vessels. The musculocutaneous nerve is cranial to the brachial artery and the median and ulnar nerves are caudal to it [2].

2. The superficial branch of the radial nerve can be palpated and blocked where it emerges at the cranial border of the lateral head of the triceps brachii in the distal aspect of the brachium [2].

To anesthetize the paw, the above two blocks may be performed. Alternatively, the radial nerve may be blocked as above and the median and ulnar nn. may be separately blocked as follows [2]:

a. Median nerve--inject caudal to the flexor carpi radialis tendon, a few centimeters proximal to the point where the cephalic vein crosses it.

b. Ulnar nerve--inject between the flexor carpi ulnaris and the extensor carpi ulnaris (ulnaris lateralis) in the distal fourth of the antebrachium. This will block the dorsal branch. The palmar branch may be blocked by directing the needle in the carpal canal just medial to the accessory carpal bone.

C. Ox

1. Dorsal branch of the ulnar n. block--this nerve may be blocked by injecting between the metacarpal bone and the interosseous muscle on the lateral side at mid-metacarpus (Fig. 5-5/24). A successful block anesthetizes the dorsal abaxial nerve of digit 4 (Fig. 5-6) [2].

2. Palmar branch of the ulnar nerve--this nerve may be blocked at mid-metacarpus between the interosseous muscle and the deep digital flexor by redirecting the needle used to block the dorsal branch of the ulnar n. (Fig. 5-5/25). A successful block partially anesthetizes the palmar abaxial nerve of digit 4 (Fig. 5-6) [2].

3. Superficial branch of the radial n. - this nerve may be blocked near mid-metacarpus by palpating it and injecting just medial to the common digital extensor tendon (Fig. 5-5/23). A successful block deadens both dorsal nerves of the third digit and the axial dorsal nerve of digit 4 (Fig. 5-6) [2].

4. Median nerve block - this nerve may be blocked by injecting between the interosseous muscle and the deep digital flexor on the medial side above mid-metacarpus (Fig. 5-5/26). A successful block deadens both palmar nerves of digit 3, the axial palmar nerve of digit 4, and partially deadens the abaxial palmar nerve of digit 4 (Fig. 5-6) [2].

References

1. Allam, M. W., D.G. Lee, F. E. Nulsen, and E. A. Fortune. 1952. The anatomy of the brachial plexus of the dog. Anat. Rec. 114(2):173-180.

2. Habel, R. E. 1981. Applied Veterinary Anatomy, second ed. Published by the author, Ithaca, New York.

3. Bowne, J. G. 1959. Neuroanatomy of the brachial plexus of the dog. Ph.D. thesis, Iowa State Univ., 1959.

4. Worthman, R. P. 1957. Demonstration of specific nerve paralyses in the dog. JAVMA 131:174-178.

5. Vaughan, L. C. 1964. Peripheral nerve injuries: an experimental study in cattle. Vet. Rec. 76:1293-1300.

6. Rooney, J. R. 1963. Radial paralysis in the horse. Cornell Vet. 53:328-338.

7. Marolt, J., V. Bego, E. Vukelic, F. Sankovic, and B. Zeskov. 1962. Untersuchungen uber funktionsstorungen des Nervus radialis und des kreislaufes in der arteria axillaris beim pferd. Dtsch. tierarztl. Wschr. 69:181-189.

8. Adams, O. R. 1974. Lameness in Horses, third ed. Lea and Febiger, Philadelphia.

9. Getty, R. 1975. Sisson and Grossman's The Anatomy of the Domestic Animals, fifth ed. W. B. Saunders, Philadelphia.

10. Sack, W. O. 1975. Nerve distribution in the metacarpus and front limb of a horse. JAVMA 167:298-305.

11. Derksen, F. J. 1980. Diagnostic local anesthesia of the equine front limb. J. Equine Pract. 2(1):41-47.

12. Getty, R., J. A. Sowa, and R. L. Lundvall. 1956. Local anesthesia and applied anatomy as related to nerve blocks in horses. JAVMA 128:583-587.

PELVIC LIMB OSTEOLOGY

The bones of the pelvic limb include the os coxae, femur, tibia and fibula, tarsal bones, metatarsal bones, phalanges, and a number of sesamoid bones. For each of these, a list of the major anatomic features that are present in most domestic mammals is given. This is followed by comparative, clinical, and developmental information. These facts should be correlated to live animals, specimens, radiographs, drawings, pictures, and verbal abstractions. Minor anatomic features with no obvious clinical significance have been intentionally omitted.

I. OS COXAE ("HEMIPELVIS")

   A. Major features [1]

   obturator foramen--the obturator nerve courses through this foramen
   acetabulum--articulates with the femoral head
       acetabular fossa--site of origin of lig. of femoral head
       lunate surface--the articular surface (half-moon shaped)
       acetabular notch--the defect in the ventral acetabular lip
   ischiatic spine--separates greater and lesser ischiatic notches
   ilium
       body--the caudal part
       wing--the cranial part
           gluteal surface--the lateral aspect where the middle gluteal
               m. and part of the deep gluteal m. attach
           sacropelvic surface--the medial aspect
               auricular surface--articulates with the sacrum
               iliac surface--lies adjacent to the internal iliac
                   vessels
               iliac crest--the cranial aspect of the wing*
                   tuber coxae--the ventral part of the iliac crest
                   tuber sacrale--the dorsal part of the iliac crest
       major (greater) ischiatic (sciatic) notch - the indentation cranial
           to the ischiatic spine
       arcuate line--an indistinct ridge on the ventromedial aspect
   ischium (pronounced iss'-ke-um)
       body--the part lateral to the obturator foramen
       ramus--the portion medial to the obturator foramen
       table--the portion caudal to the obturator foramen
       ischiatic tuberosity--attachment for the caudal thigh muscles*
       minor (lesser) ischiatic (sciatic) notch--the dorsal indentation
           caudal to the ischiatic spine
   pubis
       body--the central part
       cranial ramus--the portion which forms part of the acetabulum
       caudal ramus--the portion medial to the obturator foramen
       pecten--the cranial border formed by left and right pubes (pubises)

---

*In dairy conformation judging, the tuber coxae and ischiatic tuberosity are commonly termed "hook" and "pin," respectively.

iliopubic eminence--attachment for the pectineus m.
dorsal and ventral pubic tubercles--midline prominences
obturator sulcus--the groove at the cranial aspect of the obturator foramen through which the obturator nerve courses

pelvis as a whole (ossa coxarum, sacrum, and first caudal vertebra)
    ischiatic arch--the caudal border between ischiatic tuberosities
    pelvic symphysis--the junction of left and right ossa coxarum
        pubic symphysis--the cranial part of the pelvic symphysis
        ischiatic symphysis--the caudal part of the pelvic symphysis
    transverse diameter (of the pelvic cavity)--measured at the widest horizontal point
    vertical diameter (of the pelvic cavity)--measured from the cranial aspect of the pelvic symphysis to the dorsal wall of the pelvic cavity
    pelvic cavity--the area bounded dorsally by the vertebral column, and laterally and ventrally by the pelvis
    cranial pelvic opening (= "pelvic inlet")
    caudal pelvic opening (= "pelvic outlet")

B. Selected comparative, clinical, and developmental features

1. The os coxae of carnivores develops from 8 or more centers of ossification (Fig. 6-1) [2,3]. The main parts of the ilium, ischium, and pubis are primary centers and the acetabular bone, iliac crest, lateral and medial aspects of the ischiatic tuberosity, and a wedge-shaped area at the caudal aspect of the ischiatic symphysis develop as secondary centers. The triangularly-shaped acetabular bone is located just cranial to the acetabular fossa at the junction of the three primary centers.

2. A useful aid in radiographically differentiating feline pelvises from those of small dogs is to note that in the cat the sides of the pelvis appear nearly parallel in a V-D or D-V projection (||). Those of a dog appear to diverge ()().

3. An ox pelvis can be easily differentiated from that of a horse by noting the three-sided shape of the ruminant ischiatic tuberosity or the divided lunate surface in the ox's acetabulum (Fig. 6-2/A, B). In the small ruminants, the 3-sided feature of the ischiatic tuberosity is less evident and the lunate surface is undivided. (The ischiatic tuberosity of the pig resembles that of the ox.)

4. The pelvis is the most frequently fractured region in carnivores [4]. Conservative treatment may be used unless articular surfaces are involved or severe displacement is present. However, surgical reduction often results in faster recovery time and less lameness after healing. Some surgeons use an animal's ability to bear weight as a criterion when deciding whether to treat a fracture conservatively or surgically.

5. A midline symphyseal osteotomy is sometimes used to gain exposure in canine prostate surgery. In older animals, a T-shaped piece of bone may be removed by 3 transections: one at the cranial aspect of each obturator foramen and a third one which joins the two

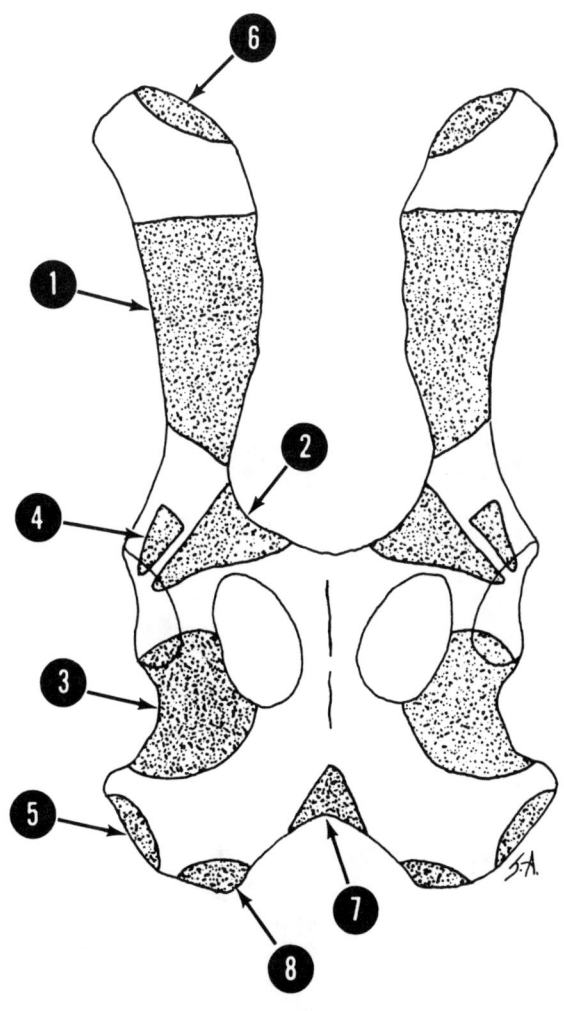

Figure 6-1

Centers of Ossification in the Canine Pelvis

	Centers	Age of Appearance*
1.	ilium	birth
2.	pubis	birth
3.	ischium	birth
4.	acetabular bone	6 weeks
5.	lateral aspect of ischiatic tuberosity	20 weeks**
6.	iliac crest	24 weeks**
7.	caudal aspect of ischiatic symphysis	24 weeks**
8.	medial aspect of ischiatic tuberosity	36 weeks**

*Data are averages based on the observations of Smith [2] and Shively [3].

**May vary by several weeks.

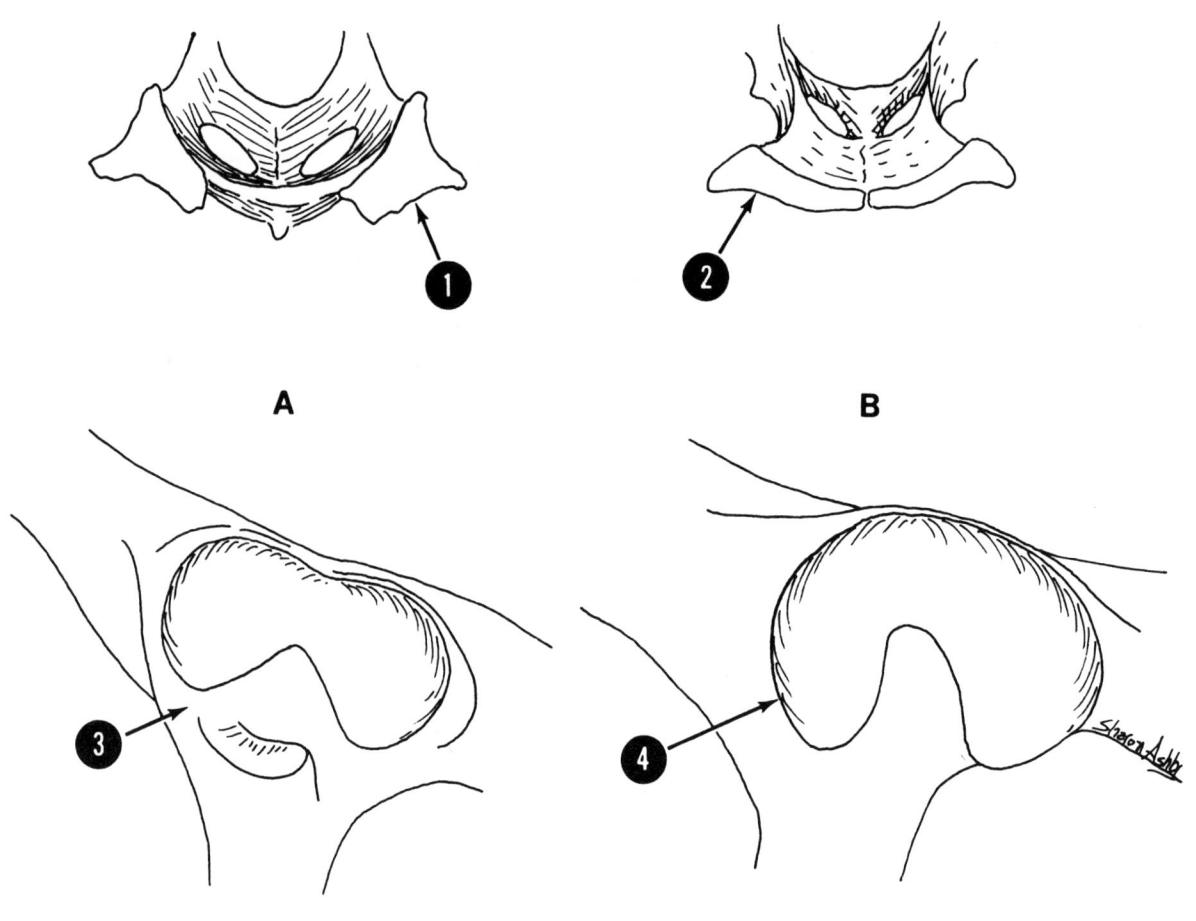

Figure 6-2

Some Comparative Features of the Pelvis in the Ox (A) and the Horse (B)

1. Three-sided shape of the bovine ischiatic tuberosity

2. "Simple" equine ischiatic tuberosity

3. Division of the lunate surface of the bovine acetabulum into a large dorsal articular surface and a small cranioventral surface by a small nonarticular area

4. Undivided lunate surface of the equine acetabulum

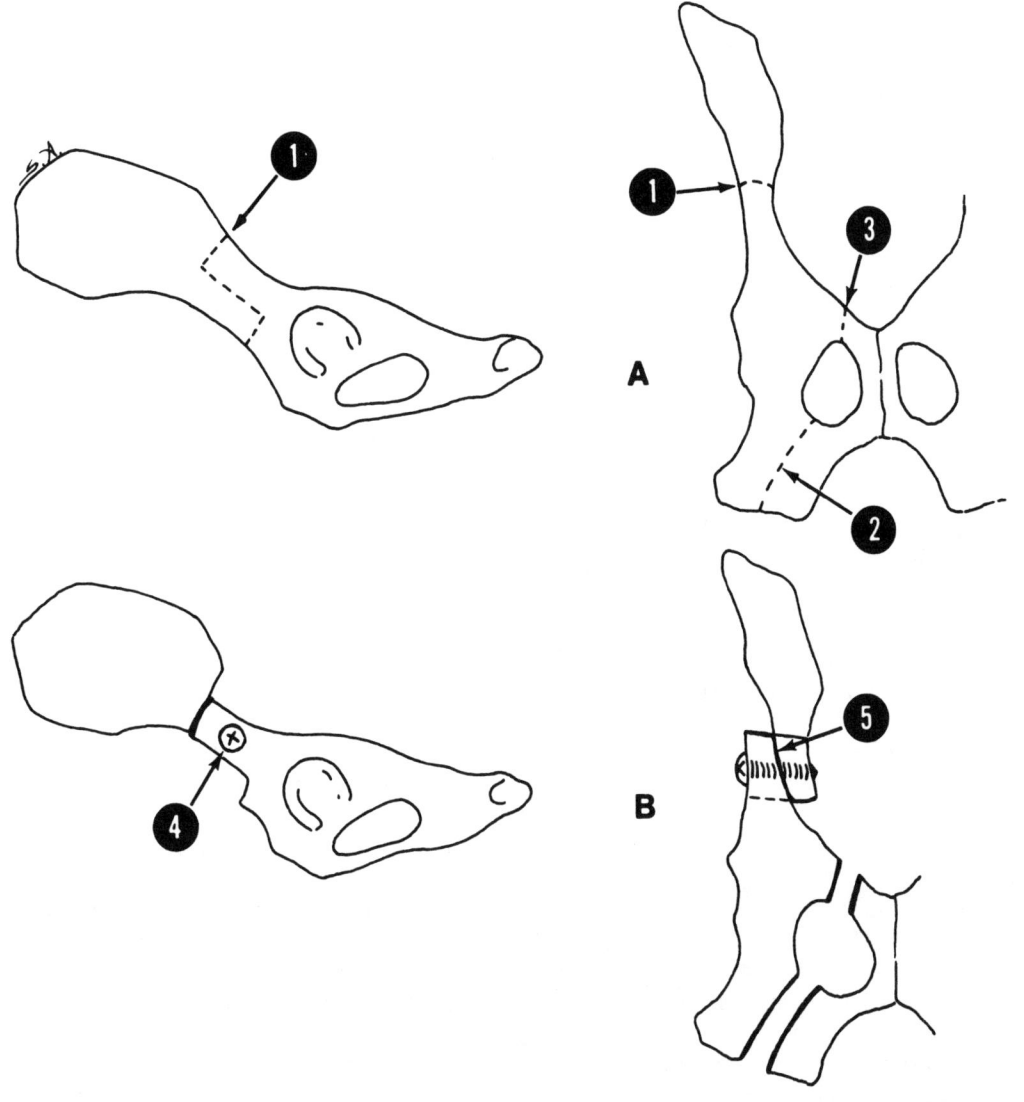

Figure 6-3

Pelvic Osteotomy as a Treatment for Canine Hip Dysplasia

    A.   Lateral and dorsal aspects to show osteotomy sites

    B.   Lateral and dorsal aspects after fixation

The purpose of this procedure is to create better coverage of the femoral head by the dorsal lip of the acetabulum. The ilium is osteotomized in a step-wedge fashion (1). The ischium is transected through the obturator foramen (2). The pubis (3) is transected in larger dogs, but in smaller dogs it may be "bent." The fragment is stabilized with a screw (4) and some surgeons add a piece of wire as well. To insure that the dorsal lip of the acetabulum rotates laterally, some remodeling of the contact area (5) may be necessary. (After Henry and Wadsworth [7].) Alternatively, a transverse osteotomy may be made at (1) (rather than a stepwise cut), and a plate used for stabilization rather than screws and wire. The plate can be torqued on its long axis to the desired angle of rotation necessary to insure coverage of the femoral head by the dorsal acetabulum [8].

foramina. The "pubic plate" is wired back in place at closure [5]. Symphysiotomy may also be used to alleviate dystocia in first calf heifers. In older cows, osseous fusion makes the approach more difficult but not impossible [6].

6. Wedge osteotomies (acetabuloplasties) to broaden the dorsal lip of the acetabulum (and thereby deepen the acetabulum) have been used experimentally to treat canine hip dysplasia, but they never became popular because success was difficult to reproduce. Pelvic osteotomies to change the angle of the acetabulum have been described [7,8]. In these procedures, the whole acetabular region is rotated laterally in order to obtain better coverage of the dorsal aspect of the femoral head (Fig. 6-3).

II. FEMUR (OS FEMORIS)

A. Major features [1]

head--articulates with acetabulum
    fovea capitis--termination of lig. of femoral head
neck--joins the head to the body
major (greater) trochanter--attachment for middle and deep gluteal mm.
    trochanteric fossa--attachment for most of the caudal hip mm.
minor (lesser) trochanter--attachment for the iliopsoas m.
third trochanter--attachment for the superficial gluteal m.
body
    medial and lateral supracondylar tuberosities--serve as attachment points for the gastrocnemius m. and the lateral one also serves as an origin for the superficial digital flexor m.
    popliteal surface--the caudal aspect of the distal femur

medial condyle--articulates with the medial condyle of the tibia
    medial epicondyle--attachment for the medial collateral ligament
lateral condyle--articulates with the lateral condyle of the tibia
    extensor fossa--attachment for the long digital extensor m.
    fossa for popliteal muscle--attachment for the popliteal m.
    lateral epicondyle--attachment for the lateral collateral lig.
trochlea--articular surface for the patella

B. Selected comparative, clinical, and developmental features

1. In the horse, the major trochanter is obviously divided into cranial and caudal parts (Fig. 6-4/1, 2), but it does not appear to be divided in other species. The horse also has a well developed third trochanter. Ruminants lack a third trochanter (they have no definitive superficial gluteal m.), and this prominence is poorly developed in the carnivores and pig. The large depression on the caudolateral aspect of the distal equine femur is the supracondylar fossa which serves as part of the site of origin for the superficial digital flexor m. Ruminants have a similar fossa (Fig. 6-4/8).

2. In the horse and ox, the medial ridge of the trochlea is significantly larger than the lateral ridge (Fig. 6-4/5, 6). In the horse,

the eminence on the proximal aspect of the medial ridge is the trochlear tubercle (Fig. 6-4/7). The patella rests on the proximal aspect of this tubercle in the resting phase of the patellar lock mechanism (see Chapter 8) [9].

3. In the dog, the femur develops from one primary center (diaphysis) and 3 or 4 secondary centers: femoral head, greater trochanter, distal epiphysis and, in larger dogs, lesser trochanter (Fig. 6-5/1-5) [10]. Fusion of the physes usually occurs at 8-12 months depending on size, breed, and the physis under consideration. Although most physes are not flat (nonplanar), the distal physis of the femur is especially undulant and this gives it an irregular "wavy" radiographic appearance. Nonplanar shapes increase the strength of the physes by enlarging the contact surface area.

4. In a ventrodorsal radiograph of a canine pelvis, the fovea capitis produces a small but usually identifiable flat area on the femoral head which should be distinguished from a pathological lesion (Fig. 6-5/8) [11,12].

5. In the horse, the femur develops from five primary centers of ossification: femoral head, greater trochanter, third trochanter, diaphysis, and distal epiphysis [13].

6. Retrograded intramedullary pins in the femurs of carnivores emerge from the bone at the trochanteric fossa (Fig. 6-5/6, 7). This fossa also serves as a natural place to start a normalgraded pin.

7. In midshaft femoral fractures, the fragments often override* because of the large muscle mass which bridges the fracture site. When overriding occurs, the distal fragment(s) is nearly always positioned (displaced) caudal to the proximal fragment(s) because the gastrocnemius and superficial digital flexor muscles rotate the distal fragment caudally (Fig. 6-6).

8. An intra-articular epiphyseal fracture of the femoral head may result in necrosis if the major vessels to the capital epiphysis, which enter around the neck, suffer disruption. The small vessels in the ligament of the femoral head are inadequate to nourish the head.

9. The greater trochanter of the femur may be osteotomized during a dorsal approach to the coxal joint (Fig. 6-5/11) [14]. This procedure, called the Gorman or transtrochanteric approach, will allow reflection of the middle gluteal, piriformis, and part of the deep gluteal mm. At closure, the greater trochanter is reattached with pins and/or wire.

---

*The term overriding implies that the fractured ends of the bone fragments have slipped past each other (i.e., they are no longer in the same transverse plane). The term displacement is used to indicate axial malalignment. Fragments can displace without overriding, but overriding always includes displacement.

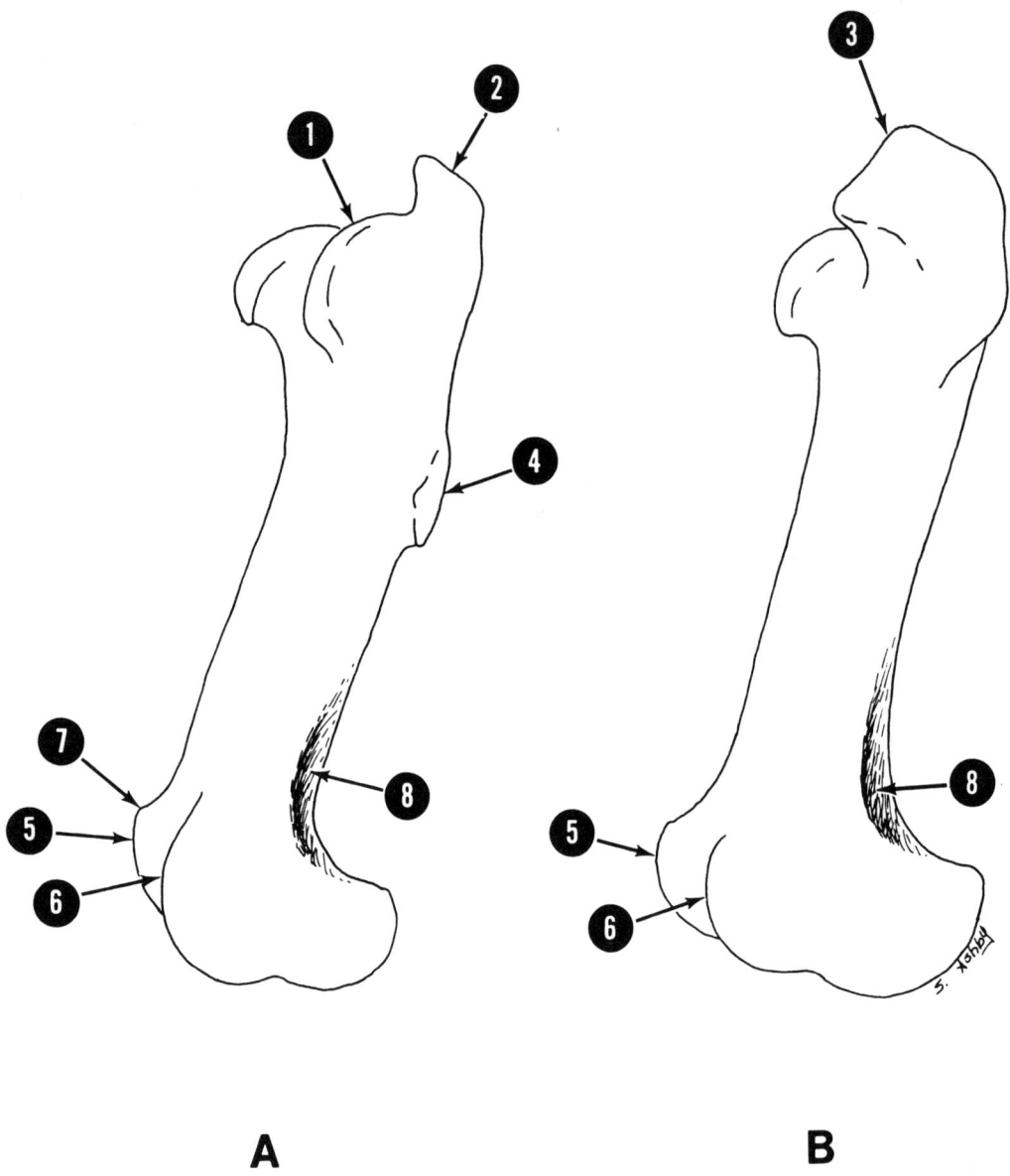

Figure 6-4

A Comparison of the Femurs of the Horse (A) and the Ox (B)
(lateral aspects of the left femurs)

1. Cranial part of greater trochanter
2. Caudal part of greater trochanter
3. Undivided greater trochanter
4. Third trochanter (absent in ox)
5. Medial ridge of femoral trochlea
6. Lateral ridge of femoral trochlea
7. Trochlear tubercle
8. Supracondylar fossa

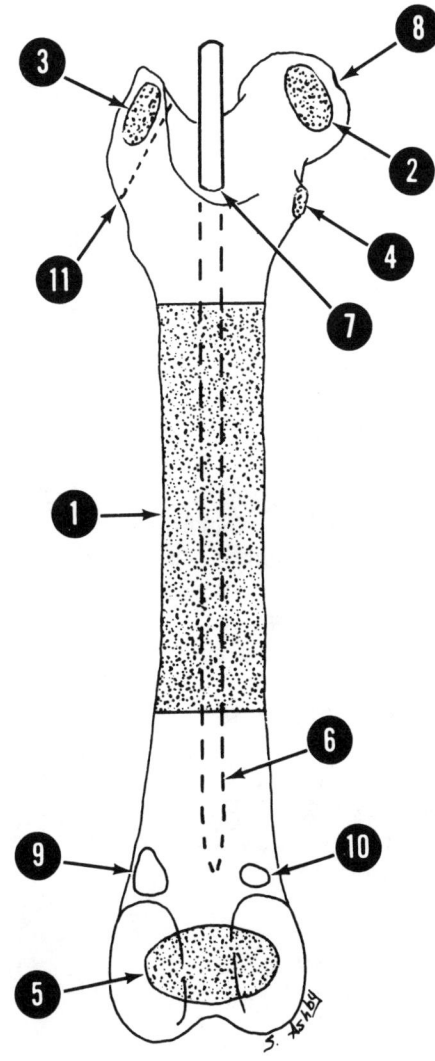

Figure 6-5

Caudal Aspect of Left Canine Femur: Clinical and Developmental Features

The positions of the primary center of ossification in the diaphysis (1) and secondary centers for the femoral head (2), greater trochanter (3), lesser trochanter (4), and distal epiphysis (5) are indicated. An intramedullary pin (6) is shown to illustrate that, when retrograded, it will emerge from the bone at the trochanteric fossa (7). Normalgraded pins may also be inserted by starting them at this location. The fovea capitis (8) produces a subtle flattened area radiographically. The sesamoid bones in the heads of the gastrocnemius m. articulate with the dorsal aspects of the femoral condyles. The lateral one (9) is a little "taller" than its medial counterpart (10). The dotted line (11) indicates the position of a trochanteric osteotomy in one of the techniques for a dorsal approach to the coxal joint.

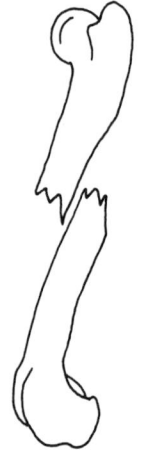

Figure 6-6

In a midshaft femoral fracture, the fragments usually override with the distal fragment displaced caudal to the proximal one. Many muscles are responsible for the overriding, including most of the caudal, cranial, and medial muscles of the thigh. The caudal displacement of the distal fragment is caused by the pull of the gastrocnemius and superficial digital flexor muscles at their origin on the distal femur. Abduction by the gluteal mm. may also cause the proximal femur to be somewhat lateral (vs. directly cranial) to the distal fragment.

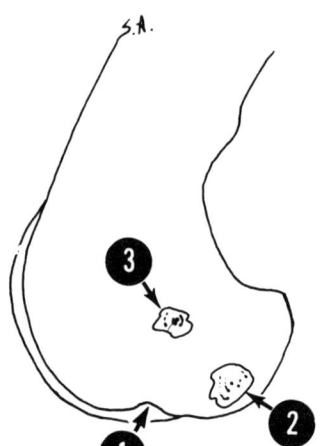

Figure 6-7

In carnivores, the extensor fossa of the lateral condyle of the femur (1) serves as a convenient radiographic marker to help differentiate the lateral condyle from the medial condyle in lateral radiographic perspectives. It appears as a notch-like radiolucency which should not be mistaken for an osseous defect. In ungulates, the medial lip of the femoral trochlea is so much larger than the lateral lip that the extensor fossa is not needed for differentiation. The fossa for the popliteus muscle (2) and the point of attachment of the lateral collateral ligament (3) are not visualized radiographically.

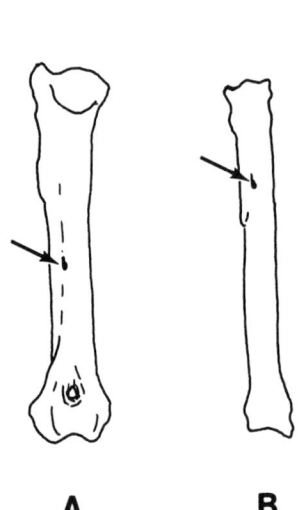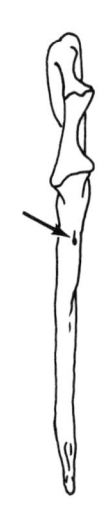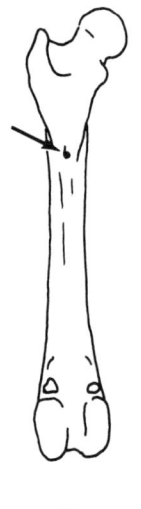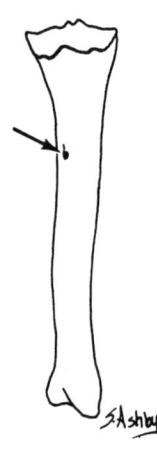

A   B   C   D   E

Figure 6-8

The Positions of the Major Nutrient Foramina (arrows) in the Five Bones Most Commonly Affected by Canine Panosteitis (all bones shown are from left limbs)

    A. Humerus (caudal aspect)   D. Femur (caudal aspect)
    B. Radius (caudal aspect)   E. Tibia (caudal aspect)
    C. Ulna (cranial aspect)

10. In carnivores the extensor fossa of the femur produces a radiolucency which should not be mistaken for a lytic lesion (Fig. 6-7). Its location on the lateral condyle often allows the medial and lateral condyles to be differentiated in ML or LM views.

11. The femur is one of the five long bones most commonly affected by canine panosteitis (eosinophilic panosteitis, enostosis, shifting leg lameness). The other most commonly affected bones are the humerus, radius, ulna, and tibia. This disease of unknown etiology is characterized by a cyclic lameness affecting one bone and then another [15]. At the time of tenderness in a given bone, there are often no radiographic signs, but a few days later the medullary cavity assumes a "cloudy" opacity, often first detectable near the position of the major nutrient foramen. In the humerus, this site is located just distal to the longitudinal midpoint of the bone and, in the other four bones, it is found at the junction of the proximal third or fourth with the rest of the bone (Fig. 6-8). The opacity is caused by endosteal new bone deposition. Radiographically, periosteal reactions may also occur with time [16]. This disease spontaneously resolves, may cycle once or several times in a given dog, and most commonly affects the German Shepherd breed. There is not a characteristic eosinophilia as was once supposed. Young dogs are affected more often than mature ones and failure to find radiographic changes in the tender limb should include follow-up films 7-10 days later and/or filming other limbs (which may currently have the radiographic changes but be clinically quiescent).

12. Articular surfaces for medial and lateral sesamoid bones of the gastrocnemius muscle are present on the dorsal (proximal) aspects of the femoral condyles in carnivores. Ungulates do not have these sesamoid bones (see Part IX, below).

III. PATELLA

A. Major features

base - the proximal aspect
apex - the distal aspect
articular surface
cranial surface

B. Selected comparative, clinical, and developmental features

1. The patella of the horse and ox has a cartilaginous process on its medial side. A patellar fibrocartilage attaches to this process which, in turn, serves as a point of attachment for the medial patellar ligament [13].

2. Chondromalacia of the patella occurs in the horse and man. It is a degeneration of the articular cartilage which results in gonitis. The cause in horses is believed to be associated with pressure related to the ligamentous attachments, and medial patellar desmotomy often reduces the lameness [17].

3. The carnivores have a variable number (2-3) of parapatellar fibrocartilages which lie adjacent to the patella. To the unfamiliar eye, these have an unusual appearance as viewed from the deep surface - a fact which might be of value during a post-mortem examination of this area.

4. In carnivores, the center of ossification for the patella appears at about 2 months of age and may be double (two centers may be present) [10].

IV. TIBIA

A. Major features

medial condyle--articulates with medial femoral condyle
lateral condyle--articulates with the lateral femoral condyle
popliteal notch--the caudal indentation between the condyles
cranial, central, and caudal intercondylar areas--the nonarticular regions between the condyles
intercondylar eminences
    medial and lateral intercondylar tubercles--serve as part of the attachment for the cruciate ligg.
extensor groove--a depression through which the tendon of the long digital extensor m. courses (as well as the peroneus tertius m. in ungulates)
body
tibial tuberosity--attachment for the patellar ligament(s)
cochlea--the distal articular surface
medial malleolus--the distal projection on the medial side

B. Selected comparative, clinical, and developmental features

1. In the carnivores and the pig, the tibia and fibula remain unfused. In the ruminants and horse, some degree of fusion occurs (Fig. 6-9, see also Part V, below).

2. In the horse, the tibia has a lateral malleolus (in addition to the medial malleolus), which consists of the distal fibula that has developmentally fused to the tibia (see Part V, below). In the other domestic mammals, the lateral malleolus retains its original identity as the distal part of the fibula.

3. In the dog, the tibia develops from one primary center (diaphysis) and 4 secondary centers: condyles, tibial tuberosity, distal epiphysis, and medial malleolus. The center for the condyles unites with the one for the tibial tuberosity at about 8 months of age, and this combined unit then unites with the diaphysis at about 11 months. The newly united regions retain a bizarre radiographic appearance for several weeks, especially between the tibial tuberosity and the diaphysis (Fig. 6-10).

4. The tibia of the horse develops from 5 primary centers of ossification: condyles, tibial tuberosity, body, medial malleolus (and distal epiphysis), and lateral malleolus (distal fibula).

V. FIBULA

   A. Major features

   head--the proximal epiphysis
   body--the diaphysis
   lateral malleolus--the distal epiphysis

   B. Selected comparative, clinical, and developmental features

   1. The generalized fibula develops from three centers of ossification: head, body, and lateral malleolus (Fig. 6-10).

   2. In the carnivores and the pig, the fibula is fully developed and does not fuse to the tibia (Fig. 6-9).

   3. In the horse and ruminants, the body of the fibula does not usually fully develop. Consequently, the head and lateral malleolus are not typically connected. In the horse, the head of the fibula remains separate, but the lateral malleolus fuses to the tibia. In the ruminants the head of the fibula fuses to the tibia, but the lateral malleolus remains separate (Fig. 6-9).

   4. In the horse, the fibula is quite variable in its development and there are instances in the literature where its proximal physis, which may not close for some time, has been clinically mistaken for a fracture [7] (Fig. 6-11).

   5. All domestic mammals have a groove on the lateral side of the lateral malleolus. In the carnivores, an additional groove is present near the caudal aspect of the lateral malleolus. Tendons of the craniolateral crural muscles pass through these grooves (see Chapter 7).

VI. TARSAL BONES

   A. Major features [1]

   talus ("tibial tarsal bone")
       body
           trochlea--articulates with the tibial cochlea
       neck
       head--distal extremity
   calcaneus ("fibular tarsal bone")
       tuber calcanei--where the common calcanean tendon attaches
       sustentaculum tali--the medial projection which supports the talus

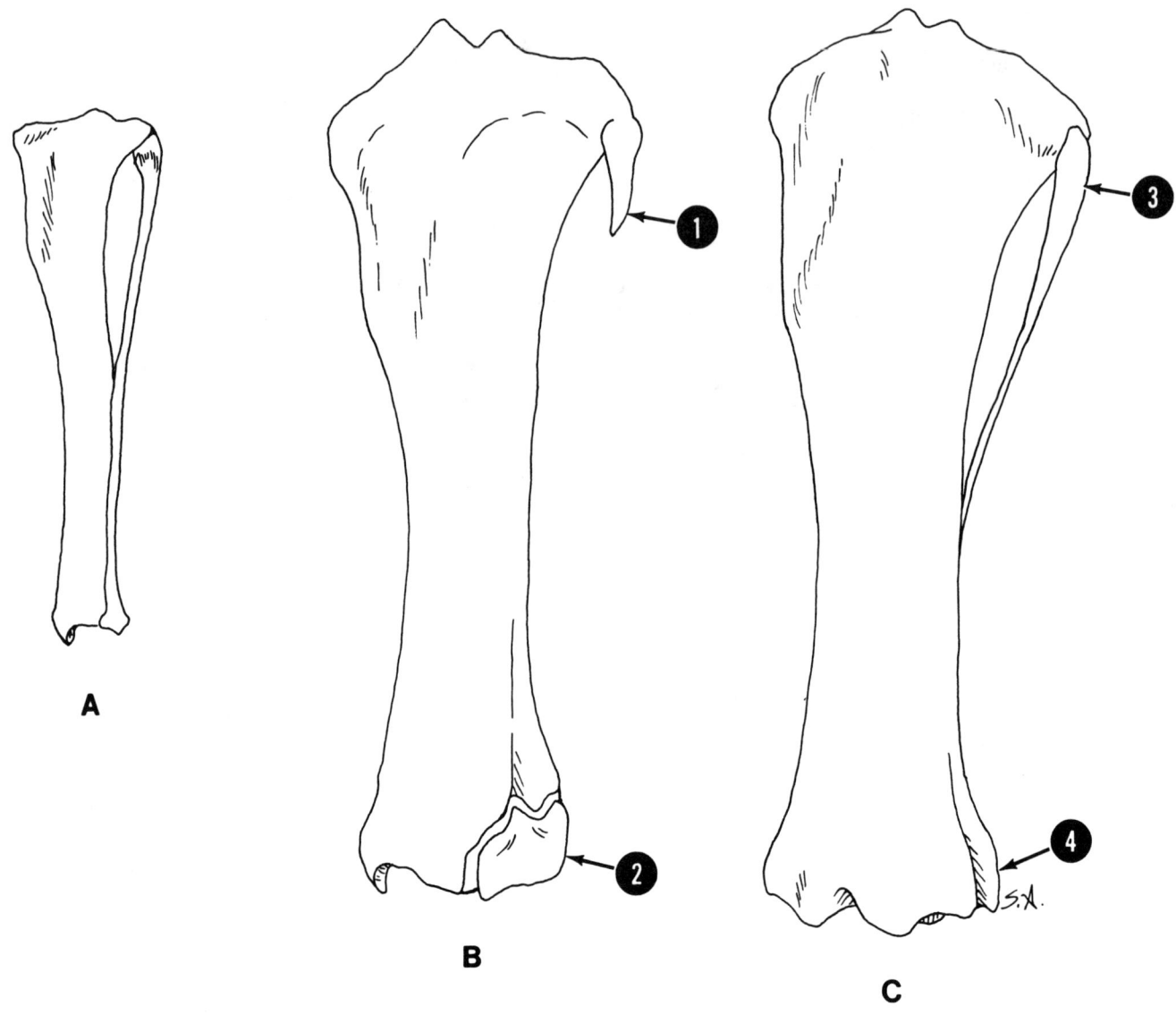

Figure 6-9

Comparison of the Tibia and Fibula in the Dog (A), Ox (B), and Horse (C) (craniolateral aspects)

A. In the dog (also in the cat and pig), the tibia and fibula remain unfused throughout their length.
B. In the ox and other ruminants, the head of the fibula (1) fuses to the tibia, the lateral malleolus (2) remains separate, and most of the fibular body fails to develop.
C. In the horse, the head of the fibula (3) remains distinct, the lateral malleolus (4) fuses to the tibia, and most of the fibular body fails to develop.

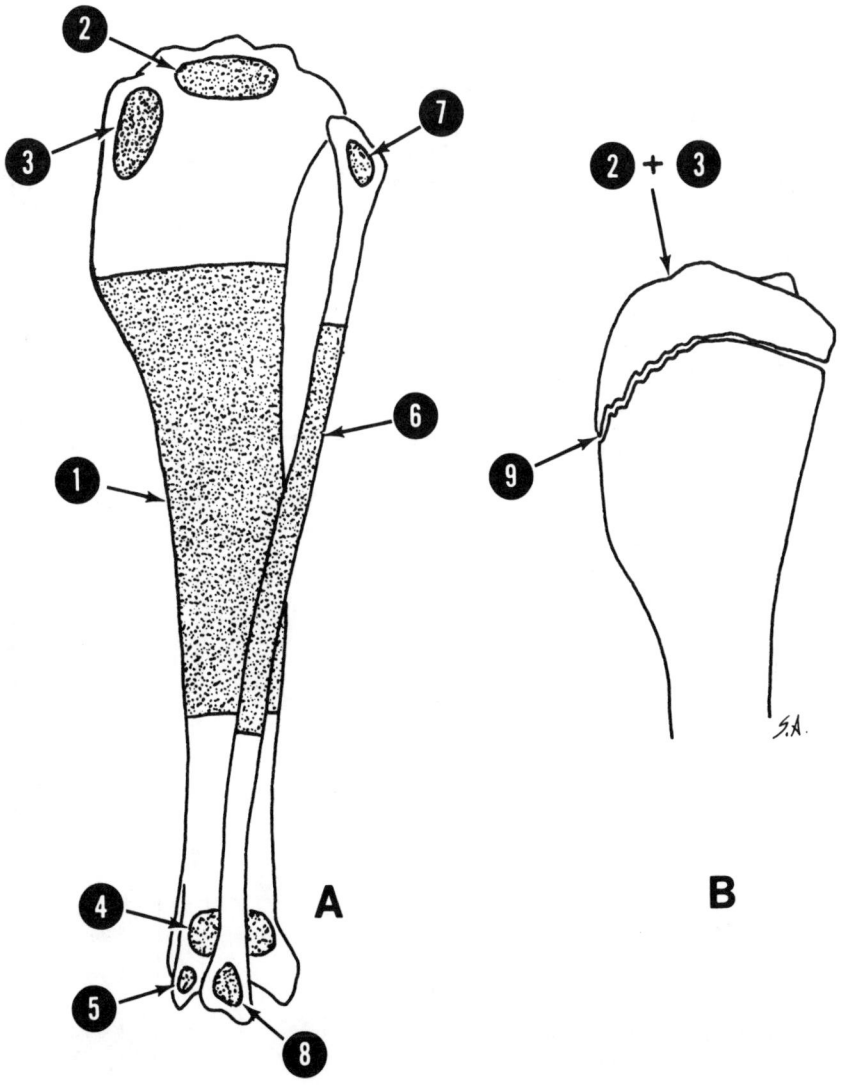

Figure 6-10

Centers of Ossification of the Tibia and Fibula of the Dog

A. Lateral aspect of both tibia and fibula
B. Lateral aspect of proximal tibia in a 10-month-old dog, showing the usual appearance near the tibial tuberosity. (The center for the condyles has already united to the center for the tibial tuberosity at this age.)

1. Primary center for the tibia
2. Secondary center for tibial condyles
3. Secondary center for tibial tuberosity
4. Secondary center for distal tibial epiphysis
5. Secondary center for medial malleolus
6. Primary center for fibula
7. Secondary center for head of fibula
8. Secondary center for lateral malleolus
9. Physis separating the fused centers for the condyles and the tibial tuberosity from the primary center of the tibia

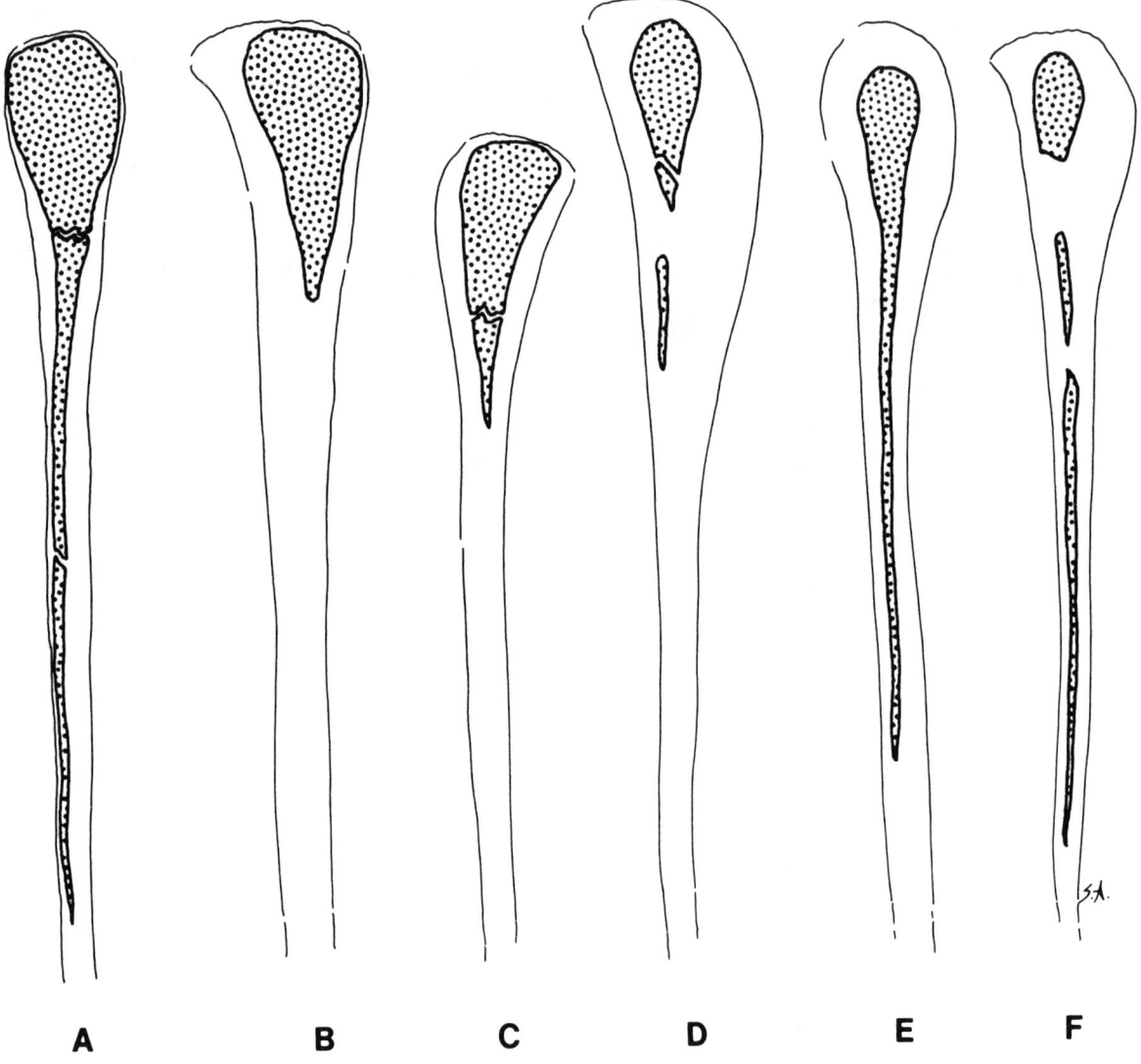

Figure 6-11

Variations in Ossification of the Proximal Equine Fibula
(drawings of radiographic images)

Age of the Animal

A - 9 years
B - 13
C - 10
D - 10
E - 9
F - 10

"Defects" in the fusion of the ossification centers occur in a large percentage of horses and may be bilaterally symmetrical. No clinical signs are actually attributable to these variations in ossification [17].

After Getty, 1975 [13]

	Commonly used abbreviations*	Official synonyms
central tarsal bone	Tc	os naviculare
first tarsal bone	T1	os cuneiforme mediale
second tarsal bone	T2	os cuneiforme intermedium
third tarsal bone	T3	os cuneiforme laterale
fourth tarsal bone	T4	os cuboideum

B. Selected comparative, clinical, and developmental features

The species specific differences in the tarsal bone patterns result from some fusions of the various bones to one another. A useful concept in remembering these specifics is to consider the generalized tarsus as consisting of seven individual bones. These seven bones can be schematically represented from the dorsal aspect of a left tarsus as shown in Fig. 6-12A. The talus and the calcaneus form the proximal row. In the distal row, the medial aspect is formed by the central tarsal bone overlying the first three tarsal bones. The lateral aspect of the distal row is formed by the fourth tarsal bone. Therefore, in the generalized tarsus, the intersection of a vertical line between the talus and calcaneus and a horizontal line just distal to the talus and calcaneus divides the tarsal skeleton into four main units (Fig. 6-12):

proximal medial unit = talus
proximal lateral unit = calcaneus
distal medial unit = central, first, second, and third tarsal bones
distal lateral unit = fourth tarsal bone

A semi-schematic comparison of the tarsal bone patterns is presented in Fig. 6-13 which more accurately represents the actual shapes of the bones than the schematic arrangements shown in Figure 6-12.

1. For orientation on the tarsus of any domestic mammal, the following general relationships may be helpful:

    a. The calcaneus serves as the point of attachment for the common calcanean tendon, and the tarsal bone just distal to it is T4.

    b. The talus articulates with the tibia and fibula, and the tarsal bone immediately distal to it is the central tarsal bone (Tc).

    c. The first, second, and third tarsal bones are distal to Tc.

    d. The fourth tarsal bone is physically as "tall" as the central and the numbered tarsal bones combined

2. The carnivores and the pig have the generalized tarsal pattern of seven separate bones (Fig. 6-12/A) [18].

---

*When using abbreviations, the context in which they are used is important. T1, for example, could also refer to the first thoracic vertebra.

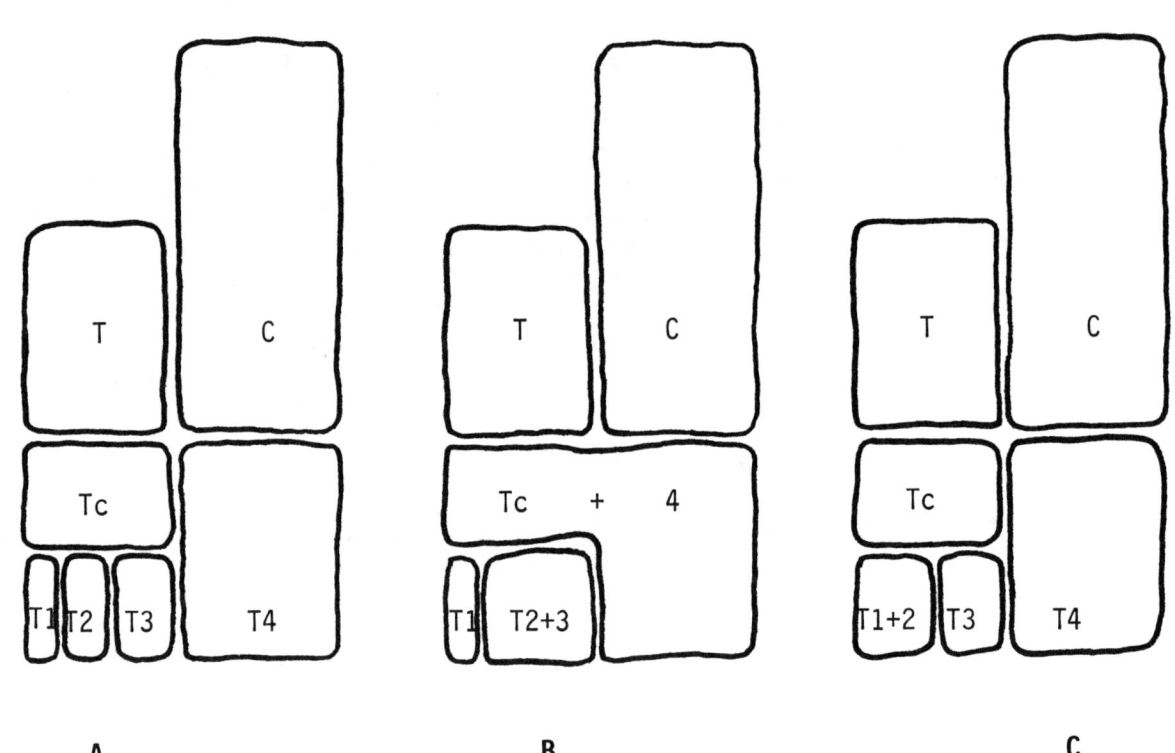

Figure 6-12

Schematic Comparison of the Tarsal Bones in the Domestic Mammals
(left tarsus, dorsal aspect)

T = talus
C = calcaneus
Tc = central tarsal bone
T1, T2, T3, T4 = first, second, third, & fourth tarsal bones

3. In the ruminants, two tarsal fusions occur. The central and fourth tarsal bones fuse and the second and third tarsal bones fuse. This results in only five separate bones. The fused entities are termed second and third tarsal bone (T2+3) and centroquartal bone (Tc+4) (Fig. 6-12/B) [19].

4. In the horse, the first and second tarsal bones are typically fused so that only 6 separate bones are present. The fused entity may be termed first and second tarsal bone (T1+2) (Fig. 6-12/C) [20].

5. It is of value radiographically to note that in the horse the distal dorsal aspect of the lateral ridge of the trochlea of the talus ends in a large, distinct notch, whereas the notch on the medial ridge is less obvious. This feature will often allow differentiation of the ridges in ML or LM perspectives.

6. The ruminants and pig have a trochlea on the head of the talus (distal trochlea) as well as on the body (proximal trochlea) [19].

7. Each tarsal bone develops from a single center of ossification except for the calcaneus which has a separate center for the tuber calcanei. (See Chapter 8 for radiographic evaluation of the tarsus.)

8. Bursitis of the hock (capped hock) is an inflammation over the tuber calcanei resulting in the formation of a subcutaneous bursa (the bursa under the tendon of the superficial digital flexor may also be involved). It occurs in horses and cattle [17,19].

VII. METATARSAL BONES

A. Major features

metatarsal bones 1-5 (the number present varies with the species)

base--the proximal epiphysis
body--the diaphysis
head--the distal epiphysis

B. Selected comparative, clinical, and developmental features

1. Five bones are present in the generalized metatarsus and they are numbered 1-5 from medial to lateral. Species differences in the metatarsal bones result from reduction in the number present and from osseous fusion. The patterns in the horse and pig are identical to those in the thoracic limbs of these species. In the carnivores, the only difference between the patterns in the thoracic and pelvic limbs is that the first metatarsal bone is even more markedly reduced than the first metacarpal bone. In ruminants, the difference is an absence of a fifth metatarsal bone.

a. The carnivores have the generalized pattern of five separate metatarsal bones (Fig. 6-13/B). The first metatarsal is markedly reduced, usually bears no digit, and is often fused to the first tarsal bone. Digits 2-5 bear weight. In the cat, the metatarsal bones are much longer than their metacarpal counterparts [18].

- b. In the ruminants, the first, second, and fifth metatarsal bones are not present, and the third and fourth bones are fused throughout their length. This fused bone is often loosely referred to as the "large metatarsal bone" or "cannon bone." It supports the third and fourth digits and has the following specific features which are homologous to those in the thoracic limb:

    (1) dorsal and plantar longitudinal grooves
    (2) proximal and distal metatarsal canals
        The proximal metatarsal canal is very small and may be absent. Even when present, it may penetrate only from the dorsal surface to the medullary cavity rather than on through the bone.
    (3) intertrochlear notch

    The separate small piece of bone on the proximal, plantaromedial aspect of Mt 3+4 (which many authors have called "metatarsal 2" or "small metatarsal bone") is the metatarsal sesamoid bone. It is associated with the interosseous muscle [19,21]. In contrast to the thoracic limb which has a fifth metacarpal bone, there is no fifth metatarsal bone (Fig. 6-13/D).

- c. The pig has no first metatarsal bone (Fig. 6-13/C). The abaxial metatarsal bones (2 and 5) are notably smaller than the axial metatarsal bones (3 and 4). All four of the metatarsal bones support digits, but only the axial digits normally bear weight. A metatarsal sesamoid bone, similar to that described in ruminants, is present. It articulates with the plantar aspect of Mt3.

- d. The horse is missing the first and fifth metatarsal bones. The second and fourth metatarsal bones are markedly reduced and are commonly known as "splint" bones, as are their thoracic limb counterparts. (This name should not be confused with the pathological condition of the interosseous ligament uniting the metatarsal bones which clinicians call "splints.") Only the large third metatarsal bone bears a digit. This bone, as well as its thoracic limb counterpart, is commonly called the "cannon bone."

2. Developmentally, metatarsal bones resemble their thoracic limb counterparts (see metacarpal bones).

3. As in the thoracic limb, the axis of the limb courses distally between the third and fourth metatarsal bones and digits, except in the horse, where it passes through the longitudinal midline of the third metatarsal bone and digit.

VIII. BONES OF THE DIGITS

The phalanges of the pelvic limb have the same features as those of the thoracic limb. The distal phalanx in the pelvic limb of the horse is longer

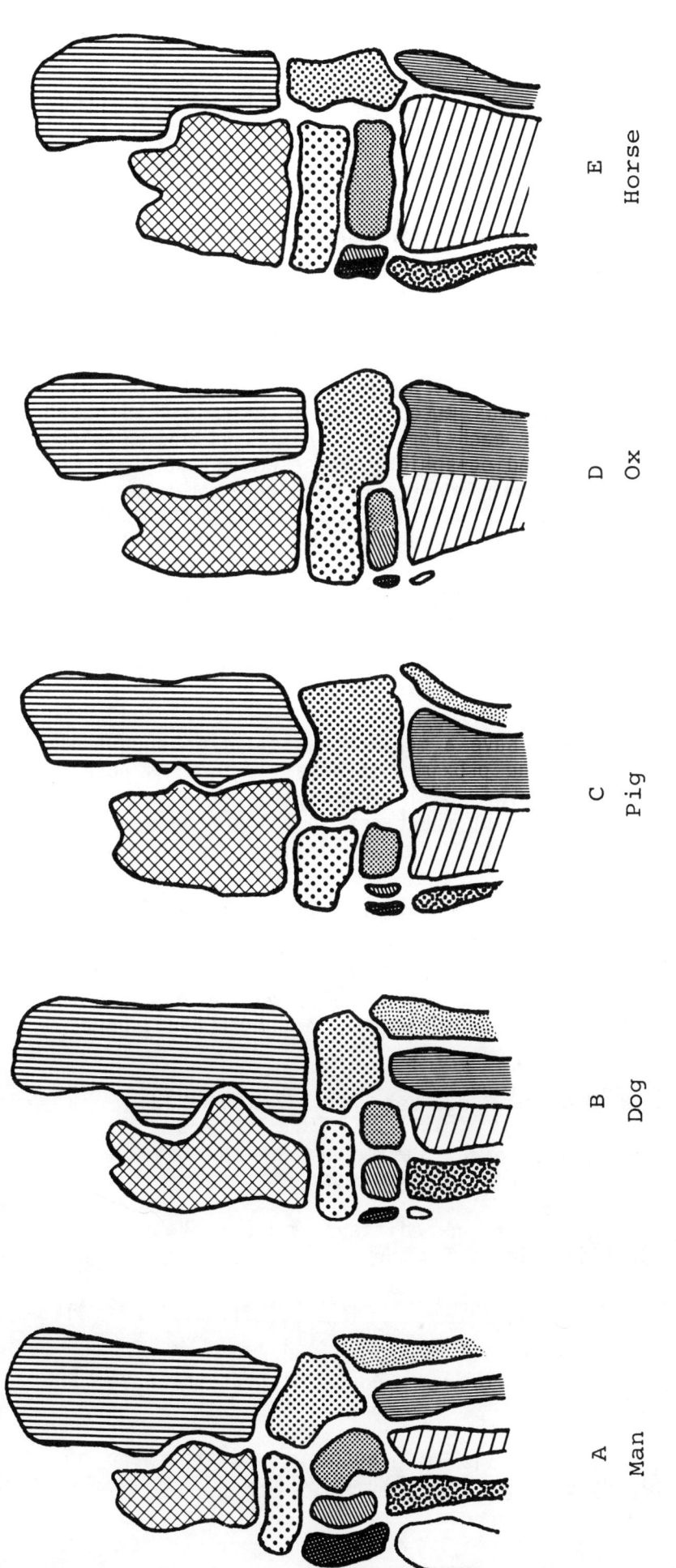

Figure 6-13

Semischematic Comparison of the Dorsal Aspects of Tarsal and Metatarsal Bones in Man, Dog, Pig, Ox, and Horse (shading indicates homology). After Nickel, Schummer, and Sieferle, 1968 [24]

and less rounded than its thoracic limb counterpart. The first digit in carnivores is usually absent.

IX. SESAMOID BONES

With the following exceptions, the sesamoid bones of the pelvic limb resemble those of the thoracic limb.

1. The patella is the largest sesamoid bone in the body. It is inserted in the tendon of the quadriceps femoris muscle.

2. In the carnivores, there is usually a sesamoid bone associated with each head of the gastrocnemius muscle. These articulate with the dorsal (proximal) aspect of each femoral condyle. It is occasionally useful to note that radiographically the sesamoid bone in the lateral head of the gastrocnemius typically sits up straighter and is "taller" than the one in the medial head. Lameness associated with fracture of one of these sesamoid bones has been reported in the dog. Carnivores also have a sesamoid bone embedded in the tendon of origin of the popliteus muscle on the caudolateral aspect of the crus just distal to the genual joint [18]. In small dogs, this latter sesamoid bone is often absent. These bones have all been termed "fabellae" in the literature and have occasional clinical significance [22,23].

3. The ruminants and the pig have a metatarsal sesamoid bone on the plantaromedial aspect of the proximal metatarsal region. As noted previously, it is embedded in the interosseous muscle and has previously been called the "small metatarsal bone" or the "second metatarsal bone" [19,21].

References

1. International Committee on Veterinary Gross Anatomical Nomenclature. 1983. Nomina Anatomica Veterinaria, third ed. Published by the Committee, Ithaca, New York.

2. Smith, R. N. 1964. The pelvis of the young dog. Vet. Rec. 76:975-979.

3. Shively, M. J. 1975. Selected Morphological Parameters of the Developing Canine Coxofemoral Joint. Ph.D. thesis, Purdue University.

4. Archibald, J. 1974. Canine Surgery, second edition. American Veterinary Publications, Santa Barbara, California.

5. Bojrab, M. J. editor 1975. Current Techniques in Small Animal Surgery. Lea and Febiger, Philadelphia.

6. Seemann, C. 1983. Ischiopubic symphysiotomy in bovine obstetrics. VM/SAC 78(2):231-236.

7. Henry, W., and P. Wadsworth. 1975. Pelvic osteotomy in the treatment of subluxation associated with hip dysplasia. JAAHA 11(5):636-643.

8. Slocum, B. 1983. "Pelvic Osteotomy: A Review of 62 Cases," paper presented at the Veterinary Orthopedic Society Convention, Waikaloa, Hawaii.

9. Habel, R. E. 1981. *Applied Veterinary Anatomy,* second ed. Published by the author, Ithaca, New York.

10. Hare, W. C. D. 1960. Radiographic anatomy of the canine pelvic limb, Part II Developing limb. JAVMA 136(11):603-611.

11. Smith, R. N. 1963. The normal and radiographic anatomy of the hip joint of the dog. J. Small Anim. Pract. 4:1-9.

12. Whittington, K., W. C. Banks, W. D. Carlson, B. F. Hoerlein, P. W. Husted, E. F. Leonard, P. L. McClave, W. H. Rhodes, and G. B. Schnelle. 1961. Report of panel on canine hip dysplasia. JAVMA 139:791-806.

13. Getty, R. 1975. *Sisson and Grossman's The Anatomy of The Domestic Animals,* fifth ed. W. B. Saunders, Philadelphia.

14. Piermattei, D. L., and R. G. Greeley. 1979. *An Atlas of Surgical Approaches to the Bones of the Dog and Cat,* second ed. W. B. Saunders, Philadelphia.

15. Ettinger, S. J. 1983. *Textbook of Veterinary Internal Medicine,* second edition. W. B. Saunders, Philadelphia.

16. Kealy, J. K. 1979. *Diagnostic Radiology of the Dog and Cat.* W. B. Saunders, Philadelphia.

17. Adams, O. R. 1974. *Lameness in Horses,* third ed. Lea and Febiger, Philadelphia.

18. Shively, M. J. 1978. Normal radiographic anatomy of the feline pelvis and rear limb. Swest Vet. 30(3):291-297, and Fel. Prac. 8(1):48-53.

19. Smallwood, J. E., and M. J. Shively. 1981. Radiographic and xeroradiographic anatomy of the bovine tarsus. Bovine Prac. 2(5):28-45.

20. Shively, M. J., and J. E. Smallwood. 1980. Radiographic and xeroradiographic anatomy of the equine tarsus. J. Equine Prac. 2(4):19-35.

21. Smith, R. N. 1956. The proximal sesamoid of the domestic ruminants. Is it the vestige of the second metatarsal? Anat. Anz. Bd. 103:241-245.

22. McCurnin, D. M. 1977. Separation of the canine fabella. VM/SAC 1438-1440.

23. Rendano, V., and T. Dueland. 1978. Variation in location of the gastrocnemius sesamoid bones (fabellae) in a dog. JAVMA 173(2):200-202.

24. Nickel, R., A. Schummer and E. Seiferle. 1968. *Lehrbuch der Anatomie der Haustiere* I. Paul Parey, Berlin.

PELVIC LIMB MYOLOGY

A general knowledge of the musculature of the pelvic limb has many applications in surgery and medicine. Some of these include orthopedic approaches, diagnosis of neuropathies, specific myopathies, and a fundamental understanding of conformation and locomotion.

The muscles of the pelvic limb can be divided into eight groups based on their general position.

      I.   Lateral muscles of the hip
     II.   Caudal muscles of the hip
    III.   Caudal muscles of the thigh
    IV.   Medial muscles of the thigh
     V.   Cranial muscles of the thigh
    VI.   Craniolateral muscles of the crus
   VII.   Caudal muscles of the crus
  VIII. Muscles of the pes

The sublumbar muscles (iliopsoas and psoas minor) could be included as a ninth group. A division of the muscles into extrinsic and intrinsic categories is not a very useful concept in the pelvic limb because the pelvic limb skeleton is directly attached to the axial skeleton through the sacroiliac joint. In the following discussion, brief references are made to the innervation of the muscles. Further details of the nerve supply are found in Chapter 9.

I.   LATERAL MUSCLES OF THE HIP (Fig. 7-1)

    The tensor fasciae latae,* the three gluteals, and the piriformis (present in carnivores only) make up this group. They act on the coxal joint causing flexion, extension, and/or abduction, and some of them have actions on the genual joint. They are innervated by the cranial and caudal gluteal nerves.

   A.   Tensor fasciae latae

       Origin: Tuber coxae.
       Termination: Fascia lata.
       Action: Tense the fascia lata (flex the coxal joint and extend the
              genual joint).

    In the carnivores, the tensor fasciae latae (t.f.l.) appears to be divided into a triangular, flat part which is positioned cranial to the greater trochanter and a fusiform part which extends down the thigh just cranial to the quadriceps femoris m. In the ungulates the t.f.l. does not appear to be divided.

---

*The names of muscles are frequently used herein without adding the term muscle.

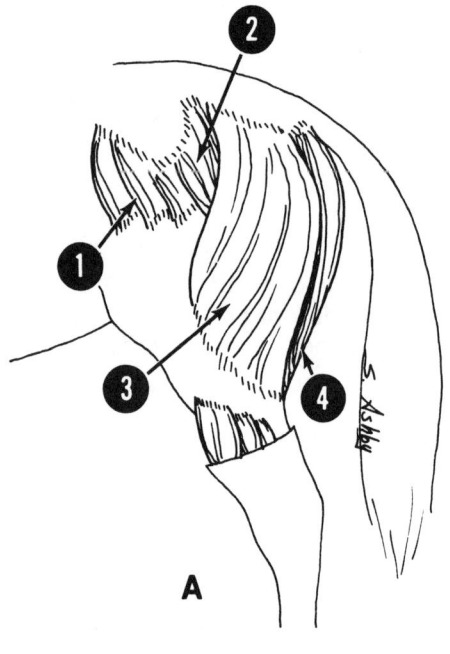
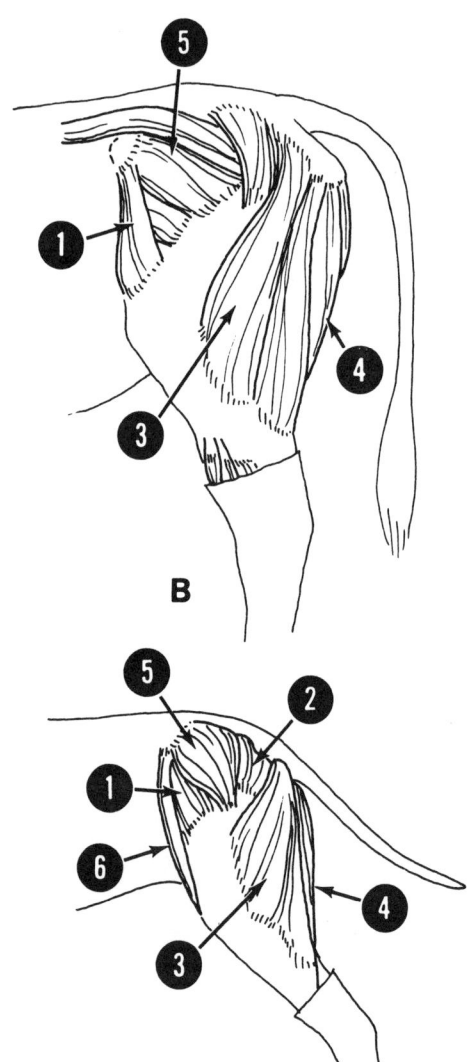

Figure 7-1

Muscles of the Rump and Thigh in the Horse (A), Ox (B), and Dog (C)

1. tensor fasciae latae m.

2. superficial gluteal m.

3. biceps femoris m. (gluteobiceps m. in ox)

4. semitendinosus m.

5. middle gluteal m.

6. cranial part of sartorius m.

The aponeurosis of the tensor fasciae latae is termed the fascia lata and is incised in the lateral approach to the femur bone. In addition to the skin and superficial fascia, it is the only structure which must be transected to expose the femoral shaft. After it has been incised, the biceps femoris is retracted caudally and the vastus lateralis is reflected cranially to reach the bone [1].

B. Superficial gluteal

Origin: Various structures dorsal to the coxal joint.
Termination: Third trochanter of the femur.
Action: Abduct the limb (may have a minor extensor action on the coxal joint, too).

The diminutive superficial gluteal muscle of carnivores overlies the caudal part of the middle gluteal m. It is located dorsocaudal to the greater trochanter of the femur in contrast to the cranioventral position of the triangular part of the tensor fasciae latae muscle with which it may be confused. A small, variably developed, and deep caudal part of the superficial gluteal muscle in the dog was mistakenly considered for many years (and in many reference books) to be the piriformis muscle (see paragraph I.D. footnote, next page) [2].

In the ruminants, the superficial gluteal muscle is fused to the biceps femoris to form the gluteobiceps muscle. There is no third trochanter on the ruminant femur.

In the horse, the superficial gluteal lies immediately caudal to and partly under the tensor fasciae latae [3]. It is partially divided into cranial and caudal bellies with the middle gluteal protruding between them.

C. Middle gluteal

Origin: On and near the gluteal surface of the ilium.
Termination: Greater trochanter of the femur.
Action: Extend the coxal joint; abduct the limb.

The middle gluteal is the largest of the gluteal muscles. It is positioned craniodorsal to the greater trochanter. In the horse, the middle gluteal partially separates the overlying superficial gluteal into the cranial and caudal bellies. In the other species, it separates the superficial gluteal from the tensor fasciae latae.

On the deep surface of the middle gluteal m., a portion separates away from the main muscle belly. In the ungulates, this is the accessory gluteal muscle. In the carnivores, this separate part is the piriformis muscle (see paragraph I.D.).

In horses, a bursa occurs between the tendon of termination of the middle gluteal m. and part of the greater trochanter. Inflammation of this bursa is termed trochanteric bursitis (whorlbone disease) and causes a lameness characterized by "dog style" locomotion (forward movement with the long axis of the body inclined to one side or the other [4]). Pain shortens the stride on the affected side, causing the hindquarters to shift (swing) toward the sound side. Affected horses may also be sensitive to pressure over the cranial part of the greater trochanter [4].

D. Piriformis muscle (present in carnivores only)

   Origin: Sacrum and first caudal vertebra.
   Termination: Greater trochanter.
   Action: Extend the coxal joint.

The piriformis muscle of carnivores lies deep and caudomedial to the middle gluteal muscle. It separates incompletely from the middle gluteal and was considered to be part of the middle gluteal muscle by many authors until recently.* The tendon of termination of the piriformis muscle blends with that of the middle gluteal m. and the two are usually manipulated together (as one unit) in dorsal approaches to the coxal joint (see deep gluteal m.).

E. Deep gluteal

   Origin: Body of ilium and ischiatic spine.
   Termination: Greater trochanter (on and near).
   Action: Abduct the limb and extend the coxal joint.

The gluteal muscles (and the piriformis m.) are the major obstacles during a dorsal approach to the coxal joint. All of these muscles may be incised near their terminations and then reconstructed at closure. Rather than perform the tenomyotomies, some surgeons prefer to osteotomize the greater trochanter (transtrochanteric or Gorman approach), and then wire or pin it back in place. The superficial gluteal and part of the deep gluteal must be transected even with a transtrochanteric approach [1].

II. CAUDAL MUSCLES OF THE HIP

The muscles which belong to this group are the obturators, the gemelli, and the quadratus femoris. They are primarily rotators and adductors of the limb. All of them terminate in or near the trochanteric fossa of the femur. They are all innervated by the sciatic nerve except for the external obturator m. which is innervated by the obturator nerve.

A. External obturator

   Origin: Ventral aspect of os coxae around obturator foramen.

---

*The small bit of muscle deep to the caudal border of the superficial gluteal in dogs, which older texts identify as piriformis m., is now considered to be a caudal slip of the superficial gluteal m. [2].

Termination: Trochanteric fossa.
Action: Adduct and rotate the limb laterally* at the coxal joint.

B. Internal obturator (absent in pig and ruminants)

Origin: Dorsal aspect of os coxae around obturator foramen.
Termination: Trochanteric fossa.
Action: Rotate the limb laterally at the coxal joint.

A true internal obturator is found only in the horse and the carnivores. In these species, the tendon of insertion passes over the lesser ischiatic notch. In the pig and the ruminants, the tendon passes through the obturator foramen and the muscle is properly designated the intrapelvic part of the external obturator. These latter animals have no muscle which is correctly termed internal obturator [5].

C. Gemelli

Origin: Lateral aspect of ischium.
Termination: Trochanteric fossa.
Action: Rotate the limb laterally at the coxal joint.

This muscle appears to be single in some species and paired in others (hence the plural name).

D. Quadratus femoris

Origin: Ventral aspect of ischium.
Termination: Proximal femur near the trochanteric fossa.
Action: Extend coxal joint; adduct and/or rotate the limb laterally at the coxal joint.

III. CAUDAL MUSCLES OF THE THIGH (Figs. 7-1, 7-2)

The caudal thigh muscles include from lateral to medial: the biceps femoris, the semitendinosus, and the semimembranosus. Functionally, they extend the coxal joint and have actions on the genual and tarsal joints as well. They are collectively and loosely known as the "hamstrings," originate on or near the ischiatic tuberosity, and are innervated by branches of the sciatic nerve.

A. Biceps femoris

Origin: On and near the ischiatic tuberosity.
Termination: Patella, tibia, and tuber calcanei.
Action: Extend the coxal, genual, and tarsal joints; flex the genual joint and abduct the leg.

In the dog, the biceps femoris originates partially from the sacrotuberous ligament (this structure is absent in cats). In the ruminants, the superficial gluteal muscle developmentally fuses to the biceps femoris and the combined muscle is called gluteobiceps. In the horse, the origin of the biceps femoris extends nearly to the dorsal midline.

---

*Lateral ("outward") rotation means the cranial aspect rotates laterally (supination). Similarly, medial ("inward") rotation implies a medial rotation of the cranial aspect (pronation).

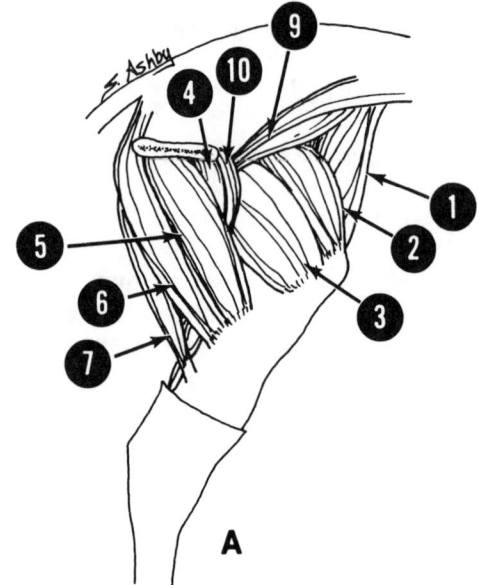

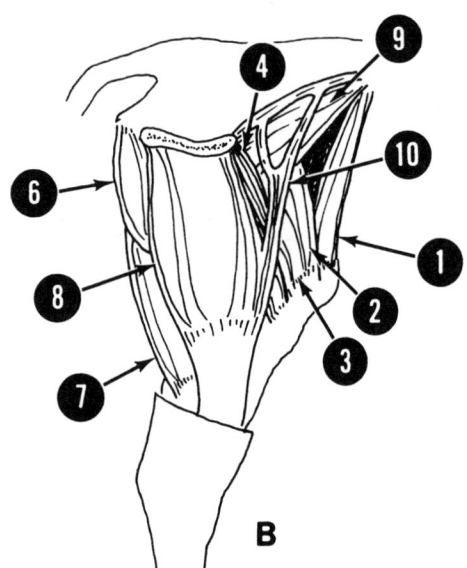

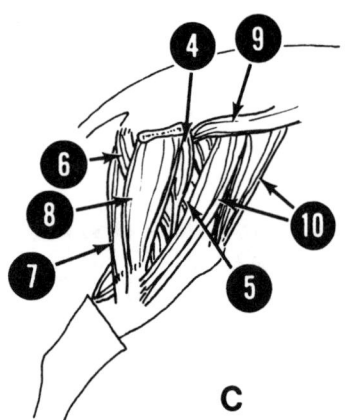

Figure 7-2

Muscles of the Medial Aspect of the Thigh in the Horse (A), Ox (B), and Dog (C)

1. tensor fasciae latae m.
2. rectus femoris m.
3. vastus medialis m.
4. pectineus m.
5. adductor m.
6. semimembranosus m.
7. semitendinosus m.
8. gracilis m. (removed in horse)
9. iliopsoas m.
10. sartorius m.

The belly of the biceps femoris (or gluteobiceps) appears to be divided into several parts (especially in large animals). In the common surgical approach to the femur bone, the biceps femoris m. is retracted caudally and the vastus lateralis m. is retracted cranially to expose the femoral body (shaft) [1]. In carnivores, the biceps femoris forms the caudoventral quarter of the orientation quadrangle around the greater trochanter.*

When using the caudal aspect of the pelvic limb of carnivores for intramuscular injections, one should recall that the sciatic nerve lies deep to the biceps femoris and caudolateral to the femur. Consequently, the needle should be directed either lateral to the nerve into the biceps femoris or medial to the nerve into the semitendinosus or semimembranosus mm. The placement to avoid is insertion of the needle into the palpable depression between the biceps femoris and semitendinosus and then directing it craniomedially. A nerve skewered by a needle rarely suffers significant damage, but if the animal lurches, the needle tip may sever all or part of the nerve. Transient or permanent nerve injury resulting from the substance injected is usually of more concern than physical damage.

B. Semitendinosus

Origin: On and near the ischiatic tuberosity.
Termination: Tibia and tuber calcanei.
Action: Extend the coxal and tarsal joints; flex the genual joint.

This muscle lies immediately medial to the biceps femoris.

C. Semimembranosus

Origin: On and near the ischiatic tuberosity.
Termination: Femur and tibia.
Action: Extend coxal joint and variable action on the genual joint.

The semimembranosus is divisible into two parts, but these may be difficult to separate--especially in the ruminants. A memory aid for the relative positions of the semitendinosus and semimembranosus is the t in -tendinosus indicates lateral and the m in -membranosus indicates medial.

In the carnivores, a small slip of muscle, the abductor cruris caudalis lies under the caudal border of the biceps femoris. It has no clinical significance.

In the horse, the caudal thigh muscles originate not only from the ischiatic tuberosity but various ones also extend up to the caudal vertebrae, broad sacrotuberous ligament, and sacroiliac ligaments. This gives the rump of the horse a full, rounded appearance (vs. the ruminants). Fibrotic

---

*Using the greater trochanter as a landmark, the superficial gluteal m. is located dorsocaudally, the middle gluteal dorsocranially, the tensor fasciae latae ventrocranially, and the biceps femoris ventrocaudally.

myopathy is a disease syndrome which affects the caudal thigh muscles in horses. It is thought to be associated with old injuries in which fibrous connective tissue replaces the skeletal muscle. Adhesions form, the gait is altered, and sometimes the lesions ossify. Myectomy of part of the involved muscle(s) improves some cases [4].

The relationship between points of attachment and the actions of muscles is very well illustrated by the caudal thigh muscles. The biceps femoris spans the three major pelvic limb joints and is broad enough to attach to structures on both the flexor and extensor surfaces of the genual joint. Therefore, not only can it act on all three joints, but it can both flex and extend the genual joint. The semitendinosus spans all three joints, but is limited to the caudal side of the genual region. Consequently, it can flex the genual joint but cannot extend it. The semimembranosus is even more limited in its attachments since it sends no tendon to the tuber calcanei. Its fewer actions reflect this more limited attachment.

IV. MEDIAL MUSCLES OF THE THIGH (Fig. 7-2)

The four muscles in this group are primarily adductors of the limb. Many of them also have some extensor or flexor action on the coxal and/or genual joints. They are innervated by the obturator nerve except for the sartorius m. which is innervated by the saphenous nerve.

A. Sartorius

> Origin: On or near the ilium.
> Termination: Medial aspect of the genual region.
> Action: Flex the coxal and genual joints (also extends the genual
> joint in carnivores).

In the horse and cat, the sartorius muscle is undivided. In the ruminants and pig, the origin of the sartorius is divided into two parts by the passage of the femoral vessels. The dog has two distinct muscle bellies (cranial and caudal) throughout the length of the muscle. In dogs and cats, the muscle may extend the genual joint as well as flex it because of the position of attachment of the cranial part of the muscle.

B. Gracilis

> Origin: Pelvic symphysis.
> Termination: Medial aspect of genual region.
> Action: Adduct the limb (may act on the coxal and genual joints in
> most species).

In the carnivores, a fascial slip from the gracilis also extends to the tuber calcanei as part of the common calcanean tendon. Consequently, in these animals the muscle also has extensor action on the tarsal joint.

C. Pectineus

> Origin: Prepubic tendon and cranial border of pubis (iliopubic
> eminence).

Termination: Body of femur.
Action: Adduct the limb (and flex the coxal joint or rotate the leg outward in some species).

The pectineus muscle has been an important structure recently in the surgical alleviation of the pain associated with canine hip dysplasia. Severance and/or removal of part of the muscle belly or tendon markedly improves the gait in some cases [6,7]. The muscle is also severed in the ventral approach to the coxal joint in carnivores [1].

The femoral triangle is located in the proximal, medial aspect of the thigh. It is bounded cranially by the sartorius muscle, caudally by the pectineus muscle and dorsally (proximally) by the body wall. In carnivores, it truly is triangular and is a convenient place to take the pulse since the femoral vessels are located within it. In large animals, it is more slitlike than triangular because the sartorius and pectineus are less divergent. Large animals have safer and more convenient places to monitor the pulse. In the horse, deep inguinal lymph nodes are found in the femoral triangle.

D. Adductor

Origin: Ventral surface of os coxae.
Termination: Caudal surface of femur bone.
Action: Adduct the limb and extend the coxal joint.

The adductor muscle is undivided in the pig and ox, but it can be divided into a smaller cranial part and a larger caudal portion in the horse and carnivores. These are named as follows:

	cranial part	caudal part
carnivores	adductor longus	adductor magnus et brevis
horse	adductor brevis	adductor magnus

V. CRANIAL MUSCLES OF THE THIGH

These muscles are represented primarily by the quadriceps group which flexes the coxal joint and extends the genual joint. The iliopsoas also flexes the coxal joint but does not act on the genual joint. These muscles are innervated by the femoral nerve.

A. Quadriceps femoris (four heads: rectus femoris, vastus lateralis, vastus intermedius, and vastus medialis)

Origin: Rectus femoris, ilium; other 3 heads, proximal femur bone.
Termination: Patella (and then to tibial tuberosity).
Action: Extend the genual joint (all heads); flex the coxal joint (rectus femoris).

In the common approach to the femur, the quadriceps femoris (vastus lateralis head) is reflected cranially after the fascia lata has been incised [1]. Note that the patella is considered to be a sesamoid in the tendon of insertion of the quadriceps femoris. The portion of the tendon which extends from the patella to the tibial tuberosity is the patellar ligament. It should not be called the "patellar tendon". In the horse and ox (but not in the small ruminants), the patellar ligament is divided into three parts: lateral patellar ligament, medial patellar ligament, and intermediate ("middle") patellar ligament. The intermediate patellar ligament of the horse and ox corresponds to the patellar ligament of other species. Protrusion of the enlarged medial ridge of the femoral trochlea (trochlear tubercle) between the medial and intermediate patellar ligaments is important in the stay apparatus of the horse (patellar lock mechanism) and in the pathological condition termed upward fixation of the patella [4]. Upward fixation is surgically relieved by desmotomy of the medial patellar ligament. This condition also affects oxen and is treated the same way. Ruminants do not have the equine ability to voluntarily lock their patellae.

B. Iliopsoas (iliacus + psoas major)

Origin: Ilium (iliacus) and lumbar vertebrae (psoas major).
Termination: Lesser trochanter.
Action: Flex the coxal joint and perhaps the joints of the vertebral column; rotate the leg outward at the hip.

VI. CRANIOLATERAL MUSCLES OF THE CRUS (Fig. 7-3)

The craniolateral muscles of the crus are primarily flexors of the tarsal joint and extensors of the digital joints. Those that originate on the femur bone can also act on the genual joint. They are innervated by the common peroneal nerve and by its superficial and deep branches.

A. Cranial tibial muscle

Origin: Lateral aspect of proximal tibia.
Termination: Proximal metatarsus.
Action: Flex the tarsal joint.

In the horse and ruminants, the tendon of termination of the cranial tibial muscle passes between branches of the peroneus tertius tendon. In the horse, the tendon of the cranial tibial m. divides to send a medial branch to the (fused) first and second tarsal bone and a distal continuation to the metatarsus. The medial branch is popularly termed the "cunean tendon" and can be palpated in the depression about 5 cm distal to the medial malleolus. It is sometimes resected to relieve the pain associated with equine tarsal osteoarthropathies ("bone spavin") [4]. There is also a bursa associated with the medial branch of the tendon and its inflammation is described as cunean bursitis [4].

B. Long digital extensor

Origin: Extensor fossa of femur.
Termination: Extensor processes of the distal phalanges.
Action: Extend the digital joints, flex the tarsal joint, and extend the genual joint.

In multidigited animals, the tendon and/or muscle belly divides for distribution to each digit. The muscle may also attach to middle and/or

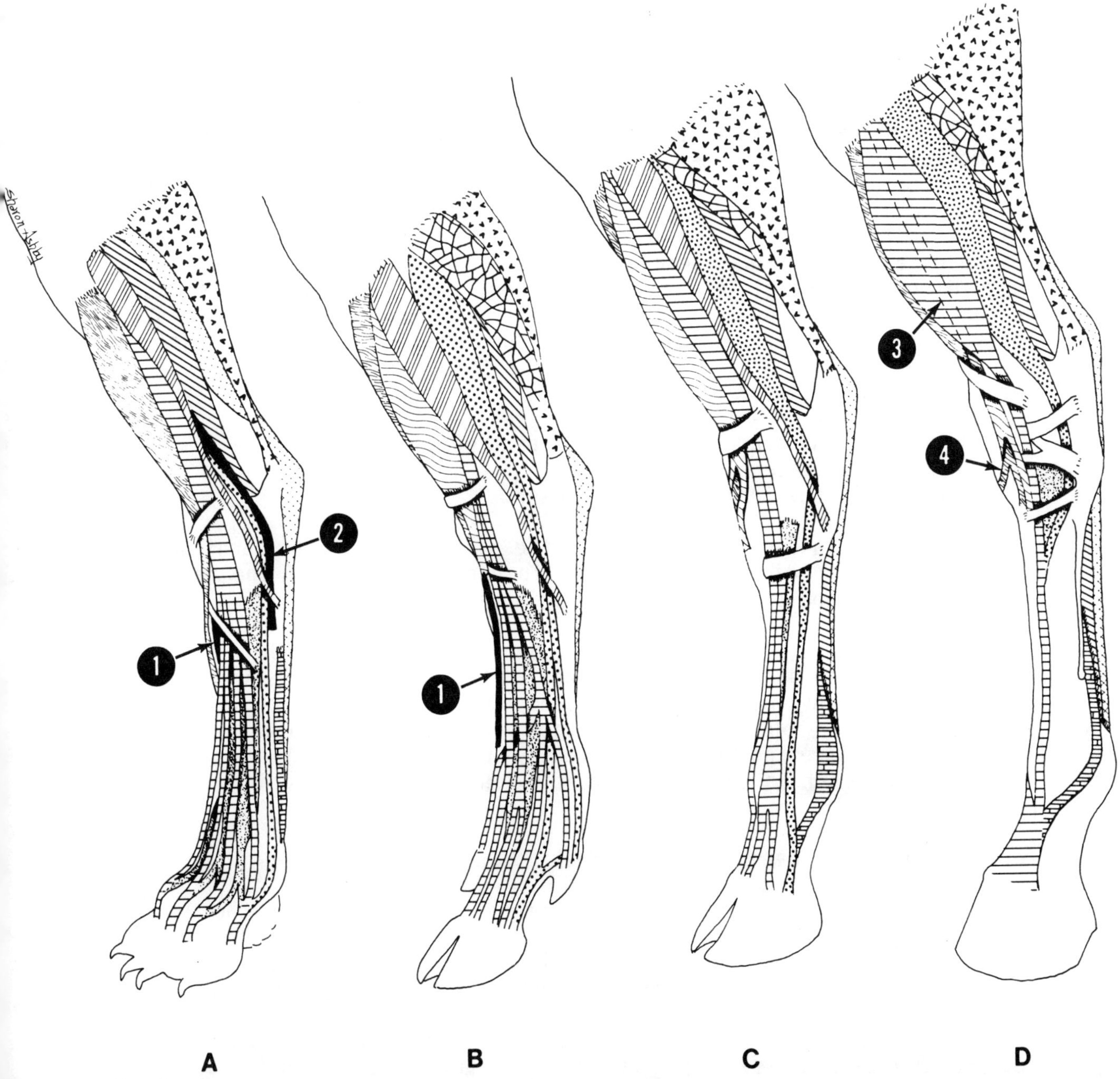

Figure 7-3
Craniolateral Crural Muscles of the Dog (A), Pig (B), Ox (C), and Horse (D)

1. Extensor hallucis longus m.
2. Peroneus brevis m.
3. Peroneus tertius m. in horse
4. Medial tendon of termination of cranial tibial m. in horse ("cunean tendon")

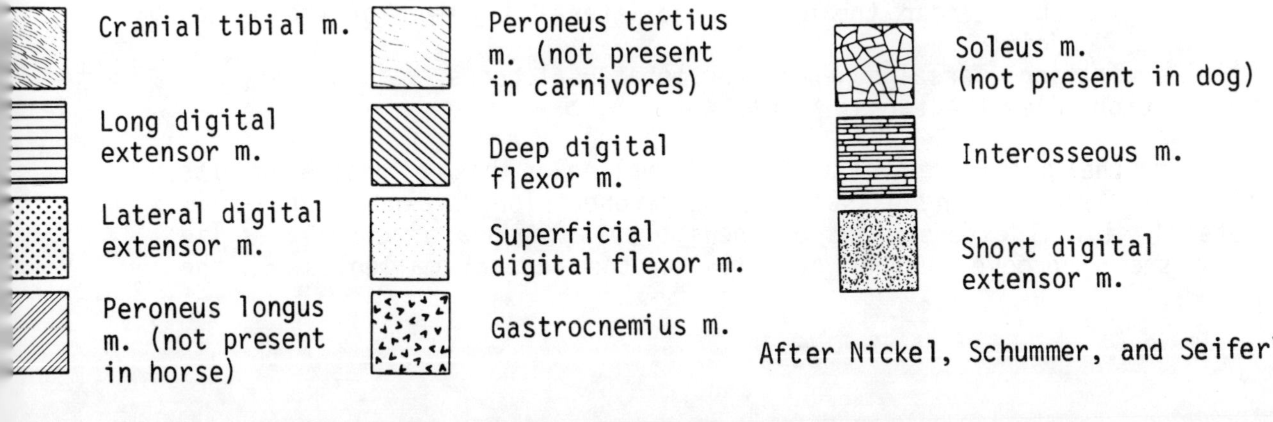

Cranial tibial m.

Long digital extensor m.

Lateral digital extensor m.

Peroneus longus m. (not present in horse)

Peroneus tertius m. (not present in carnivores)

Deep digital flexor m.

Superficial digital flexor m.

Gastrocnemius m.

Soleus m. (not present in dog)

Interosseous m.

Short digital extensor m.

After Nickel, Schummer, and Seiferle, 1968

proximal phalanges in some species. In the ox, there are two bellies and the medial belly sends a tendon only to the medial weight-bearing digit (digit 3), but the tendon of the lateral belly divides for distribution to both digits. As in the thoracic limb, the medial belly has been called "medial digital extensor." Because it attaches to the femur, the long digital extensor has been repositioned as a surgical treatment for ruptured cranial cruciate ligament in dogs, but the technique is not currently popular [10]. Its attachment at the extensor fossa is, however, a useful orientation marker during surgery of the genual joint.

C. Lateral digital extensor

>Origin: On and near the proximal aspect of the fibula.
>Termination: Lateral digit(s).
>Action: Aid the long digital extensor.

The tendon is distributed only to the fifth digit in the carnivores and to the fourth digit in ruminants. In pigs, a branch of the tendon goes to digit 4 and another one is distributed to digit 5.

In the horse, the tendon can be palpated above the lateral malleolus and also distal to the tarsus. In the region of the tarsus, it is lost in the heavy retinacula. The tendon unites with the long digital extensor tendon about a third of the way down the metatarsus. The lateral digital extensor is surgically resected in some cases of "stringhalt," which is an involuntary flexion of the tarsal joint during movement [4].

D. Peroneus tertius (absent in carnivores)

>Origin: Extensor fossa of the femur (in common with the long digital extensor).
>Termination: Base of the metatarsal bone(s) and some tarsal bones.
>Action: Flex the tarsal joint and extend the genual joint.

This muscle is entirely tendinous in the horse and is part of the reciprocal apparatus (see paragraph VII.C.). It is passive in its action and causes simultaneous flexion of the tarsal joint whenever the genual joint is flexed [11]. Rupture of the peroneus tertius can be diagnosed in a horse if the tarsal joint can be extended while the genual joint is flexed. In the ruminants, the peroneus tertius muscle is fleshy, covers much of the cranial tibial muscle, and is partially fused to the long digital extensor.

E. Peroneus longus (absent in the horse)

>Origin: On or near the lateral collateral ligament of the genual joint.
>Termination: Tarsal bones and/or metatarsal bones.
>Action: Flex the tarsal joint.

In the carnivores, the lateral malleolus has a groove on its lateral aspect for the passage of the peroneus longus tendon. The small lateral digital extensor and peroneus brevis tendons of carnivores lie in a second groove further caudally on the lateral malleolus. In the horse, only one groove is present on the lateral side (for passage of the lateral digital extensor). In the ruminants, the lateral digital extensor and the peroneus longus both pass through a single groove. Heavy retinacula are present in all species to hold these tendons in place.

In the sheep, pig, and carnivores, a small extensor digit I (hallucis) longus is present [9]. The carnivores also have a peroneus brevis* which lies adjacent to part of the lateral digital extensor [2].

VII. CAUDAL MUSCLES OF THE CRUS

The five caudal crus muscles are primarily extensors of the tarsal joint and flexors of the digital joints. Those that attach to the femur also flex the genual joint. In differentiating these muscles, examine their points of attachment. The two digital flexors are the only ones which continue distally to the phalanges. As in the thoracic limb, the superficial digital flexor extends distally only as far as the middle phalanges and the deep digital flexor courses on to the distal phalanges. These muscles are innervated by the tibial nerve.

A. Gastrocnemius (medial and lateral heads)

Origin: Medial and lateral supracondylar tuberosities of the femur (or their general area).
Termination: Tuber calcanei of the calcaneus.
Action: Extend the tarsal joint; flex the genual joint.

The carnivores have a sesamoid bone embedded in the tendon of origin of each head of the gastrocnemius m. These articulate with facets on the proximal aspects of the femoral condyles. In mid-shaft femoral fracture, the caudal pull of the gastrocnemius and superficial digital flexor mm. on the distal femur is supposedly the major force which rotates the distal fragment caudally so that the position of the proximal fragment is cranial and that of the distal fragment is caudal after overriding occurs. Rupture of the gastrocnemius is fairly common in cattle.

B. Soleus (absent in dog)

Origin: Head of fibula (lateral femur in pig).
Termination: Tendon of lateral head of gastrocnemius muscle.
Action: Assist the gastrocnemius muscle in extension of the tarsal joint.

The soleus and the two heads of the gastrocnemius are collectively termed the triceps surae. The soleus is absent in the dog, but it is present in the cat.

C. Superficial digital flexor

Origin: Supracondylar fossa or lateral supracondylar tuberosity.

---

*Species specificity of the three peroneus muscles is as follows: horse--p. tertius (only); ruminants and pig--p. tertius and p. longus; carnivores--p. longus and p. brevis.

Termination: Tuber calcanei of calcaneus and middle phalanges.
Action: Flex the genual and digital joints; extend the tarsal joint.

In all species, the tendon of the superficial digital flexor twists around the medial side of the tendon of the gastrocnemius so that it (s.d.f.) can gain the superficial position necessary for it to continue distally after attachment to the sides of the tuber calcanei. In the cat, the portion between the tuber calcanei and the digits has a fleshy part and is known as the short digital flexor muscle. In multidigited species, the tendon divides, as in the thoracic limb, to send a branch to each digit. These tendons also form collars near the metatarsophalangeal joints through which the deep digital flexor tendon branches pass as they did in the thoracic limb.

In the horse, the muscle is almost entirely tendinous, and it attaches to the distal aspect of the proximal phalanx (as well as to the proximal aspect of the middle phalanx) as it did in the thoracic limb to help prevent dorsal buckling of the proximal interphalangeal joint. No accessory ligament is associated with the superficial digital flexor muscle of the equine pelvic limb.

In the horse, the proximal part of the superficial digital flexor muscle (i.e., the part between the femur and calcaneus) and the peroneus tertius muscle (both of which are largely tendinous) form the so called "reciprocal" apparatus which causes the genual and tarsal joints to move synchronously (i.e., when the genual joint extends, the tarsal joint must also extend because of the superficial digital flexor m. and similarly when the genual joint flexes, the tarsal joint must also flex because of the peroneus tertius m.). In both instances, the action at the tarsal joint is passively caused by the tendon-like character of the involved muscle. The superficial digital flexor component of the reciprocal apparatus also functions in the "stay" apparatus [11].

A bursa is present between the tendon of the superficial digital flexor m. and the tuber calcanei. In the horse, at least, a separate subcutaneous bursa may also occur. Either or both of these may be involved in "capped hock."

The common calcanean tendon refers to the aggregated tendons in the distal crus which attach to the tuber calcanei. Included are the tendons of the triceps surae (calcanean or "Achilles" tendon) plus those of the superficial digital flexor, biceps femoris, semitendinosus, and in the carnivores, the gracilis. The common calcanean tendon occasionally ruptures in the horse, and thus affected animals cannot bear weight on the limb [4].

In large animals, caudal presentations at birth may present obstetrical problems if the tarsi enter the birth canal first since traction on them in the flexed position will not allow the genual joints to extend sufficiently for delivery. If attempts to turn the fetus are not successful and a C-section is not indicated, severing the common calcanean tendon may allow the legs to be presented with the tarsal joints flexed and the genual joints extended. In this manner, the fetus may be delivered without further fetotomy or surgery to the dam [12].

Spastic paresis is a disease of cattle characterized by spastic contraction of the superficial digital flexor and gastrocnemius muscles. In some cases, other muscles are also involved. C.N.S. lesions have not been found [8].

D. Deep digital flexor

This muscle consists of three heads in the ungulates and two heads in the carnivores (see discussion below). The names for the heads of the deep digital flexor are:

1. tibialis caudalis (caudal tibial muscle) = "superficial head"
2. lateral digital flexor = "flexor hallucis [digiti I] longus" = "deep head"
3. medial digital flexor = "flexor digitorum longus" = "medial head"

Origin: Caudal aspect of the tibia and fibula.
Termination: Distal phalanges.
Action: Flex the digital joints and extend the tarsal joint.

The largest and most powerful head of the deep digital flexor (d.d.f.) is the lateral digital flexor. Its tendon passes over the sustentaculum tali of the calcaneus. The tendon of the caudal tibial muscle follows this same route in ungulates and the two join as they continue distally on the plantar aspect of the tarsus. In the carnivores, the caudal tibial muscle is vestigial, inserts into the fascia near the tarsus, and is not considered to be a part of the d.d.f. In all species, the tendon of the medial digital flexor passes through a groove on the caudal aspect of the medial malleolus and joins the other component(s) of the d.d.f. at the distal aspect of the tarsus. The tendon of the deep digital flexor is distributed like that of the thoracic limb (i.e., a branch to each major digit).

A synovial sheath is associated with the d.d.f. tendon in the region of the flexor canal of the tarsus ("tarsal sheath"). Tenosynovitis of this sheath is clinically termed "thorough-pin" and produces a swelling on the medial aspect of the tuber calcanei just dorsal to the common calcanean tendon [4].

In the horse, an accessory ("check") ligament is usually present. It consists of a fibrous continuation of the tarsal joint capsule and joins the tendon of the deep digital flexor at about mid-metatarsus [13].

E. Popliteus

Origin: Popliteal fossa.
Termination: Proximal caudal aspect of tibia.
Action: Flex the genual joint.

Although the major part of the belly of the popliteus muscle is on the caudomedial aspect of the tibia, its proximal part courses obliquely to originate on the laterally positioned popliteal fossa of the femur.

The popliteus muscle of the cat and of larger dogs has a sesamoid bone in its tendon of origin. Avulsion of the origin of the popliteus muscle has been reported in carnivores. It may be confirmed radiographically by noting distal displacement of the sesamoid bone of the popliteus muscle.

Various extensor and flexor retinacula are present near the tarsus to hold the crural muscle tendons in position. There are different numbers and arrangements of these in the various species, but the differences are not clinically significant.

VIII. MUSCLES OF THE PES

There are no important differences between the muscles of the pes and those of the manus except for the presence of a short digital extensor muscle located on the dorsal aspect of the tarsus or metatarsus. Tendons from this small muscle join the other digital extensors. The interosseous m. ("suspensory ligament" in the horse) is essentially identical to that of the thoracic limb.

There are a number of minor muscles present in some of the domestic animals which have not been included in this discussion. They include many tiny muscles associated with the digits and various others such as the articularis (capsularis) coxae, the articularis genus, and the gluteo-femoralis [5].

References

1. Piermattei, D. L., and R. G. Greeley. 1979. An Atlas of Surgical Approaches to the Bones of the Dog and Cat, second ed. W. B. Saunders, Philadelphia.

2. Evans, H. E. and G. C. Christensen. 1979. Miller's Anatomy of the Dog, second ed. W.B.Saunders, Philadelphia.

3. Getty, R. 1975. Sisson and Grossman's The Anatomy of the Domestic Animals, fifth ed. W. B. Saunders, Philadelphia.

4. Adams, O. R. 1974. Lameness in Horses, third ed. Lea and Febiger, Philadelphia.

5. International Committee on Veterinary Gross Anatomical Nomenclature. 1983. Nomina Anatomica Veterinaria, third ed. Published by the Committee, Ithaca, New York.

6. Cardinet, G. H., M. M. Guffy, and L. J. Wallace. 1974. Canine hip dysplasia; Effects of pectineal tenotomy on the coxofemoral joints of German Shepherd dogs. JAVMA 164:591-598.

7. Cardinet, G. H., M. M. Guffy, and L. J. Wallace. 1974. Canine hip dysplasia: effects of pectineal myectomy on the coxofemoral joints of Greyhound and German Shepherd dogs. JAVMA 165:529-532.

8. Amstutz, H. E., editor 1980. Bovine Medicine and Surgery, second ed. American Veterinary Publications, Inc., Santa Barbara, California.

9. Nickel, R., A. Schummer, and E. Seiferle. 1968. *Lehrbuch der Anatomic der Haustiere.* Band I. Paul Parey, Berlin.

10. Roush, J., B. Hohn, and M. DeAngelis. 1970. Evaluation of transplantation of the long digital extensor tendon for correction of anterior cruciate ligament rupture in dogs. JAVMA 156(3):309-312.

11. Shively, M. J. 1982. Functional and clinical significance of the reciprocal apparatus. *Eq. Prac.* 4(1):5-6 (Anatomist's Notebook Series).

12. Habel, R. E. 1981. *Applied Veterinary Anatomy,* second ed. Published by the author, Ithaca, New York.

13. Shively, M. J. 1983. Functional and clinical significance of the check ligaments. *Equine Prac.* 5(2):37-42.

8

PELVIC LIMB ARTHROLOGY

The major joints of the pelvic limb in domestic mammals consist of the sacroiliac joint, coxal ("coxofemoral") joint, genual ("stifle") joint, tarsal ("hock") joint, and digital joints. The pelvic limb differs from the thoracic limb in having a direct connection to the axial skeleton through the sacroiliac joint. All of the major pelvic limb joints are synovial (although the sacroiliac joint is partly fibrocartilaginous).

I. SACROILIAC JOINT

   A. General features

   The pelvis is angled 30-45° from the horizontal (varying with species and breed) at its junction with the sacrum. The sacroiliac joint is partly synovial and partly fibrocartilaginous, and is capable of very little movement. It is stabilized by three sets of ligaments, named according to their general location in relation to the joint [1]:

   1. Ventral sacroiliac ligg.
   2. Dorsal sacroiliac ligg.
   3. Interosseous sacroiliac ligg.

   The interosseous sacroiliac ligaments consist of fibrocartilage which lies between and unites some parts of the ilial and sacral wings.

   B. Comparative and clinical considerations

   1. In the ungulates, the ventral sacroiliac ligaments surround the whole joint including its dorsal aspect. In these species, the dorsal sacroiliac ligament refers to the strong sheet attaching to the tuber sacrale and the sacral spines (Figs. 8-1B/2 and 8-1C/2).

   2. The dog (but not the cat) has a sacrotuberous ligament in addition to the dorsal, ventral, and interosseous sacroiliac ligaments [2]. The sacrotuberous ligament is a band joining the sacrum and first caudal vertebra to the ischiatic tuberosity (Fig. 8-1A).

   3. The ungulates have a broad sacrotuberous ("sacrosciatic") ligament which is a sheet of connective tissue joining the sacrum and the first two caudal vertebrae to the ilium, ischiatic spine, and the ischiatic tuberosity. The openings which it leaves at the greater and lesser ischiatic notches are the greater and lesser sciatic foramina which serve as vascular and neural passageways. The caudal free border of the broad sacrotuberous ligament corresponds to the sacrotuberous ligament of the dog (Fig. 8-1B, C) [2].

   4. Unilateral luxations of the sacroiliac joint cannot occur without simultaneous pelvic fracture(s). However, unilateral fractures <u>can</u> occur without concurrent luxations.

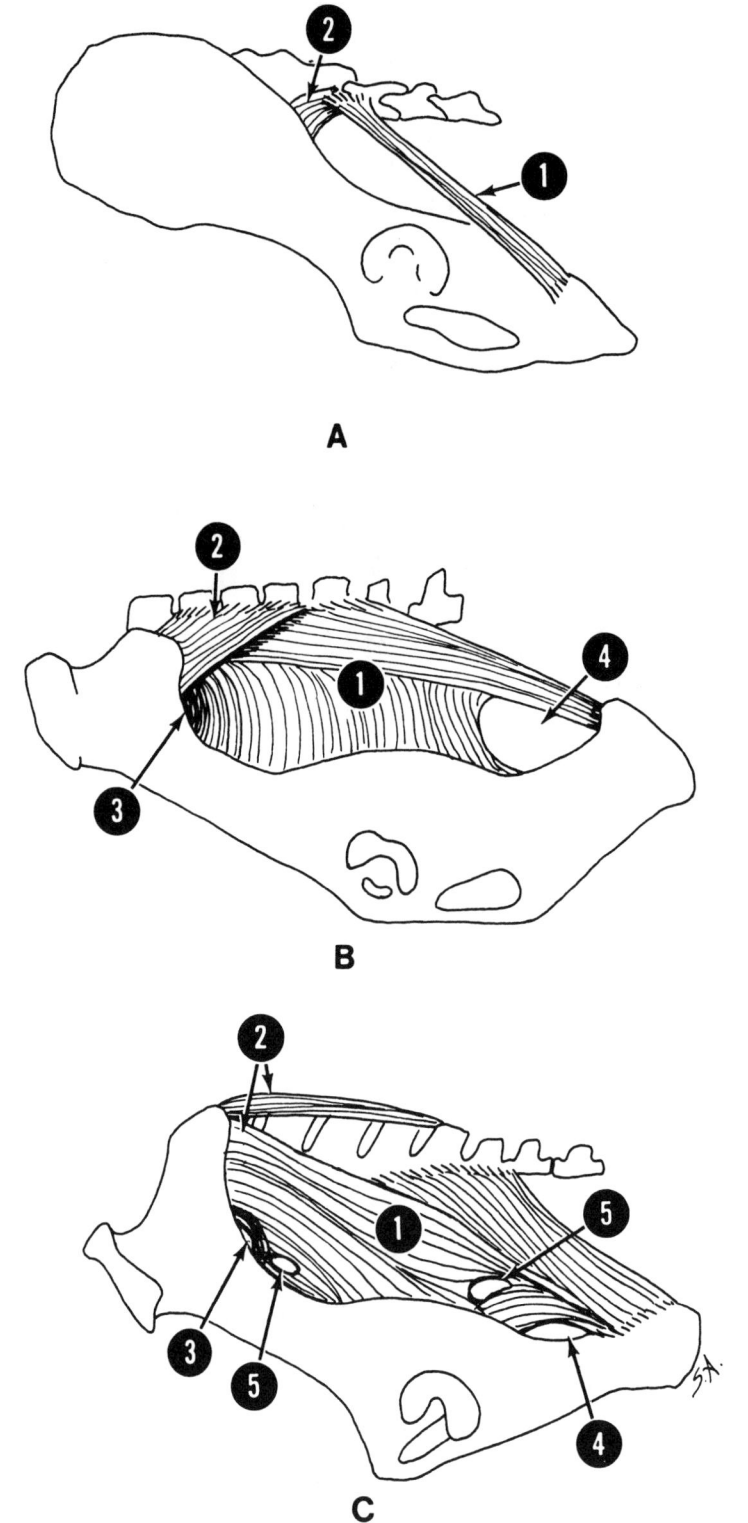

Figure 8-1

Ligaments Associated with the Sacroiliac Joint
(lateral aspect of a dog [A], ox [B], and horse [C]).

1. sacrotuberous lig. (dog); broad sacrotuberous lig. (ox, horse)
2. dorsal sacroiliac lig.
3. greater sciatic foramen
4. lesser sciatic foramen
5. foramina for vessels and nerves (horse)

II. COXAL JOINT ("COXOFEMORAL JOINT," "HIP JOINT")

A. General features

The coxal joint is a classic ball and socket articulation involving the head of the femur and the acetabulum. It has no collateral ligaments and depends on three other anatomic components for its integrity:

1. the ligament of the femoral head which originates in the acetabular fossa and terminates on the fovea capitis of the femoral head,
2. the joint capsule,
3. the pelvic muscle mass.

The defect in the ventral aspect of the acetabular lip caused by the acetabular notch is filled in by the transverse acetabular ligament. This ligament has no role in maintaining the integrity of the coxal joint in any species except possibly the horse (see below) [3].

B. Comparative and clinical considerations

1. In the horse, the ligament of the femoral head attaches not only in the acetabular fossa, but also to the os coxae just cranioventral to the acetabulum. Horses also have an accessory ligament of the femur [4]. This ligament is a strong band of connective tissue from the prepubic tendon* that perforates the origin of the pectineus m. and the transverse acetabular ligament to enter the joint. It attaches to the head of the femur in the fovea capitis, adjacent to the ligament of the femoral head (Fig. 8-2). Because the transverse acetabular ligament binds it down as it courses through the acetabular notch, it may contribute to coxal joint stability [3].

2. The ligament of the femoral head in ruminants is small and sometimes absent. This is one of several probable reasons why coxal luxations occur more frequently in cattle than in horses [3]. Others include lack of an accessory ligament, a shallower acetabulum and a flatter femoral head, and a less complete dorsal lip (border) of the acetabulum [5].

3. Coxal luxations can occur dorsally, ventrally, cranially, and caudally, but the most common direction is craniodorsally [6,7]. Intrapelvic luxation is sometimes applied to impaction fractures which drive the femoral head medially through the acetabulum [6].

---

*The prepubic tendon is the connective tissue which lies just cranial to the pubic bones and serves as the point of termination for the rectus abdominis muscles. It may be considered to be the central part of the larger cranial pubic ligament--the transversely oriented connective tissue which joins the cranial border (pecten) of one pubis to its contralateral counterpart. Both the prepubic tendon and the cranial pubic ligament should be differentiated from the symphyseal tendon ("subpelvic tendon") which is ventral to the pelvic symphysis and serves as the medial tendon of origin for the gracilis and adductor muscles [1].

Table 8-1

Synoviocentesis Techniques for the Equine Pelvic Limb

Coxal joint--insert the needle horizontally into the notch at the cranial aspect of the base of the greater trochanter. Advance the needle medially along the dorsal aspect of the femoral neck several centimeters until synovium is encountered.

Genual joint:

    Medial sac of femorotibial joint--insert the needle horizontally in the distal aspect of the depression between the medial collateral ligament and the medial patellar ligament.

    Lateral sac of femorotibial joint--insert the needle in the distal aspect of the space between the lateral patellar ligament and the lateral collateral ligament. Alternatively, the needle can be directed adjacent (either cranial or caudal) to the long digital extensor tendon as it courses through the extensor groove of the tibia.

    Femoropatellar joint--insert the needle near the center of the space between the lateral and intermediate patellar ligaments. Alternatively, the needle may be inserted between the medial and intermediate patellar ligaments.

Tarsal joint:

    Tarsocrural joint--insert the needle into the center of the area bounded by the medial malleolus (proximally), the "cunean" tendon (distally), the medial collateral ligament (plantarly), and the medial saphenous vein (dorsally). In simpler terms, this locus can be found about 3 cm proximal to the cunean tendon, just plantar to the medial saphenous vein.

    Centrodistal ("distal intertarsal") joint--insert the needle at the T-shaped junction of the central tarsal bone with the third tarsal bone and the fused first and second tarsal bones. Direct the needle plantarolaterally.

    Tarsometatarsal joint--insert the needle on the medial side about 12 mm distal to the site for injection of the centrodistal joint. These joints can also be injected plantarolaterally between the fourth tarsal bone and fourth metatarsal bones.

    Tendon sheath of the long digital extensor muscle--maximally flex the tarsal joint to cause the tendon sheath to stand out. Insert the needle into it a few centimeters proximal to the tarsus on the cranial aspect of the limb.

    Subcutaneous calcanean bursa--press or stretch the skin over the tuber calcanei to cause the bursa to bulge, and insert the needle into it.

    Tarsal sheath of the deep digital flexor muscle--insert the needle along the deep digital flexor tendon as it courses over the sustentaculum tali.

Table 8-1 (Continued)

Synoviocentesis Techniques for the Equine Pelvic Limb

Calcanean bursa of the superficial digital flexor muscle--insert the needle horizontally along the medial border of the common calcanean tendon about 5 cm proximal to the tuber calcanei. Direct the needle laterally.

Bursa of the calcanean tendon--with the limb not bearing weight, insert the needle through the superficial digital flexor tendon over the tuber calcanei.

Note: For injection techniques further distally, see Table 3-1.

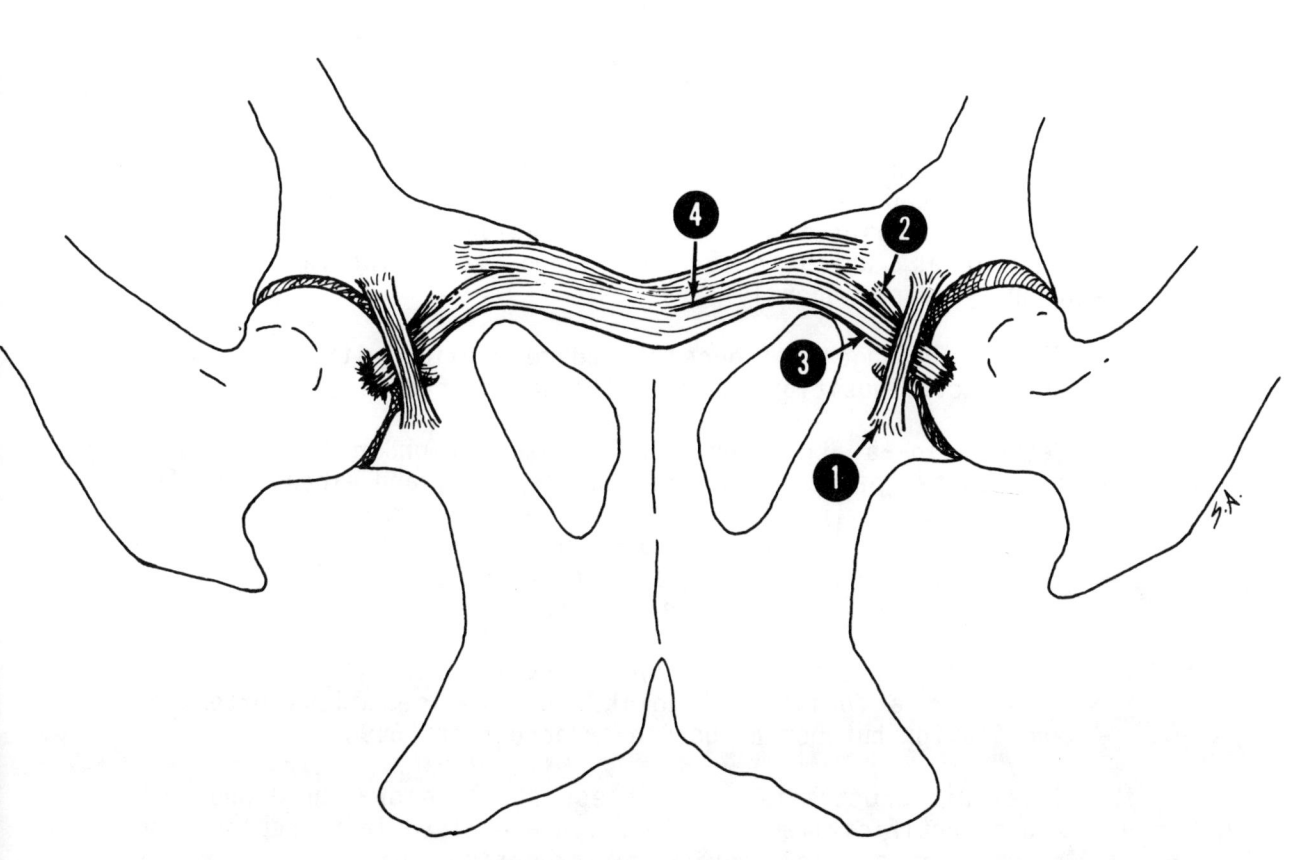

Figure 8-2

Equine Coxal Joints (ventral aspect)

1. transverse acetabular lig.
2. lig. of femoral head (in the horse its proximal attachment extends beyond the craniolateral aspect of the acetabular fossa)
3. accessory lig. of femur bone
4. prepubic tendon (central part of the cranial pubic ligament)

There are several physical ways to assess luxation of the coxal joints in small animals. One is to compare the relative positions of the greater trochanters and the ischiatic tuberosities on each side. Another is to lay the animal on its back, pull the limbs caudally, and compare leg lengths. In a craniodorsal luxation (the femoral head is cranial and dorsal to the acetabulum), the affected leg appears to be shorter. Finally, a thumb can be inserted between the greater trochanter and ischiatic tuberosity. If the thumb is forced out of this depression when the limb is rotated outward (supinated), the joint is intact [6]. These manipulations may be facilitated by general anesthesia. The weight of the animal and the craniodorsal pull of the middle and deep gluteal mm. are biomechanical factors which may cause the femoral head to luxate craniodorsally more often than in other directions.

4. In carnivores, a number of methods have been used to correct coxal luxations. First, the luxation is reduced manually or surgically, and then one of several methods is used to maintain reduction. Craniodorsal luxations are reduced manually, if possible, by applying distal tension on the limb with the femur rotated externally (i.e., with the cranial part of the femur rotated laterally or supinated). With pressure on the greater trochanter, the femoral head can usually be felt to "snap" into place and reduction is completed with medial rotation (pronation). Some of the techniques which have been used to maintain stability (temporarily or permanently) are:

   a. Flexion bandage--a figure 8 bandage applied with the limb in an abducted position and with the joints flexed [6].

   b. DeVita pin--a Steinmann pin is inserted under the ischiatic tuberosity, passed over the femoral neck, and embedded in the ilium [6,8]. It is left in place 1-3 weeks and, in this position, it prevents recurrence of dorsal luxations. One criticism of this technique is that the pin is placed blindly and one risks injury to the sciatic nerve.

   c. External pin (Kirschner) splint--a complex series of pins, bars, and a "universal" joint. This device allows extension and flexion but not adduction or abduction [6,9].

   d. Total hip prosthesis--a stainless steel femoral head and neck and an artificial acetabulum which are glued in to replace the natural ones. This device is expensive and the surgery is complex.

   e. Knowles' toggle pin--a hole is drilled through the base of the greater trochanter, up the femoral neck, out the femoral head, and extended through the wall of the acetabular fossa into the pelvic cavity. The toggle pin is inserted through the hole into the pelvic cavity and the femur is held tightly in place with heavy suture attached to the toggle pin [3,10]. A modification of this technique has been reported in which an open approach is used and the hole is drilled in the femur from the fovea capitis laterally [11]. This allows more anatomic placement of the suture "ligament." Modifications in the toggle pin have also been reported [12].

    f.   Suturing the remnants of the joint capsule is a good technique for maintaining reduction if they can be found. Extensive soft tissue damage may render the capsule unidentifiable.

As a salvage procedure, ostectomy of the femoral head and neck may be used to treat coxal luxations.

5.   The coxal joint of carnivores may be surgically approached in several ways to reduce luxations, repair fractures, remove the femoral head and neck, etc. Three of the major techniques will be briefly considered [6,13]:

    a.   Dorsal approach. The gluteal muscles (and the piriformis m.) may be transected near their terminations on the greater and third trochanters (gluteal tenomyotomy) and then sutured at closure. Some surgeons prefer to osteotomize the greater trochanter (transtrochanteric osteotomy) to free the middle and deep gluteals and the piriformis muscle, and then wire it in place at closure. The dorsal approach has the advantage of excellent total exposure, but it is more traumatic than the craniolateral or ventral approach.

    b.   Ventral approach. A T-shaped skin incision is made in the fold of the groin with the stem of the T extending distally over the pectineus muscle. The pectineus is transected and the joint is approached by reflecting the iliopsoas m. cranially and the adductor caudally. Branches of the deep femoral vessels are bothersome near the joint and may require ligation. Although the exposure is more limited than in a dorsal approach, the ventral approach has some advantages in femoral head and neck ostectomies because all structures dorsal to the hip are left intact for postoperative stability.

    c.   Craniolateral (lateral) approach. The tensor fasciae latae m. is reflected cranially by severing its caudal attachment. The coxal joint is then approached between the rectus femoris and vastus lateralis mm. This technique is the least traumatic of the three considered here, but it affords relatively poor exposure unless the origin of the vastus lateralis is partially reflected from the femoral neck and third trochanter. This approach is the one most commonly used for femoral head and neck ostectomies [14].

6.   When retrograding an intramedullary pin in the femur, there are six possible manipulations of the coxal joint which can be made as the pin emerges from the femur at the trochanteric fossa:

    extension or flexion
    adduction or abduction of the leg at the hip
    medial or lateral rotation of the leg at the hip.

The manipulations used should insure that the pin will miss (remain lateral to) the sciatic nerve (which passes dorsally over the femoral neck). Of the six possibilities, adduction is the most important, and abduction should definitely be avoided since it tends to point the emerging pin directly at the nerve. In addition, either the normal position of the leg or some medial rotation (rotation of the cranial part of the thigh medially, i.e., pronation) is helpful to keep the trochanteric fossa lateral to the nerve. Lateral rotation (supination) moves the trochanteric fossa caudally and medially and should definitely be avoided. Although many surgeons believe otherwise, neither extension nor flexion is significant in missing the nerve. It is true that flexion of the joint places the emerging pin closer to the nerve, but without concurrent abduction and/or lateral rotation, moderate flexion does not endanger the nerve. Some surgeons advocate extension since it keeps the emerging pin parallel to the nerve. However, when the joint is extended, the pin also has to penetrate a greater thickness of the gluteal muscles to emerge, and the stump that remains when the pin is ultimately cut is longer than necessary and irritates the tissues around it. Therefore, since other manipulations guarantee the safety of the sciatic nerve, a normal or slightly flexed position of the joint seems advantageous [3].

7. Canine hip dysplasia (CHD) is a clinically important developmental disease syndrome of young dogs. Its etiology is uncertain and it is characterized by joint laxity and pain. Radiographically, the features include shallow acetabula* and/or flattened femoral heads, "wedging" of the coxal joint space** caused by subluxation, and osteophyte development around the margins of the articular surfaces. For diagnostic radiographs, the pelvis must be parallel to the table (not tilted to the right or left), and the femora must be rolled "in" to center the patellae on them. CHD may be treated conservatively; by pectineal tenotomy or myotenectomy [15,16]; by femoral head and neck ostectomy; or by attempting to increase the acetabular coverage of the femoral head through pelvic osteotomies [17,18] (Fig. 6-3), or intertrochanteric varus osteotomies [19].

8. Pelvic "tilt" in a V-D radiograph of a carnivore pelvis can be assessed by examining the obturator foramina and ilial wings for symmetry [20]. If the pelvis is tilted, the "up" acetabulum will appear deeper,* and the "up" obturator foramen will appear larger in diameter than the "down" ones, respectively. However, the "down" ilial wing will appear broader than the "up" one. These differences are not caused by magnification factors related to the distance of the subject from the film. Instead, they are related to different

---

*"Depth" of the acetabulum is subjectively or quantitatively assessed on a V-D projection as the distance between the dorsal acetabular lip ("rim") and what appears to be the bottom of the acetabular fossa.

**"Wedging" of the coxal joint space occurs when the shadow of the dorsal aspect of the femoral head is not parallel to the cranial aspect of the acetabular lip on a V-D projection.

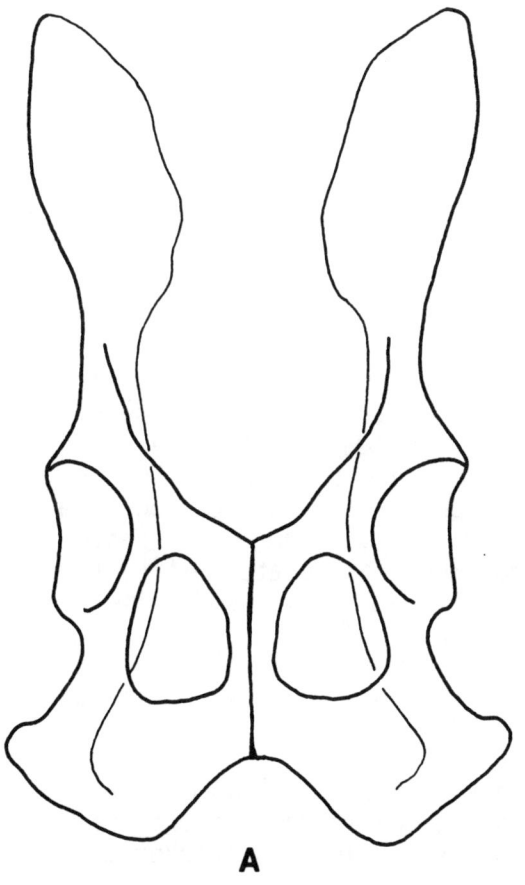
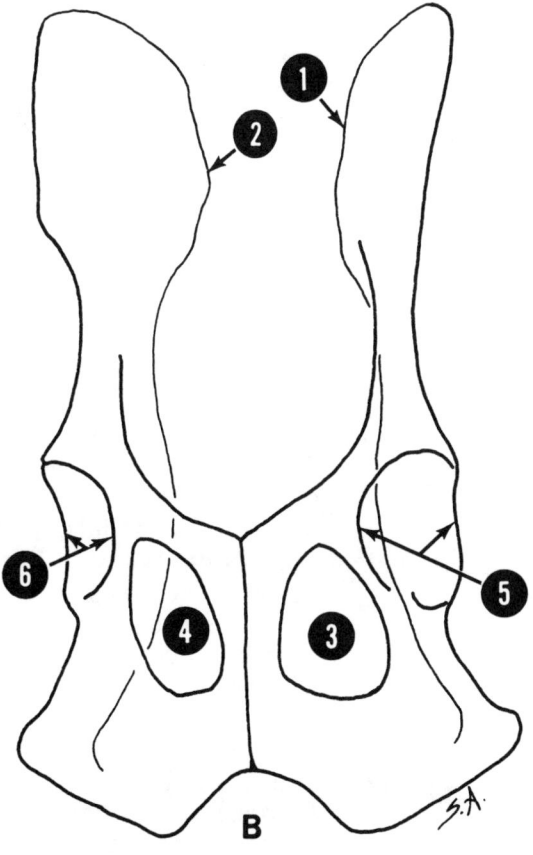

Figure 8-3

Indications of Obliquity in a V-D Radiograph of a Canine Pelvis

A. Untilted pelvis

The ilial wings, obturator foramina, and acetabula are symmetrical.

B. Pelvis tilted to the dog's right

The "up" ilial wing (1) is narrower than the "down" one (2). In addition, the "up" obturator foramen (3) appears larger than the "down" one (4), and the "up" acetabulum (5) appears deeper than the "down" one (6).

perspectives of the left and right sides which can best be appreciated by looking at the ventral aspect of an os coxae and rolling it from side to side (Fig. 8-3).

9. Aseptic necrosis (Legg-Calve-Perthe's disease) of the femoral head is a disease of young dogs of some of the smaller breeds. Its etiology is unknown, but it is believed to be a circulatory disturbance (disruption) resulting in demineralization. Pain is the clinical manifestation [21].

10. Femoral head and neck ostectomies are often used to improve severe cases of CHD, aseptic necrosis of the femoral head, or severe fractures of the proximal femur and/or acetabulum [22]. The false (fibrous) joint which forms following surgery gives stability and many dogs are markedly improved by this procedure. Smaller dogs are better candidates than larger ones because they do better postoperatively. The clinical improvement associated with the surgery results from removal of the pain associated with bone to bone contact. Consequently, a smooth stump left on the femur is helpful. Some surgeons have advocated moving part of the deep gluteal muscle belly (or biceps femoris m.) to insure a soft tissue buffer between the os coxae and femur [23].

11. The cartilaginous extension of the acetabular lip (labrum acetabulare) often discussed by surgeons is not developed in carnivores. In fact, the cartilage at the lip is not significantly thicker than that on the lunate surface [15].

12. Arthrocentesis of the coxal joint in horses has been described (Table 8-1).

III. GENUAL JOINT ("STIFLE JOINT")

A. General features

The genual joint is the most complex joint in the body. It consists of the femorotibial joint and the femoropatellar joint [1].

1. The femorotibial joint occurs between the condyles of the femur, the condyles of the tibia, and the interposed medial and lateral meniscal fibrocartilages (menisci). It has the following stabilizing ligaments (Fig. 8-4).

    a. medial ("tibial") collateral ligament--originates on the medial epicondyle of the femur and terminates on the proximal, medial tibia.

    b. lateral ("fibular") collateral ligament--originates on the lateral epicondyle of the femur and terminates on the head of the fibula.

    c. cranial ("anterior" or "lateral") cruciate ligament--originates on the lateral wall of the intercondylar fossa of the femur (medial side of the lateral condyle) and terminates on the cranial intercondylar area of the tibia.

d. caudal cruciate ("posterior" or "medial") ligament--originates on the craniomedial wall of the intercondylar fossa of the femur (lateral side of the medial condyle) and terminates on the caudal intercondylar area of the tibia.

e. The ligaments associated with the menisci also help to stabilize the joint--especially the unpaired meniscofemoral ligament which attaches the lateral meniscus to the femur. The abaxial surfaces of the menisci are attached to the joint capsule. The meniscal ligaments include (Fig. 8-4):

   (1) cranial (tibial) ligament of the lateral meniscus--attaches the cranial aspect of the lateral meniscus to the tibia.

   (2) caudal (tibial) ligament of the lateral meniscus--attaches the caudal aspect of the lateral meniscus to the tibia.

   (3) cranial (tibial) ligament of the medial meniscus--attaches the cranial aspect of the medial meniscus to the tibia.

   (4) caudal (tibial) ligament of the medial meniscus--attaches the caudal aspect of the medial meniscus to the tibia.

   (5) meniscofemoral ligament--attaches the caudal aspect of the lateral meniscus to the femur near the caudal part of the medial condyle. This ligament has also been termed "femoral ligament of the lateral meniscus" and is the only ligament which attaches either meniscus to the femur.

2. The femoropatellar joint occurs between the articular surface of the patella and the trochlea of the femur. The ligaments associated with this joint include:

   a. lateral femoropatellar ligament--attaches to the lateral border of the patella and to the lateral epicondyle of the femur. This ligament and its medial counterpart are regional thickenings in the fibrous joint capsule and may be difficult or impossible to grossly identify.

   b. medial femoropatellar ligament--attaches to the medial border of the patella and to the medial epicondyle of the femur. This ligament and its lateral counterpart are sometimes called "fabellopatellar" ligaments in carnivores.

   c. patellar ligaments--extend between the patella and the tibial tuberosity. Actually, these are a continuation of the tendinous insertion of the quadriceps femoris muscle distal to the patella. In the carnivores, pig, and small ruminants, a single band is present and it attaches to the tibial tuberosity. In the horse and the ox, three ligaments extend from the patella to the tibial tuberosity (Fig. 8-5):

Figure 8-4

Ligaments of the Equine Genual Joint

A. Isolated menisci from the left genual joint (caudal aspect)

1. lateral meniscus
2. cranial tibial lig. of lateral meniscus
3. caudal tibial lig. of lateral meniscus
4. meniscofemoral lig.
5. medial meniscus
6. cranial tibial lig. of medial meniscus
7. caudal tibial lig. of medial meniscus
8. cranial cruciate lig.
9. caudal cruciate lig.

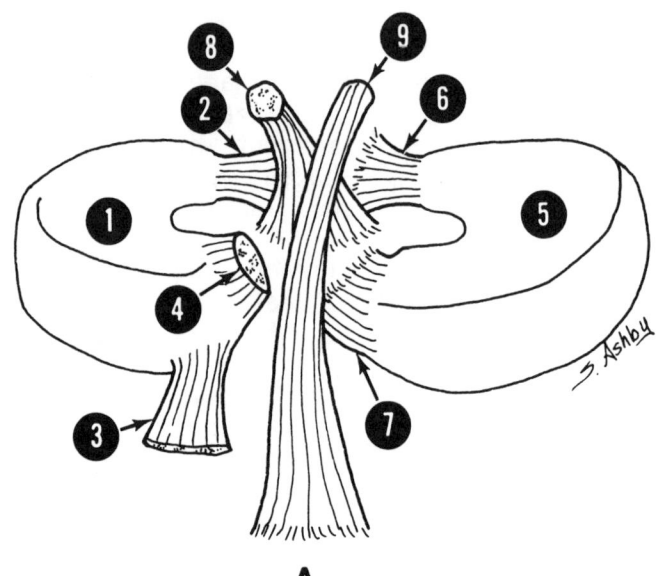

B. Caudal aspect of left joint

1. lateral collateral lig.
2. cranial cruciate lig.
3. meniscofemoral lig.
4. caudal tibial lig. of lateral meniscus
5. caudal cruciate lig.
6. medial collateral lig.

After Getty, 1975 [4]

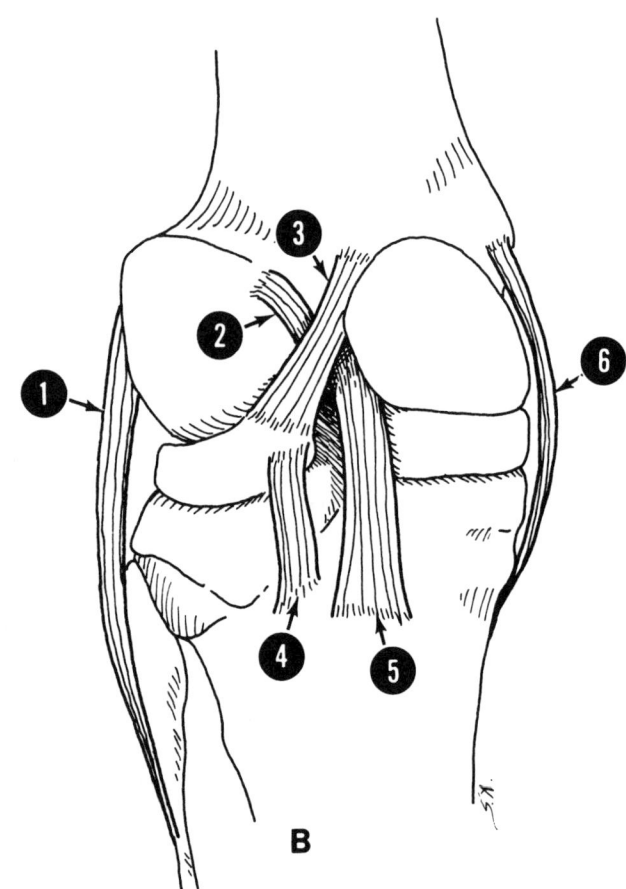

(1) intermediate ("middle," "straight") patellar ligament--corresponds to the single patellar ligament of other species
(2) medial patellar ligament
(3) lateral patellar ligament

B. Comparative and clinical considerations

1. The carnivores have a sixth meniscal ligament which connects the cranial extremities of the medial and lateral menisci. It is termed the transverse ("intermeniscal") ligament of the genual joint [1].

2. The enlarged proximal aspect of the medial ridge of the femoral trochlea in horses (trochlear tubercle) can be voluntarily forced between the medial and intermediate patellar ligaments to help the animal to stand with reduced muscular effort (part of the stay apparatus). With the patella "hung" on the medial ridge of the trochlea, the stifle is locked in an extended position that requires essentially no muscular effort to maintain. Pathological (involuntary) "catching" of this mechanism is termed "upward fixation of the patella" and is surgically corrected by severing the medial patellar ligament (medial patellar desmotomy) [24]. This obliterates (at least for a time) the patellar lock mechanism in that limb.

3. Cruciate ligaments ruptured from trauma are commonly encountered in small animals. The cranial ("anterior") drawer sign is commonly used to assess the integrity of the cranial cruciate ligament which frequently is ruptured when the caudal cruciate ligament is still intact.* The caudal cruciate ligament may rupture, too, but nearly always does so with concurrent disruption of the cranial cruciate ligament and/or a collateral ligament. A number of specialized repair techniques for ruptured cranial cruciate ligaments have been used [25]. For many years, Paatsama's method of inserting a strip of fascia lata through holes drilled in the femur and tibia (simulating the natural ligament) was popular [26]. Two other methods which have been used are imbrication of the joint capsule [27] and the "over-the-top procedure." In this latter procedure, a strip of fascia lata and patellar ligament, including a wedge of the patella, is dissected free proximally but left attached to the tibial tuberosity. The free end is then passed caudally between the femoral condyles and "over the top" of the caudal aspect of the lateral femoral condyle. Sutured down to soft tissue in this position, it forms a substitute for the cruciate ligament [28].

---

*An avulsion of the tibial tuberosity may also result in a cranial ("anterior") drawer sign if the tibial attachment of the cranial cruciate ligament is included in the avulsed fragment. The cranial drawer sign is a noticeable ability to subluxate the joint from its normal position to one in which the tibia is slightly further cranial (relative to the femur). The manipulation is done with the joint in moderate flexion [2]. A caudal drawer sign is present when the caudal cruciate ligament is ruptured.

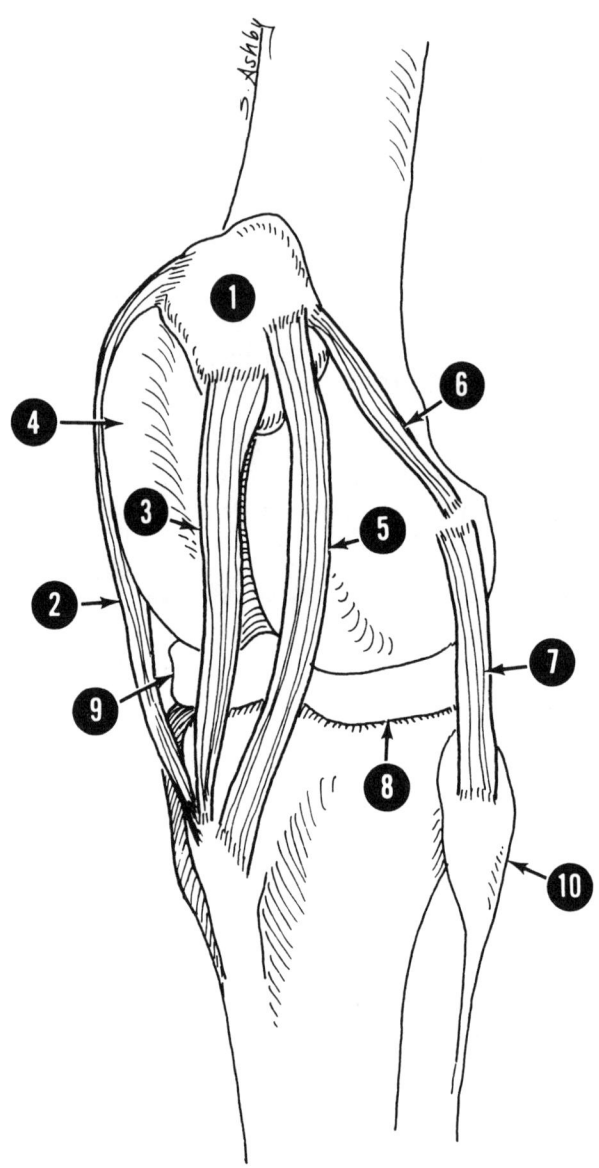

Figure 8-5

Ligaments of the Equine Genual Joint
(craniolateral aspect)

1. patella
2. medial patellar ligament
3. intermediate ("middle") patellar ligament
4. enlarged medial ridge of femoral trochlea
5. lateral patellar ligament
6. lateral femoropatellar ligament
7. lateral collateral ligament
8. lateral meniscus
9. medial meniscus
10. fibula

After Getty, 1975 [4]

4. In the carnivores, the sesamoid bone in each head of the gastrocnemius muscle should be identified in radiographs of the genual joint. The sesamoid bone in the popliteus muscle may be absent in small dogs, but is typically present in cats. An obsolete name for any of these three sesamoid bones is "fabella" (plural, "fabellae").

5. The "infrapatellar fat" is the adipose tissue located deep to the patellar ligament(s) under the synovial membrane of the joint. Its removal during arthrotomies was formerly advocated by surgeons to increase visualization of other structures, but more recent studies have indicated that it may play a role in supplying blood vessels to the cranial cruciate ligament [29]. Radiographic "loss" of the infrapatellar fat shadow refers to increased opacification (density) of its normal silhouette and usually indicates inflammatory changes in the joint.

6. The menisci are often damaged by trauma which may cause ruptures or tears of various types. Consequently, they should be examined (as much as is possible) for signs of injury whenever cruciate ligament repairs are performed. Removal of part or all of a damaged meniscus will often improve an animal clinically. It has been shown that if removed, menisci tend to reform--although the new ones are not as anatomically complete as their predecessors [30]. The medial meniscus is damaged in dogs much more frequently than the lateral one because it is subjected to more trauma from the femoral and tibial condyles during a "drawer" action than the lateral meniscus. Removal of the medial meniscus is accomplished by approaching the joint through a parapatellar incision and then freeing the meniscus by [31]:

    a. transecting the transverse ligament and the cranial tibial ligament of the medial meniscus near the cranial extremity of the meniscus where they are combined,

    b. dissecting the abaxial surface free from the joint capsule,

    c. severing the caudal tibial ligament of the medial meniscus. This step requires a small, pointed blade and the tibia and femur may have to be levered apart.

7. Ruptured collateral ligaments are repaired using wires and screws or transplanted fascia. Avulsion of an attachment may be repaired with a screw, wire, or pin. External splintage is usually applied [32].

8. In the horse, the genual joint cavity is divided into three sacs: the medial and lateral femorotibial sacs and the femoropatellar sac. It is clinically significant that the femoropatellar sac usually communicates with the medial femorotibial sac and sometimes (about 25%) communicates with the lateral femorotibial sac. Direct communication between the medial and lateral femorotibial sacs is rare in horses [2]. If one sac is infected, all three should be

considered infected, but each should be treated individually. Arthrocentesis of the genual joint may be performed in several loci adjacent to the patellar ligaments (Table 8-1). The femoropatellar joint may be punctured by a needle on either side of the intermediate patellar ligament. The medial part of the femorotibial joint may be penetrated just caudal to the medial patellar ligament. Similarly, the lateral part of the femorotibial joint, which is often anatomically distinct, may be penetrated caudal to the lateral patellar ligament [24]. Similar techniques may be used in cattle.

9. Luxation of the patella is seen in both large and small animals and is very common in small dogs. The patella may displace medially or laterally. In dogs, medial luxations are more common in small breeds and are usually congenital [32,33]. Lateral luxations occur more commonly in larger dogs and are often developmental and associated with genu valgum [32]. Many techniques are available for correction and some surgeons will combine 2 or 3 of them in one operation [6,34].

   a. Chondroplasty of the femoral trochlea--physically deepen it by removing the cartilage [33]. In younger dogs, a cartilage flap can be elevated and bone removed from under the flap [32]. Another recently introduced procedure involves sawing out and replacing a wedge of cartilage and bone [35].

   b. Imbrication of the joint capsule and/or reinforcement of the femoropatellar ligament on the opposite side--this tends to hold the patella in the trochlear groove of the femur [33,36,37].

   c. Osteotomy and translocation of the tibial tuberosity--this moves the attachment of the patellar ligament and helps keep the patella centered in the trochlear groove of the femur [33].

   d. Femoropatellar desmotomy--to release ("free") the patella on the affected side [38].

   e. Femoral and/or tibial (de-rotational) osteotomy--to correct abnormal torsions or curvatures of the shaft [6].

   f. Patellectomy--a last resort.

   Of these various techniques, the first three are the most popular and the others are rarely used.

10. The standard surgical approach to the genual joint in carnivores is a parapatellar incision. After the skin is cut, the joint capsule is incised just lateral or medial to the patellar ligament. Proximal and distal extensions of this incision and flexion of the joint will allow the patella to be luxated for good exposure [13].

IV. TIBIOFIBULAR ARTICULATIONS

The tibiofibular articulations vary considerably among the species of domestic mammals because of the variations in the development of the fibula. They include proximal and distal tibiofibular joints. A fibrous interosseous membrane fills in most of the space between the tibia and fibula. The horse and the ruminants have a fibular head and lateral malleolus, but they are missing most of the fibular body.

A. Proximal tibiofibular joint

1. In the horse, pig, and carnivores, the head of the fibula articulates with the lateral, proximal tibia by a synovial joint. Cranial and caudal ligaments of the head of the fibula attach it to the tibia.

2. In the ruminants, the head of the fibula typically fuses to the tibia.

B. Distal tibiofibular joint

1. In the horse, the lateral malleolus fuses to the tibia.

2. In the ruminants, pig, and carnivores, a synovial joint lies between the distal, lateral tibia and the lateral malleolus. Cranial and caudal tibiofibular ligaments support the joint.

V. TARSAL JOINT

A. General features

1. Like the carpal joint, the tarsal joint is a composite articulation made up of several individual articulations (Fig. 8-6).

    a. The tarsocrural joint is located between the tibia and fibula and the proximal row of the tarsal bones. It is popularly but incorrectly termed the "tibiotarsal" or "talocrural" joint [38]. Most of the movement ascribed to the tarsal joint occurs at the tarsocrural component, especially in the horse and carnivores.

    b. Intertarsal joints occur between individual tarsal bones side to side as well as from proximal to distal. Four of these have specific designations as follows [1]:

        (1) Talocalcaneal joint--the articulation between the talus and the calcaneus. Several articular facets may be involved.

        (2) Talocalcaneocentral joint--the joint primarily between the talus and the central tarsal bone. "Calcaneus" was included in the name because the joint cavity also extends between the talus and calcaneus.

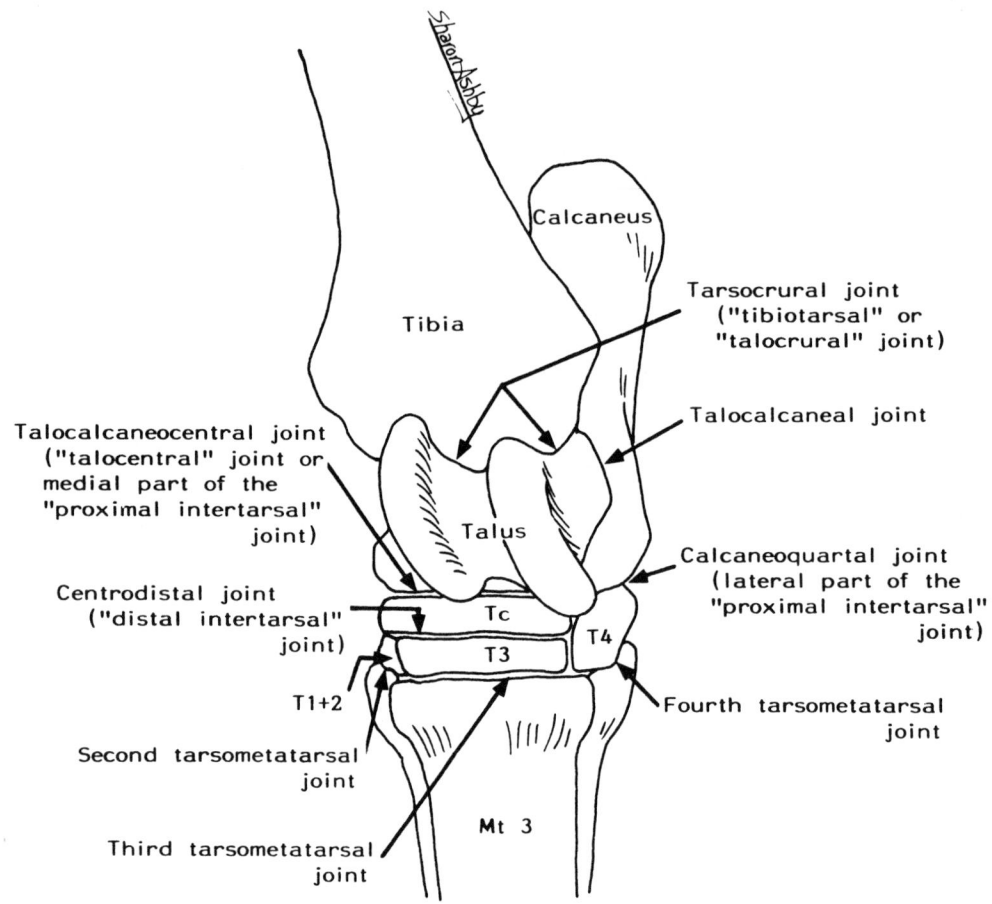

Figure 8-6A

Dorsolateral Schematic View of the Skeleton of a Left Equine Tarsus.

(Proper names for the various joints are indicated and obsolete synonyms are listed in quotes.)

    Tc = central tarsal bone

    T1+2 = fused first and second tarsal bones

    T3 = third tarsal bone

    T4 = fourth tarsal bone

    Mt3 = third metatarsal ("cannon") bone

From Shively, 1982 [39]

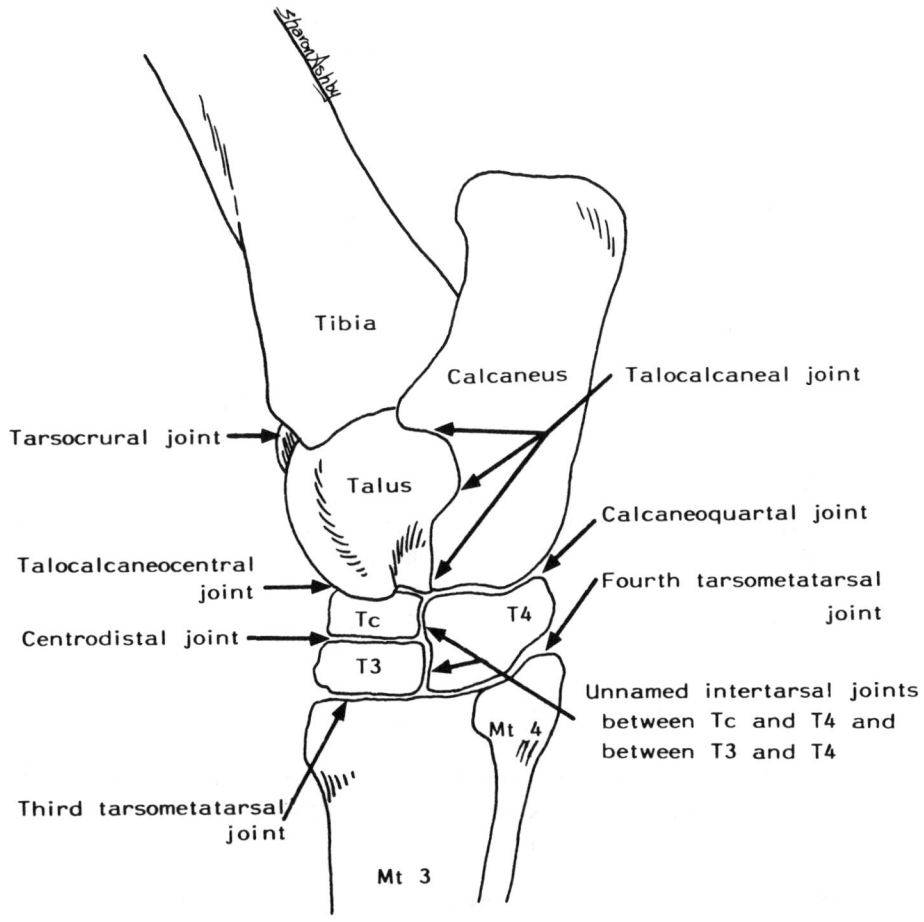

Figure 8-6B

Lateral View of the Skeleton of a Left Equine Tarsus.

(Proper names for the various joints are indicated.)

    Tc = central tarsal bone

    T3 = third tarsal bone

    T4 = fourth tarsal bone

    Mt3 = third metatarsal ("cannon") bone

    Mt4 = fourth metatarsal ("lateral splint") bone

From Shively, 1982 [39]

- (3) Calcaneoquartal joint--the joint between the calcaneus and the fourth tarsal bone. This joint and the talocalcaneocentral joint have been collectively and popularly termed "proximal intertarsal joint." This is an unofficial but useful term although, technically, it is a misnomer since the talocalcaneal joint (also an intertarsal joint) is located further proximally [39].

- (4) Centrodistal joint--the joint between the central tarsal bone and the distal row of the tarsal bones. This joint has been popularly but unofficially termed "distal intertarsal joint." Technically, it is not the most distal of the intertarsal joints [39].

There are no specific nomina for the intertarsal joints between T1 and T2, T2 and T3, T3 and T4, or Tc and T4.

c. The tarsometatarsal joint(s) are articulations between the distal tarsal bones and the metatarsal bones. They are numbered according to their metatarsal components.

2. There are numerous ligaments associated with the tarsal joint complex. The major ones include the following [1]:

a. Medial ("tibial") collateral ligament

- (1) Long part--originates on the medial malleolus and terminates on the medial (number varies with species) metatarsal bones.

- (2) Short part(s)--named specifically according to the various bones they join.

b. Lateral ("fibular") collateral ligament

- (1) Long part--attaches to the lateral malleolus and to the lateral metatarsal bones.

- (2) Short part(s)--named specifically according to the various bones they join.

In addition to these collateral ligaments, numerous individual ligaments are present which join individual tarsal bones and anchor the tarsal bones to the metatarsal bones. They have little specific clinical significance and there is considerable species variation. Several ligaments bind the calcaneus to other structures further distally. One of the better developed of these is the long plantar ligament located on the plantar aspect of the calcaneus [4]. It joins the calcaneus (and fourth tarsal bone) to the base of the fourth metatarsal bone.

B. Comparative and clinical considerations

1. In the ruminants and pig, the tarsocrural joint is formed by articulations between tibia, fibula, talus, and calcaneus. In the horse and carnivores, the calcaneus is not involved.

2. In the pig and ruminants, the "proximal intertarsal joint" has more mobility than it does in the other domestic species. This is related to the presence of a distal trochlea (as well as a proximal one) on the talus.

3. "Curb" is an equine malady defined as an enlargement along the plantar aspect of the calcaneus due to the inflammation and thickening of the long plantar ligament [24].

4. Severe injuries to the tarsal joint complex may necessitate arthrodesis. "Minor" injuries such as malleolar fractures are often successfully treated with pins, wires, and/or screws. Surgical approaches to these areas are relatively simple procedures [6,13].

5. There are 3 synovial "pouches"* associated with the tarsocrural joint of horses and these are located on the dorsomedial, medioplantar, and lateroplantar aspects of the joint [2].

    (1) Dorsomedial pouch--bounded by the medial malleolus, medial ("cunean") tendon of the cranial tibial m., tendon of the peroneus tertius m., and the long part of the medial collateral ligament. This is the preferred site for arthrocentesis of the tarsocrural joint and the needle is inserted plantar to the cranial branch of the medial saphenous vein.

    (2) Medioplantar pouch--positioned between the long part of the medial collateral ligament and the deep digital flexor tendon at the level of the medial malleolus.

    (3) Lateroplantar pouch--between the calcaneus and the lateral malleolus.

6. The question often arises as to which of the divisions of the equine tarsal joint complex communicate. Usually, all of the proximally located joints (tarsocrural, talocalcaneal, talocalcaneocentral, and calcaneoquartal) share a common synovial cavity; the centrodistal joint is distinct; and the three tarsometatarsal joints share one cavity. However, in occasional horses, the proximal joints have been shown to communicate with the centrodistal joint and sometimes also with the tarsometatarsal joints [40]. Injection technique for these joints and related structures in the horse are noted in Table 8-1. Similar techniques can be used in the ox.

---

*The term "pouch" is used to indicate areas where the capsule is not limited by bones or tendons and is, therefore, free to expand. Pouch does not imply internal divisions. The term "sac" is used to indicate an internal division (complete or incomplete) of the joint cavity. Some authors do not follow this usage.

7. "Spavin" is a broadly defined term usually used to indicate some form of equine tarsal arthropathy. The spavin test consists of a short period (2-3 minutes) of acute flexion of the tarsal joint. This will often accentuate the lameness during the first few steps after the leg is released [24].

   a. Bog spavin--(also termed hydroarthrosis) is distension of the three synovial pouches associated with the tarsocrural joint. The greatest enlargement is usually dorsomedially.

   b. Bone spavin--tarsal osteoarthritis which may result in ankylosis of the "distal intertarsal" and tarsometatarsal joints. "Jack spavin" is an especially large form of bone spavin, and "high spavin" is used to imply higher (more proximal) involvement ("proximal intertarsal joint" or tarso-crural joint). Cunean tenotomy may alleviate the clinical signs in some cases, and arthrodesis may improve others.

   c. Blind (occult) spavin--a tarsal lameness with no palpable or radiological changes.

   d. Blood spavin--no commonly accepted definition exists. The term is often used to refer to enlargement of venous channels near the tarsus.

8. Four standard radiographic views are commonly made of the tarsus for a "complete" evaluation. These include dorsoplantar (DP), lateromedial (LM), dorsoplantar lateromedial oblique (DPLMO), and dorsoplantar mediolateral oblique (DPMLO). In addition, a latero-medial view of the flexed tarsus (LMF) and a dorsoplantar view of the calcaneus and talus with the tarsus flexed (DPF) may be required to illustrate certain lesions [41,42].

9. Selected radiographic features of the tarsus may be of value clinically:

   a. The carnivores have a proximal "spur" on the lateral aspect of the base of the fifth metatarsal bone which may mimic an osteophyte [43].

   b. In carnivores, the second tarsometatarsal joint is significantly proximal to its lateral counterparts. This gives the tarsometatarsal joints a "stairstep" appearance on dorsoplantar projections, and superimposes a transverse pseudo-fracture line across the third tarsal bone on ML or LM projections [43].

   c. In dorsoplantar projections of canine tarsi, the third tarsal bone often appears to be split vertically because of the cleft between the plantar aspects of T3 and T4 [43].

   d. In lateral projections of canine tarsi, the "distal inter-tarsal" joint appears as two radiolucencies: a proximal one between Tc and T3, and a distal one between Tc and T2 [43].

e. In ruminants, the metatarsal sesamoid bone ("small metatarsal bone") should not be mistaken for a lesion [42].

f. Radiographic changes associated with spastic paresis in cattle include increased concavity of the dorsal aspect of the proximal part of the calcaneus and widening of the epiphyseal cartilages (physes) of the tuber calcanei and distal tibia [42].

g. Osteochondritis dissecans lesions have been reported in rapidly growing bulls, involving the cranial aspect of the intermediate ridge of the tibial cochlea. This area is well visualized by a DPLMO view [42].

h. In horses, the medial and lateral ridges of the trochlea tali can be distinguished on lateral views because the lateral one has a larger "notch" at its distal aspect. The lateral one is usually projected further dorsally, too, but slight obliquity can affect this distinction. In cattle, the lateral ridge of the trochlea extends further proximally than the medial ridge [41].

i. In the horse, the torus tarseus (chestnut) can cause a confusing shadow on DPLMO projections. Even though it is located on the medial aspect of the limb, it is positioned far enough plantarly to be visible [40]. This same view is valuable for evaluating distention of the dorsomedial pouch of the tarsocrural joint as seen in tarsal hydroarthrosis ("bog spavin").

j. The ossification center for the tuber calcanei fuses to the rest of the calcaneus at 16-24 months of age in horses and at about 3 years of age in cattle [41,42].

10. A number of conformational defects of the limb are partially or wholly associated with the tarsus. In a horse, for example, the metatarsus should be vertically oriented and in line with the caudal aspect of the hip (Fig. 8-7A). Animals in which the tarsus is exceptionally angled (flexed) are termed "sickle-hocked" or said to have "curby" conformation (Fig. 8-7B). Those with very straight tarsi (and genual joints) are termed "post-legged" or "straight behind" (Fig. 8-7C). Viewed from the caudal aspect, the limbs should be straight and parallel (Fig. 8-8A). Horses in which the tarsal joints deviate medially (especially at the tubera calcanei) are said to be "cow-hocked" (Fig. 8-8B).

The intermetatarsal joints, metatarsophalangeal joints, proximal interphalangeal joints, and distal interphalangeal joints resemble the homologous joints of the thoracic limb.

VI. EQUINE STAY APPARATUS

The so-called "stay apparatus" of the horse consists of a collection of of appendicular structures which allow a horse to stand with reduced muscular effort [44,45]. The structures involved are composed of fibrous connective tissue

Figure 8-7

Lines and Angulations of the Equine Pelvic Limb (lateral aspect)

A. Normal

B. "Sickle-hocked" ("curby" conformation)

C. "Post-legged" ("straight behind")

From Shively, 1982 [47]

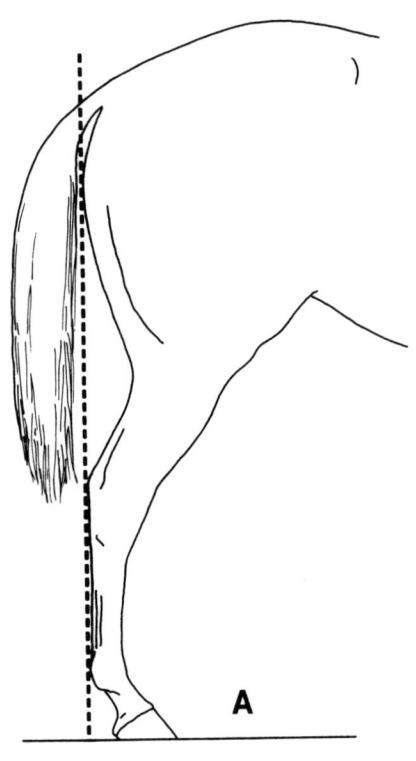
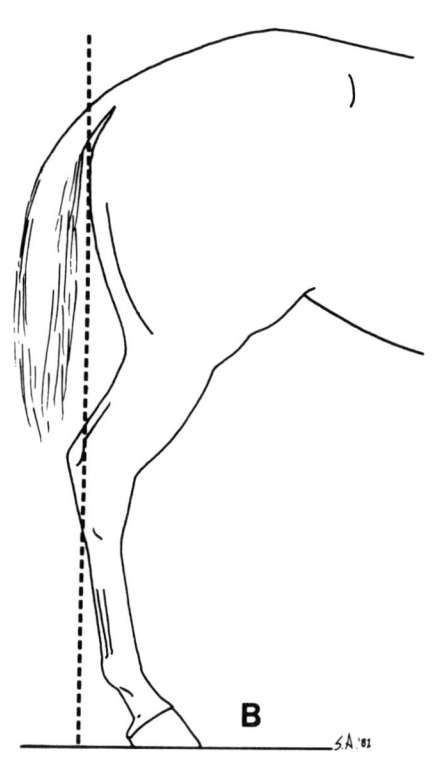
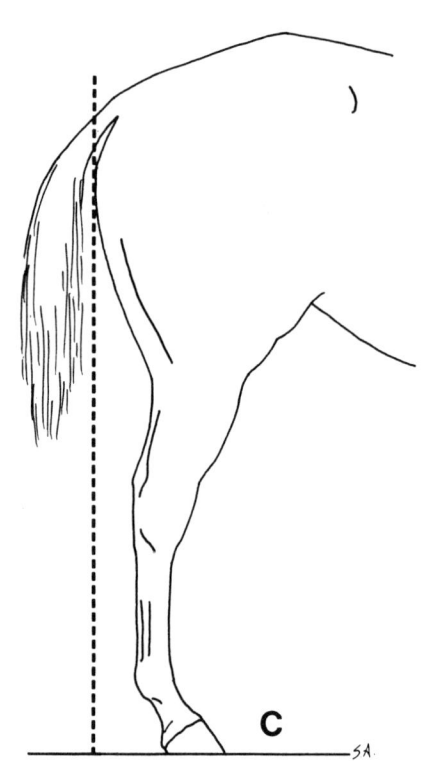

Figure 8-8

Lines and Angulations of the Equine Pelvic Limb
(caudal aspect)

A. Normal

B. "Cow-hocked"

From Shively, 1982 [47]

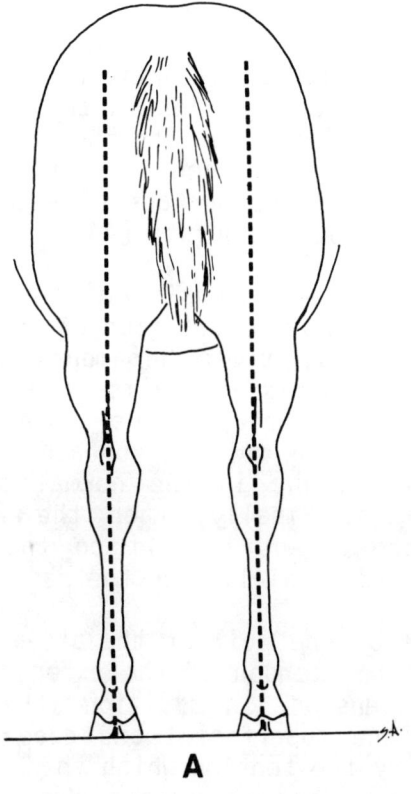
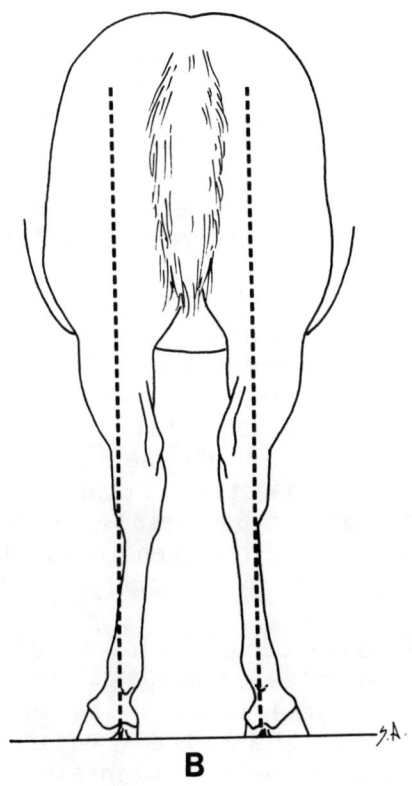

(tendons, ligaments, deep fascia) and they resist the gravitational tendency toward joint collapse. The stay apparatus includes the following (Figs. 8-9 and 8-10):

A. Structures peculiar to the thoracic limb
1. connective tissue of the serratus ventralis m.
2. tendon of biceps brachii m.
3. lacertus fibrosus
4. collateral ligaments of the cubital joint
5. accessory ligaments of superficial and deep digital flexor muscles
6. tendinous portions of ulnaris lateralis and flexor carpi ulnaris muscles

B. Structures peculiar to the pelvic limb
1. patellar lock mechanism
2. reciprocal apparatus (extensor portion)
3. fibrous band portion of gastrocnemius
4. accessory ligament of the deep digital flexor m.

C. Structures present in both limbs
1. interosseous muscle
2. "distal sesamoidean" ligaments
3. palmar (plantar) ligaments of proximal interphalangeal joint

When a horse is at rest, a large percentage of its weight is transferred to the scapulae through the fibrous connective tissue of the serratus ventralis muscles. Gravitational forces tend to flex the shoulder joints until the tendinous cores of the biceps brachii muscles are stretched taut. Tension in the tendinous portion of each biceps muscle then resists further flexion of the shoulder joints and passively supports them. Pressure and friction between the intermediate tubercle of each humerus and the indentation of the deep surface of each biceps tendon also help to prevent further flexion of the shoulder joints [44].

A number of structures are involved in passive extension of the cubital joint. The collateral ligaments attach caudal to the axis of rotation of the joint. Consequently, once the joint is maximally extended, these ligaments must be stretched to flex the joint. The tendons of the ulnaris lateralis, flexor carpi ulnaris, and superficial digital flexor also attach to the humerus caudal to the axis of rotation of the cubital joint. Each of these muscles contains a large amount of connective tissue which is stretched tight in the normal standing position and thus helps to extend the cubitus. Finally, when the foot is weight-bearing, the tendinous attachment of the biceps brachii on the radius assists cubital extension by pulling proximally (and cranially) on the radius [44].

Passive carpal joint extension is effected by the pull of the biceps tendon on the lacertus fibrosus. This puts tension on the tendon of the extensor carpi radialis muscle which helps maintain carpal extension. In addition, the interosseous muscle and the accessory ligaments of the superficial and deep digital flexor muscles help to maintain carpal extension by the tension which they place on the caudal and palmar aspect of the radius, carpus, and metacarpus during weight bearing [44].

The digital joints are supported by the interosseous muscles (i.e., suspensory ligaments), distal sesamoidean ligaments, and by the accessory (i.e., "check") ligaments and their associated superficial and deep digital flexor

Figure 8-9

Schematic Representation of the Thoracic Limb Components of the Equine Stay Apparatus

1. tendon of serratus ventralis
2. tendon of biceps brachii
3. lacertus fibrosis
4. collateral lig. of cubital jt.
5. extensor carpi radialis
6. tendon of common digital extensor
7. extensor branch from interosseous m.
8. interosseous m.
9. deep digital flexor
10. accessory lig. of 9
11. superficial digital flexor
12. accessory lig. of 11

The distal sesamoidean ligg. are not illustrated here (see Chapter 3).

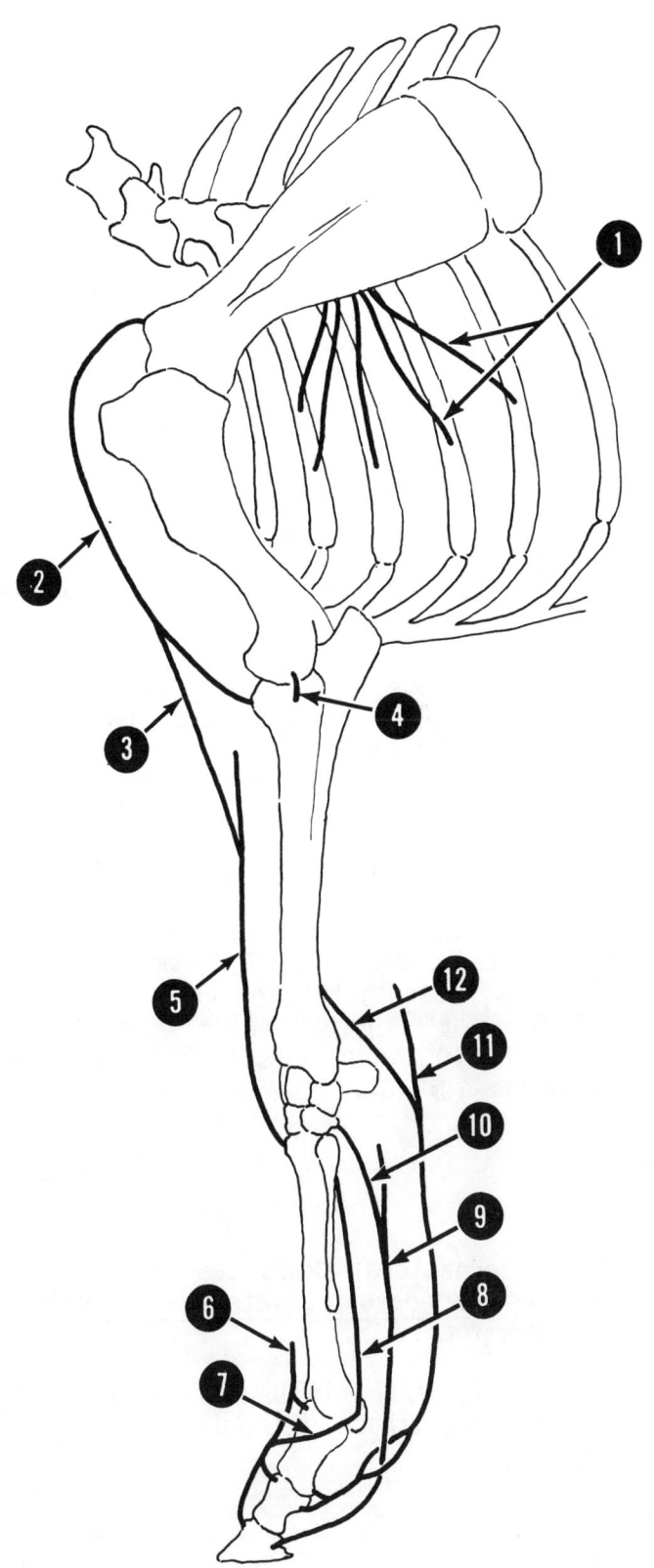

tendons. All of these structures are involved in supporting the metacarpophalangeal joint. The proximal interphalangeal joint is supported by the digital flexor tendons and the straight sesamoidean ligament as well as by the palmar ligaments (which are peculiar to this joint). The distal interphalangeal joint actually flexes during weight-bearing and can be disregarded in this discussion [45].

In the pelvic limb, no specific structures are directly involved in locking the coxal joint, but the patellar lock mechanism does so indirectly by locking the genual joint. The patellar lock mechanism is brought into effect by extending the genual joint. The patella is then rotated medially by the sartorius and/or gracilis muscles, and the trochlear tubercle on the medial ridge of the femoral trochlea is forced between the medial and intermediate patellar ligaments. With the patella thus "hooked" over the trochlear tubercle, the genual joint is locked in extension because the patella cannot glide distally in the trochlea (which it must do for flexion to occur). To unlock the patella, the quadriceps is contracted slightly to raise the patella and then the biceps femoris and/or tensor fasciae latae are contracted slightly to rotate the patella laterally and re-center it in the femoral trochlea. Because the horse's weight must be partially shifted to the opposite limb during initiation of the patellar lock, only one limb may be locked at any given moment. A horse with one patella "locked" stands with the pelvis tilted toward the locked side. The opposite limb is relaxed, and the contralateral toe rests on the ground surface. Even though it appears that locking the limb precludes the need for muscular activity in the limb, the horse soon tires and switches supporting limbs. Which muscles are active and tire in this situation remains unknown [45].

Locking the genual joint through the patellar lock mechanism also passively locks the tarsal joint in extension via the superficial digital flexor component of the reciprocal apparatus. (Some authors indicate that a fibrous band in the gastrocnemius is also involved.) The superficial digital flexor of the horse has a strong tendinous core. It attaches to the distal, caudal femur and also to the calcaneus (before continuing on to the digits). With the genual joint locked in extension, the superficial digital flexor tendon is passively pulled taut at its attachment on the calcaneus. This keeps the tarsal joint extended and resists the gravitational forces which tend to flex (collapse) it. The peroneus tertius muscle (tendinous in the horse) forms the "flexor" part of the reciprocal apparatus but plays no role in the stay apparatus [46].

The digital joints of the pelvic limb are supported by structures similar to those in the thoracic limb. No accessory ligament of the superficial digital flexor muscle is present, but the tendinous nature of the muscle apparently obviates the need for the ligament. (The tendinous nature of the muscle from its calcaneal attachment to its phalangeal insertions accomplishes the same purpose as would an accessory ligament.)

References

1. International Committee on Veterinary Gross Anatomical Nomenclature. 1983. Nomina Anatomica Veterinaria, third ed. Published by the Committee, Ithaca, New York.

2. Habel, R. E. 1981. Applied Veterinary Anatomy, second ed. Published by the author, Ithaca, New York.

Figure 8-10

Schematic Representation of the Pelvic Limb Components of the Equine Stay Apparatus and Reciprocal Apparatus

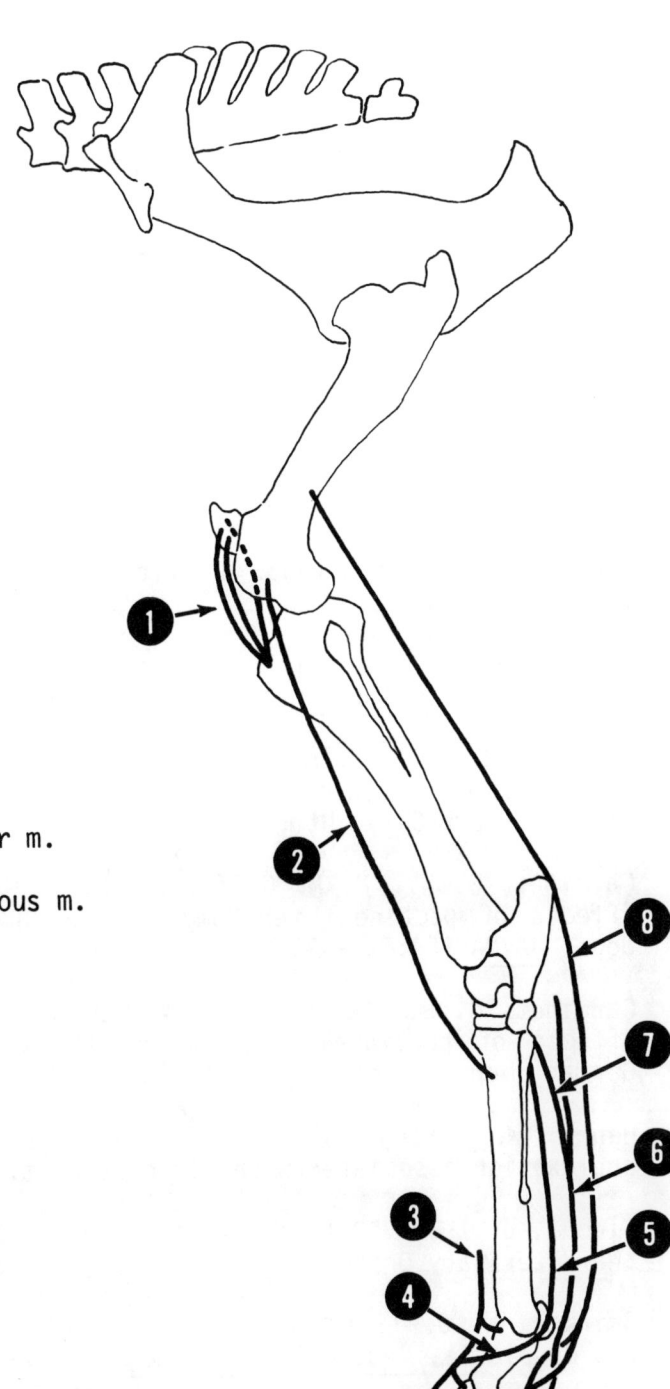

1. patellar ligg.
2. peroneus tertius m.
3. tendon of long digital extensor m.
4. extensor branch from interosseous m.
5. interosseous m.
6. deep digital flexor m.
7. accessory lig. of 6
8. superficial digital flexor m.

The distal sesamoidean ligg. are not illustrated here (see Chapter 3).

3. Shively, M. J. 1982. Twenty more veterinary anatomic lies, half truths, and misleading statements. Jour. Vet. Med. Ed. 9(1):20-21.

4. Getty, R. 1975. Sisson and Grossman's The Anatomy of the Domestic Animals, fifth ed. W. B. Saunders, Philadelphia.

5. McFarland, L. Z. 1970. Veterinary Surgical Anatomy. Department of Veterinary Anatomy, University of California, Davis.

6. Archibald, J., ed. 1974. Canine Surgery, second edition. American Veterinary Publications, Santa Barbara, California.

7. Alexander, J. W. 1982. Coxofemoral luxations in the dog. Comp. Cont. Ed. Prac. Vet. 4(7):575-582.

8. DeVita, J. 1952. A method of pinning for chronic dislocation of the hip joint. Proc. Book of the 89th Ann. Mtg. of the AVMA 89:191-192.

9. Olsen, M. L. 1957. Multiple fractures of the pelvis. In Canine Surgery, fourth ed., pp 733-734. American Veterinary Publications, Inc., Evanston, Illinois.

10. Knowles, A. J., J. O. Knowles, and R. P. Knowles. 1953. An operation to preserve the continuity of the hip joint. JAVMA 123:508-515.

11. Piermattei, D. L. 1963. A technic for surgical management of coxofemoral luxations. Sm. Anim. Clin. 3:373-386.

12. Piermattei, D. L. 1965. Fabrication of an improved toggle pin. VM/SAC 60(4):384-389.

13. Piermattei, D. L., and R. G. Greeley. 1979. An Atlas of Surgical Approaches to the Bones of the Dog and Cat, second ed. W. B. Saunders, Philadelphia.

14. Shively, M. J. 1982. A survey of selected orthopedic procedures in the pelvic limb. Paper presented at the annual meeting of the Veterinary Orthopedic Society, Park City, Utah.

15. Cardinet, G. H., M. M. Guffy, and L. J. Wallace. 1974. Canine hip dysplasia; Effects of pectineal tenotomy on the coxofemoral joints of German Shepherd dogs. JAVMA 164:591-598.

16. Cardinet, G. H., M. M. Guffy, and L. J. Wallace. 1974. Canine hip dysplasia; Effects of pectineal myectomy on the coxofemoral joints of Greyhound and German Shepherd dogs. JAVMA 165:529-532.

17. Henry, W., and P. Wadsworth. 1975. Pelvic osteotomy in the treatment of subluxation associated with hip dysplasia. JAAHA 11(5):636-643.

18. Slocum, B. 1983. "Pelvic Osteotomy: A Review of 62 Cases." Paper presented at the Veterinary Orthopedic Society Convention, Waikaloa, Hawaii.

19. Brinker, W. O. 1971. Corrective osteotomy procedures for treatment of canine hip dysplasia. Vet. Clinic N. Amer. 1:467-477.

20. Stunkard, J. A., A. E. Schwichtenberg, and T. P. Griffin. 1969. Evaluation of hip dysplasia in German Shepherd dogs. Mod. Vet. Pract. 50:40-44.

21. Ettinger, S. J. 1983. Textbook of Veterinary Internal Medicine, second ed. W. B. Saunders, Philadelphia.

22. Gendreau, C., and A. J. Cawley. 1977. Excision of the femoral head and neck: The long-term results of 35 operations. JAVMA 13:605-608.

23. Dueland, R., J. Trotter, and J. Beryon. 1980. Mediale verlagerung des tiefen glutaeus muskels bei der femurkopfresektion. Klientierpraxis 25(7):389-392.

24. Adams, O. R. 1974. Lameness in Horses. third ed. Lea and Febiger, Philadelphia.

25. Arnoczky, S. and J. Marshall. 1977. The cruciate ligaments of the canine stifle: an anatomical and functional analysis. Am. J. Vet. Res. 38:1807-1814.

26. Paatsama, S. 1952. Ligament injuries in the canine stifle joint. Thesis, Helsinki Veterinary College, Selsinki, Finland.

27. DeAngelis, M., and R. E. Law. 1970. A lateral retinacular imbrication technique for the surgical correction of anterior cruciate ligament rupture in the dog. JAVMA 157(1):79-84.

28. Arnoczky, S., G. Tarvin, J. Marshall and B. Saltzman. 1979. The over-the-top procedure: A technique for anterior cruciate ligament substitution in the dog. JAAHA 15(3):283-290.

29. Arnoczky, S., R. Rubin, and J. Marshall. 1979. Microvasculature of the cruciate ligaments and its response to injury. An experimental study in dogs. J. Bone Jt. Surg. 61A(8):1221-1229.

30. DeYoung, D. J., G. L. Flo, and H. Tvedten. 1980. Experimental medial meniscectomy in dogs undergoing cranial cruciate ligament repair. JAAHA 16(5):639-645.

31. Flo, G. L., and D. J. DeYoung. 1978. Meniscal injuries and medial meniscectomy in the canine stifle. JAAHA 14:683-689.

32. Bojrab, M. J. ed. 1975. Current Techniques in Small Animal Surgery. Lea and Febiger, Philadelphia.

33. DeAngelis, M., and R. B. Hohn. 1970. Evaluation of surgical correction of canine patellar luxation in 142 cases. JAVMA 156(5):587-594.

34. Vierheller, R. C. 1959. Surgical correction of patellar ectopia in the dog. JAVMA 134(1):429-433.

35. Boone, E. G., R. B. Hohn, and S. E. Weisbrode. 1983. Trochlear recession wedge technique for patellar luxation: An experimental study. JAAHA 19(5):735-742.

36. Flo, G. F. and W. O. Brinker. 1970. Fascia lata overlap procedure for surgical correction of recurrent medial luxation of the patella in the dog. JAVMA 156:595-599.

37. Herron, M. R. 1969. Medial luxation of the canine patella--a simple technic for surgical correction. Mod. Vet. Prac. 57(7):30-33.

38. Lacroix, J. V. 1930. Recurrent luxation of the patella in dogs. North Am. Vet. 11:47-48.

39. Shively, M. J. 1982. Correct anatomic nomenclature for the joints of the equine tarsus. Equine Prac. 4(4):9-12.

40. Brown, M. P. and K. Valko. 1980. A technique for intra-articular injection of the equine tarsometatarsal joint. VM/SAC 75(2):265-270.

41. Shively, M. J., and J. E. Smallwood. 1980. Radiographic and xeroradiographic anatomy of the equine tarsus. Equine Prac. 2(4):19-35.

42. Smallwood, J. E. and M. J. Shively. 1981. Radiographic and xeroradiographic anatomy of the bovine tarsus. Bovine Prac. 2(5):28-45.

43. Shively, M. J. 1979. "Anatomy of the canine tarsus, Part I: bones, muscles, nerves, vessels." Paper presented at the Conference of the Veterinary Orthopedic Society, Vail, Colorado.

44. Worthman, R.P. 1966. The stay apparatus of the horse. Version adopted by the American Association of Veterinary Anatomists at this annual meeting, July 1966.

45. Sack, W. O. 1982. The stay apparatus of the horse's hind limb. Printed notes of a lecture given at the preconvention seminar of the American Association of Veterinary Anatomists, Snowbird, Utah.

46. Shively, M. J. 1979. Twenty-four veterinary anatomic fibs, half-truths, and misleading statements. Jour. Vet. Med. Ed. 6(3):182-187.

47. Shively, M. J. 1982. Equine-English dictionary: Part I, Standing conformation. Equine Pract. 4(5):10-27.

9

PELVIC LIMB ANGIOLOGY

Knowledge of the vascular pattern of the pelvic limb has clinical applications in routine venipunctures, special radiographic procedures, indwelling catheter insertions, and numerous surgical procedures. The presence of collateral circulation often negates the need for any particular vessel, and in a normal, healthy dog, even the femoral vessels may be ligated with no or only transient ill effects [1]. However, preservation of vascular integrity where possible is an important surgical principle to optimize healing and maintain orientation in the surgical field.

The major arterial channel supplying the pelvic limb includes (from proximal to distal) the femoral, popliteal, cranial tibial, and dorsal pedal arteries [2]. As noted in the thoracic limb (Chapter 4), the landmarks for the regional name changes of this main channel and its first order branches are of primary significance. These are relatively constant regardless of species (Fig. 9-1). From various branchings and anastomoses of these vessels, the metatarsal arteries and the proper digital arteries arise. The following discussion is limited primarily to the major vessels of the pelvic limb and does not involve minor vessels or the numerous unnamed muscular branches. The significant variations in the various species have been cited.

Arteries of the Pelvic Limb (Fig. 9-1)

I. FEMORAL ARTERY

The femoral artery is the most proximal segment of the major vascular channel supplying the pelvic limb. It is the extra-abdominal continuation of the external iliac artery and begins at the point where that vessel passes through the abdominal wall (vascular lacuna). Some authors consider it to begin immediately distal to the origin of the deep femoral artery. (This difference is academic because the two sites are very close to each other.) The femoral artery courses down the medial side of the thigh, and its proximal portion lies within the femoral triangle. It enters the femoral triangle in the pig and ruminants by passing through the origin of the sartorius muscle, and in carnivores and the horse by coursing caudal to the sartorius. In the carnivores, its position in the femoral triangle is a convenient place to check the pulse. Further distally, the femoral artery passes laterally and caudally into the thigh musculature.

The femoral artery is frequently used as a catheterization site for angiocardiography because of its superficial position on the medial aspect of the thigh. It is of concern during any procedures involving the medial thigh, but it is not a vital structure [1]. After the origin of the (distal) caudal femoral artery, the femoral artery is continued as the popliteal artery. The major branches of the femoral a. include the following:

A. Lateral circumflex femoral artery

This vessel is counterpart to the medial circumflex femoral artery (which is a branch of the deep femoral artery). It courses distally between the rectus femoris and vastus medialis mm. to supply the thigh musculature.

Figure 9-1

Schematic Pattern of the Major Arteries of the Pelvic Limb
(medial aspect)

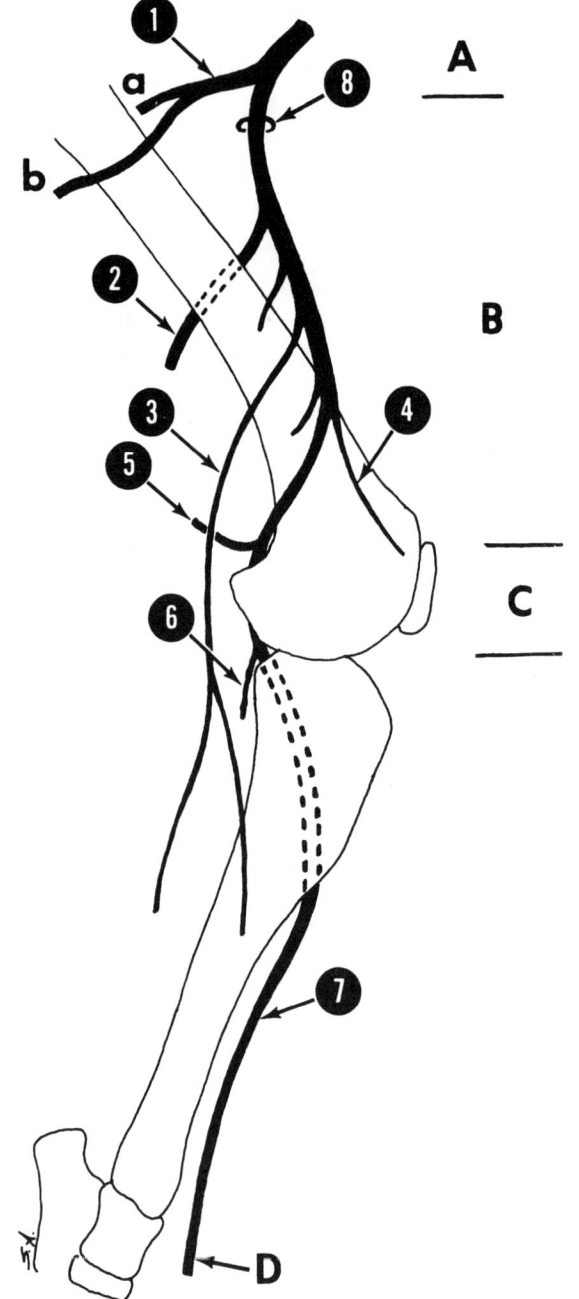

A. Branches of the external iliac a.
    1. Deep femoral a.
        a. pudendoepigastric trunk
        b. medial circumflex femoral a.
B. Branches of the femoral a.*
    2. Lateral circumflex femoral a.
    3. Saphenous a.
    4. Descending genicular a.
    5. Caudal femoral a.
C. Branches of the popliteal a.
    6. Caudal tibial a.
    7. Cranial tibial a.
D. Dorsal pedal a.

*The proximal extent of the femoral artery is marked by the vascular lacuna (8) where the external iliac artery passes through the abdominal wall. Unlabeled branches of the femoral artery are muscular branches with no specific designation in the ungulates. In the carnivores, the larger two of these are the proximal and middle caudal femoral aa.

B. Saphenous artery

The saphenous artery is a branch of the femoral artery which arises proximal to the genual joint, remains superficial, and courses distally to contribute to the digital vascular supply. It divides into a cranial branch and a caudal branch in the horse and carnivores, but it does not make this division in the pig and ox [3].

C. Descending genicular artery

This small vessel is distributed to structures around the genual joint.

D. Caudal femoral artery

This artery is distributed primarily to the musculature of the caudal thigh and caudal crus (see paragraph E.2. below). It is the largest of the muscular branches of the femoral artery and arises near the genual joint.

E. The following species specific variations may be of interest:

1. The carnivores have a superficial circumflex iliac artery which arises near or in common with the lateral circumflex femoral artery [3]. It supplies the sartorius, tensor fasciae latae, and part of the quadriceps femoris mm.

2. The carnivores have proximal and middle caudal femoral arteries as well as a larger distal caudal femoral artery. This latter vessel corresponds to the caudal femoral a. of other species. In the ungulates, unnamed muscular branches may be present in similar loci and correspond to the proximal and middle caudal femoral aa.

3. The nutrient artery of the femur in the horse may arise directly from the femoral artery, or it may be a branch of the caudal femoral artery.

II. POPLITEAL ARTERY

The popliteal artery is the continuation of the femoral a. which courses between the heads of the gastrocnemius m. For all practical purposes, the locus of name-change may be considered to be the origin of the distal caudal femoral artery. The popliteal artery supplies a number of small, named branches to structures near the genual joint, but these branches are not clinically significant. It terminates by dividing into the cranial and caudal tibial arteries. The cranial tibial a. is larger than the caudal tibial a. and is the main vascular channel of the crus.

III. CRANIAL TIBIAL ARTERY

The cranial tibial artery passes craniolaterally through the interosseous space between the tibia and fibula, and then courses distally between the craniolateral muscles of the crus and the tibia. It supplies a number of small, named branches to crural structures, and is continued at the level of the tarsocrural articulation as the dorsal pedal artery.

IV. DORSAL PEDAL ARTERY

The dorsal pedal artery is the continuation of the cranial tibial artery distal to the tarsocrural joint. It courses across the flexor (dorsal) aspect of the tarsal joint and in the ungulates it sends a perforating branch between the tarsal bones (perforating tarsal a.) to join the plantar digital supply.* The dorsal pedal a. then forms the dorsal metatarsal arteries and, in the horse, the single third dorsal metatarsal a. continues through the interosseous space between Mt3 and Mt4 (distal perforating branch) to the plantar aspect of the midmetatarsus (see digital arteries). In dogs, the dorsal pedal artery is one of several vessels which may be used during surgery to monitor the pulse. (The brachial, lingual, common carotid, and femoral aa. may also be used.)

V. DIGITAL ARTERIES

The general patterns and terminology of the digital vessels parallel those of the thoracic limb (see Chapter 4). Superficial vessels in the metatarsal region are termed common digital arteries, and are present on the dorsal and/or plantar aspects of the limb (dorsal and plantar common digital arteries). The common digital arteries are numbered 1-4, depending on which metatarsal skeletal components they parallel (a first common digital artery occupies the area between Mt1 and Mt2, a second common digital artery is found between Mt2 and Mt3, etc.). Deeper vessels in the metatarsal region which parallel the common digital arteries are termed metatarsal arteries and are also numbered from medial to lateral [2]. The common digital arteries and the metatarsal arteries both contribute to the formation of the proper digital arteries (dorsal and plantar; axial and abaxial; 1-4). As in the thoracic limb, the details of the digital arterial supply have very little clinical application in the carnivores and pig. The horse and ox are each distinctive enough to warrant separate descriptions.

Horse

In the horse (Fig. 9-2), the major arterial channel distal to the tarsometatarsal joints is the third dorsal metatarsal artery. It is the direct continuation of the dorsal pedal a., distal to the tarsus, and is positioned dorsolaterally. About halfway down the metatarsus, it courses plantarly and passes between Mt3 and Mt4 to continue on the plantar aspect of the metatarsus. As it courses between Mt3 and Mt4, it becomes the distal perforating branch (Fig. 9-2/12). It is susceptible at this level to trauma from fractures of Mt4. A few centimeters further distally, it divides into the medial and lateral digital aa. (Fig. 9-2/13,14) which are distributed to the digit in the same manner as their thoracic limb counterparts.

In addition to the vasculature described above, the caudal branch of the saphenous artery divides into the medial and lateral plantar aa. at the level of the tarsocrural joint (Fig. 9-2/7,8). The medial and lateral plantar aa. are also properly termed the second and third plantar common digital aa. An

---

*In the carnivores, the perforating branch of the second dorsal metatarsal a. is homologous to the perforating tarsal aa. of ungulates.

S-shaped anastomosis from the caudal tibial artery provides additional input into these channels. The lateral plantar artery gives rise to a deep plantar arch which receives additional input from the perforating tarsal a. and supplies the second and third plantar metatarsal aa. As in the thoracic limb, the medial and lateral plantar aa. are superficially positioned and the medial and lateral plantar metatarsal aa. are deep. Distally, these vessels contribute to the digital supply by anastomosing with the medial and lateral digital aa. or with the distal perforating branch of the third dorsal metatarsal a.

Ox

In the ox (Fig. 9-3), as in the horse, the continuation of the dorsal pedal artery, distal to the tarsus, is the third dorsal metatarsal a. It courses distally in the dorsal longitudinal groove of Mt3+4 and gives rise to the distal perforating branch (Fig. 9-3/5) which courses through the distal metatarsal canal. At this level, the parent vessel becomes the third dorsal common digital a. (Fig. 9-3/6). It courses between the digits and anastomoses with the third plantar common digital a. (see below).

On the plantar aspect of the limb, the saphenous artery divides at the level of the tarsus into the medial and lateral plantar aa. (Fig. 9-3/8,9). Anastomotic branches from these join the perforating tarsal a.* in forming the three small deeply located plantar metatarsal aa. (Fig. 9-3/11,12,13). Similar branches from the medial and lateral plantar aa. anastomose with the distal perforating branch which courses through the distal metatarsal canal. Near the distal metatarsus, the medial plantar a. divides into the second and third plantar common digital aa. (Fig. 9-3/14,15). The second plantar common digital artery supplies the axial plantar proper a. of digit 2 and the abaxial plantar proper a. of digit 3. The third plantar common digital a. anastomoses with the third dorsal common digital a. in the intertrochlear notch. From these, the axial plantar proper aa. of digits 3 and 4 arise. The fourth plantar common digital a. (Fig. 9-3/16) is the direct continuation of the lateral plantar a. It supplies the abaxial plantar proper a. of digit 4 and the axial plantar proper a. of digit 5. A number of branches from the plantar proper digital aa. arise which course to the dorsal aspect of the digits.

Veins of the Pelvic Limb

Most of the veins of the pelvic limb parallel arterial channels and assume the same name as their arterial counterparts. The superficial venous channels which can be identified medially and laterally in the crus are the medial and lateral saphenous veins and their branches. The lateral saphenous vein is larger than the medial saphenous vein in the dog and ox, while the medial vein is larger in the cat and horse.

---

*At the emergence of the plantar aspect of the pes, the bovine perforating tarsal a. is termed the third proximal perforating branch. Dorsally, this vessel enters the tarsal canal by penetrating between T2+3 and TC+4 (actually it passes between the T3 and T4 components of these bones). Plantarly, it emerges from an unnamed canal near the proximal end of Mt3+4 (Fig. 9-3).

Figure 9-2

Major Arteries of the Equine Pes (left limb)

    A.   Dorsal aspect

    B.   Plantar aspect

1. Cranial tibial a.
2. Dorsal pedal a.
3. Perforating tarsal a. (entering the tarsal canal)*
4. Third dorsal metatarsal a.
5. Caudal tibial a.
6. Caudal branch of saphenous a.
7. Medial plantar a. (second plantar common digital a.)
8. Lateral plantar a. (third plantar common digital a.)
9. Deep plantar arch
10. Medial (second) plantar metatarsal a.
11. Lateral (third) plantar metatarsal a.
12. Distal perforating branch (of third dorsal metatarsal a.)
13. Lateral digital a. (lateral plantar proper digital a.)
14. Medial digital a. (medial plantar proper digital a.)

*The tarsal canal is a neurovascular passageway between the third and fourth tarsal bones. It does not transmit tendons (in contrast to its thoracic limb counterpart, the carpal canal).

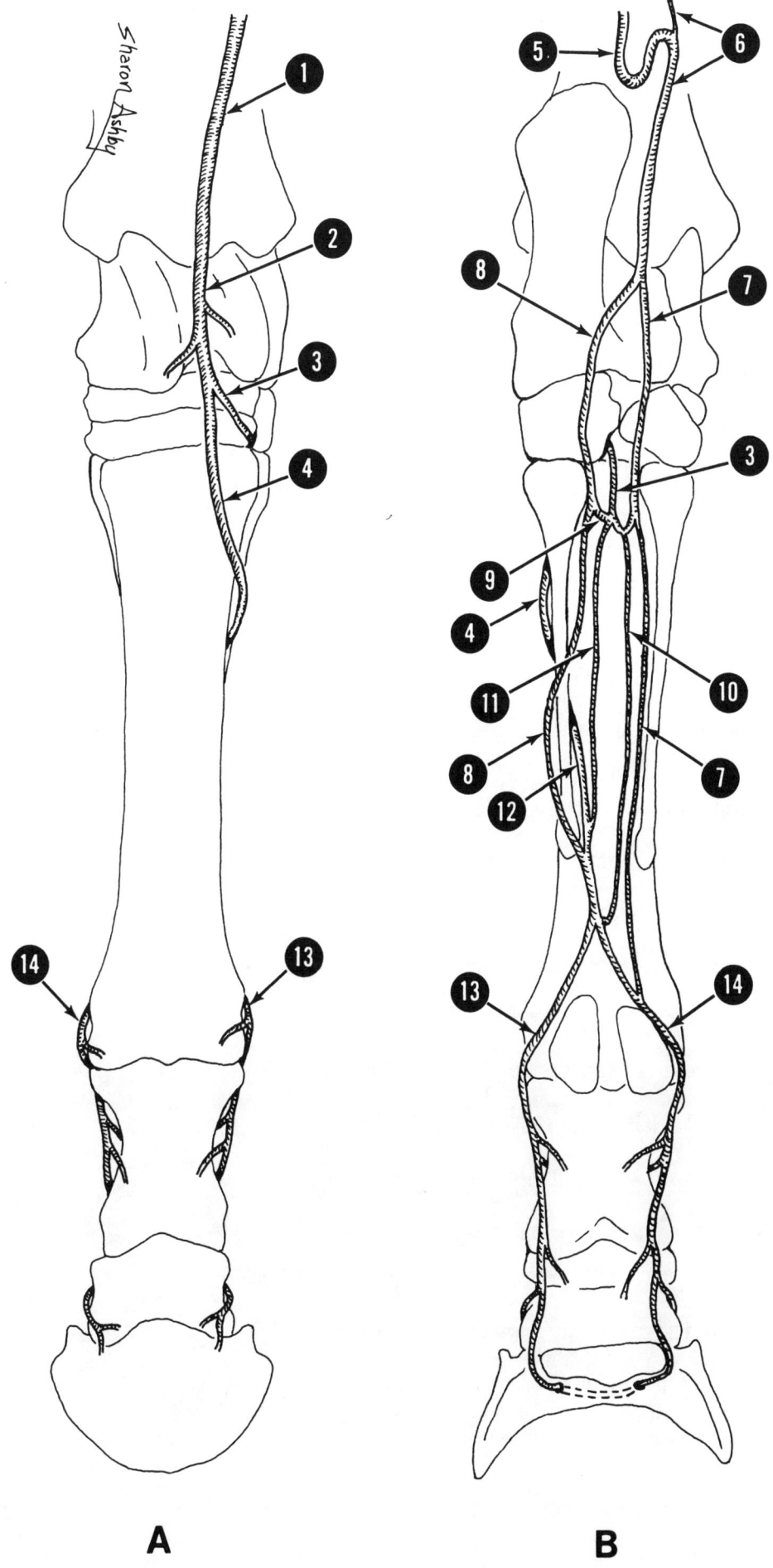

A   B

Figure 9-3

Major Arteries of the Bovine Pes (left limb)

    A.   Dorsal aspect

    B.   Plantar aspect

1. Cranial tibial a.
2. Dorsal pedal a.
3. Perforating tarsal a.
4. Third dorsal metatarsal a.
5. Distal perforating branch
6. Third dorsal common digital a.
7. Saphenous a.
8. Lateral plantar a.
9. Medial plantar a.
10. Third proximal perforating branch (this is the name of the plantar emergence of the perforating tarsal a.--number 3 above)
11. Second plantar metatarsal a.
12. Third plantar metatarsal a.
13. Fourth plantar metatarsal a.
14. Second plantar common digital a.
15. Third plantar common digital a.
16. Fourth plantar common digital a.
17. Axial plantar proper a. of digit 2
18. Abaxial plantar proper a. of digit 3
19. Axial plantar proper aa. of digits 3 and 4
20. Abaxial plantar proper a. of digit 4
21. Axial plantar proper a. of digit 5

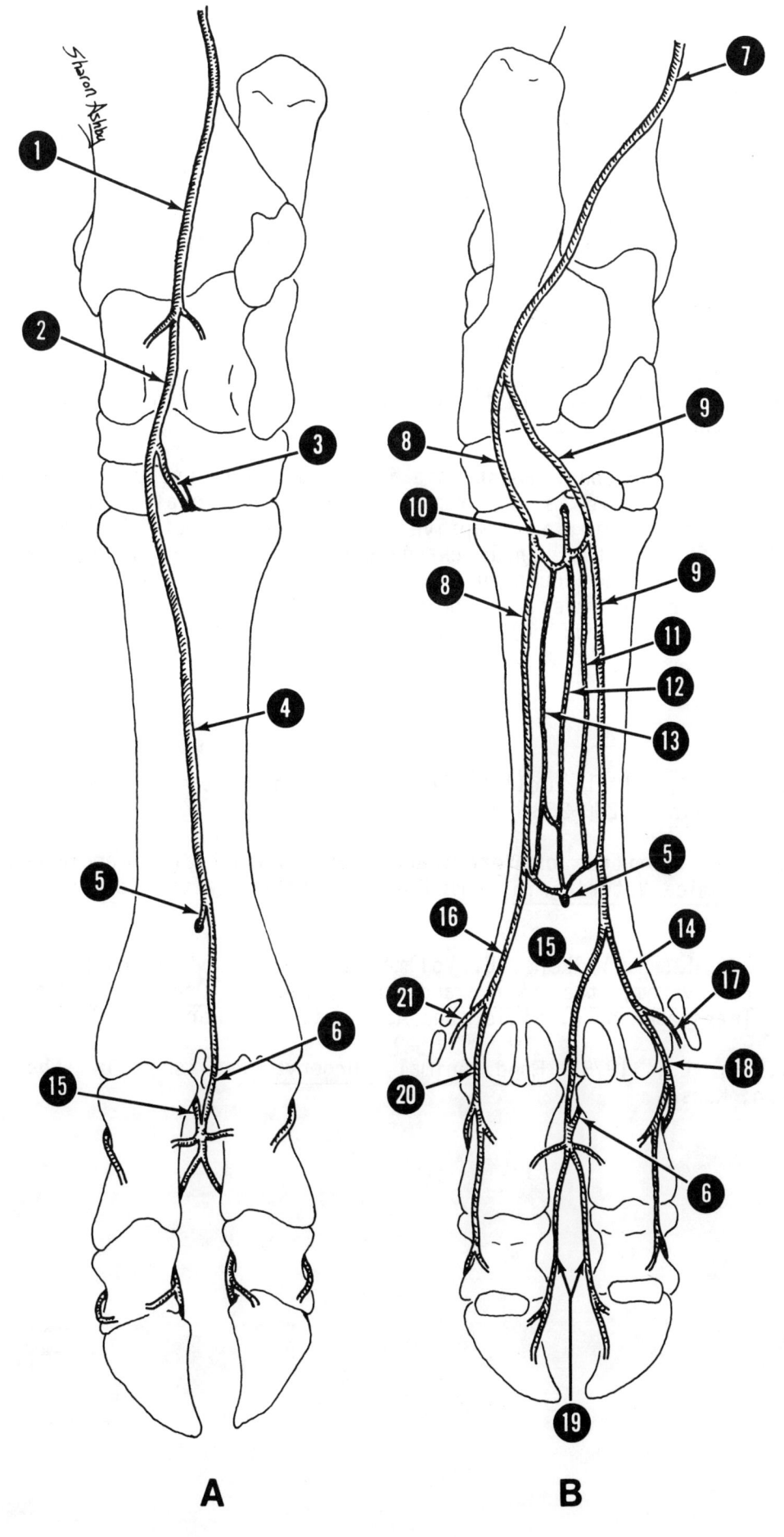

The lateral saphenous vein in the dog is often used for venipunctures if the cephalic vein cannot be used. It is sometimes difficult to thread because it is bound so loosely in the subcutaneous tissues. In the cat, the medial saphenous v. (femoral v. if very proximal) may be used for venipunctures. In both the dog and cat, these alternate sites are poor choices for blood sampling because of their small caliber. The external jugular vein or cephalic vein is usually used instead.

In the horse, the large vein which crosses the superficial aspect of the medial branch of the tendon of insertion of the cranial tibial muscle ("cunean" tendon) is the cranial branch of the medial saphenous v. The segment of it distal to the tarsus is the largest vein of the metatarsus (dorsal common digital vein 2).

Intravenous regional anesthesia is occasionally useful in surgeries of the distal limb. This is performed by injecting local anesthetic into a distal vein and holding it "captive" with a tourniquet [4]. The effect is improved by forcing the venous channels empty with a tight elastic bandage before putting on the tourniquet and before injecting the anesthetic. The venipuncture for the injection, however, should be made before emptying the veins since they are difficult to thread when collapsed.

References

1. Cummings, B. C., 1961. Collateral circulation of the canine pelvic limb. Small Anim. Clin. 1:260-268.

2. International Committee on Veterinary Gross Anatomical Nomenclature, 1983. Nomina Anatomica Veterinaria, third ed. Published by the Committee, Ithaca, New York.

3. Schummer, A. H., H. Wilkens, B. Vollmerhaus, and K. H. Habermehl. 1981. The Circulatory System, the Skin, and the Cutaneous Organs of the Domestic Mammals. Translated by W. Siller and A. Wight. Paul Parey, Berlin.

4. Noordsy, J. L., 1978. Food Animal Surgery. Published by the author, Manhattan, Kansas.

PELVIC LIMB NEUROLOGY

I. LUMBOSACRAL PLEXUS

The lumbosacral plexus is formed by the ventral branches of the lumbar and sacral spinal nerves. The ventral branches of the first three or four pairs of the lumbar nerves are distributed primarily to the abdominal wall and are given specific names as follows [1]:

Nerve	Animals with six pairs* of lumbar nn. (horse, ox)	Animals with seven pairs* of lumbar nn. (carnivores)
L1	iliohypogastric n.	cranial iliohypogastric n.
L2	ilioinguinal n.	caudal iliohypogastric n.
L3	genitofemoral and lateral cutaneous femoral nn.	ilioinguinal n.
L4	--------------------	genitofemoral and lateral cutaneous femoral nn.

Of these four, the ones most significant in local or regional anesthesia for standing flank surgery are the ventral branches of L1, L2, and the last thoracic spinal nerve (see Chapter 18). The other nerves derived from the lumbosacral plexus are the named nerves which are distributed primarily to the pelvic limb. As with the brachial plexus in the thoracic limb, the pattern of the lumbosacral plexus varies among species and individuals [2]. Therefore, no attempt will be made to equate exactly which segments of the cord give rise to which named derivatives.

II. MAJOR NERVES OF THE PELVIC LIMB (Figs. 10-1, 10-2, 10-3)

Most of the nerves which supply the pelvic limb are derivatives of the lumbosacral plexus. In addition to the named branches of the first four lumbar nerves noted above, these derivatives include:

A. femoral n.
B. obturator n.
C. cranial gluteal n.
D. caudal gluteal n.
E. caudal cutaneous femoral n.
F. caudal clunial nn.
G. ischiatic (sciatic) n.
  1. tibial n.
  2. common peroneal nerve
H. pudendal n.
I. caudal rectal nn., branch to the coccygeal m., branch to the levator ani m.

Of these, the femoral and obturator nerves are generally considered to be derivatives of the lumbar segment of the lumbosacral plexus and the others form the sacral component [1]. However, parts of several may have some caudal

---

*Pigs, sheep, and goats may have either six or seven pairs of lumbar nn. corresponding to their individual vertebral formulae.

lumbar input. The most clinically important nerves of the pelvic limb are the femoral, obturator, and ischiatic nerves (including the common peroneal n. and the tibial n. which are branches of the ischiatic nerve). Approximate lumbosacral fiber contributions to these nerves are as follows (as presented by Habel [3]):

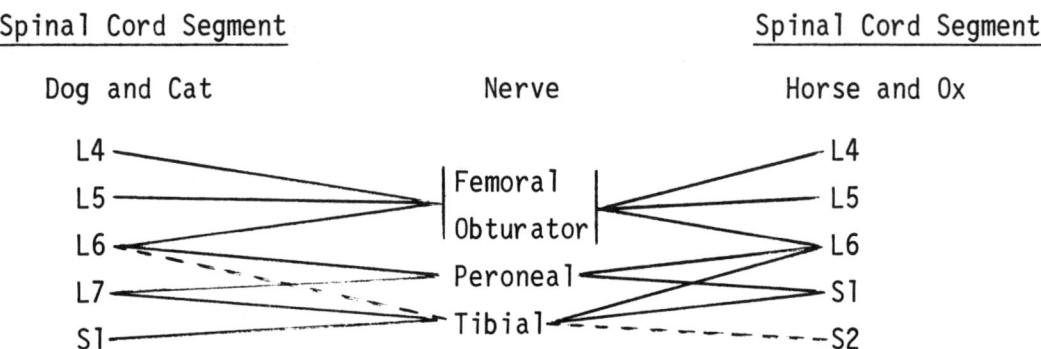

As in the thoracic limb, a working knowledge of the nerves of the pelvic limb should include the muscle groups they supply, the general areas of cutaneous distribution, and their location in regard to major muscles and bony prominences. This knowledge will aid in the diagnosis of neuropathies, will help prevent iatrogenic nerve damage during surgical procedures, and is necessary to perform and interpret diagnostic and surgical nerve blocks.

A. Femoral Nerve

The femoral nerve supplies the cranial thigh muscles (quadriceps femoris and iliopsoas). Its superficial branch (the saphenous n.) supplies the sartorius muscle and is distributed cutaneously to the medial side of the limb. The main part of the femoral nerve enters the quadriceps femoris between the rectus femoris and vastus medialis heads, and its saphenous nerve branch continues distally in a subcutaneous position. Femoral nerve disruption results in passive flexion of the genual joint and inability to bear weight on the limb. There is also a sensory deficit on the medial aspect of the limb because of loss of the saphenous nerve [3,4].

B. Obturator Nerve

The obturator nerve passes through the obturator foramen. It supplies most of the medial thigh muscles (all but the sartorius) as well as the external obturator m. The intrapelvic portion of the obturator nerve is susceptible to contusion injuries during parturition (especially in ruminants) and is cited as one cause of post-parturient "downer-cows" [5]. These animals may recover uneventfully. Contrary to popular belief, they are often able to stand, but they have difficulty rising from a prone position. An experimental study has indicated that the sciatic nerve may also be involved and that the contusion during parturition may involve lumbosacral components of both nerves [6]. The obturator nerve has generally been considered to have no cutaneous distribution, but a small cutaneous branch to the medial thigh has been described [7]. In carnivores, the part supplying the gracilis is subject to injury in pectineal myotomies or myectomies. Section of the obturator nerve in dogs produces an inability to prevent abduction when on a slick surface [4].

C. Cranial Gluteal Nerve

The cranial gluteal nerve passes through the greater ischiatic foramen (notch in carnivores). It supplies the middle and deep gluteals and the tensor fasciae latae. It has no cutaneous distribution. Surgeons should preserve this nerve during approaches to the hip which involve gluteal tenomyotomies.

D. Caudal Gluteal Nerve

The caudal gluteal nerve courses through the greater ischiatic foramen (notch in carnivores). It supplies the superficial gluteal muscle, and in some species it also supplies the piriformis, parts of the biceps femoris, semitendinosus, and parts of the other gluteal muscles. It has no cutaneous distribution except that in some species the caudal cutaneous femoral n. may arise from it.

E. Caudal Cutaneous Femoral Nerve

The caudal cutaneous femoral nerve is a branch of the lumbosacral plexus, but it may arise in common with the pudendal, ischiatic, or caudal gluteal nn. in various species. It is sensory over the caudal thigh region.

F. Caudal Clunial Nerves

The caudal clunial nerves (from the sacral part of the lumbosacral plexus) are closely associated with the caudal cutaneous femoral n. and are cutaneously distributed. They are too small for gross differentiation and have no clinical significance other than supplying small cutaneous dermatomes. (The cranial and middle clunial nerves are not branches of the lumbosacral plexus--they are derived from <u>dorsal</u> branches of the lumbar and sacral spinal nerves.)

G. Ischiatic (Sciatic) Nerve

The ischiatic nerve is the largest nerve arising from the lumbosacral plexus. It emerges through the greater ischiatic foramen (ischiatic notch) and passes dorsally over the coxal joint and then courses distally on the caudolateral aspect of the thigh, deep to the biceps femoris. Proximal to the genual joint, it divides into the tibial and common peroneal nerves. The ischiatic nerve supplies the caudal thigh muscles and the caudal hip muscles (except the external obturator). Disruption of the proximal part of the sciatic nerve results in paralysis of the caudal thigh muscles and all muscles distal to the genual joint. The limb does not collapse because the femoral nerve is intact to the quadriceps femoris muscle, but the tarsus is unstable [4]. To insure

Figure 10-1

Nerves of the Canine Pelvic Limb (medial aspect)

1. Ventral branches of L5-7
2. Ventral branches of S1-3
3. Cranial gluteal nerve
4. Caudal gluteal nerve
5. Pelvic nerve
6. Caudal rectal nerve
7. Caudal cutaneous femoral nerve
8. Perineal nerve
9. Pudendal nerve
10. Sciatic nerve
11. Muscular branches of the sciatic nerve
12. Tibial nerve
13. Common peroneal nerve
14. Caudal cutaneous sural nerve
15. Lateral plantar nerve
16. Medial plantar nerve
17. Superficial peroneal nerve
18. Saphenous nerve (caudal branch)
19. Deep peroneal nerve
20. Saphenous nerve
21. Femoral nerve
22. Obturator nerve

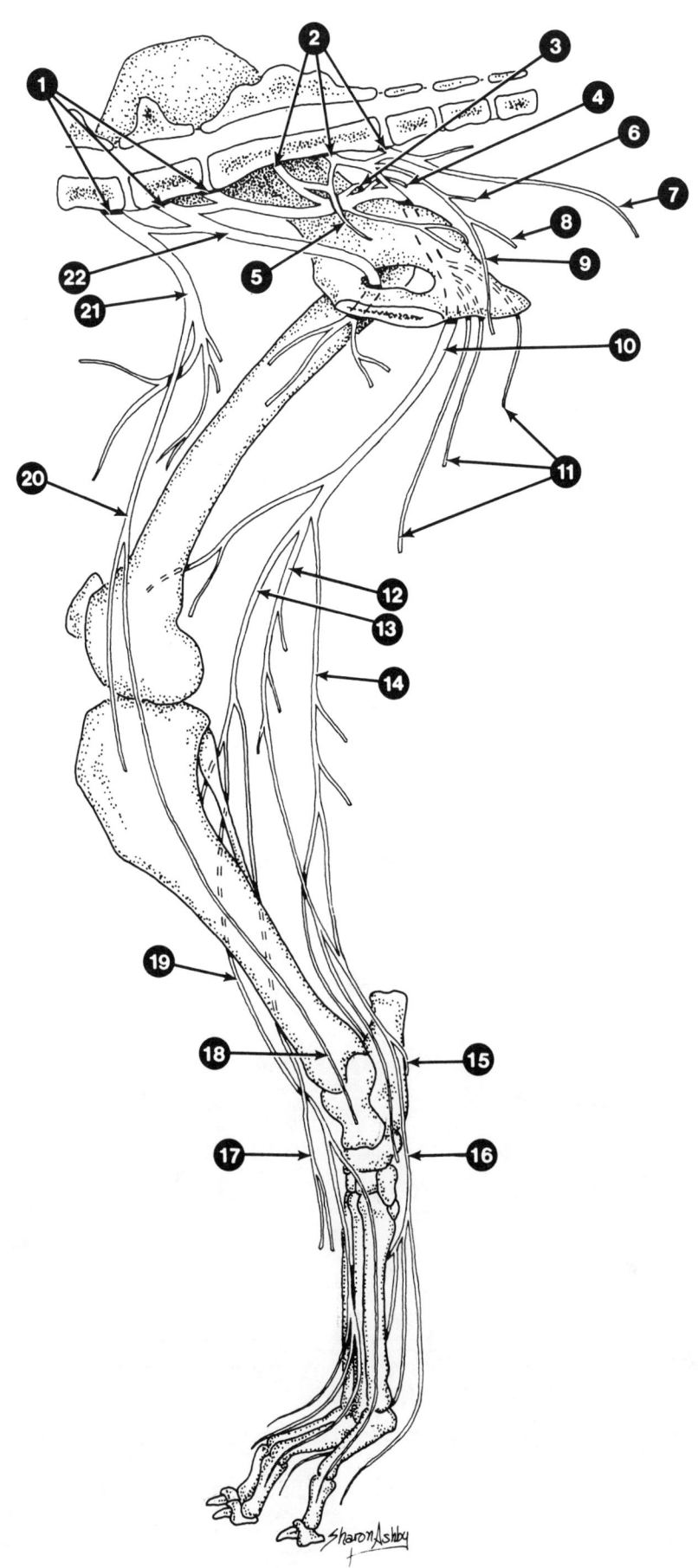

Figure 10-2

Nerves of the Equine Pelvic Limb (medial aspect)

1. Ventral branch of L6
2. Ventral branches of S1-4
3. Caudal rectal nerve
4. Cutaneous branch of caudal rectal nerve
5. Branches to external anal sphincter m.
6. Pudendal nerve
7. Deep perineal nerve
8. Dorsal nerve of penis (clitoris)
9. Preputial (mammary) branch of pudendal nerve
10. Pelvic nerve
11. Sciatic nerve
12. Muscular branches of sciatic nerve
13. Femoral nerve
14. Cranial gluteal nerve
15. Obturator nerve
16. Branches of femoral nerve to quadriceps femoris m.
17. Saphenous nerve
18. Common peroneal nerve
19. Tibial nerve
20. Caudal cutaneous sural nerve
21. Superficial peroneal nerve
22. Deep peroneal nerve
23. Lateral plantar nerve (plantar common digital n. 3)
24. Medial plantar nerve (plantar common digital n. 2)
25. Dorsal metatarsal nerve 2
26. Deep branch of lateral plantar nerve
27. Communicating branch
28. Medial (second) plantar metatarsal nerve
29. Medial plantar (proper) digital nerve
30. Dorsal branch of medial plantar digital nerve

Used with permission of Dr. J. E. Smallwood

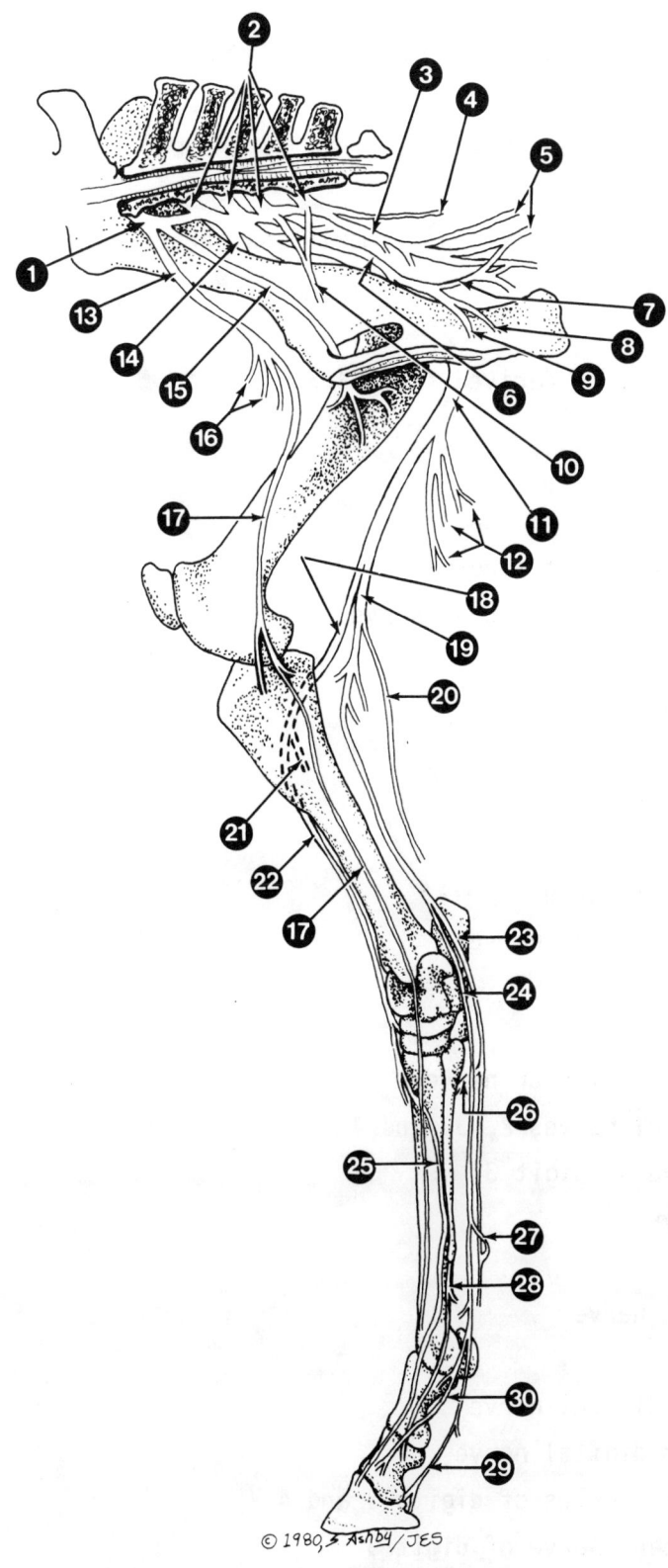

Figure 10-3

Nerves of the Bovine Pelvic Limb (medial aspect)

1. Roots of the lumbosacral plexus derived from L5 and L6
2. Femoral nerve
3. Branches of femoral n. to quadriceps femoris and sartorius mm.
4. Saphenous nerve
5. Obturator nerve
6. Roots of the sacral plexus derived from S1-S5
7. Cranial gluteal nerve
8. Caudal rectal nerve
9. Pudendal nerve
10. Proximal cutaneous branch of pudendal nerve
11. Distal cutaneous branch of pudendal nerve
12. Deep perineal nerve
13. Dorsal nerve of penis (clitoris)
14. Sciatic nerve
15. Muscular branches of sciatic nerve
16. Tibial nerve
17. Caudal cutaneous sural nerve
18. Muscular branches of tibial nerve
19. Lateral plantar nerve
20. Medial plantar nerve
21. Deep branch of lateral plantar nerve
22. Plantar common digital nerves 2, 3, and 4
23. Abaxial plantar nerve of digit 3
24. Common peroneal nerve
25. Muscular branches
26. Superficial peroneal nerve
27. Deep peroneal nerve
28. Third dorsal common digital nerve
29. Second dorsal common digital nerve
30. Axial dorsal (proper) nerves of digits 3 and 4
31. Abaxial dorsal (proper) nerve of digit 3

Used with permission of Dr. J. E. Smallwood

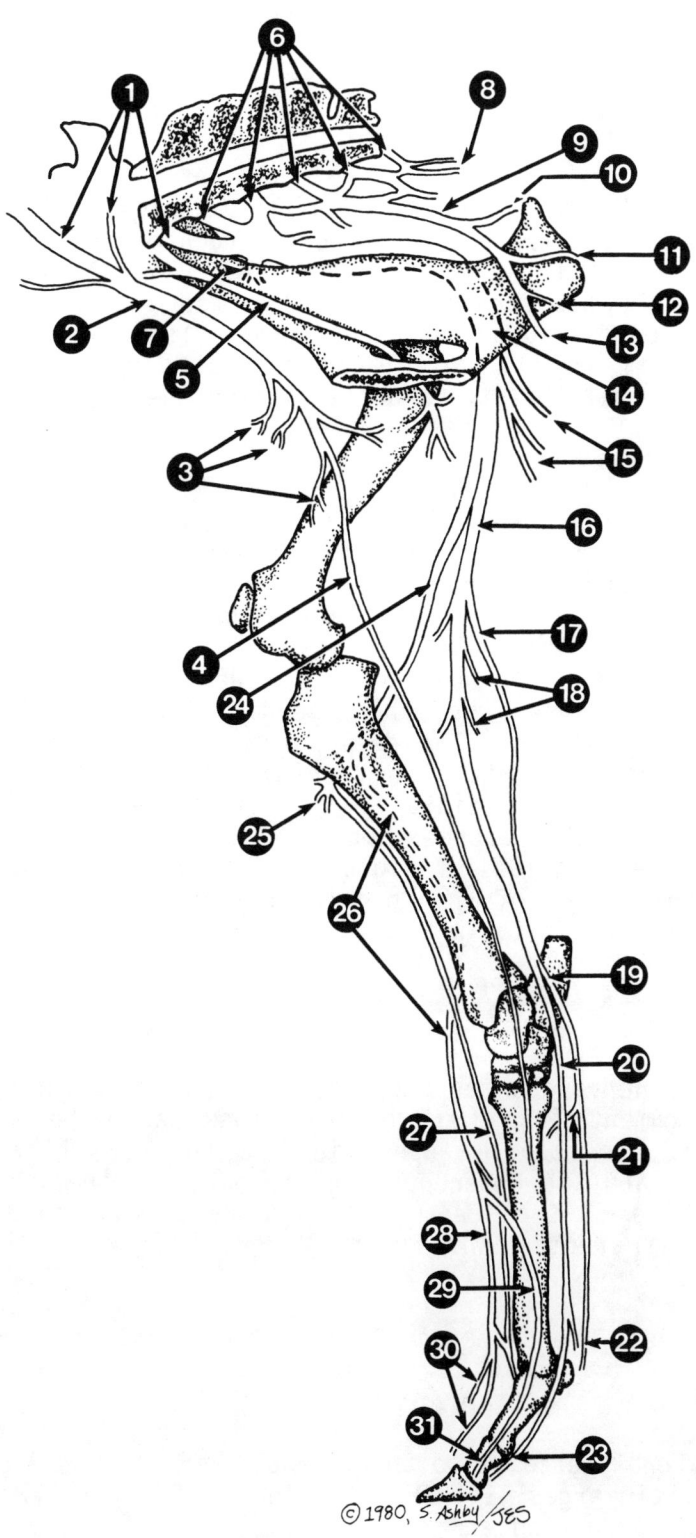

that a retrograded pin emerging at the trochanteric fossa of the femur does not injure the sciatic nerve, the limb should be adducted, and the cranial aspect of the thigh should be rolled medially (internally rotated or pronated) [8].* During its course down the caudolateral thigh, the sciatic nerve lies deep to the biceps femoris m. and it is susceptible to injury from misplaced intramuscular injections.

1. Tibial nerve

   The tibial nerve courses caudally to enter the caudal crus muscles between the two heads of the gastrocnemius. It supplies the caudal muscles of the crus** and is sensory to the skin over the caudal crus and plantar pes. A major named branch of the tibial nerve is the caudal cutaneous sural nerve. Disruption of the tibial nerve (proximal to its muscular branches) causes a drop at the tarsal joint and inability to actively flex the digital joints [4].

2. Common peroneal nerve

   The common peroneal nerve courses cranially to supply the craniolateral crus muscles and is sensory to the skin over the craniolateral crus and dorsal pes. It supplies several muscular and cutaneous branches including the lateral cutaneous sural nerve (see Part IV below). The main distal continuations of the common peroneal nerve are the deep peroneal nerve (which is primarily distributed to muscles) and the superficial peroneal nerve (which is primarily cutaneous). The deep peroneal nerve courses distally in close association with the cranial tibial a. The superficial peroneal nerve courses distally in a more superficial position. Disruption of the peroneal nerve (proximal to its muscular branches) results in loss of digital extension and the animal often stands on the dorsum of the knuckled digits. The animal may learn to compensate by "flipping" the foot as happens in low radial paralysis [4].

H. Pudendal Nerve

   The pudendal nerve courses caudally in close association with the sacrotuberous ligament (dog [9]) or the broad sacrotuberous ligament (ungulates [10]). Its major branches include the dorsal nerve of the penis or clitoris and the cutaneously distributed perineal nn. It also sends some branches to the scrotum and mammary glands and it may give rise to the caudal rectal nn. Pudendal nerve block is discussed in Chapter 15.

I. Caudal Rectal Nerves, Branch to the Coccygeal Muscles, and Branch to the Levator Ani

---

*Some surgeons prefer to extend the joint so that the pin will course approximately parallel to the nerve as it emerges. Either extension or flexion will work, and neither is as important as adduction and pronation. (See the discussion of this subject in Chapter 8, paragraph II.B.6.)

**When unmodified, the term crus refers to the portion of the pelvic limb between the genual joint and the tarsus. This use of crus is not to be confused with portions of the diaphragm, penis, and clitoris which bear the same name.

The caudal rectal nerves supply the external anal sphincter, and they may also supply some other branches to the anal region. In some species, these nerves have a small cutaneous distribution [10]. The caudal rectal nn. can be damaged in anal sac resections, resulting in paresis or paralysis of the external anal sphincter m. The branches to the coccygeal and levator ani mm. originate from the sacral nerves directly in the dog [9], but in the ungulates they are combined with the caudal rectal nn.

The nerves which supply the tail are the caudal nerves. They do not technically belong to the lumbosacral plexus since they are derived from the caudal segments of the spinal cord.

III. NERVE SUPPLY TO THE PES

The specific details of the nerves in the pes have little clinical application in the carnivores and pig. In the horse and ox, the patterns vary sufficiently to warrant separate descriptions.

A. Nerve Supply to the Pes of the Horse (Fig. 10-4)

The major nerve supply to the tarsus, metatarsus, and digit of the horse is derived from the tibial and peroneal nerves. Additionally, the saphenous nerve has some distribution to this region.

The tibial nerve divides proximal to the tarsus into the medial and lateral plantar nerves (second and third plantar common digital nerves - Fig. 10-4/9,10) [10]. These large nerves are homologous to the medial and lateral palmar nerves of the thoracic limb. They pass through the flexor canal and course distally down the metatarsus on either side of the flexor tendons. In the proximal metatarsus, the lateral plantar nerve supplies a deep branch (Fig. 10-4/11) which is distributed to the interosseous m. and also gives rise to the small medial and lateral plantar metatarsal nerves. In the distal metatarsus, a communicating branch (smaller and less consistent than that in the thoracic limb) courses superficially and obliquely across the flexor tendons from the medial plantar nerve to the lateral plantar nerve (Fig. 10-4/14). At the metatarsophalangeal joints, the medial and lateral plantar nerves become the medial and lateral plantar (proper) digital nerves. The term proper is often dropped in everyday usage. These digital nerves have dorsal branches similar to their thoracic limb counterparts. In fact, the whole pattern of distribution is very similar to that of the thoracic limb. The plantar nerves and plantar metatarsal nerves of the pelvic limb are homologous to the palmar nerves and palmar metacarpal nerves of the thoracic limb; the deep branch of the lateral plantar nerve is homologous to the deep branch of the lateral palmar nerve (or more properly, deep branch of the ulnar nerve, etc.). For the details of distribution of these nerves, see the appropriate section on thoracic limb neurology. The plantar nerves supply slightly less of the digit than their thoracic limb counterparts and the difference is partly due to the distal extent of the dorsal metatarsal nerves (see below).

On the dorsum of the pes, branches of the superficial peroneal n. ramify over the dorsal and lateral aspect of the metatarsus as far distally as the metatarsophalangeal joint (Fig. 10-4/1). The deep

Figure 10-4

Nerves of the Equine Pes (left limb)

    A. Dorsal aspect

    B. Plantar aspect

1. Superficial peroneal nerve
2. Deep peroneal nerve
3. Caudal cutaneous sural nerve
4. Saphenous nerve
5. Branch of deep peroneal nerve which accompanies perforating tarsal artery
6. Medial (second) dorsal metatarsal nerve
7. Lateral (third) dorsal metatarsal nerve
8. Tibial nerve
9. Medial plantar nerve
10. Lateral plantar nerve
11. Deep branch of lateral plantar nerve
12. Medial plantar metatarsal nerve
13. Lateral plantar metatarsal nerve
14. Communicating branch
15. Medial plantar (proper) digital nerve
16. Lateral plantar (proper) digital nerve
17. Dorsal branch of medial plantar (proper) digital nerve
18. Dorsal branch of lateral plantar (proper) digital nerve
19. Muscular branch to interosseous m.

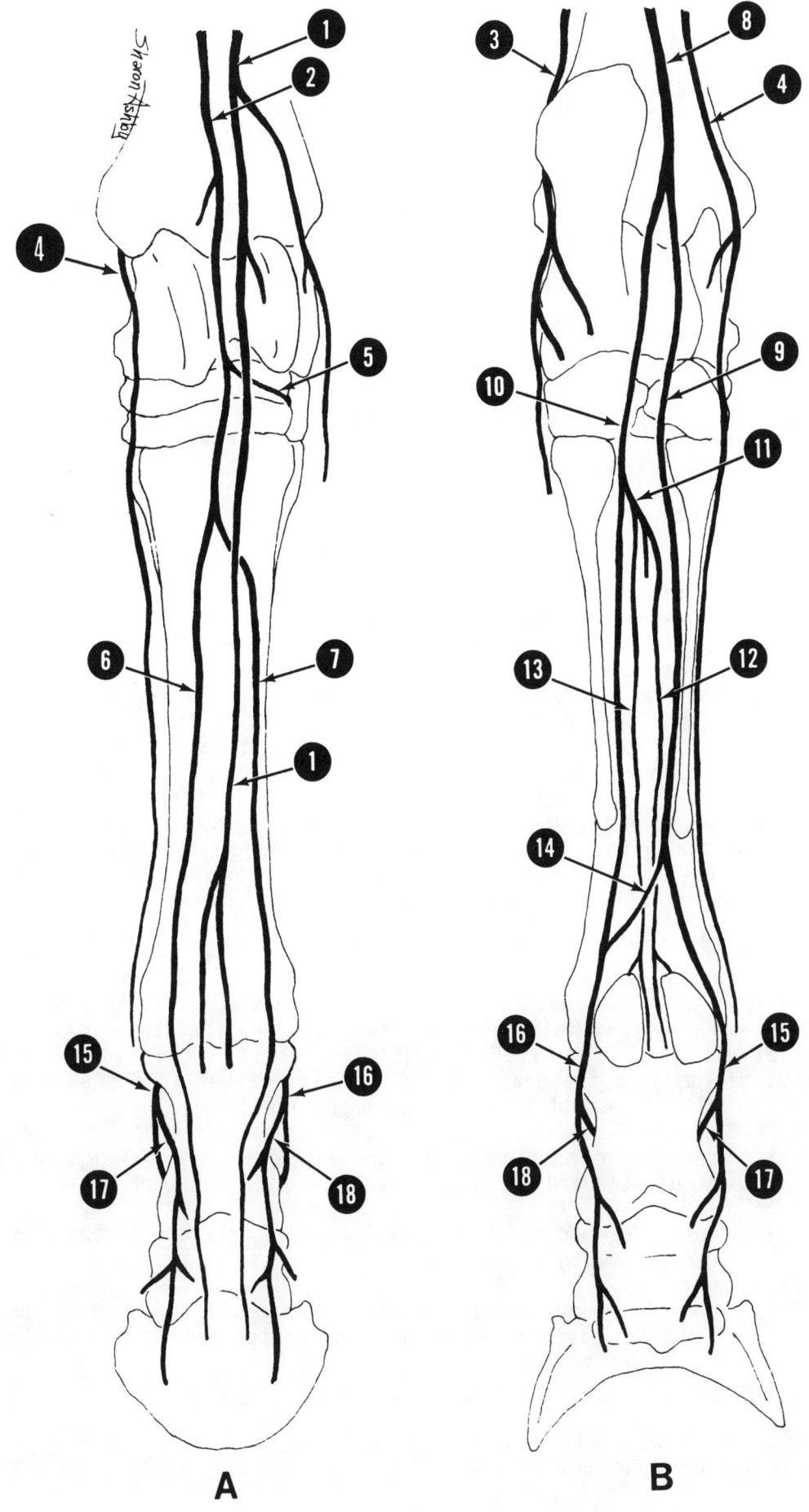

peroneal nerve supplies some branches to tarsal structures including a branch which accompanies the perforating tarsal artery. It also divides near this point into the medial and lateral dorsal metatarsal nerves. (Fig. 10-4/6,7). The medial dorsal metatarsal nerve courses distally on the dorsomedial aspect of the metatarsus closely applied to the third metatarsal bone. It continues distally to the coronary region where it innervates the dorsal part of the laminar and coronary corium, and it may communicate with the medial plantar metatarsal nerve. The lateral dorsal metatarsal nerve follows the third dorsal metatarsal artery distally until the artery penetrates to the plantar side. From this level, it continues distally, unaccompanied, on the lateral aspect of the metatarsus in a manner similar to its medial counterpart. These dorsal metatarsal nerves innervate the dorsal parts of the interphalangeal joints.

The only nerve yet undescribed which is distributed to the pes is the saphenous nerve which continues down the medial aspect of the metatarsus as far as the metatarsophalangeal joint (Fig. 10-4/4).

B. Nerve Supply to the Pes of the Ox (Fig. 10-5)

Proximal to the tarsus, the tibial nerve divides into the medial and lateral plantar nerves (Fig. 10-5/15,16). These course distally on the plantar aspect of the metatarsus adjacent to the flexor tendons. In the proximal metatarsus, the lateral plantar nerve gives rise to a deep branch which supplies the interosseous muscle. (Fig. 10-5/17). Further distally the lateral plantar nerve becomes the fourth plantar common digital nerve. The major distal continuation of this nerve is the abaxial plantar proper nerve of digit 4, but it also gives rise to a small plantar proper nerve to digit 5.* The medial plantar nerve divides in the distal metatarsus into the second and third plantar common digital nerves (Fig. 10-5/19,20). The second plantar common digital nerve divides into a small plantar proper nerve to digit 2* and an abaxial plantar proper nerve to digit 3. The third plantar common digital nerve divides into the axial plantar proper nerves of digits 3 and 4.

On the dorsal aspect of the pes, the superficial peroneal nerve gives rise to the dorsal common digital nerve 4 (Fig. 10-5/3) and about mid-metatarsus the remaining nerve trunk divides into the dorsal common digital nerves 2 and 3 (Fig. 10-5/4,5). These three common digital nerves divide into the dorsal proper digital nerves in the same manner as on the plantar aspect of the limb. Specifically:

1. dorsal common digital nerve 2 supplies a dorsal proper nerve of digit 2 and an abaxial dorsal proper nerve of digit 3.

2. dorsal common digital nerve 3 divides into axial dorsal proper nerves of digits 3 and 4.

3. dorsal common digital nerve 4 divides into a dorsal proper nerve of digit 5 and an abaxial dorsal proper nerve of digit 4.

---

*Since digits 2 and 5 have only one plantar proper nerve, the modifying <u>axial</u> is not necessary to its designation.

To summarize the digital nerve supply, all of the plantar digital nerves are derivatives of the tibial nerve and all of the dorsal digital nerves are derivatives of the peroneal nerve. There are, however, some communications between dorsal and plantar nerves.

The deep peroneal nerve continues distally down the metatarsus as the third dorsal metatarsal nerve (Fig. 10-5/6). It sends communicating branches through the intertrochlear notch to the plantar proper nerves of digits 3 and 4. Some dorsal-plantar communicating branches are present on some of the other digital nerves as well.

Branches of the saphenous nerve are distributed to the plantaromedial aspect of the proximal metatarsus and branches of the caudal cutaneous sural nerve are distributed to the plantarolateral aspect. These do not contribute to the digital innervation.

IV. SENSORY DERMATOMES OF THE PELVIC LIMB (Fig. 10-6)

As in the thoracic limb, familiarity with the sensory dermatomes is of value in the diagnosis of neuropathies and in checking the effectiveness of surgical and diagnostic nerve blocks. Junctions of one dermatome with another are not precise and considerable overlap occurs in some areas. Only three direct branches of the lumbosacral plexus are given a cutaneous designation: lateral cutaneous femoral n., the caudal cutaneous femoral n., and the caudal clunial nn. The other cutaneous nerves which supply the pelvic limb are derivatives of larger nerves that have other (motor) distributions. The major cutaneous nerves of the pelvic limb and their origins are listed below. The areas of their distribution vary somewhat among the species, but basic generalities are present (Fig. 10-6) [10].

A. Lateral cutaneous femoral n.--from the lumbosacral plexus (lumbar part)

B. Caudal cutaneous femoral n.--from the lumbosacral plexus (sacral part)

C. Cranial clunial nn.*--from the lateral parts of the dorsal branches of lumbar nerves

D. Middle clunial nn.*--from the lateral parts of the dorsal branches of sacral nerves

E. Caudal clunial nn.*--from the lumbosacral plexus (sacral part)

F. Cutaneous branch of the saphenous n. - from the saphenous nerve which is, in turn, a branch of the femoral nerve. The saphenous nerve also has a muscular branch which supplies the sartorius m.

G. Lateral cutaneous sural n.--from the common peroneal nerve

H. Cutaneous branches of the superficial peroneal n.

---

*The clunial nerves are distributed to the dorsal and dorsolateral aspect of the lumbar and gluteal regions and to the caudal aspect of the thigh.

Figure 10-5

Nerve Supply to the Pes of the Ox (left limb)

    A.   Dorsal aspect

    B.   Plantar aspect

1. Superficial peroneal nerve
2. Deep peroneal nerve
3. Fourth dorsal common digital nerve
4. Second dorsal common digital nerve
5. Third dorsal common digital nerve
6. Third dorsal metatarsal nerve
7. Dorsal proper nerve of digit 2
8. Abaxial dorsal proper nerve of digit 3
9. Axial dorsal proper nerves of digits 3 and 4
10. Abaxial dorsal proper nerve of digit 4
11. Dorsal proper nerve of digit 5
12. Tibial nerve
13. Saphenous nerve
14. Caudal cutaneous sural nerve
15. Medial plantar nerve
16. Lateral plantar nerve
17. Deep branch of lateral plantar nerve
18. Fourth plantar common digital nerve
19. Third plantar common digital nerve
20. Second plantar common digital nerve
21. Plantar proper nerve of digit 2
22. Abaxial plantar proper nerve of digit 3
23. Axial plantar proper nerves of digits 3 and 4
24. Abaxial plantar proper nerve of digit 4
25. Plantar proper nerve of digit 5
26. Injection site for blocking the branches of the superficial peroneal n. The third dorsal metatarsal nerve may be blocked through the same cutaneous puncture.
27. Injection sites for blocking the medial and lateral plantar nn.

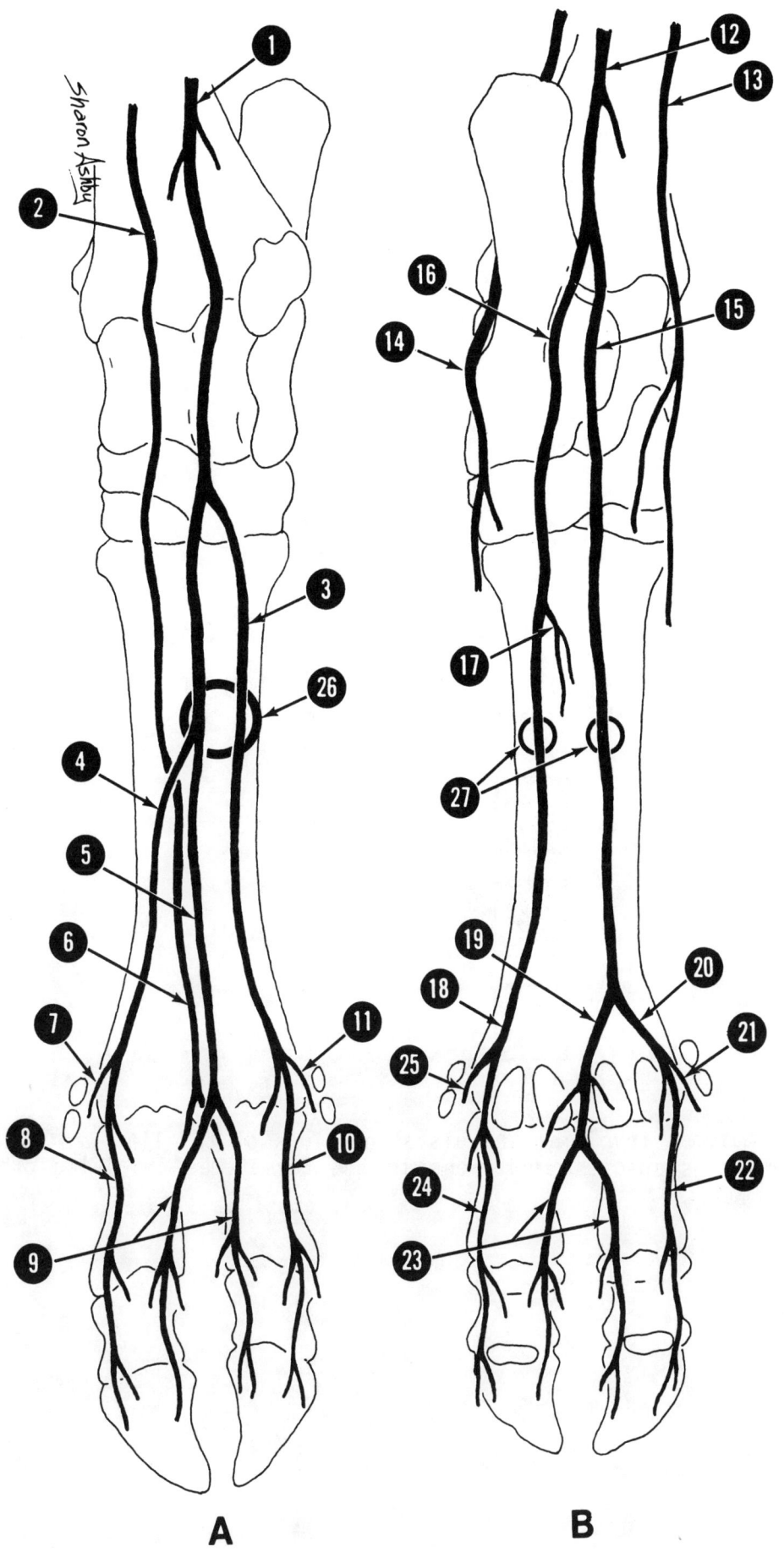

Figure 10-6

Cutaneous Dermatomes of the Pelvic Limbs of the Horse (A), Ox (B), and Dog (C).

(Lateral aspects are illustrated at the left of the figure
and medial aspects are shown at the right.*)

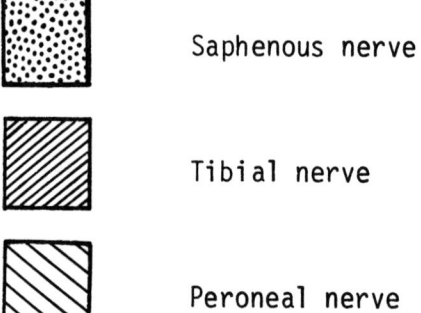

Saphenous nerve

Tibial nerve

Peroneal nerve

*Only the dermatomes involving the distal portions of the limb are shown because there are numerous species variations in the dermatomes involving other nerves further proximally.

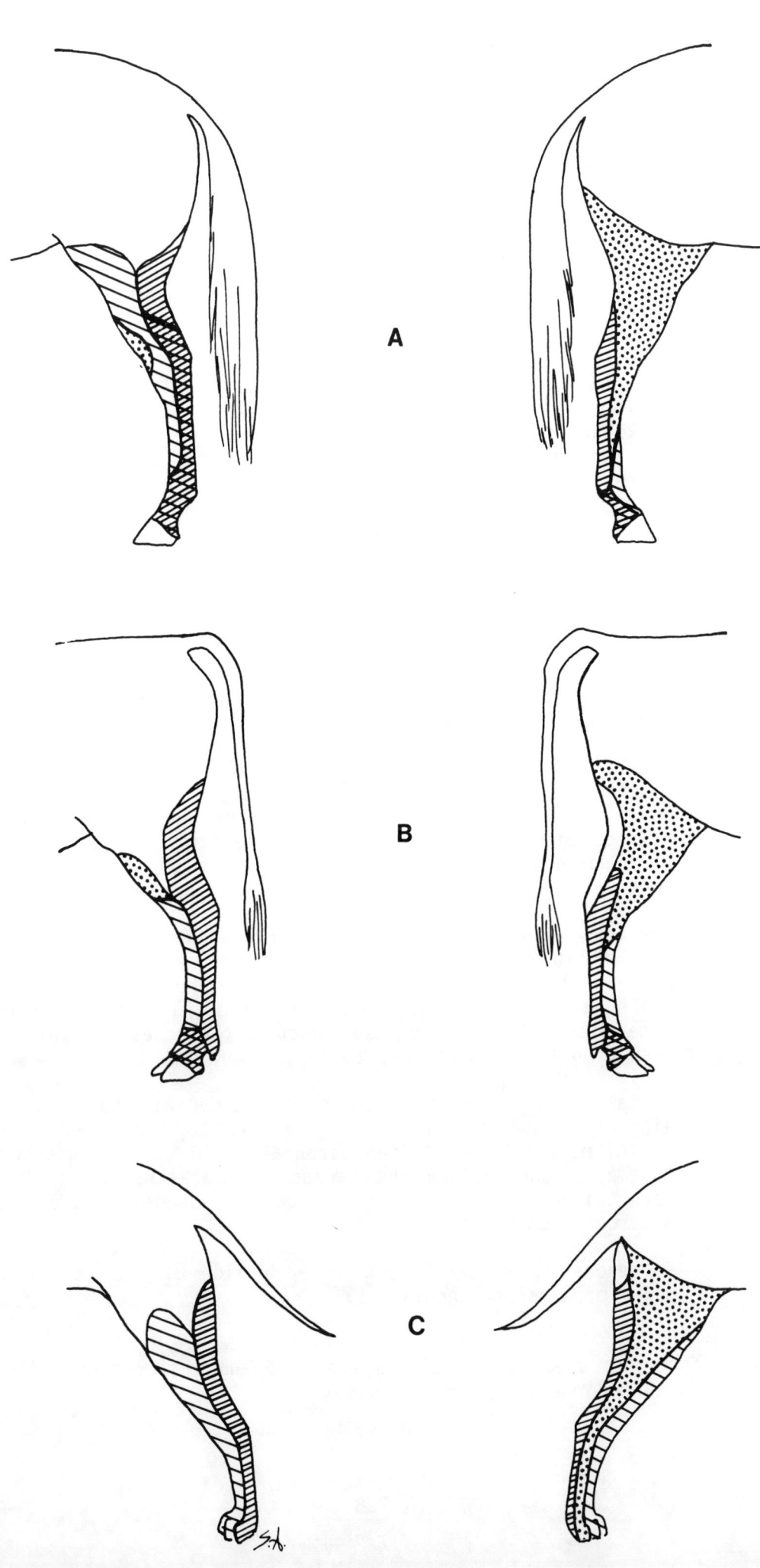

I. Caudal cutaneous sural n.--from the tibial nerve

J. Other cutaneous branches of the tibial nerve

There are also numerous small cutaneous branches associated with the pudendal and caudal rectal nerves that may be partially distributed to the proximal aspect of the pelvic limb. The nerves which supply the digits are all derivatives of the peroneal and tibial nerves.

V. DIAGNOSTIC AND SURGICAL NERVE BLOCKS

Local and regional nerve blocks on the pelvic limb are frequently and routinely performed in horses but relatively rarely in other species. A few selected blocks and their uses will be considered. An excellent discussion of this subject has been presented by Dr. Habel [3] and his commentary is summarized here.

A. Horse

1. Plantar digital block--this block is done in the same manner and has the same effect as the palmar digital block of the thoracic limb. The medial and lateral plantar digital nerves are blocked.

2. Plantar block--this block is done in a similar manner and has essentially the same effect as the palmar block of the thoracic limb. As in the thoracic limb, not only are the medial and lateral plantar nn. blocked, but also the medial and lateral plantar metatarsal nn. which emerge at the distal ends of the second and fourth metatarsal bones. Additionally, the medial and lateral dorsal metatarsal nn. (derived from the deep peroneal nerve) must be blocked if anesthesia of the whole digit is desired. These may be blocked by infiltrating on the sides of the third metatarsal bone 2-3 cm dorsal to the distal ends of Mt2 and 4 [3].

3. Peroneal n. block--both the superficial and deep branches may be blocked 10 cm proximal to the tarsocrural joint in the groove between the long and lateral digital extensors. The same cutaneous puncture can be used to block both nerves. This block should not be done diagnostically because muscular branches are also blocked, resulting in an iatrogenic locomotor deficit.

4. Tibial n. block--inject on the caudomedial aspect of the deep digital flexor tendon 10 cm proximal to the tuber calcanei. A tibial n. block and a deep peroneal n. block will anesthetize the foot.* To anesthetize the tarsus and metatarsus, the superficial peroneal n., the saphenous n., and the caudal cutaneous sural n. must be blocked also.

5. Saphenous n. block--inject on each side of the medial saphenous vein, proximal to the tarsus.

---

*The equine "foot" as used here includes the hoof and its contents. There is no official designation for this anatomic concept.

6. Caudal cutaneous sural n. block--inject on the caudolateral aspect of the common calcanean tendon just proximal to the tuber calcanei.

As in the thoracic limb, specific desensitization of joints is more effectively done by intra-articular injection of a local anesthetic than by regional nerve blocks.

B. Dog [3]

1. Tibial nerve block--palpate the nerve and inject at the caudomedial aspect of the deep digital flexor m., a few centimeters proximal to the tuber calcanei. It lies cranial to the common calcanean tendon directly on the deep digital flexor.

2. Saphenous nerve block--inject at the caudomedial aspect of the proximal end of the tibia.

3. Peroneal nerve block--inject in the depression between the long digital extensor and the peroneus longus near the longitudinal midpoint of the crus. Inject superficially for the superficial peroneal nerve and deeply (near the bone) for the deep peroneal nerve.

By performing all three blocks as noted above, the pes can be anesthetized.

C. Ox [3]

1. Superficial peroneal n. block--the branches of the superficial peroneal n. may be blocked by injecting on either side of the large dorsal branch of the lateral saphenous vein proximal to the mid-metatarsus (Fig. 10-5/26).

2. Deep peroneal n. block--the distal continuation of the deep peroneal nerve (third dorsal metatarsal nerve) may be blocked through the same skin puncture used for the branches of the superficial peroneal nerve. The needle is passed deeply between the extensor tendons. Alternately, this nerve can be blocked near the metatarsophalangeal joint.

3. Medial and lateral plantar nn. block--the medial and lateral plantar nerves may be blocked on the medial and lateral sides of the flexor tendons proximal to the mid-metatarsus (Fig. 10-5/27).

By performing all three of these blocks, the digits (but not the metatarsus or metatarsophalangeal joints) can be anesthetized. The metatarsus is supplied by unblocked branches which arise proximal to the blocking level, and deeper branches of the nerves (also unblocked) supply the joints.

References

1. International Committee on Veterinary Gross Anatomical Nomenclature. 1983. <u>Nomina Anatomica Veterinaria,</u> third ed. Published by the Committee, Ithaca, New York.

2. Fletcher, T. F. 1970. Lumbosacral plexus and pelvic limb myotomes of the dog. Am. J. Vet. Res. 31:35-41.

3. Habel, R.E. 1981. Applied Veterinary Anatomy, second ed. Published by the author, Ithaca, New York.

4. Worthman, R. P. 1957. Demonstration of specific nerve paralyses in the dog. JAVMA 131:174-178.

5. Vaughan, L. C. 1964. Peripheral nerve injuries: An experimental study in cattle. Vet. Rec. 76:1293-1300.

6. Cox, V. S., J. E. Breazile, and T. R. Hoover. 1975. Surgical and anatomic study of calving paralysis. Am. J. Vet. Res. 36:427-430.

7. Budras, K. D. 1972. Zur homologisierung der mm. adductores und des m. pectineus der haussaugetiere. Zbl. Vet. Med. 1:73-91.

8. Shively, M. J. 1982. Twenty more veterinary anatomic lies, half truths, and misleading statements. Jour. Vet Med. Ed. 9(1):20-21.

9. Evans, H. E., and G. C. Christensen. 1979. Miller's Anatomy of the Dog, second ed. W. B. Saunders, Philadelphia.

10. Getty, R. 1975. Sisson and Grossman's The Anatomy of the Domestic Animals, fifth ed. W. B.Saunders, Philadelphia.

ABDOMEN

I. ABDOMINAL TOPOGRAPHY

The abdomen may be divided into several major divisions, each of which has subdivisions as noted below (Fig. 11-1A) [1].

cranial abdominal region--consists of the xiphoid region ventrally and the left and right hypochondriac regions further laterally.
middle abdominal region--consists of the umbilical region ventrally and the left and right lateral abdominal regions further laterally.
caudal abdominal region--consists of the pubic region ventrally and the left and right inguinal regions further laterally.

This concept of abdominal topography is used less frequently (especially in carnivores) than a division into quadrants by the median plane and a transverse plane through the umbilicus (Fig. 11-1B). The principal location of the major abdominal organs according to quadrants is noted in table 11-1.

II. LATERAL AND VENTRAL ABDOMINAL WALL

The dorsal abdominal wall is reinforced by the vertebral column, but the lateral and ventral abdominal wall is formed primarily by four pairs of muscles. Contraction of these muscles increases the intra-abdominal pressure and may play a functional role in urination, defecation, vomition, and parturition. They also help maintain the normal posture by flexing the vertebral column.

A. Muscles forming the abdominal wall (Fig. 11-2)

1. External abdominal oblique--originates on the ribs and lumbar fascia and terminates by forming an aponeurosis which blends into the linea alba. The fibers of the belly are oriented caudoventrally and terminate several centimeters from the ventral midline where the aponeurosis begins. The caudal free border of the external abdominal oblique courses from the tuber coxae to the prepubic tendon and is properly termed the inguinal ligament.

2. Internal abdominal oblique--originates on the tuber coxae and lumbar fascia and terminates by forming an aponeurosis which blends into the linea alba. The fibers of the belly are oriented cranioventrally and, like those of the external abdominal oblique, terminate several centimeters from the ventral midline where the aponeurosis begins.

3. Transversus abdominis m.--originates from the ribs, lumbar fascia, and tuber coxae and terminates by forming an aponeurosis which continues to the ventral midline to join the linea alba. The fibers of the transversus abdominis are oriented dorsoventrally.

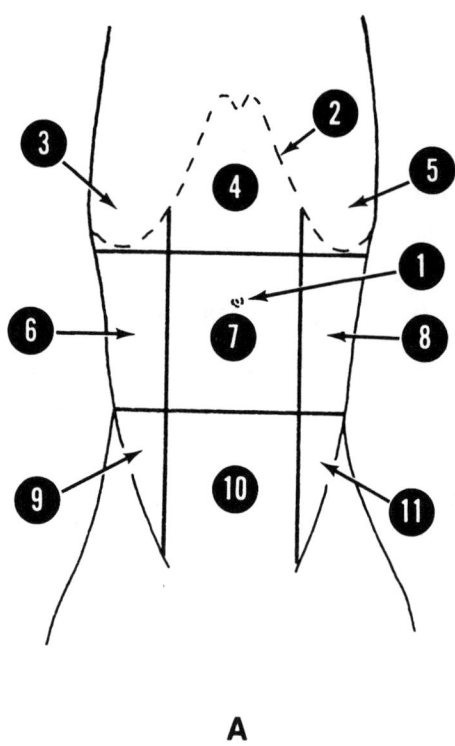
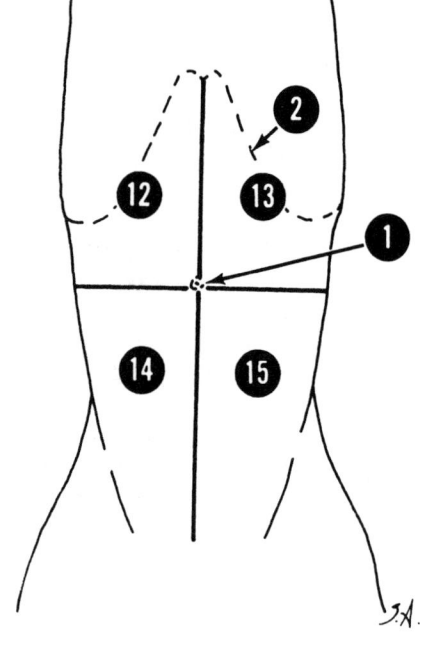

A

B

Figure 11-1

Division of the Abdomen into Subparts

A. By <u>NAV</u> regions [1]
B. By <u>quadrants</u>

1. umbilicus
2. costal arch
3. right hypochondriac region
4. xiphoid region
5. left hypochondriac region
6. right lateral abdominal region
7. umbilical region
8. left lateral abdominal region
9. right inguinal region
10. pubic region
11. left inguinal region
12. right cranial quadrant
13. left cranial quadrant
14. right caudal quadrant
15. left caudal quadrant

Table 11-1

Location of the Major Abdominal Organs by Quadrants

Right cranial quadrant = RCr
Left cranial quadrant = LCr
Right caudal quadrant = RCd
Left caudal quadrant = LCd

Organ	Quadrant
Cardia of stomach	LCr
Pylorus	RCr
Descending duodenum	RCr and RCd
Ascending duodenum (1)	LCr and LCd
Jejunum	all four quadrants
Cecum (2)	RCd
Ascending colon (3)	RCr
Transverse colon	RCr and LCr
Descending colon (1)	LCr and LCd
Left kidney (1,4)	LCr and LCd
Right kidney (4)	RCr and RCd
Pancreas (5)	RCr and RCd
Liver (6)	RCr and LCr
Spleen	LCr
Left suprarenal gland	LCr
Right suprarenal gland	RCr
Urinary bladder	RCd and LCd

Notes:

1. In the ruminants, the physical presence of the rumen in the abdomen displaces several organs to the right of the median plane that would normally be found to the left. These include the ascending duodenum, descending colon, and left kidney.

2. In the pig, the cecum is found primarily to the left of the median plane.

3. In the ungulates, the ascending colon is found in other or additional quadrants. In ruminants, it is displaced to the right by the rumen and is found in both right cranial and right caudal quadrants. In the horse, it occupies all four quadrants (large colon). In the pig, it occupies the middle of the abdominal cavity.

4. The cranial extremities of the kidneys may be located in cranial quadrants and the caudal extremities in caudal quadrants -- hence two quadrants were noted for each kidney.

5. The left lobe of the pancreas may extend into the LCr quadrant in some species.

6. A larger portion of the liver is usually located in the RCr quadrant, but a significant portion of it extends across the midline in all species except the ruminants.

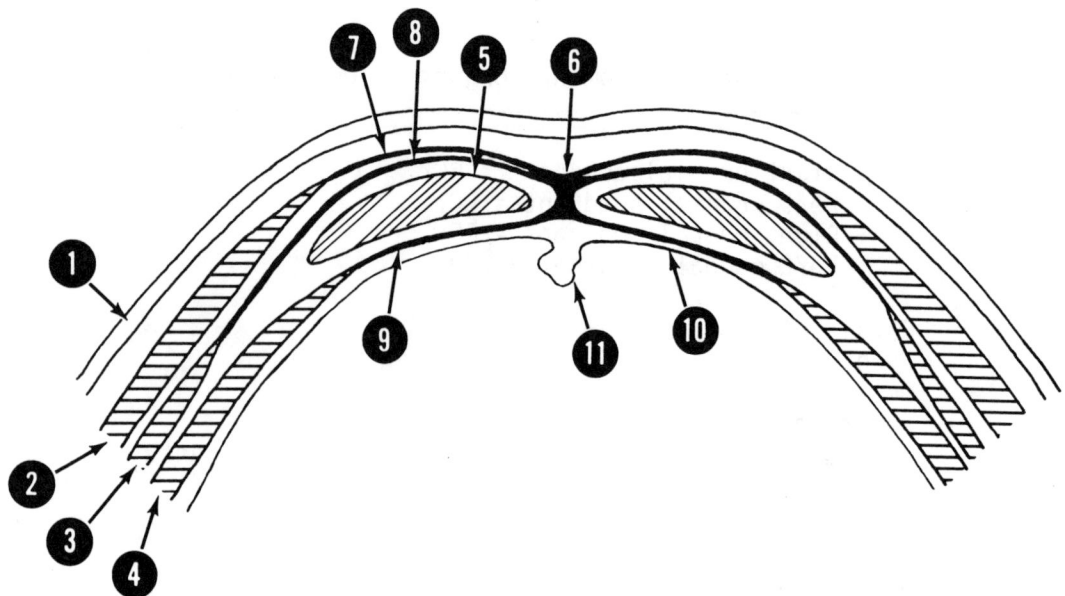

Figure 11-2

Transverse Section of the Ventral Abdominal Wall
(oriented with the animal in dorsal recumbancy)

1. Skin
2. External abdominal oblique m.
3. Internal abdominal oblique m.
4. Transversus abdominis m.
5. Rectus abdominis m.
6. Linea alba
7. Aponeurosis of external abdominal oblique m.
8. Aponeurosis of internal abdominal oblique m.
9. Aponeurosis of transversus abdominis m.
10. Parietal peritoneum
11. Falciform ligament

The sheath of the rectus abdominis m. = 7, 8, and 9 (the external lamina = 7 + 8; the internal lamina = 9 and part of 8 in some places)

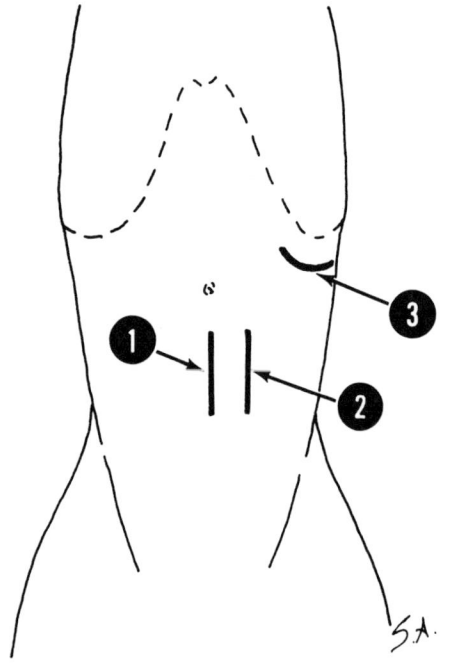

Figure 11-3

Incision Lines in the Abdominal Wall

1. Ventral midline incision
2. Paramedian incision
3. Paracostal incision

4. Rectus abdominis m. - originates from the caudal sternum and terminates on the pubis as the prepubic tendon. The rectus is ensheathed by the aponeuroses of the other abdominal wall muscles. The aponeuroses which course superficially over the rectus (primarily those of the external and internal abdominal oblique mm.) form the external lamina of the sheath of the rectus abdominis.* Those aponeuroses which course deep to the rectus (primarily that of the transversus abdominis but also, in some species, part of the internal abdominal oblique) form the internal lamina of the sheath of the rectus abdominis.

B. Comparative and clinical considerations regarding the abdominal wall

1. In carnivores, the internal lamina of the sheath of the rectus muscle is very difficult to identify in the caudal part of the abdomen because most of the aponeurosis of the transversus abdominis muscle courses superficially to the rectus abdominis [2].

2. Directional orientation of the muscle fibers is a useful identification criterion during paralumbar or paracostal laparotomies. However, in large animals the difference in their directional orientations near the paralumbar fossa is not as great as might be expected. Further ventrally, the fibers assume their characteristic directions.

3. In a ventral midline incision, the linea alba is severed and no muscle fibers are cut (Fig. 11-3/1). It is one of the most popular incisions for routine laparotomies because closure is greatly simplified and it is relatively atraumatic. In very small dogs and cats, the linea alba is so narrow that it is quite easy for a surgeon to accidentally incise too far to the left or right, resulting in an unintentional paramedian entry along part of the incision. These incisions may have linea alba on one side and the exposed edge of the rectus abdominis with the laminae of its sheath on the other side. In carnivores, the falciform ligament, along with the fat embedded within it, is routinely trimmed away during the entry to avoid its accidental inclusion in the suture line during closure (its presence may delay healing and contribute to a dehiscence). Usually three lines of sutures are used for closure: linea alba, subcutaneous tissue, and skin. Although the peritoneum has little, if any, holding power, and is not considered important to include in the closure, it usually is included because of its adherence along the edges of the incision. In male domestic mammals (except the cat), the prepuce must be reflected to one side for a caudal ventral midline incision.

4. A paramedian incision is made parallel and lateral to the midline (Fig. 11-3/2). Once the external lamina of the rectal sheath is

---

*Each rectus abdominis muscle is enveloped by a single sheath (rectal sheath) consisting of two laminae (internal and external). However, the external lamina is commonly called "superficial" or "ventral sheath," and the internal lamina is commonly called "deep" or "dorsal sheath." These common names incorrectly imply a plurality.

incised, the fibers of the rectus may be bluntly separated longitudinally to expose and incise the internal lamina. This type of paramedian incision which actually goes through the rectus abdominis, is sometimes called a perrectus incision [3]. Alternately, if the incision in the external lamina is near the midline, the whole rectus muscle may be retracted laterally to incise the internal lamina. (This avoids the necessity of separating the muscle fibers.) Closure, in either case, may be accomplished with four suture lines: internal lamina of rectal sheath (including peritoneum), external lamina of rectal sheath, subcutaneous tissue, and skin. Alternately, only 3 suture lines may be used by incorporating both laminae of the rectal sheath in one line. The rectus itself is not sutured in either case. The paramedian incision takes more time but results in a more secure closure than a ventral midline incision.* A paramedian incision made lateral to the rectus abdominis is termed a pararectus incision.

5. Paracostal incisions are made parallel to the caudal ribs (Fig. 11-3/3). The fibers of the abdominal obliques and transversus abdominis muscles may be separated longitudinally by layer ("grid" incision) or they may be severed parallel to the skin incision. This approach is often used for adrenalectomies to treat Cushing's syndrome and may be of value in repair of some diaphragmatic hernias.

6. Paralumbar or flank incisions are made similarly to paracostal incisions, but are positioned further caudally.

7. Umbilical hernias (omphaloceles) in young animals are quite common and some species have a hereditary predisposition. In puppies and foals, small hernias may correct themselves with time, but large ones may require surgery. In large animals a variety of corrective procedures have been employed (overlap and sutures, meshes, clamps). In pigs, umbilical hernias are not as likely to spontaneously regress [4].

III. PERITONEUM (EPIPLOON) AND PERITONEAL CAVITY

The peritoneum is the serous membrane lining the abdominal cavity and covering the abdominal organs. It consists of a layer of mesothelium with a thin, connective tissue backing. The peritoneal cavity is the potential space bounded by this lining membrane. Except for a small volume of fluid, nothing is within the peritoneal cavity except aberrant ova (and sperm) in the female which may occasionally pass through the opening of the ovarian bursa to gain entry into the main part of the peritoneal cavity [5].

A. Anatomical features

---

*It is true that the linea alba is the strongest single area for closure of an incision. However, in introductory surgical laboratories, paramedian closures (with two lines of suture in dense connective tissue) suffer fewer post-operative dehiscences than ventral midline incisions. There is some evidence that, in experienced hands, closure of the internal lamina is unnecessary.

1. Peritoneum

    There are two major divisions of peritoneum based on their location:

    a. Visceral peritoneum--covers the surfaces of the visceral abdominal organs.* (Opinions vary as to whether the peritoneum on nonvisceral organs such as the aorta and spleen should be classified as visceral or parietal.)

    b. Parietal peritoneum--lines the wall of the abdominal cavity. This includes all peritoneum which is not directly on a visceral abdominal organ. The parietal peritoneum is continuous with the visceral peritoneum through a number of connecting segments. All of these consist of two layers fused together and are named and positioned as follows:

        (1) greater omentum--joins the greater curvature of the stomach to the dorsal body wall. Its subparts include:
            superficial wall--attaches to the greater curvature of the stomach (abomasum and left longitudinal groove of rumen; Fig. 11-4).
            deep wall--attaches to the dorsal body wall (right longitudinal groove of rumen - Fig. 11-4).
            gastrophrenic lig.--attaches stomach to diaphragm
            gastrosplenic lig.--attaches stomach to spleen
            phrenicosplenic [splenorenal] lig.--attaches the spleen to the diaphragm or left kidney (varies among species).
        (2) lesser omentum--joins the lesser curvature of the stomach and the duodenum to the liver. The portion of it which joins the stomach and liver is called the gastrohepatic lig. The part which joins the liver and duodenum is the hepatoduodenal lig.
        (3) mesoduodenum--suspends the rest of the duodenum (see hepatoduodenal lig.)
        (4) mesentery--suspends the jejunum and ileum
            root--the initial part which attaches to the dorsal body wall
            mesojejunum
            mesoileum
        (5) mesocolon
        (6) mesorectum
        (7) falciform lig. of the liver--a cranial remnant of the ventral mesentery between the umbilicus and the liver (this should be differentiated from the round ligament of the liver which is surrounded by the falciform lig. and represents the vestigial umbilical vein).

---

*Visceral organs are those that belong to the visceral body systems (digestive, urogenital, and respiratory). Criteria which distinguish the visceral body systems include a tubular design, a mucous membrane lining, and one or more openings at the body surface. The systems which do not have these characteristics are considered to be somatic systems (musculoskeletal, circulatory, endocrine, nervous, and integumentary systems). Some authors, however, also consider the organs of the circulatory and endocrine systems to be viscera.

(8) left and right triangular ligg. and coronary lig. of the liver--The coronary and triangular ligaments are reflections of peritoneum from the diaphragm to the liver. The triangular ligg. reflect to the right and left lobes and the coronary lig. attaches centrally around the caudal vena cava.
(9) hepatorenal lig.
(10) median lig. of the urinary bladder--a caudal remnant of the ventral mesentery between the umbilicus and the urinary bladder.
(11) lateral ligg. of the urinary bladder--these folds of peritoneum should be differentiated from the round ligaments of the bladder (remnants of the umbilical aa.) which they surround.
(12) broad lig. of uterus--the fold of peritoneum that suspends the female reproductive organs. This should be differentiated from the round lig. of the uterus which is a remnant of the female gubernaculum. It has three named subparts:
- mesometrium
- mesosalpinx
- mesovarium

Most of the broad ligament (mesometrium) supports the uterus. The mesovarium is the part which supports the ovary and should be differentiated from the visceral peritoneum on the ovarian surface. The mesosalpinx is the portion of the broad ligament which forms the lateral wall of the ovarian bursa and suspends the uterine tube ("oviduct").
(13) suspensory ligg. of the ovaries
(14) mesorchium - the peritoneum which suspends the testis. It surrounds and is fused to the vessels and nerves of the spermatic cord.
(15) mesoductus deferens - the peritoneum which suspends the ductus deferens

2. Peritoneal cavity

The peritoneal cavity is the space within the abdominal cavity between the parietal peritoneum and the visceral peritoneum. It has a number of named subdivisions and diverticula:

a. omental bursa--a subdivision of the peritoneal cavity between the two walls of the greater omentum. It communicates with the rest of the peritoneal cavity through the epiploic foramen - a small passageway located between the caudal vena cava and the portal vein.

b. ovarian bursa--a subdivision of the peritoneal cavity around the ovary. It is connected to the rest of the peritoneal cavity by the opening of the ovarian bursa.

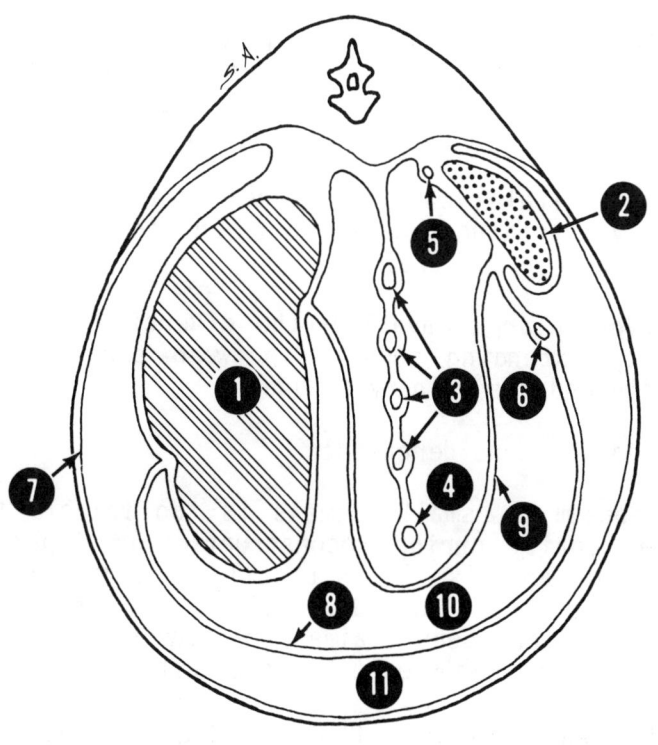

Figure 11-4

Schematic Representation of a Tranverse
Section through an Ox at the Level of T-13
(as viewed from the caudal aspect)

1. rumen
2. liver
3. spiral colon
4. small intestine
5. ascending duodenum
6. descending duodenum
7. parietal peritoneum
8. superficial wall of greater omentum
9. deep wall of greater omentum
10. omental bursa
11. main part of the peritoneal cavity

After Sisson and Grossman, 1953 [6]

c. testicular bursa--a homologue of the ovarian bursa located between the epididymis and the testis.

d. rectogenital excavation --the diverticulum of the peritoneal cavity extending caudally between the rectum and reproductive viscera. The portion of it which extends up along each side of the rectum is the pararectal fossa.

e. vesicogenital excavation--the diverticulum of the peritoneal cavity extending caudally between the urinary bladder and the reproductive viscera.

f. pubovesicular excavation--the diverticulum of the peritoneal cavity extending caudally between the floor of the pelvic cavity and the urinary bladder.

B. Surgical and medical considerations

1. The peritoneum in small animals is too friable to suture as an individual entity during reconstruction of laparotomy incisions. Even in large animals, it is usually included with other layer(s) rather than sutured individually. Improper or careless closure of the peritoneum has been claimed to delay healing and is considered to be a factor in dehiscence by some authors [3].

2. It is frequently stated that nothing is within the peritoneal cavity except a small amount of serous fluid. However, at ovulation, ova break through the visceral peritoneum on the ovarian surface and enter the ovarian bursa. They are then normally picked up by the infundibulum. Occasionally, they pass by the infundibulum and "sneak" out through the opening of the ovarian bursa into the major part of the peritoneal cavity. There they die or, if they have been fertilized, they may (rarely) establish an ectopic pregnancy. Reliable reports of ectopic pregnancies in domestic species are lacking.

3. Intestinal herniation and entrapment through the epiploic foramen is possible but it is very rare.

4. The yellow, distended nature of the falciform ligament is caused by fat between its two layers. The falciform ligament is routinely trimmed away during midline celiotomies in carnivores to prevent accidental inclusion in the closing suture line which could delay healing and contribute to a dehiscence [3].

IV. STOMACH AND ABOMASUM

The stomach is located directly caudal to the liver and part of it contacts the diaphragm. The abomasum of ruminants has essentially the same features as the stomach of the other domesticated species.

A. General features (Fig. 11-5):

parietal and visceral surfaces
greater and lesser curvatures

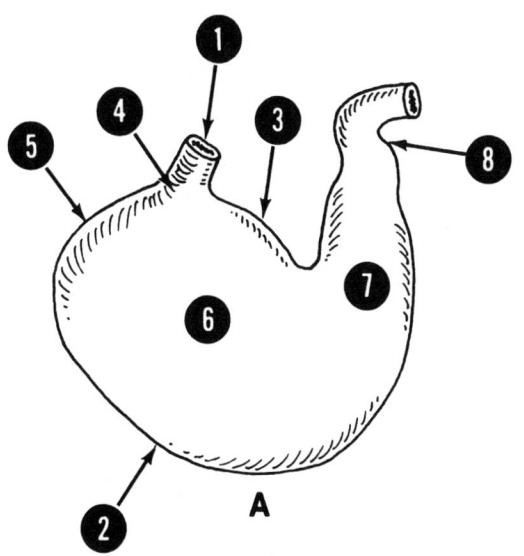
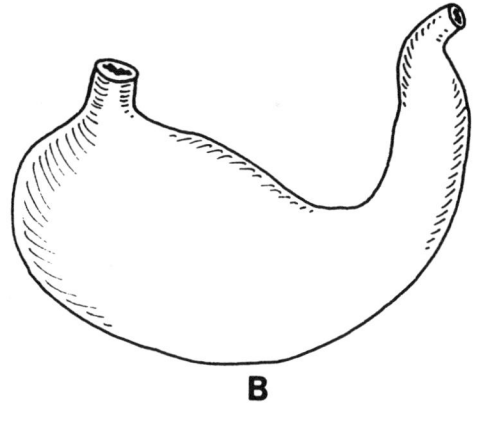
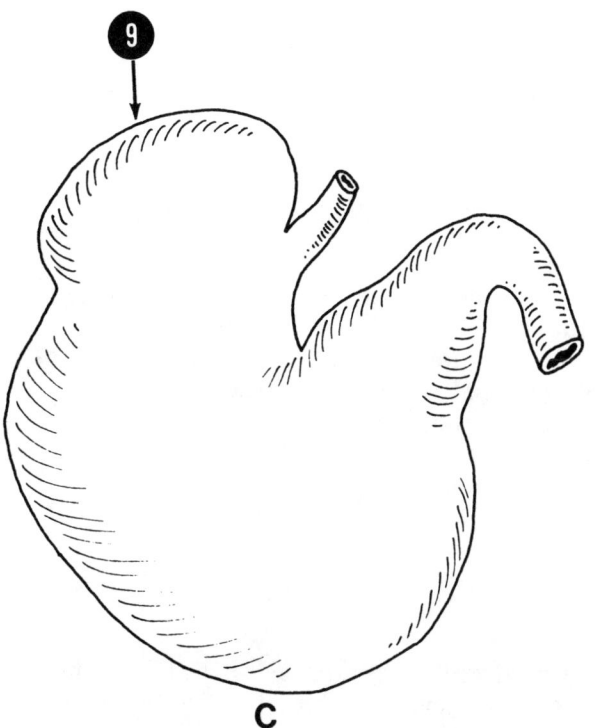
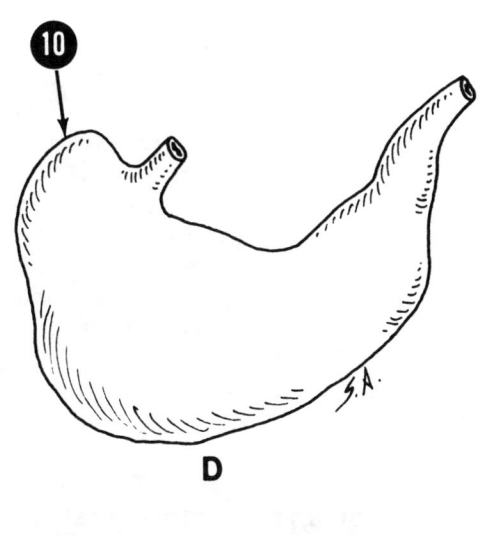

Figure 11-5

Stomachs of the Dog (A), Cat (B), Horse (C), and Pig (D)
(parietal surface)

1. esophagus
2. greater curvature
3. lesser curvature
4. cardiac part (cardia)
5. fundus
6. body
7. pyloric part
8. pylorus
9. blind sac (saccus cecus)--horse only
10. gastric diverticulum--pig only

cardiac part--around the opening of the esophagus (does not apply to abomasum)
    cardiac ostium--the opening of the esophagus into the stomach
fundus--the part which protrudes cranial to the level of the cardia
body--the major portion of the stomach
pyloric part--the portion which narrows to join the duodenum
    pyloric antrum--the cone-shaped initial portion of the pyloric part
    pyloric canal--the cylindrical continuation of the pyloric part
pylorus--the junction with the duodenum
    pyloric ostium--the passageway into the duodenum

The various histologic glandular regions of the stomach (proper gastric glands, pyloric glands, and cardiac glands) do not exactly correspond to the named gross regions of the stomach. The proper gastric glands have parietal and chief cells which produce hydrochloric acid and digestive enzymes, respectively. The other glands (pyloric and cardiac) produce mucus only.

B. Comparative features

1. The pig and ruminants have a projection from the wall of the pylorus termed the torus pyloricus. It is poorly developed in young animals.
2. The pig has a diverticulum associated with its fundus.
3. The fundus of the horse is very extensive and projects considerably above the level of the cardia. The proper name for this portion of the equine stomach is saccus cecus (blind sac). It is homologous to the ruminoreticulum of ruminants [1].
4. In the horse, the junction of the nonglandular mucosa from the esophagus with the glandular mucosa of the stomach occurs in the body of the stomach rather than at the cardia. This junction is marked by the margo plicatus, an irregular, raised ridge.
5. Like the horse, the pig has a nonglandular part of the mucosa located near the cardia. It is an elongated strip which extends into and partially lines the gastric diverticulum.
6. The mucosa of the abomasum of ruminants is arranged in spiral folds.

C. Surgical and medical considerations

1. The torus pyloricus of pigs and ruminants has no clinical significance, but it may be mistaken for an obstructive lesion by those unfamiliar with it.

2. For gastrotomies, a site should be selected which avoids the major vessels along the lesser curvature (left and right gastric vessels) and greater curvature (left and right gastroepiploic vessels) (Fig. 11-10).

3. The abomasum occasionally displaces to the left side (commonly) or to the right side (rarely). It may be surgically replaced by suturing it in position directly (abomasopexy) or indirectly (omentopexy). A few cases of abomasal torsion requiring similar corrections have also been reported [4].

4. Gastric torsion and/or distension are emergency problems in dogs which often occur after meals and exercise, especially in large breeds. Surgical intervention and manual reduction may be necessary. A gastrocentesis in the umbilical region at the point of greatest distension may be indicated [7].

5. "Bots" (larval _Gastrophilus_ spp.) are often found in equine stomachs and most species seem to prefer the nonglandular areas of the mucosa.

6. Submucosal myotomies may be performed in carnivores to relieve stenoses near the cardia or pylorus [3].

V. RUMINANT FORESTOMACH* (Fig. 11-6)

The forestomach of ruminants (proventriculus) includes the rumen, reticulum, and omasum.

A. Rumen

The rumen is the largest compartment of the forestomach and may contain 50-60 gallons of ingesta and gas in a large dairy cow [9]. It occupies most of the left half of the abdominal cavity.

1. Surface topography [1,9]

   parietal (on the left) and visceral (on the right) surfaces
   dorsal and ventral curvatures
   cranial and caudal extremities
   right and left longitudinal grooves--horizontally oriented linear
     surface indentations along the parietal and visceral surfaces
   right and left accessory grooves--branches from the longitudinal
     grooves
   cranial and caudal grooves--indentations which connect the left
     longitudinal groove to the right longitudinal groove
   dorsal and ventral coronary grooves--indentations extending dor-
     sally and ventrally from the caudal aspects of the longitudinal
     grooves
   ruminoreticular groove--the indentation between the rumen and
     reticulum (may be confused with the reticular groove--see
     reticulum)
   insula ruminis (officially present on the right side only)--the
     ruminal surface between the right longitudinal groove and the
     right accessory groove

2. Internal features

---

*Dr. Habel offers this comment in his _Applied Veterinary Anatomy_ [8]: "No domestic animal has more than one stomach. The ruminants have one stomach with four compartments. No part of the stomach develops from the esophagus. The terms monogastric and polygastric, frequently encountered in the literature, are nonsense."

Figure 11-6

Rumen, Reticulum, Omasum, and Abomasum of an Ox

- A. Parietal surface (with cutaway to illustrate lumen)
- B. Visceral surface
    1. esophagus
    2. reticulum
    3. ruminoreticular groove
    4. ruminoreticular fold
    5. cranial groove
    6. cranial pillar
    7. cranial sac (atrium of rumen)
    8. ventral sac
    9. caudal groove
    10. caudal pillar
    11. caudoventral blind sac
    12. caudodorsal blind sac
    13. dorsal sac
    14. ruminoreticular ostium
    15. reticular groove
    16. abomasum
    17. duodenum
    18. omasum
    19. right longitudinal groove
    20. (right) dorsal coronary groove
    21. (right) ventral coronary groove
    22. right accessory groove
    23. insula ruminis

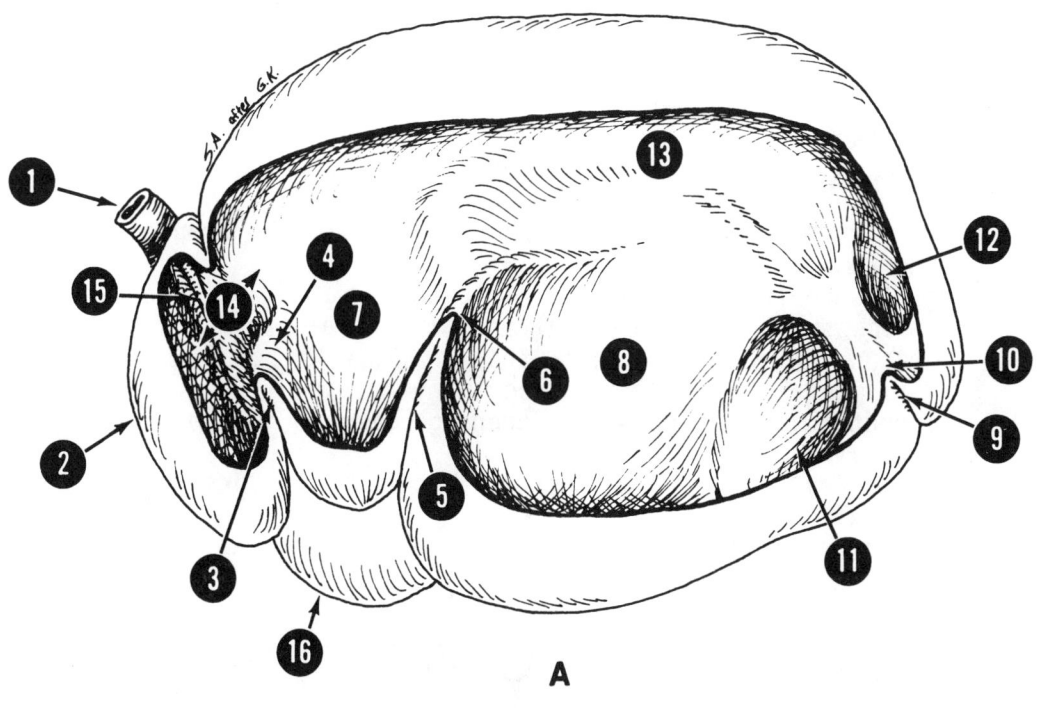

A

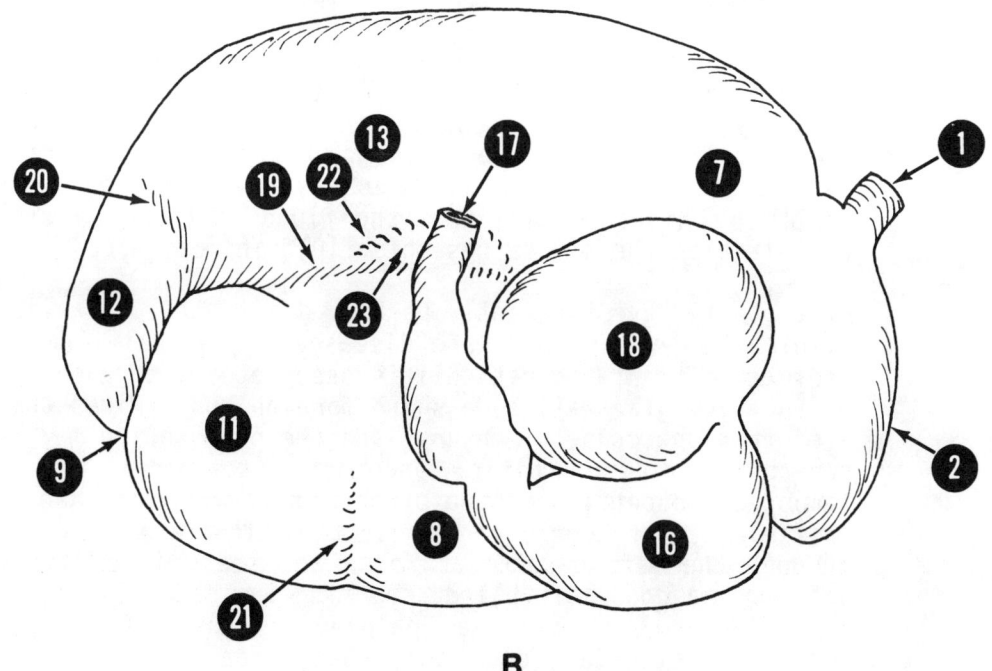

B

cranial pillar--an internal septum corresponding to the cranial groove
caudal pillar--an internal septum corresponding to the caudal groove
ruminoreticular fold--an internal septum corresponding to the ruminoreticular groove. Internal pillars corresponding to each of the other external grooves (right and left longitudinal pillars, dorsal and ventral coronary pillars, etc.) are also present
dorsal sac--the portion dorsal to the longitudinal grooves
    caudodorsal blind sac--the continuation of the dorsal sac caudal to the dorsal coronary grooves
atrium (cranial sac)--the portion cranial to the cranial pillar of the rumen.
ventral sac--the portion ventral to the longitudinal grooves
    recessus ruminis--cranial end of ventral sac
        caudoventral blind sac--the continuation of the ventral sac caudal to the ventral coronary groove
ruminoreticular ostium--the opening between the rumen and the reticulum
intraruminal ostium--the opening between the dorsal sac and the ventral sac
papillae--the mucosal projections of various shapes and sizes

3. Surgical and medical considerations

  a. Ruminal paracentesis (trocarization) is indicated in cases of acute tympany in which passage of a stomach tube does not relieve the gas. The trocar is forced through the center of the paralumbar fossa and angled ventrally through the wall of the dorsal sac of the rumen [4].

  b. The rumen may be palpated through the left paralumbar fossa. Contractions occur at about 30-second intervals and may be visually documented by examining the paralumbar fossa. When the animal is eating, the rumen may contract about three times per minute. On percussion, the gas in the upper third can easily be distinguished from the fluid further ventrally. On auscultation the sounds resemble fluid in motion [8].

  c. Rumenotomies are frequently performed in cattle to relieve the clinical signs of "hardware disease," a general term usually indicating traumatic reticulitis associated with a perforation of the reticular wall by a sharp foreign body. Wires and nails are often the cause of injury, and the perforation may lead to peritonitis, pericarditis, pneumonia, abscesses, or cardiac tamponade, depending on the other organs involved. Many "cure" themselves. If surgery is elected, the approach is made through the left paralumbar fossa and the wall of the dorsal sac or caudodorsal blind sac is incised. To reach the reticulum, the surgeon can palpate the cranial pillar, then the ruminoreticular fold, and finally feel the characteristic mucosa of the reticulum. As in boxing, a long reach is advantageous.

d. Rumen fistulas are sometimes surgically established to experimentally study rumen physiology. A routine paralumbar rumenotomy is performed and then the edges of the skin incision are sutured to the edges of the ruminal incision.

B. Reticulum

The reticulum is morphologically and physiologically so closely related to the rumen that the two are frequently considered as the ruminoreticulum. The reticulum has a volume of only a few gallons [9].

1. Anatomical features

   diaphragmatic and visceral surfaces
   greater and lesser curvatures
   reticulo-omasal ostium (contains unguiculiform papillae)
   reticular crests and cells--the ridges and depressions of the "honeycombed" mucosa
   reticular groove--the reticular portion of the gastric groove*

2. Surgical and medical considerations

   a. The position of the reticulum immediately adjacent to the diaphragm allows penetrating foreign bodies to cause a myriad of problems, depending on the direction they travel and the organs they injure. Magnets have been placed in the reticulum (orally) to collect metal objects and keep them from penetrating the wall [4].

   b. The reticulum cannot be palpated but can be auscultated at the ventral ends of the left sixth or seventh intercostal spaces. Liquid and gas in motion can be heard at intervals of about one per minute. Two palpable rumen contractions usually occur between reticular contractions. A grunt of pain may occur in association with reticular contractions in cases of traumatic reticulitis [8].

C. Omasum

1. Anatomical features

---

*The gastric groove of the ruminant stomach extends from the cardia through the lesser curvature of the reticulum, base of the omasum, and on into the abomasum. It is customarily divided into three segments corresponding to the compartment of the stomach complex through which it passes: reticular groove, omasal groove, abomasal groove. It closes reflexly in young animals during suckling to form a tubular channel to transport milk directly to the abomasum. In adults, the gastric groove does not close except in response to pharmacologic levels of certain salts. It can be closed iatrogenically by oral administration of a 0.4 molar copper sulfate solution (sheep) or a 10% $NaHCO_3$ solution (cattle). Closure usually lasts less than 10 seconds [10]. In the adult, the groove plays no role in deglutition, regurgitation, or eructation [11].

> parietal and visceral surfaces
> curvature and base
> omasoabomasal ostium
> laminae (about 100 are present in the ox, about 80 in the sheep)
> omasal groove--the omasal portion of the gastric groove

    2. Surgical and medical considerations

        a. The dull sound of the omasum on percussion (right side) cannot be distinguished from the liver. It can be palpated through the wall of the rumen during a rumenotomy, but is "hidden" under the rib cage externally. Auscultation does not yield valuable information [8].

        b. If traumatic peritonitis involves the omasum, pain may be elicited by manual pressure on the ventral part of the right seventh to ninth intercostal spaces and in the right hypochondriac region [8].

VI. SMALL INTESTINE (Fig. 11-7)

The small intestine includes the duodenum, jejunum, and ileum. Other than total lengths and positions of the duodenal papillae, these do not have major morphological differences among the various domestic species.

A. Major features

    1. duodenum--extends from the pylorus to the jejunum

> cranial part--the portion which extends cranially from the pylorus
> cranial duodenal flexure--the area where the cranial part turns to course caudally
> descending part--the portion of the duodenum which courses caudally on the right of the root of the mesentery
> caudal duodenal flexure--the portion which turns to the left to course caudal to the root of the mesentery
> ascending part--the portion which courses cranially on the left side of the root of the mesentery
> duodenojejunal flexure--the portion which turns caudally to be continued by the jejunum
> major duodenal papilla--the projection on which the bile duct and pancreatic duct (if present) open
> minor duodenal papilla--the projection on which the accessory pancreatic duct (if present) opens

    2. jejunum--the longest part of the small intestine

    3. ileum--the shortest segment of small intestine. Arbitrarily, it may be grossly differentiated from the jejunum by the proximal extent of the antimesenteric fold of the peritoneum which joins the colon (ileocecal fold) [9].
> ileal ostium--the opening of the ileum into the large intestine (often called "ileocolic valve") [12]

B. Comparative features

1. The ruminants, horse, and pig have a sigmoid loop in the cranial part of the duodenum [9].

2. The horse has a dilatation in the cranial part of its duodenum termed the duodenal ampulla [9].

3. In the cat and horse, a hepatopancreatic ampulla is present surrounding the major duodenal papilla [9].

4. The jejunum varies in length from 1 m or less in the cat to as much as 50 m in the ox [9].

5. The ileal ostium joins the cecum in the horse and empties into the ascending colon in all other domestic animals.*

C. Clinical considerations

1. Enterotomies are performed primarily for the removal of foreign bodies.

2. Intestinal resection and anastomosis may be indicated in some cases of intussusception, necrosis caused by foreign bodies, torsion, or volvulus. Anastomoses may be done end to end, side to side, or end to side. The vascular integrity of the part not resected is very important and all discolored tissue is usually removed. Further insurance regarding the blood supply is gained by transecting obliquely and leaving the mesenteric border of the cut edge longer than the antimesenteric border in the two ends to be rejoined [3].

3. Volvulus of the small intestine may occur in several species. It may require manual reduction or surgical resection.

VII. LARGE INTESTINE (Fig. 11-7)

The large intestine includes the cecum, colon, rectum, and anal canal [1].

A. Cecum

1. General features

   base--the initial portion which joins the colon
   body
   apex--the free, blind end

2. Comparative features

   a. The cecum is shortest in the cat and is increasingly longer in the dog, pig, ruminants, and horse.

   b. In the horse there are two openings into the cecum, the ileal ostium and the cecocolic ostium. In all other domestic animals the ileal ostium opens into the colon.*

---

*Some developmental studies have indicated that the initial part of the equine cecum near the base is, in fact, colon. Considered in this manner, the horse has the same general pattern as the other domestic species, (i.e., the ileum actually enters the colon) [9].

Figure 11-7

Schematic Perspective of the Intestinal Arrangement in the Dog (A), Pig (B), Ox (C), and Horse (D) (right lateral aspect)

1. pylorus of stomach
2. descending duodenum
3. caudal duodenal flexure
4. ascending duodenum
5. duodenojejunal flexure
6. jejunum
7. ileum
8. cecum
9. transverse colon
10. descending colon
11. rectum
12. anus

Specific parts of the ascending colon in the pig (B) and ox (C)

13. proximal loop (ox only)
14. centripetal turns of spiral loop
15. central flexure of spiral loop
16. centrifugal turns of spiral loop
17. distal loop

Specific parts of the ascending colon in the horse (D)

18. right ventral colon
19. sternal flexure
20. left ventral colon
21. pelvic flexure
22. left dorsal colon
23. diaphragmatic flexure
24. right dorsal colon

Modified from Nickel, Schummer, Seiferle, and Sack, 1973 [9])

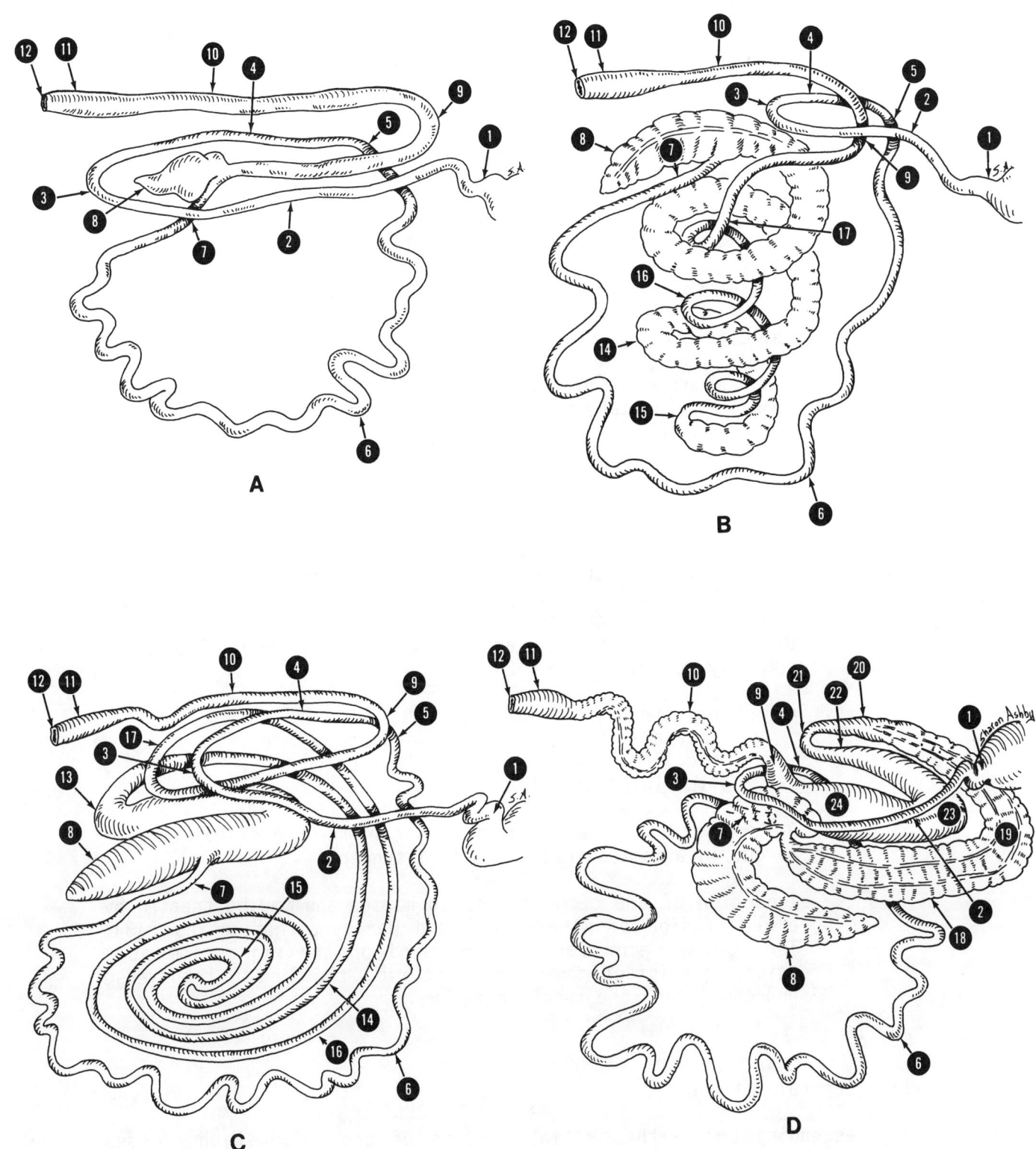

251

c. In the carnivores, pig, and ruminants, the ileal ostium appears to be a convenient place to divide the cecum from the colon. In reality, however, the ileum actually empties into the colon and the cecum is a diverticulum from the initial part of the ascending colon. This is more easily observed in the carnivores than in the pig or ruminants.

d. In the pig and horse, the cecum has sacculations (haustra) because of the longitudinal smooth muscle bands (teniae) in its wall.

e. The cecum of the horse is very large. Its base lies in the right paralumbar fossa and its apex extends cranially on the midline to nestle between the right and left ventral colons.

3. Clinical considerations

a. Surgical removal of the cecum (typhlectomy) in carnivores is sometimes indicated by cecal impaction, dilation, or inversion. Before the development of efficient drugs, it was also an accepted treatment for whipworm infestation. Ablation may still be indicated when medical treatment fails [3].

b. Intussusceptions, most common in carnivores, occasionally involve the cecum and/or the intestine near it. If caught early, before vascular strangulation and necrosis, they may be manually reduced without intestinal resection. The intussusception usually consists of an invagination of a proximal part of the intestine into an adjacent distal part. The types commonly described are [12]:

    ileal--involves ileum only
    ileocecal--ileum invaginates into cecum
    ileocolic--ileum invaginates into colon
    colic--involves colon only

A "retrograde" intussusception is one where a distal segment of gut invaginates into a proximal segment.

c. Impaction of the cecum occurs in horses and may be treated by oral infusion of mineral oil and parasympathomimetics [13]. The equine cecum can be trocarized on the right side at a point equidistant from the last rib, the lumbar transverse processes, and the tuber coxae [8].

B. Colon

1. General features

    ascending colon--the initial portion of the colon which courses cranially. Most of the differences in the intestinal patterns of the domestic species are related to variations in its arrangement and degree of development (see comparative features).

right colic flexure--the junction of ascending colon and transverse colon. Generally used in reference to the carnivores.
transverse colon--the portion of the colon which courses from right to left cranial to the root of the mesentery.
left colic flexure--the junction of the transverse colon with the descending colon.
descending colon--connects the transverse colon to the rectum.

2. Comparative features

   a. In the horse, the ascending colon is often called the large colon* and has the following specific subparts:

	number of teniae	sacculations
right ventral colon	4	+
sternal flexure	4	+
left ventral colon	4	+
pelvic flexure	transition area	-
left dorsal colon	1	-
diaphragmatic flexure	transition area	-
right dorsal colon	3	-

   These are listed in the order that ingesta would encounter them and are named by their location. The right and left dorsal colons are located dorsal to their respective ventral colons, and the diaphragmatic flexure overlies the sternal flexure. On the basis of diameter, the right dorsal colon is the largest segment and the pelvic flexure and initial part of the left dorsal colon are the smallest. The terminal part of the right dorsal colon is a "stomachlike dilatation" sometimes termed the ampulla coli [1,9].

   Longitudinal bands of smooth muscle (teniae), like those in the cecum, are present in the wall of the colon. In the ventral colons** (and descending colon) these are very well developed and draw up the wall to form sacculations (haustra). Less well-developed bands on the dorsal colons** do not cause the formation of haustra. Knowledge of the numbers of bands on various parts of the large intestine has some clinical applications (see paragraph B.3).

   b. In the ruminants, the ascending colon has the following parts:

   proximal loop
   spiral loop

---

*One should be careful to differentiate large colon, used in the horse to refer to the ascending colon, from large intestine (which incudes the cecum, colon, rectum, and anal canal).
**When used alone, the term ventral colon(s) refers collectively to the right ventral colon, sternal flexure, and left ventral colon. Similarly, the term dorsal colon(s) refers collectively to the left dorsal colon, diaphragmatic flexure, and right dorsal colon.

                centripetal turns (going in toward the central flexure)
                central flexure
                centrifugal turns (coming back out from the central flexure)
            distal loop

        The spiral loop is nearly planar (a flat coil).

   c. In the pig, the ascending colon has the same basic parts as that of the ruminants. However, the proximal loop is absent, the distal loop is subtle, and the spiral loop is arranged in an inverted, cone-shaped coil with the central flexure down at the apex. The centripetal turns form the outside of the coil and spiral clockwise (as viewed dorsally) down to the central flexure. The centrifugal turns are inside of these and spiral back up in a counterclockwise direction. The centripetal turns are sacculated because of the teniae and are larger in diameter than the centrifugal turns [9].

   d. The short, unmodified ascending colon of the carnivores has no subparts.

   e. The descending colon of the horse is often called the small colon (colon tenue) [1]. It is very long (much longer than it has to be to connect the transverse colon and rectum), and has well-developed bands and sacculations.

   f. Although there are numerous differences in the ascending colons of the various domestic species, some general rules of intestinal arrangement hold true for any species:

       (1) the descending duodenum and ascending colon are on the right side of the root of the mesentery. (In the horse, the ascending colon is so large that parts of it are found on both sides).

       (2) the ascending duodenum and the descending colon are on the left side of the root of the mesentery. (In the ox, the rumen displaces the descending colon to the right side of the abdomen.)

       (3) the transverse colon passes from right to left cranial to the root of the mesentery.

3. Clinical considerations

    a. Knowledge of the number of bands in various parts of the equine large intestine has some value in surgery, necropsy, and rectal palpation. The number 444,132 gives the total number on the cecum, right ventral colon, left ventral colon, left dorsal colon, right dorsal colon, and descending colon, respectively. One or more teniae may be visually obscured by mesentery and intestinal ligaments and some are so poorly developed that they are difficult to palpate or are positioned where they cannot be palpated. Of most significance in palpation is the differentiation of descending colon (2 well-developed bands plus haustra), pelvic flexure (1 well-developed band), and small intestine (no bands).

In regard to the number of teniae on the flexures, the sternal flexure has 4 teniae as do the other parts (left and right) of the ventral colon. The pelvic flexure is a region of transition from 4 bands (LVC) to 1 band (LDC) and most authors consider it to have 1. The diaphragmatic flexure is another region of transition from 1 (LDC) to 3 (RDC). Finally, the transverse colon is also a region of transition from 3 (RDC) to 2 (small colon).

    b. In addition to the cecum, there are two other regions of the equine large intestine that are likely to impact: the pelvic flexure and the right dorsal colon. All three of these areas are associated with a change in diameter (from large to small).

    c. The descending colon of carnivores is normally on the left side of the abdomen, and ingesta in its lumen forms a useful radiographic marker in VD or DV perspectives of the abdomen. Sometimes it gets displaced by a distended or diseased urinary bladder or other organ.

C. Rectum

The rectum is the terminal portion of the intestine which continues into the pelvic cavity. In the horse, dog, and ox, it dilates terminally to form the rectal ampulla. The major clinical value of the rectum is its use in palpation. Rectal prolapses occur in several species and may require surgical resection.

D. Anal canal

The anal canal is the short terminal portion of the alimentary canal. Its external opening is the anus and histologically it has three regional zones based on the type of lining epithelium (columnar, intermediate, and cutaneous zones). Specialized glands are found in this region in some animals [9]:

1. anal glands (present in some form in all domestic mammals)--these are clinically quiescent and release their secretion into the intermediate zone of the anal canal. Some sources have considered these glands to be absent in cats, but they are, in fact, present.

2. circumanal glands (present in dogs)--these are modified sebaceous glands located in the skin surrounding the anus. They occasionally become neoplastic and this condition presents clinically as a perianal adenoma.

3. glands of the paranal sinuses (present in dogs and cats)--these are located within the wall of each paranal sinus (anal sac). They release their secretion into the paranal sinuses and each sinus serves as a collecting and storage reservoir for the secretion of

the glands in its wall. The single excretory duct of each of the two sinuses opens onto the ipsilateral aspect of the cutaneous zone of the anal canal. It is the paranal sinuses that become impacted and/or inflamed which, in some cases, necessitates their manual expression and/or surgical removal. Since the glands of each paranal sinus are located within its walls, surgical resection of the sinuses also removes their glands. Clinically, the term "anal glands" is often incorrectly used to refer to the anal sacs.

VIII. LIVER (Fig. 11-8)

The liver is located directly caudal to the diaphragm. It is one of the few organs of the body which receives both arterial and venous blood [5].

A. General features

diaphragmatic surface--adjacent to the diaphragm
    groove of the vena cava--the indentation which partially surrounds the caudal vena cava
visceral surface--adjacent to the stomach
right, left, dorsal, and ventral borders
fossa of the gallbladder
round lig. (lig. teres) of the liver--the vestige of the umbilical vein
hepatic porta--the area where the portal vein, hepatic artery, and biliary ducts enter and leave the liver
esophageal impression--the indentation formed by the esophagus
lobes [9]:
    left lobe--the part of the liver to the left of a line from the esophagus to the round ligament. In some species, the left lobe is divided into left lateral and left medial lobes (see comparative features below)
    right lobe--the part of the liver to the right of a line from the caudal vena cava to the fossa for the gallbladder. In some species, the right lobe is divided into right lateral and right medial lobes (see comparative features below).
    caudate lobe--the part of the liver between the left and right lobes and dorsal to the hepatic porta. The caudate lobe has a caudate process (caps end of right kidney) and, in some species, a papillary process (protrudes into the lesser curvature of the stomach).
    quadate lobe--the part of the liver between the left and right lobes and ventral to the hepatic porta.

B. Comparative features

1. In the ruminant liver, very few fissures are present to aid the differentiation of the various liver lobes. In addition, the large forestomach causes a 90° rotation of the liver so that the left lobe is positioned ventrally.

2. In the carnivores, the following additional divisions of the four basic lobes are present:

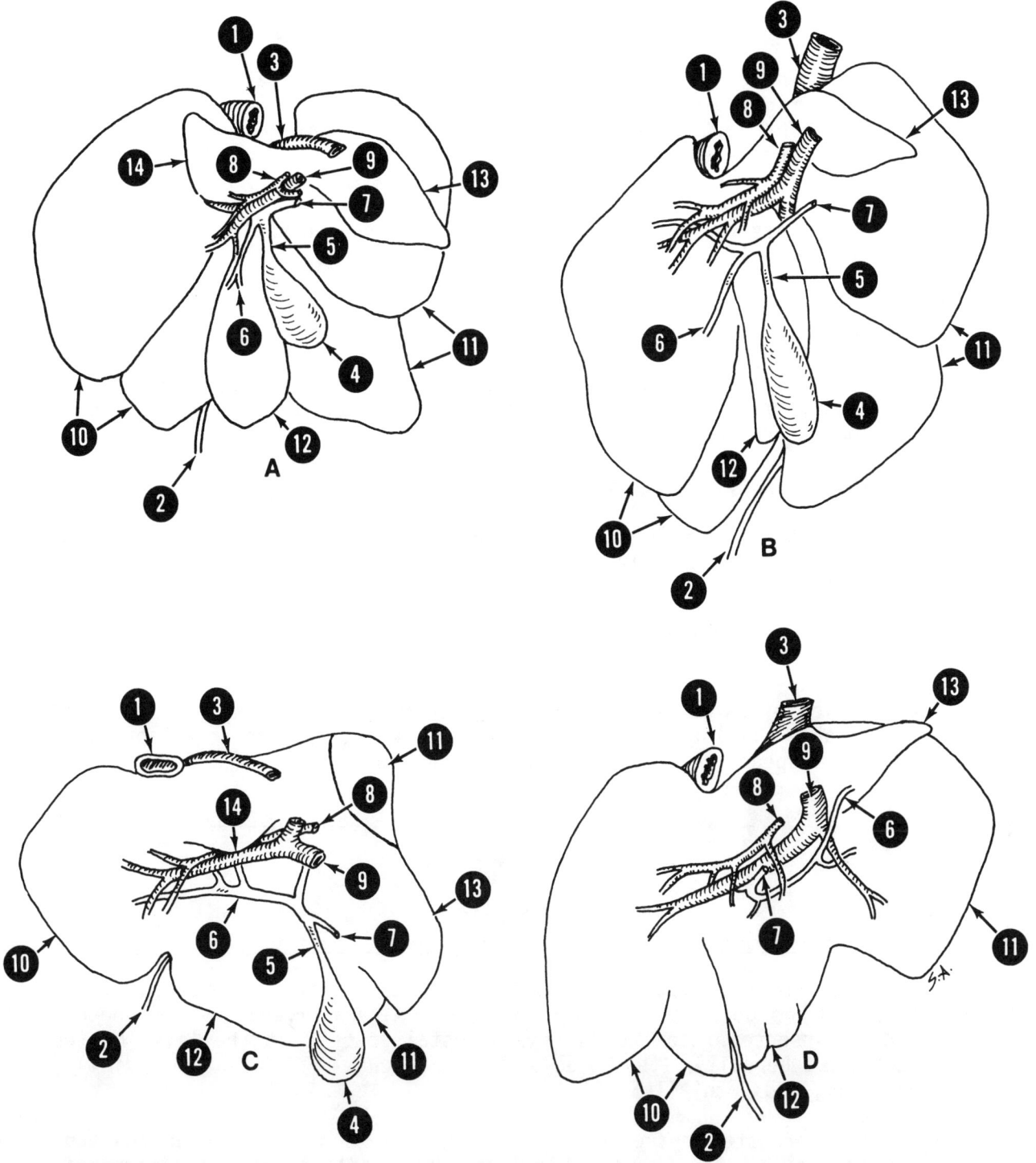

Figure 11-8

Livers of the Dog (A), Pig (B), Ox (C), and Horse (D) (visceral surfaces)

1. esophagus
2. round ligament of liver
3. caudal vena cava
4. gallbladder
5. cystic duct
6. hepatic duct(s)
7. bile duct
8. hepatic a.
9. portal v.
10. left lobe (lateral and medial in dog, pig, and horse)
11. right lobe (lateral and medial in dog and pig)
12. quadrate lobe
13. caudate process of caudate lobe
14. papillary process of caudate lobe (dog and ox only)

After Nickel, Schummer, Seiferle, and Sack, 1973 [9]

        a. The right lobe is divided into a right lateral lobe and a right medial lobe.
        b. The left lobe is divided into a left lateral lobe and a left medial lobe.
        c. The caudate lobe is divided into a caudate process that caps the right kidney and a papillary process that extends into the lesser curvature of the stomach. The caudate lobe of the ox is similarly divided, but the papillary process is very small.

    3. The liver of the pig resembles that of the carnivores except that there is no papillary process on the caudate lobe.

    4. The liver of the horse resembles that of the carnivores except that the right lobe remains undivided and, like the pig, there is no papillary process on the caudate lobe.

C. Surgical and medical considerations

    1. Partial hepatectomy may be indicated to alleviate the problems resulting from traumatic rupture of the liver. A large portion of the liver may be removed with no ill effects since it has marked regenerative capabilities. Intestinal segments may be translocated to cover and help revascularize a ruptured or severed liver. Hemorrhage and bile peritonitis are major concerns.

    2. Liver biopsies are routinely performed to assess hepatic functions (Table 11-2) In carnivores, some surgeons prefer to do a laparotomy to inspect the whole liver when taking a biopsy.

Table 11-2

Liver Biopsy Sites

Horse:	right intercostal space 12 at the level of a line between the tuber coxae to the point of the shoulder [14]. Alternatively, a 20-cm needle can be inserted into the left intercostal space 8 at the level of the deltoid tuberosity (the needle in this case is directed medially, dorsally, and cranially) [8].
Ox:	right intercostal space 10 or 11, about 1/4 of the length of the bony rib ventral to the vertebral column. The needle is inserted perpendicularly to the body surface [15]. In young calves (under 4 weeks of age), the relatively larger liver may be reached caudal to the last rib. In older calves, the liver may be biopsied in the eleventh or twelfth intercostal space [8].
Dog:	a midventral incision is made under local or general anesthesia just caudal to the xiphoid process. A finger is inserted to fix the left lobe against the abdominal floor. The biopsy needle is inserted through a separate stab incision [16].

IX. GALLBLADDER

The gallbladder is positioned between the right lobe and the quadrate lobe of the liver. It is not present in the horse.

A. General features

fundus
body
neck
cystic duct--the channel to and from the neck of the gallbladder
hepatic ducts--the grossly visible biliary channels leaving the lobes of the liver
bile duct--the single biliary channel which courses through the hepatoduodenal ligament and opens into the duodenum at the major duodenal papilla

B. Comparative features (Fig. 11-8):

1. In the pig and in the ruminants, the hepatic ducts unite to form a common hepatic duct which then joins the cystic duct to form the bile duct.

2. In the horse, which lacks a gallbladder, no cystic duct is present, and the distal part of the common hepatic duct which continues on to the duodenum is usually called the bile duct.

3. In the carnivores, several hepatic ducts separately enter the cystic duct which becomes the bile duct after the entry of the last hepatic duct.

4. In the carnivores, ox, and sheep, some of the bile enters the gallbladder through small hepatocystic ducts. These ducts penetrate the wall of the gallbladder in places where it is in contact with the liver [9].

5. Species variation in the location of the major duodenal papillae [9]:

dog and pig--2 to 6 cm distal to the pylorus
cat--3 cm distal to the pylorus (in hepatopancreatic ampulla)
ruminants--at sigmoid loop of duodenum (30-40 cm distal to pylorus in small ruminants and 50-70 cm distal to pylorus in ox)
horse--12-15 cm distal to pylorus (in hepatopancreatic ampulla)

C. Surgical and medical considerations

1. Surgery involving the gallbladder is rarely done in domestic animals because cholelithiasis and other diseases of the gallbladder are rarely diagnosed. Rupture of the bile duct may be treated by anastomosing the ruptured ends or by ligation of the duct and anastomosis of the gallbladder to the duodenum (cholecystoduodenostomy). Rupture of a hepatocystic duct may be treated with ligation of that duct [3].

2. Post mortem examination of the biliary ducts is routinely done during meat inspection of ruminants to detect liver fluke infestations. The ducts appear smooth and greenish if normal, thickened and brownish if infected with Fasciola hepatica, and a black pigment will be present if Fascioloides magnum is involved.

X. PANCREAS

The pancreas is closely associated with the duodenum. It develops by evaginating from the primitive gut as two (dorsal and ventral) budding primordia that remain connected to it by secretory ducts. Either the dorsal or the ventral primordium may regress during development so that in some species the pancreas is a definitive development of only one of the primordia and has only one duct (cat, pig, ruminants). In other species, regression does not occur and both ducts remain reflecting the double origin of the pancreas (dog, horse). The duct of the ventral primordium is the pancreatic ("Wirsung's") duct which opens at the major duodenal papilla. The duct of the dorsal primordium is the accessory pancreatic ("Santorini's") duct which opens on the minor duodenal papilla [9].

A. General features

body--the part that lies against the cranial part of the duodenum.
left lobe--the part which extends from the body to the left.
right lobe--the part which extends from the body to the right along the descending duodenum.
pancreatic duct
  and/or
accessory pancreatic duct

B. Comparative features

1. In some domestic mammals (carnivores, ruminants), the portal vein indents the body to form a pancreatic notch (incisura pancreatis). In the others (pig, horse) the body completely encircles the portal vein to form a pancreatic ring (anulus pancreatis).

2. Species differences in the body and lobes (for purists)

   a. In the carnivores, the pancreas is U-shaped with a centrally placed body adjacent to a bend in the cranial part of the duodenum.

   b. In the ruminants, the body is relatively small, the right lobe is long, and the left lobe is wide.

   c. In the pig, the right lobe is small and the left lobe is large.

   d. The pancreas of the horse has a large body, a small right lobe, and a long left lobe.

3. Species differences in the definitive pancreatic ducts:

	ventral primordium persists (pancreatic duct)	dorsal primordium persists (accessory pancreatic duct)
dog	+ (occasionally -)	+
cat	+	- (20% +)
pig	-	+
ox	- (occasionally +)	+
sheep & goat	+	-
horse	+	+

4. The pancreatic ducts are often confused with the duodenal papillae on which they open. For clarification:

   a. The bile duct always opens at the major duodenal papilla and since all domesticated mammals have a bile duct, all have a major duodenal papilla.

   b. The pancreatic duct, if present (see paragraph X.B.3 above), also opens at the major duodenal papilla (see paragraph IX.B.5 for the location of this papilla).

   c. The accessory pancreatic duct, if present (see paragraph X.B.3 above), opens at the minor duodenal papilla. Its location relative to the major duodenal papilla is noted below [9]:

   horse--on the same level as the major duodenal papilla but on the opposite wall of the duodenum
   carnivores and pig--a few centimeters distal to the major duodenal papilla
   ox--about 30 cm distal to the major duodenal papilla.

   d. Species which lack an accessory pancreatic duct (small ruminants and most cats) do not have a minor duodenal papilla.

5. It is confusing to some individuals that the accessory pancreatic duct of the dog is consistently present and is larger than the pancreatic duct (which may be absent). Several variations of the pancreatic ducts in dogs have been reported and these sometimes have significance in partial pancreatectomies.

C. Surgical considerations:

1. If the normal pancreas must be manipulated, it should be handled with extreme gentleness to avoid iatrogenic pancreatitis.

2. Surgical removal of part or all of the pancreas is sometimes indicated because of neoplasia. In carnivores, where this surgery is most likely to be done, one should be aware of the positions of the pancreatic ducts relative to the body and lobes, because a functional connecting duct should be left intact in partial pancreatectomies [17]. Otherwise, the whole pancreas should be removed. The pancreatic duct leaves the middle of the body and the accessory pancreatic duct is located at the junction of the body and the right lobe (Fig. 11-9). If the right lobe is removed, the pancreaticoduodenal artery, which courses through it, should be preserved by gently peeling the pancreatic tissue away from the duodenum. If the vessel cannot be preserved, the descending duodenum should be resected [3]. In a study of 50 dogs, 42 were found to have 2 pancreatic ducts, 4 had only an accessory duct, and 4 had 3 ducts [18].

XI. SPLEEN

In all domestic mammals the spleen is flattened in shape and is located adjacent to the left abdominal wall.

A. General features

parietal surface
visceral surface
cranial border
caudal border
dorsal extremity
ventral extremity
hilus

B. Comparative features

1. In the pig, horse, and carnivores, the hilus is an elongated groove on the visceral surface. In the ruminants, the hilus is a focal indentation near the dorsal border.

2. In the ox, pig, horse, and carnivores the spleen is elongated and, in the horse, it is noticeably wider near its dorsal extremity than at its ventral extremity.

3. In the sheep and goat, the spleen is triangular or rectangular in shape.

C. Medical and surgical considerations

1. In dogs, the spleen often has suspicious looking, focal discolorations along its borders. These are usually nodular hyperplasias or siderotic plaques with no clinical significance. Two or three separate spleens are occasionally encountered in clinically normal carnivores.

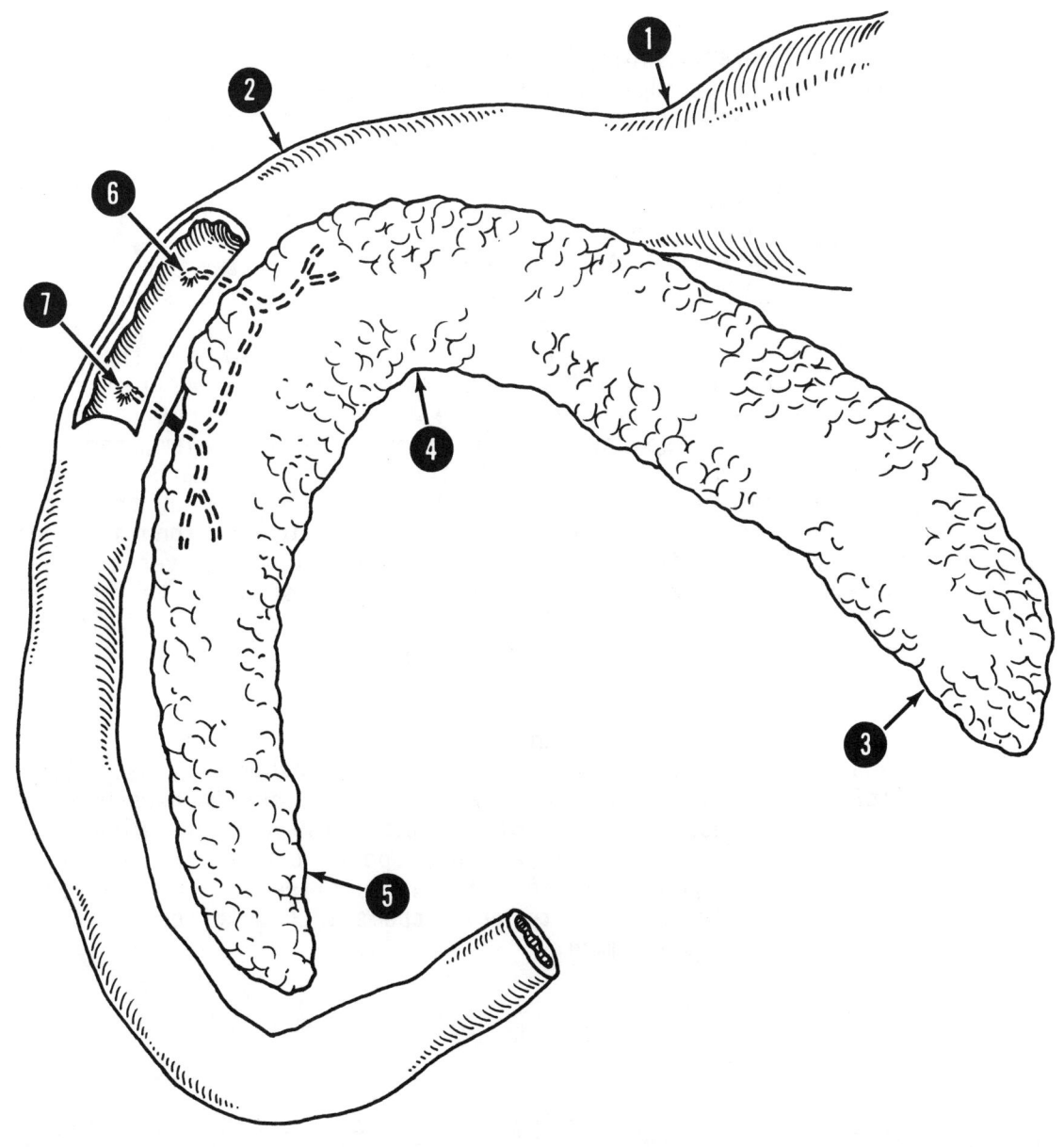

Figure 11-9

The Location of the Pancreatic Ducts in the Dog

1. pylorus
2. descending duodenum
3. left lobe of pancreas
4. body of pancreas
5. right lobe of pancreas
6. pancreatic duct (opening on major duodenal papilla)
7. accessory pancreatic duct (opening on minor duodenal papilla)

2. In carnivores, splenectomies are common surgical procedures indicated by neoplasia, traumatic rupture of the spleen or torsion of the splenic pedicle. Splenectomies are also done to aid the study of some blood diseases (feline infectious anemia). The pattern of the splenic vessels is clinically significant because the main splenic a. not only sends several branches into the elongated hilus, but it also sends a number of continuations through the gastrosplenic ligament to the greater curvature of the stomach (short gastric arteries)*. The anatomic significance of this is that one cannot effect hemostasis during a splenectomy by simply ligating the main splenic a. (and vein) and then removing the spleen, because retrograde hemorrhage will occur through the short gastric aa. (which will be disrupted when the gastrosplenic ligament is broken down). To circumvent this problem, the branches of the splenic vessels, which enter the hilus, are ligated, the gastrosplenic ligament is disrupted near the spleen, and the short gastric arteries are left intact (Fig. 11-10). It should be pointed out that the integrity of the short gastric vessels is not necessary for adequate circulation to the stomach. In fact, if the spleen has no tumors and is markedly congested, the main splenic artery may be injected with epinephrine (to cause it to contract and thus conserve blood) and then ligated [3].

3. In ruminants, splenectomies are sometimes done experimentally (anaplasmosis research). The gastric branches of the splenic a. (left and right ruminal aa.) arise several centimeters proximal to the spleen and so the single continuation of the splenic artery which enters the hilus at a single point can be tied off with one ligature. The gastrosplenic ligament is extremely short--especially near the proximal extremity where the spleen is directly applied to the surface of the rumen.

References

1. International Committee on Veterinary Gross Anatomical Nomenclature. 1983. Nomina Anatomica Veterinaria, third ed. Published by the Committee, Ithaca, New York.

2. Evans, H. E., and G. C. Christensen. 1979. Miller's Anatomy of the Dog, second ed. W. B. Saunders, Philadelphia.

3. Archibald, J., ed. 1974. Canine Surgery, second edition. American Veterinary Publications, Santa Barbara, California.

---

*Anatomy texts frequently show a major continuation of the splenic a. as the left gastroepiploic a. which follows the greater curvature of the stomach. However, in gross dissections, the gastroepiploic vessel often cannot be identified until at least halfway around the greater curvature, and direct connections between it and the splenic a. are difficult to observe.

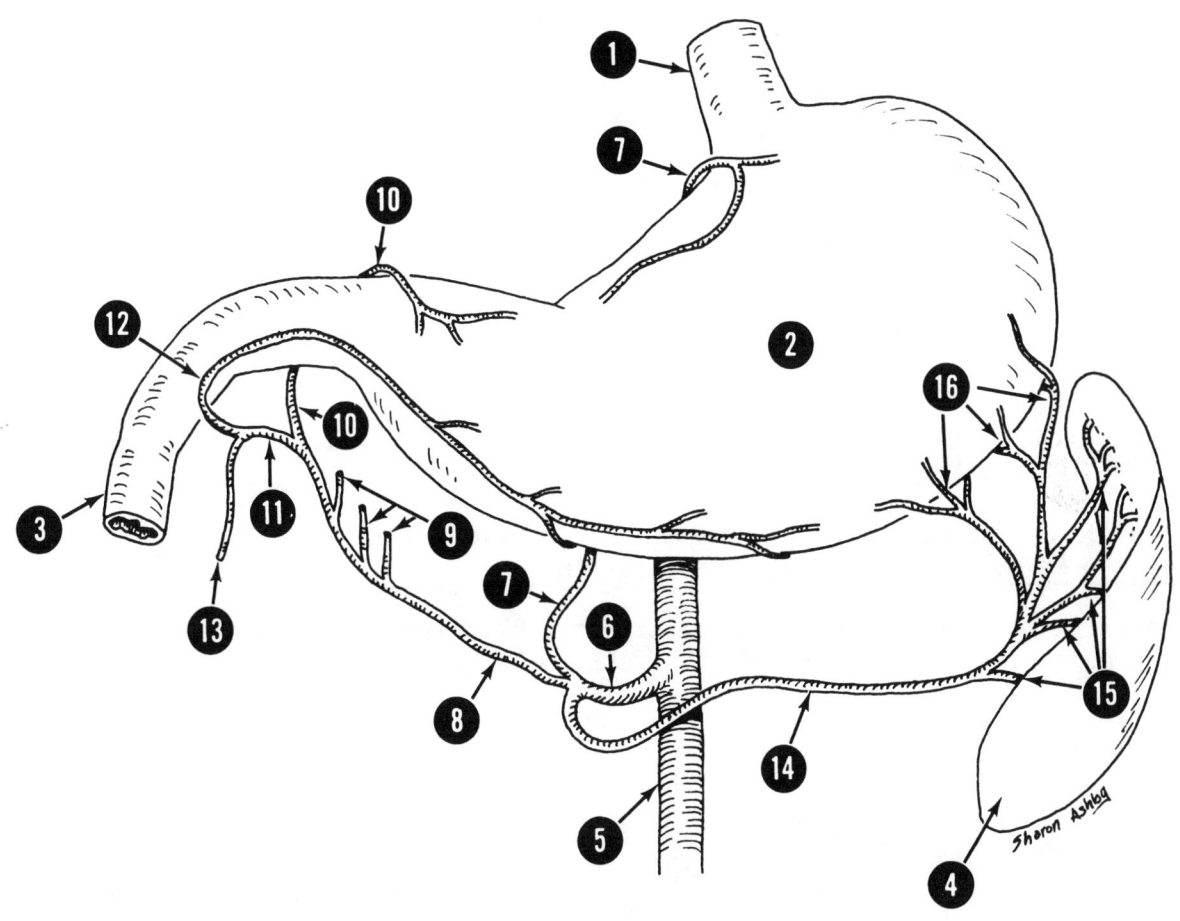

Figure 11-10

Blood Supply of the Stomach and Spleen of a Dog (ventral aspect)

1. esophagus
2. body of stomach
3. descending duodenum
4. spleen (parietal surface, ventral extremity)
5. abdominal aorta
6. celiac a.
7. left gastric a.
8. hepatic a.
9. branches of hepatic a. to liver
10. right gastric a.
11. gastroduodenal a.
12. right gastroepiploic a.
13. cranial pancreaticoduodenal a.
14. splenic a.
15. branches of splenic a. to spleen
16. short gastric aa.

The short gastric a. (16) nearest to the duodenum is frequently termed left gastroepiploic a., but grossly it is difficult or impossible to follow it to any connection with the rest of the gastroepiploic vasculature along the greater curvature.

4. Oehme, F. W., and J. E. Prier. 1974. *Textbook of Large Animal Surgery*. Williams and Wilkins, Baltimore.

5. Shively, M. J. 1979. Twenty-four anatomic fibs, half-truths, and misleading statements. *Jour. Vet. Med. Ed.* 6(3):182-187.

6. Sisson, S., and J. Grossman. 1953. *The Anatomy of the Domestic Animals* fourth ed. W. B. Saunders, Philadelphia.

7. Kirk, R., ed. 1977. *Current Veterinary Therapy* VI. W. B. Saunders, Philadelphia.

8. Habel, R. E. 1981. *Applied Veterinary Anatomy*, second ed. Published by the author, Ithaca, New York.

9. Nickel R., A. Schummer, E. Seiferle, and W. Sack. 1973. *The Viscera of the Domestic Mammals*. Verlag Paul Parey, Berlin.

10. Jones, L., N. Booth, and L. McDonald, eds. 1977. *Veterinary Pharmacology and Therapeutics*. Iowa State University Press, Ames, Iowa.

11. Williams, E. I. 1955. A study of reticulo-ruminal motility. *Vet. Rec.* 67:907-911.

12. McFarland, L. Z. 1970. *Veterinary Surgical Anatomy*. Department of Veterinary Anatomy, University of California, Davis.

13. Blood, D. C., J. A. Henderson, and O. M. Radostits. 1979. *Veterinary Medicine*, fifth ed. Lea and Febiger, Philadelphia.

14. Gibbons, W. J. 1966. *Clinical Diagnoses of Diseases of Large Animals*. Lea and Febiger, Philadelphia.

15. Udall, R. H., R. G. Warner, and S. E. Smith. 1952. A liver biopsy technique for cattle. *Cornell Vet.* 42:25-27.

16. Osborne, C. A., J. B. Stevens, and V. Perman. 1969. Needle biopsy of the liver. JAVMA 155:1605-1620.

17. Dingwall, J. S., and W. McDonnel. 1972. Partial pancreatectomy in the dog. JAAHA 8:86-92.

18. Nielsen, S. W., and E. J. Bishop. 1954. The duct system of the canine pancreas. *Amer. J. Vet. Res.* 15:266-271.

THORAX

I. THORAX AND THORACIC CAVITY

The thorax is the cranial portion of the trunk and is positioned between the neck and abdomen. The thoracic cavity is the space within the thorax and it contains the thoracic organs, the pleurae, and the pleural cavities. The pleurae are the serous membranes that line the left and right pleural cavities which are, in turn, located within the thoracic cavity. Each pleural cavity is a closed body cavity containing nothing but a small amount of serous fluid. It is an important concept that the organs within the thoracic cavity are invaginated into the pleural cavities but are not inside of them.

A. General features [1]

   cranial thoracic opening ("thoracic inlet")--the opening formed by the vertebral column, the first pair of ribs, and the sternum
   caudal thoracic opening--the opening at caudal end of the thoracic cavity which is normally sealed by the diaphragm
   costal arch--the palpable structure formed by the costal cartilages of several of the caudal ribs which articulate with each other
   intercostal space--the space between adjacent ribs, occupied by the external and internal intercostal mm.
   endothoracic fascia--the connective tissue lining the thoracic cavity
   pleural cavities (left and right; Fig. 12-1)
   pleurae--the serous membranes lining the pleural cavities and covering the surface of the thoracic organs
      pulmonary pleura--the pleura on the surface of each lung (= "visceral" pleura)
      parietal pleura--all pleura which is not on the surface of a lung
         mediastinal pleura--the pleura on the mediastinum
            pericardiac pleura--the pleura on the pericardium
         costal pleura--the pleura lining the thoracic wall
         diaphragmatic pleura--the pleura on the diaphragm
   costodiaphragmatic recess--the potential space between the ribs and diaphragm caused by the convexity of the diaphragm
   pulmonary ligaments--reflections of pleurae from the caudal lobes of the left and right lungs to the mediastinum
   mediastinum--the partition between left and right pleural cavities; it may be divided into cranial, caudal, dorsal, ventral, and middle parts
   plica vena cava--the fold of pleura around the caudal vena cava
   mediastinal recess--the area between the mediastinum and the plica vena cava (occupied by the accessory lobe of the right lung)

B. Comparative and clinical features

   1. The line of pleural reflection is where the costal pleura reflects off the thoracic wall and onto the diaphragm to become the diaphragmatic pleura. It closely coincides with the attachment of the diaphragm to the ribs. This line parallels the basal border of

Figure 12-1

Transverse Section of the Thorax through the Heart to Show
the Relationship of the Serous Membranes and Cavities
to the Major Thoracic Organs (caudal aspect)

1. Thoracic wall
2. Left lung
3. Right lung
4. Heart
5. Aorta, azygos vein, and thoracic duct
6. Esophagus
7. Parietal (specifically costal) pleura
8. Pulmonary ("visceral") pleura
9. Parietal (specifically pericardiac mediastinal) pleura
10. Left pleural cavity
11. Right pleural cavity
12. Parietal lamina of serous pericardium
13. Visceral lamina of serous pericardium (epicardium)
14. Pericardial cavity

The serous membranes are adherent to the structures they cover. In addition, the pericardiac mediastinal pleura (9) is adherent to the parietal pericardium (12).

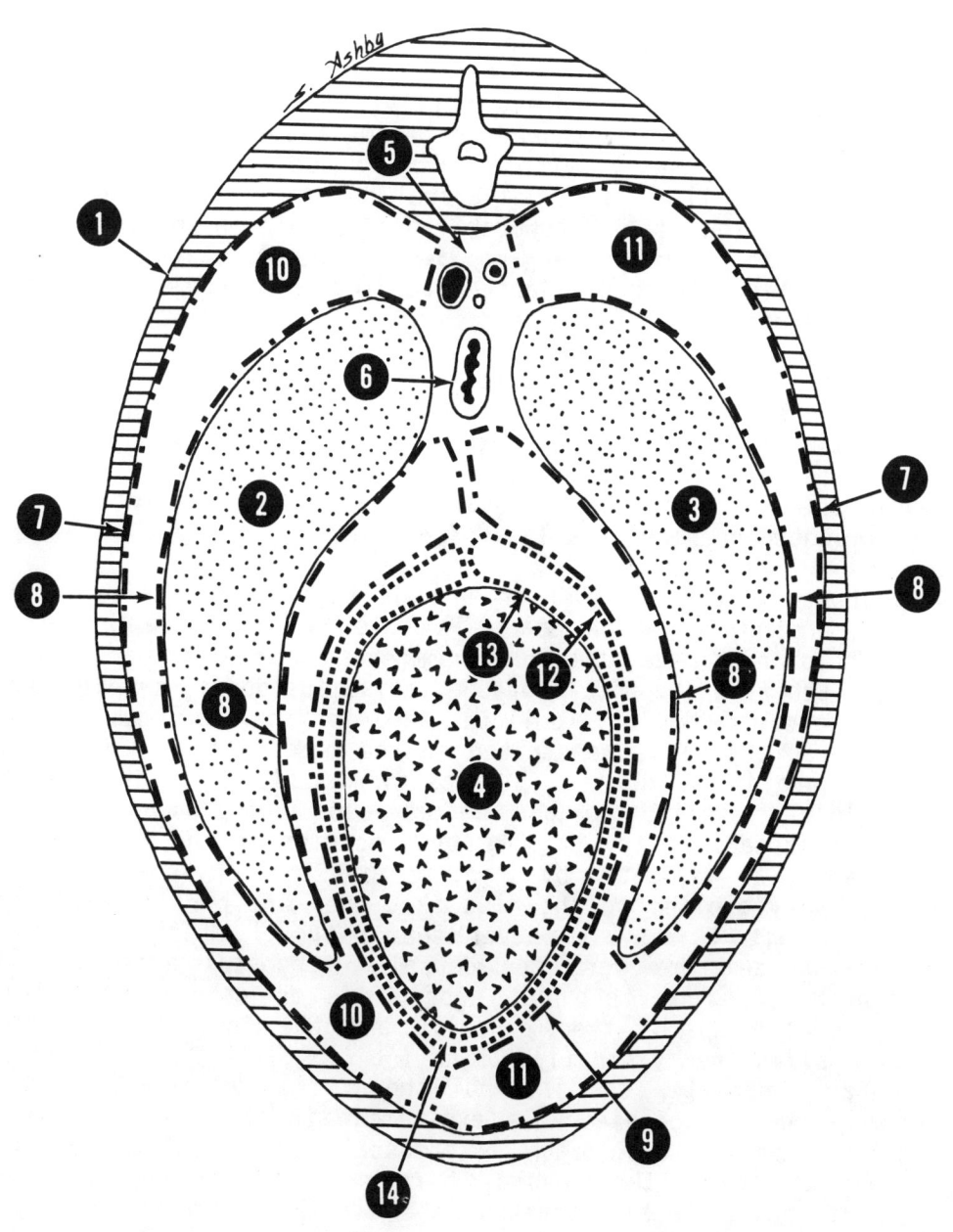

the lung, but remains slightly caudoventral to it because the basal border of the lung does not completely invade the costodiaphragmatic recess.

2. The mediastinum is formed by all of the structures between the left and right pleural cavities. Although several organs are included (trachea, esophagus, heart, etc.), in some places the mediastinum is formed only by the right and left mediastinal pleurae. Perforations (fenestrations) ranging from 1 mm in diameter on down to microscopic sizes have been reported in carnivores, horses, and sheep. These do not occur in the ox, goat, or pig, or in the young of any animal [2]. Theoretically, these could allow a unilateral pneumothorax or pyothorax to become bilateral. In horses, inflammatory processes apparently close these openings, and it has also been shown that acute unilateral pneumothorax is not fatal to dogs [2]. To be safe, however, one should probably consider any traumatic pneumothorax to be bilateral. Cattle have a thick mediastinum and can tolerate standing unilateral thoracotomies with no respiratory assistance.*

3. There are a number of muscles associated with the thorax, but most of them have little clinical significance. The external and internal intercostal muscles bridge the intercostal spaces and can be differentiated by the orientation of their fibers (the external muscles are oriented caudoventrally and the internal ones are oriented cranioventrally).

4. Thoracotomies are most often made through an intercostal incision. Depending on which space is entered, and how high or low the incision is made, the surgeon may be required to partially transect or separate the fibers of the latissimus dorsi, serratus ventralis, external abdominal oblique, and/or the scalenus muscles. The thoracic wall is penetrated in the middle of an intercostal space to avoid the dorsal intercostal vessels (and nerves) which are closely applied to the caudal aspect of each rib [3]. It is unnecessary to try to make the incision in the caudal part of the space, as advocated by some, because the nerves and vessels are so closely applied to the ribs that they are partially protected. In fact, it is hard to sever them without actually trying [4]. If transected, however, the dorsal intercostal arteries will bleed profusely from both cut ends since the aorta (or costocervical trunk) supplies them dorsally and the internal thoracic artery supplies them ventrally. If an intercostal incision is extended too far ventrally, the internal thoracic artery may be severed, and this causes considerable excitement in the surgery suite. Toward its ventral end, each intercostal artery splits and sends one branch along the cranial border of its respective rib. These arterial branches anastomose with the internal thoracic artery independent of each other.

---

*When the terms "complete" or "incomplete" are used in reference to the mediastinum, the reference is usually to the animal's ability to tolerate unilateral pneumothorax. This does not necessarily correlate with the presence or absence of fenestrations.

5. A rib may be resected to gain additional exposure in an intercostal thoracotomy [3]. This procedure is not usually needed in small animals, but may be necessary to establish drainage in cases of traumatic pericarditis in cattle. The periosteum is split with an elevator, and a section of rib is removed. The rib reforms (with time following closure) from osteogenic cells in the periosteum.

6. A midsternal thoracotomy (mediastinotomy) may be done on the ventral midline using either bone cutters or a sternum splitting mallet and osteotome. In some animals, a scalpel blade may be sufficient [3]. This approach is preferred for some specialized surgeries involving the heart and may be advantageous in the repair of some diaphragmatic hernias. The internal thoracic vessels should be avoided.

7. Transthoracic (sternum transecting) incisions may also be used for thoracotomies, but the internal thoracic vessels must be ligated. These incisions are rarely used.

8. To regain the vacuum in the pleural cavity (-ies) when closing the thoracic wall, the lungs are maximally inflated by the anesthetist during the last part of the closure. Further air can be withdrawn after the surgery by thoracentesis. A valved chest drainage tube may also be sutured in place for this purpose. Residual air in the pleural cavities is resorbed with no ill-effects.

II. TRACHEA, BRONCHI, AND LUNGS

The trachea divides into the two (left and right) principal ("primary") bronchi. Each principal bronchus further arborizes as it enters the ipsilateral lung. There are two lungs in all domestic mammals (left and right).

A. Basic features [1]

   tracheal cartilages--hyaline cartilages which maintain luminal patency
   tracheal (trachealis) muscle--the smooth muscle which bridges the (dorsal) open ends of the tracheal cartilages
   tracheal bifurcation--the division into principal bronchi
       tracheal carina--the ridge between the openings of the principal bronchi
   principal bronchi (left and right)--the major air ducts to the lungs
   lobar bronchi--branches of each principal bronchus (="secondary" bronchi)
   segmental bronchi--branches of lobar bronchi (="tertiary" bronchi)
   bronchioles--branches of bronchi which contain no cartilage
   base of a lung--the caudal aspect (Fig. 12-2)
   apex of a lung--the cranial aspect
   costal surface of a lung--the surface adjacent to the ribs
   medial surface--the surface adjacent to the mediastinum
   diaphragmatic surface--the surface adjacent to the diaphragm
   dorsal border of a lung--the dorsal edge of the lung
   acute border
       ventral border--the ventral edge of the lung between the apex and the basal border

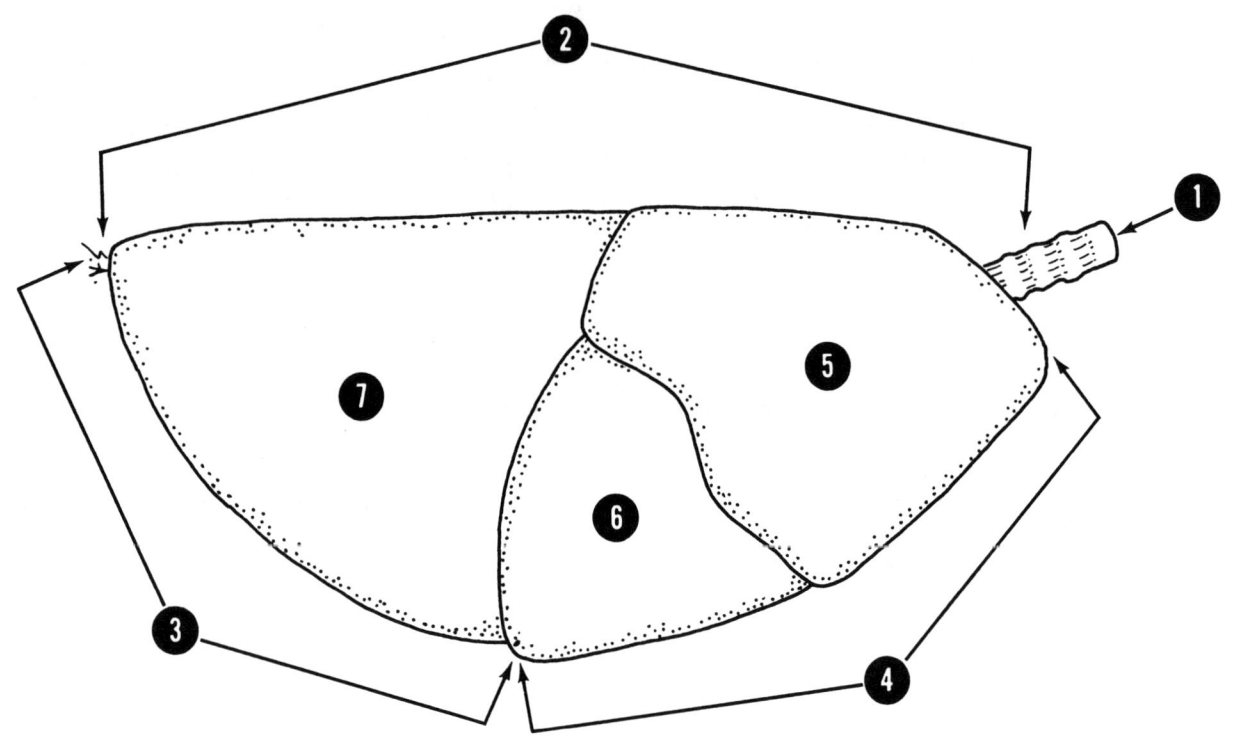

Figure 12-2

Right Lung of a Dog (costal surface)

1. Trachea
2. Dorsal border
3. Basal border
4. Ventral border (3 + 4 = acute border)
5. Cranial lobe
6. Middle lobe
7. Caudal lobe

        basal border--the caudoventral edge of the lung which lies adjacent to the diaphragm

right cardiac notch \
left cardiac notch   } areas where the interlobar fissures (see below) are wide and allow the pericardium to be in direct contact with the thoracic wall

cranial lobe
    cranial part
    caudal part
middle lobe (right lung only)
caudal lobe
accessory lobe (right lung only)
interlobar fissures--indentations between adjacent lobes

B. Comparative features

1. In all domestic species, the left lung has 2 lobes (cranial and caudal) and, in all but the horse, the right lung has four lobes (cranial, middle, caudal, and accessory). The horse lacks a middle lobe on the right lung (Fig. 12-3) [1,5].

2. In all species but the horse, the cranial lobe of the left lung is further divided into two parts: cranial and caudal.

3. In ruminants, the cranial lobe of the right lung is also divided into cranial and caudal parts.

4. Obsolete terms for the cranial, middle, and caudal lobes of the right lung are "apical," "cardiac," and "diaphragmatic" lobes, respectively. These same three obsolete terms have also been used for the three major divisions of the left lung (cranial part of the cranial lobe, caudal part of the cranial lobe, and caudal lobe). The accessory lobe has been called "intermediate" or "azygos" lobe.

5. In the ruminants and pig, a tracheal bronchus arises cranial to the tracheal bifurcation. The tracheal bronchus supplies the cranial lobe of the right lung.

C. Surgical and medical considerations

1. Collapse of the trachea with a resultant respiratory distress syndrome is a disease syndrome of small dogs. Radiographic examination at both maximal inspiration and expiration may be necessary to visualize the lesion (narrowed segment of the trachea). The collapse usually occurs as a dorsoventral flattening near the thoracic inlet. Some cases require fluoroscopy to demonstrate the lesions. Most cases respond to symptomatic treatment, but several surgical corrections have been described. Hepatomegaly is present (for some obscure reason) in a high percentage of cases [6].

2. The two major indications for removing a lung or lung lobe are trauma and neoplasia. The major anatomical structures of concern are the branch of the bronchial tree and the branches of the

Figure 12-3

Lungs of Dog (A), Pig (B), Ox (C), and Horse (D)
(dorsal aspect)

1. Trachea

2. Cranial lobe of left lung (has cranial and caudal parts in all but the horse)

3. Caudal lobe of left lung

4. Cranial lobe of the right lung (has cranial and caudal parts in ruminants)

5. Middle lobe of right lung (not present in horse)

6. Caudal lobe of right lung

7. Accessory lobe of right lung (position is indicated by dotted lines)

8. Tracheal bronchus to right cranial lobe (present in pig and ruminants only)

After Nickel, Schummer, Seiferle, and Sack, 1973 [5]

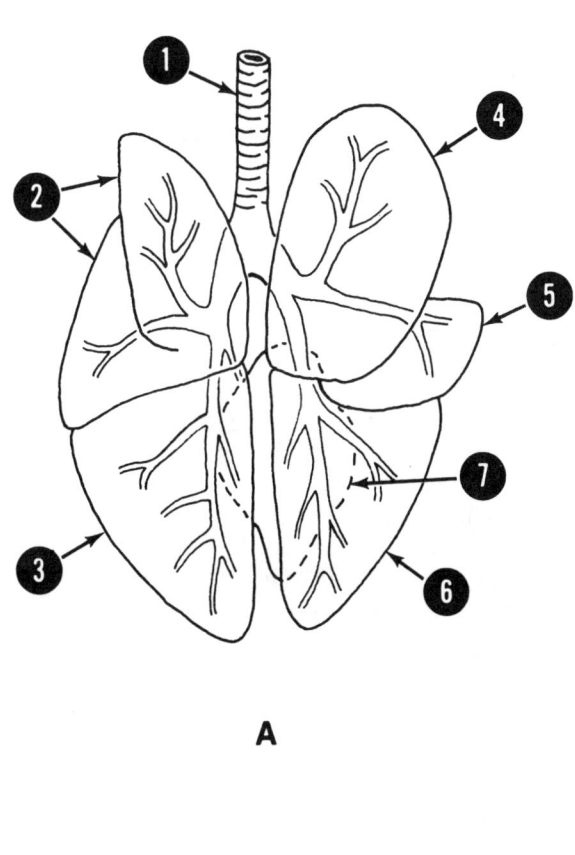

A

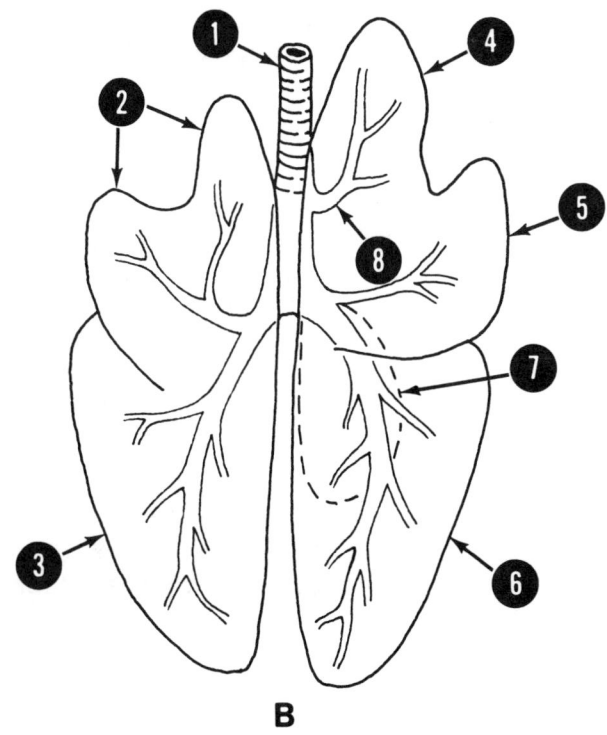

B

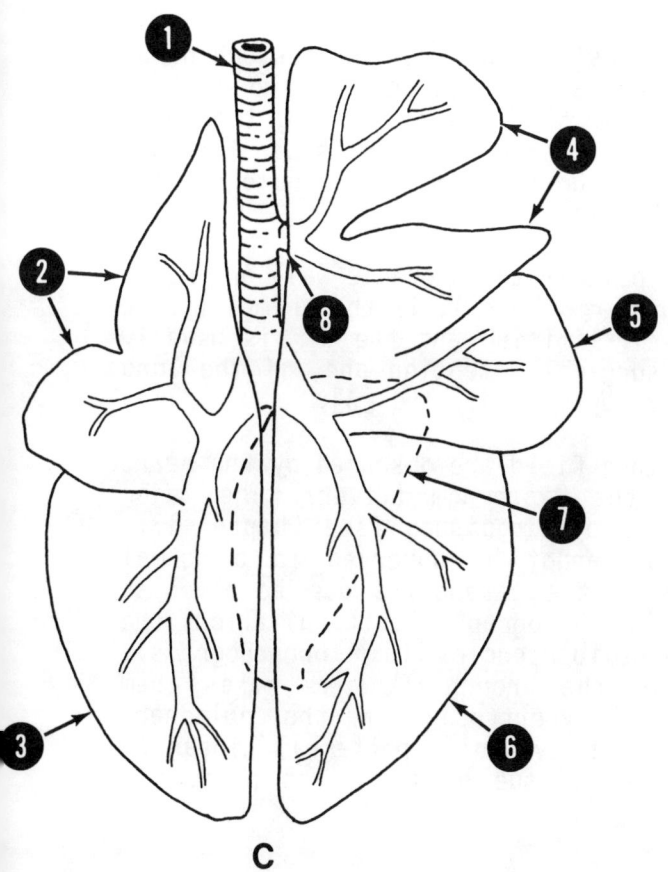

C

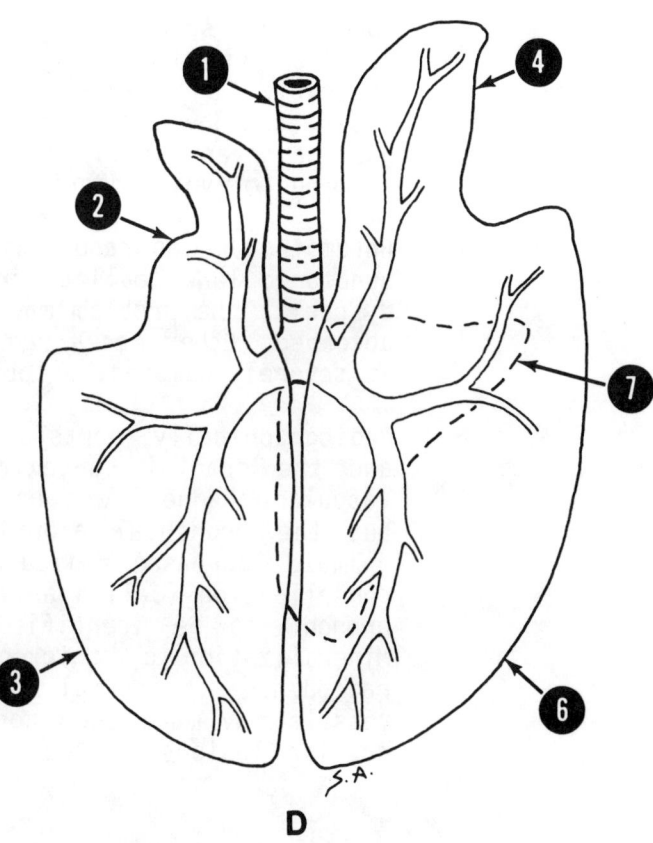

D

275

pulmonary artery and vein. These must be collectively or individually ligated. In larger animals, oversewing the end of the bronchus may effect better closure [3]. In smaller animals (and cats), this is a tedious and unnecessary procedure if no leaks are observed after bronchial ligation.

3. The cardiac notches of the lung are not usually given consideration during cardiocentesis. Although they represent clefts between lobes where the heart is in close contact with the thoracic wall, there are other factors more important than whether one misses or hits the lung with the needle (see heart and pericardium, Part III).

4. Auscultation of normal lungs yields very little sound. The area on the thorax where the lung field can be ausculted is somewhat limited by the thoracic limb, especially in large animals. The general area is a triangle bounded by the caudal border of the triceps brachii (cranially), a line from the caudal angle of the scapula to the tuber coxae (dorsally), and a curved line (concave ventrally) from the olecranon to the dorsal end of the next to the last intercostal space (caudoventrally) [2].

5. Percussion of the lung field is an art that requires considerable practice to develop proficiency. The sound produced by striking with a finger or percussion hammer is derived from three sources [2]: the noise of the impact, the sound of vibration of the thoracic wall, and the resonance of the underlying air-filled cavity. The sound varies from flat to resonant, depending on the character of the underlying organs.

6. Thoracentesis for diagnosis or drainage is done in an intercostal space. The space is punctured just dorsal to the costochondral junction (in the cranial intercostal spaces, one may go further ventrally) and midway between the ribs. In performing thoracentesis, the line of diaphragmatic attachment (which is parallel but just caudoventral to the line of pleural reflection) should be kept in mind to avoid entering the abdominal cavity [2].

7. Pneumothorax can result from a hole in the thoracic wall or from a punctured lung (bullet, fractured rib, etc.). If the animal is not dyspneic, the problem may be self-limiting and the air is usually absorbed. Other cases require surgical attention and, if the lung is severely damaged, a lobectomy may be indicated [3].

8. Radiographically, parts of the lung field are obscured by the heart and the cranial convexity of the diaphragm (liver). The major vascular channels can usually be distinguished (see Chapter 13), but the bronchial arborization cannot be observed in a normal animal. Increased radiodensity of the parenchyma due to alveolar consolidation (called an alveolar radiographic pattern) allows the bronchi to be identified as radiolucencies (air bronchograms). Mineralization or thickening of the bronchial walls makes them radiodense (bronchial pattern). Hypertrophy of the pulmonary vessels may make them more obvious (vascular pattern). Linear or nodular lesions in the connective tissue of the lungs produce a

myriad of changes referred to collectively as interstitial patterns [7]. Radiographs of diseased lungs usually show a mixture of two or more of the four patterns noted above. Alveolar and interstitial patterns are the ones most commonly observed.

III. HEART AND PERICARDIUM

In most domestic mammals, the heart is located from about the second or third to the fifth or sixth intercostal space and extends dorsally from the sternum about two-thirds of the distance toward the vertebral column. The heart lies essentially on the midline, but the apex (free, pointed end) is inclined caudally, ventrally, and to the left.

A. Basic features [1]

base--the craniodorsal aspect where the great vessels enter and leave
apex--the caudoventral, free end
paraconal (left) interventricular groove--located cranioventrally
subsinusal (right) interventricular groove--located caudodorsally
coronary groove--the fat-filled indentation separating the atria from the ventricles
pericardium--the membrane around the heart which has a fibrous outer part and a serous inner part
    fibrous--the connective tissue between the mediastinal pleura and the pericardium, which may form identifiable ligaments in some species or individuals (sternopericardiac lig. and phrenico-pericardiac lig.)
    serous--the serous membrane around the heart
        parietal lamina--the outer portion of the serous pericardium; continuous at the base of the heart with the visceral lamina
        visceral lamina (= epicardium)--the serous membrane covering the myocardium
pericardial cavity--the space between the parietal and visceral laminae of the serous pericardium
myocardium --the muscle of the heart
right atrium--receives systemic veins
    pectinate mm.--irregular bundles of myocardium lining the atrium
    vena caval sinus--the area where the venae cavae enter (including the openings of the cranial vena cava, caudal vena cava, and the coronary sinus)
    right auricle--the blind-ended portion of the atrium
    intervenous tubercle--the ridge between the openings of the cranial and caudal venae cavae
    fossa ovalis--the depression caudal to the intervenous tubercle where the foramen ovale was located
interatrial septum--the partition between the left and right atria
right ventricle--receives the outflow from the right atrium
    right atrioventricular [tricuspid] valve
        angular cusp--the cranial cusp (not present in carnivores)
        parietal cusp--the cusp adjacent to the free (lateral) wall
        septal cusp--the cusp adjacent to the interventricular septum
    chordae tendineae--fibrous cords which anchor the free edges of the cusps

                papillary mm.--evaginations of the myocardium which anchor the
                    chordae tendineae
                conus arteriosus--the funnel-shaped outflow tract of the right
                    ventricle (proximal to the pulmonary valve)
                valve of the pulmonary trunk (pulmonary valve)
                trabecula septomarginalis--a band ("moderator band") of myocardium
                    traversing the lumen
                trabeculae carneae--irregular bundles of myocardium which project
                    into the lumen
            left atrium--receives several pulmonary veins
                left auricle--the blind-ended portion of the atrium
                valve of the foramen ovale--a thin flap of tissue over the opening
                    of the foramen ovale
                openings of pulmonary veins
            left ventricle--receives the outflow from the left atrium
                left atrioventricular [mitral, biscuspid] valve
                    parietal cusp--the caudal cusp
                    septal cusp--the cranial cusp
                chordae tendineae--see right ventricle
                papillary mm.--see right ventricle
                aortic valve
                trabeculae carneae--see right ventricle
            interventricular septum--the partition between right and left ventricles

B. Physiological and comparative considerations

1. Because of the torqued orientation of the heart within the thorax, the right and left ventricles are positioned almost cranially and caudally, respectively (rather than right and left) [8].

2. In all domestic animals, a connective tissue "skeleton" in the heart separates the more delicate atria from the more massive ventricles. This contains some cartilage in all animals and, in the ox and older horses, two bones (ossa cordi) are present as well [8].

3. The right atrioventricular valve of carnivores has only two major (parietal and septal) cusps--although smaller cusps may be found at the extremities of these major ones.

4. The left ventricular wall is much thicker than the right ventricular wall (except in fetuses and neonates where they are about equal in thickness). This difference reflects the fact that the left side is a high-pressure system, whereas the right side is a relatively low-pressure system. The left ventricle extends down to the apex, but the right one does not. The lumen of the left ventricle is cone-shaped, whereas the right ventricular lumen is flattened and wraps around the former.

5. The specialized conducting system of the heart is part of the myocardium and is not a gross anatomical entity. It includes the sinoatrial node where the impulse for contraction initiates, the atrioventricular node and fascicle, and the left and right conducting crura.

6. In cats, the heart is positioned 1-2 intercostal spaces further caudally than in dogs.

C. Clinical considerations

1. In cardiac auscultation, the first sound is caused by (or at least associated with) closure of the A-V valves. The second sound is caused by closure of the semilunar valves (aortic and pulmonary valves) [2]. Ventricular contraction (systole) occurs between the first and second sounds and ventricular relaxation (diastole) occurs between the second and first sounds. The intraventricular pressure, caused by the ventricular contraction, causes the A-V valves to close and the semilunar valves to open. During ventricular diastole, the semilunar valves close from aortic and pulmonary trunk back-pressure, and the A-V valves open when the intra-atrial pressure from venous return exceeds the intra-ventricular pressure. It is possible that gravitational pull on the intra-atrial blood may also be a factor in opening the A-V valves.

2. A heart murmur is an abnormal sound associated with the turbulent flow of blood. By definition, they can be ausculted but they cannot be demonstrated radiographically [4]. However, angiography can often be used to demonstrate the cause of a murmur. A murmur during ventricular contraction could be caused by a leak (insufficiency) in an A-V valve (which is supposed to be closed) or by a narrowing (stenosis) in a semilunar valve (which is supposed to be open). Conversely, a murmur during ventricular diastole could be caused by a stenosis of an A-V valve (which should be open) or by an inssuficiency of a semilunar valve (which should be closed). The temporal relationship of valvular murmurs to the cardiac cycle is summarized below [2]:

valvular pathology	murmur should occur during
atrioventricular insufficiency	systole
atrioventricular stenosis	diastole
aortic or pulmonary insufficiency	diastole
aortic or pulmonary stenosis	systole

Of the various valvular conditions, left AV insufficiency is the most common and has been reported to occur in a large proportion (up to 40%) of the canine population [6]. Three types of aortic stenoses have been reported (supravalvular, valvular, and subvalvular), depending on the location of the offending fibrosis [6]. Pulmonic insufficiency and left A-V stenosis are rare.

3. Once it has been decided that a murmur is systolic (between the first and second heart sounds) or diastolic (between the second and first sounds), the problem of determining the exact cause becomes an anatomic one of locating where (which valve) the murmur is heard

the loudest. This point, called the PMI (point of maximal intensity), is usually located at the auscultation site of the offending valve. Because various thoracic structures influence the conduction of sound from the heart valves to the thoracic wall, the PMI's for various valves do not correspond precisely to the anatomic locations of the valves. General positions for auscultation of specific valves for all species are summarized below [2]:

Valve	Position for Auscultation*
Left A-V	low in the left fourth or fifth intercostal space (about the level of the olecranon)
Aortic	high in the left fourth intercostal space (just below a horizontal line passing through the shoulder joint)
Pulmonic	low in the left third intercostal space
Right A-V	low in the right third to fifth intercostal space

4. The two most common nonvalvular murmurs are those associated with patent ductus arteriosus (PDA) and interventricular septal defects (ISD). The typical murmur produced by patent ductus is often called a machinery murmur and is continuous. It is loudest on the left side, between the P and the A. The one associated with an interventricular septal defect is a systolic murmur and is loudest on the right side near the sternum. ISDs are very common in terriers and in larger dogs. A subaortic stenosis may cause a similar murmur [9].

5. Auscultation of the feline heart is confounded by the small size of the heart, the high heart rate, and also by purring. Purring may be diminished or eliminated by digital pressure dorsal to the larynx. Feline heart disease has been reviewed by Tilley [10].

6. Percussion of the heart may be used to determine if the heart is enlarged. The area of absolute cardiac dullness demarcates the area where the pericardium is in contact with the thoracic wall. It gives a flat sound on percussion. The area of relative cardiac dullness is more difficult to pinpoint [2].

---

*In practice, one does not count spaces and measure for the PMI. Instead, the stethoscope head is placed in the approximate location and moved as needed to maximize the sound. A memory aid for the left side is $P^A M$--$3^4 5$, where P, A, and M represent the pulmonary, aortic, and mitral valves, the numbers indicate intercostal spaces, and the staggered positions represent "high" or "low" within an intercostal space.

7. In cardiocentesis, either the right or left ventricle can be used. Some veterinarians prefer to puncture the left side because its thicker wall may close the puncture wound better and its lumen (circular on transverse section) is easier to hit than that of the right ventricle (flattened on transverse section). The left side has a further advantage when blood is collected because the higher systolic pressure will bleed the animal faster. To puncture the left ventricle, palpate for the strongest ventricular contractions on the left thoracic wall (at about the lower left fifth intercostal space) and direct the needle toward the opposite shoulder. A burst of ectopic beats may accompany the penetration of the ventricular wall. If these persist, the needle should be withdrawn and an adjacent site should be penetrated [11]. The left ventricle can be penetrated from the right side by passing the needle through the right ventricle and the interventricular septum [12].

8. Stenoses of the pulmonary and aortic valves often cause poststenotic dilations (aneurysms) because of the turbulent flow. These can be visualized by angiography [6].

9. Dirofilariasis causes enlargement of the right ventricle and pulmonary trunk where the adult worms reside. The enlargement is due to the increased pressure required to pump blood through the pulmonary vasculature because of inflammation of the vascular intima. The pulmonary arteries are also grossly enlarged and have increased tortuosity. Adult heartworms may be surgically removed by incisions in the right atrium, right ventricle, and/or pulmonary trunk [3]. However, most cases are treated medically.

10. In a V-D radiograph* of a normal canine thorax, the heart is normally about two-thirds the width of the thoracic cavity. It assumes an egg-shaped outline with the base wider than the apex. A slight cant of the apex to the left is normal. In a V-D projection, the sternum and vertebral column should be superimposed; if not, the animal was accidentally tilted (obliqued). The base of the pulmonary trunk is represented by the portion of the cardiac shadow from about 12:30 to 1:30 o'clock. The left atrium is found from 1:30 to 3:00. (In dogs it may not actually form part of the border unless it is enlarged [13].) The left ventricle is located from 3:00 to 6:00 and the part of the shadow from 6:00 to 11:30 is right ventricle (Fig. 12-4). The mediastinum normally obscures cardiac shadows from about 11:30 to 12:30. Enlargement of the right atrium may be seen at 11:00 to 12:00. All of these "times" may vary by 30 minutes to an hour due to individual and breed variations in cardiac orientation.

---

*Dorsoventral projections have actually been found to be of more value than V-D views in interpreting the heart because the shape and position are more consistent. Regardless of how the exposure was made, however, thoracic films should always be viewed in the same way (most commonly, in a V-D perspective with the animal's right to the viewer's left). Similarly, lateral views should always be viewed from the same perspective (most commonly, with the head to the left) whether they are left-right laterals or right-left laterals [13].

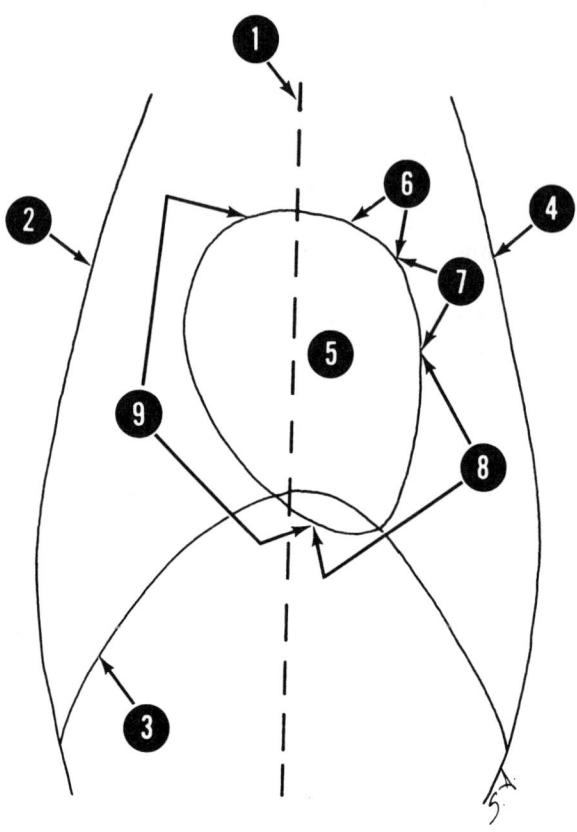

Figure 12-4

Prominent Radiographic Shadows in a V-D Perspective of a Canine Thorax

1. The midline - where one should ideally find the superimposed shadows of the sternum and the vertebral column*
2. Right thoracic wall
3. Diaphragm
4. Left thoracic wall
5. Heart

Approximate position of structures in the cardiac silhouette

6. Pulmonary trunk
7. Left atrium (auricle of left atrium)
8. Left ventricle
9. Right ventricle

*Often the animal will be tilted slightly to one side or the other and superimposition of the sternum and vertebral column will not be present.

After Habel, 1981 [2]

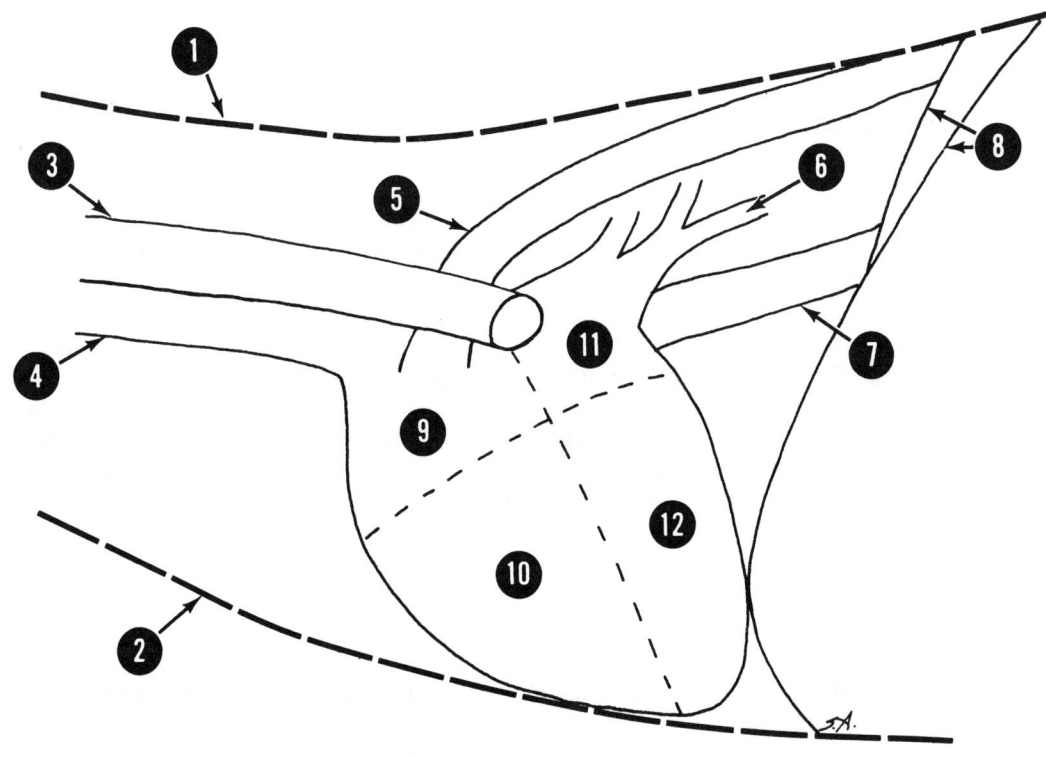

Figure 12-5

Prominent Radiographic Shadows in a Lateral
Perspective of a Canine Thorax

1. Dorsal limit of thoracic cavity
2. Ventral limit of thoracic cavity
3. Trachea (at its caudal extent is an end-on view of a principle bronchus)
4. Cranial vena cava
5. Aorta (its apparent "origin" from 9 is caused by superimposition)
6. Pulmonary veins
7. Caudal vena cava
8. Crura of diaphragm

Approximate position of the heart chambers in the cardiac silhouette

9. Right atrium
10. Right ventricle
11. Left atrium
12. Left ventricle

After Habel, 1981 [2]

11. In a lateral perspective of the thorax, the apex of the heart is obliqued ventrocaudally. The right ventricle comprises most of the ventral portion of the cranial border of the cardiac shadow, and the left ventricle is most of the ventral portion of the caudal border (including the apex). The right atrium is the craniodorsal part of the shadow and the left atrium is the caudodorsal part (Fig. 12-5). The heart should extend about two-thirds of the distance from the sternum to the vertebral column. Cardiac enlargement may be assessed by dorsal displacement of the tracheal shadow, toward the vertebral column (from which it should normally diverge). Right ventricular enlargement is indicated by increased sternal contact. Left ventricular enlargement is indicated by a straightened caudal border.

12. Anatomic changes associated with specific enlargements of various chambers may be observed radiographically [13]:

    a. right atrium--elevation of trachea, loss of the cranial "waist" of the heart, and enlargement of the 9-11 o'clock border (lateral perspective).

    b. right ventricle--increased sternal contact, elevation of the trachea amd elevation of the caudal vena cava (lateral view), and rounding of the right border (V-D view).

    c. left atrium--elevation of the distal trachea and in the dog (but not in the cat) the left principal bronchus appears dorsal to the right one (lateral perspective); enlargement of the heart at 2-3 o'clock (V-D view).

    d. left ventricle--caudal border of the heart appears straighter (lateral perspective); the apex may shift to the right of the midline and the left ventricular border may appear rounded (V-D view).

13. Limited open-heart surgery may be performed by inflow venous occlusion. In this technique, flow in the cranial and caudal vena cavae (and sometimes in the azygos vein as well) is temporarily stopped by tension on umbilical tape or heavy suture loops which have been passed around them. The surgeon has about $2\frac{1}{2}$ - 3 minutes to work before brain damage occurs [14]. However, if the work is not finished, the heart can be allowed to pump a short time and the venous occlusion can again be applied. This technique will allow pulmonary stenosis correction, but more sophisticated open heart techniques (such as repair of an interventricular septal defect) require heart-lung bypass machines and/or hypothermic techniques. Using hypothermia, a heart can be stopped for over 20 minutes with no (detectable) brain damage in dogs [15].

14. A left intercostal thoracotomy at the fourth or fifth intercostal space is used in correcting pulmonary stenosis in carnivores [3]. After inflow venous occlusion (VO), a right ventriculotomy or a pulmonary arteriotomy is performed and the stenosis can be relieved with a valvulotome [3]. Preferably, however, a larger incision is made to allow direct visual assessment of the valve leaflets. Fused

edges may be reseparated or, if individual leaflets are unrecognizable, the connective tissue ring can be incised from its free margin to the wall of the pulmonary trunk to create new leaflets. The insufficiency that this may produce is less serious than the original pulmonary stenosis. Two or three preplaced, untied, inverting mattress sutures over the incision line will allow the surgeon using VO to temporarily close the incision (by pulling the sutures tight) and allow the heart to pump. These sutures are ultimately used for final closure of the cardiotomy.

15. A left intercostal thoracotomy, at about the fourth intercostal space, is also used in correcting a patent ductus arteriosus [3]. The ductus is isolated by careful dissection between the aorta and pulmonary trunk and then ligated with nonabsorbable suture material or divided and oversewn [3].

16. The pericardium may be left unsutured after open heart surgery or only loosely approximated. This insures that a cardiac tamponade will not occur. Cardiac tamponade results from a luminal filling deficit due to pressure from fluid accumulation in the pericardial cavity. It may be caused by hemorrhage or may be due to a collection of purulent fluid as in some cases of traumatic pericarditis in cattle. The pressure of the fluid prevents the heart from filling with blood during diastole.

17. The heart suffers a number of developmental anomalies which may present as clinical problems.* Some of these include:

    a. Anomalies of the atrial septum

        (1) Probe patency of the foramen ovale--the foramen ovale in many otherwise normal individuals fails to permanently close. No interatrial shunting (or an insignificant amount) seems to occur. This does not have clinical significance and should be recognized as "normal" at necropsy.

        (2) Interatrial septal defect and/or clinically patent foramen ovale. Two types of septal defects are recognized: ostium primum defects (ventral part of septum) and ostium secundum defects (upper part of septum) [6]. These anomalies may allow considerable interatrial shunting.

        (3) Common atrium--the interatrial septum fails to develop and there are usually other defects in the heart.

    b. Interventricular (ventricular) septal defect - this produces a characteristic systolic murmur.

    c. Tetralogy of Fallot--this anomaly consists of a pulmonary stenosis, a ventricular septal defect, over-riding aorta (over both ventricles), and hypertrophy of the right ventricle.

---

*Abnormalities of the great vessels are considered in Central Angiology (Chapter 13).

d. Transposition of the great vessels--the aorta originates from the right ventricle and the pulmonary trunk from the left ventricle.

e. Persistent truncus arteriosus--the pulmonary trunk and aorta are a common trunk for a short distance beyond the heart.

f. Valvular stenoses--developmental or acquired strictures.

g. Valvular atresia--the valve(s) fail to develop properly.

h. Dextrocardia--this condition, where the heart is angled to the right, is often associated with situs inversus of the other thoracic organs.

i. Ectopia cordis--this condition, where the heart is on the surface of the chest, is usually caused by an embryologic failure of midsternal closure.

IV. DIAPHRAGM (Fig. 12-6)

The diaphragm is a skeletal muscle that forms a septum between the thoracic and abdominal cavities in mammals.

A. Major features [1]

lumbar part--the dorsal part
    right crus   include fleshy portions as well as the
    left crus   tendinous parts that attach to the lumbar vertebrae
costal part--the lateral part
sternal part--the ventral part
aortic hiatus--passageway for the aorta, thoracic duct, and azygos vein
esophageal hiatus--passageway for the esophagus and vagal nerve trunks
vena caval foramen ("caval foramen")--passageway for the caudal vena cava
central tendon--the V-shaped aponeurotic central portion
cupula --the cranial aspect of the convexity of the diaphragm

B. Functional and medical considerations

1. The diaphragm is markedly convex on its cranial aspect. During contraction, it lowers the intrapleural pressure by becoming flatter and increasing the length of the thorax. As a result, air rushes down the trachea and inflates the lungs. Expiration is primarily a passive process, resulting from the elasticity of the fibers in the pulmonary parenchyma and also from the surface tension of the fluid lining the alveoli. Although some other thoracic muscles (including the intercostal mm.) may aid respiration, the contraction of the diaphragm and the natural tendency for the lungs to shrink are the two major factors.

2. The concave nature of the caudal aspect of the diaphragm allows the abdominal viscera to extend cranially and invaginate into the caudal aspect of the rib cage. This is why liver biopsies in some

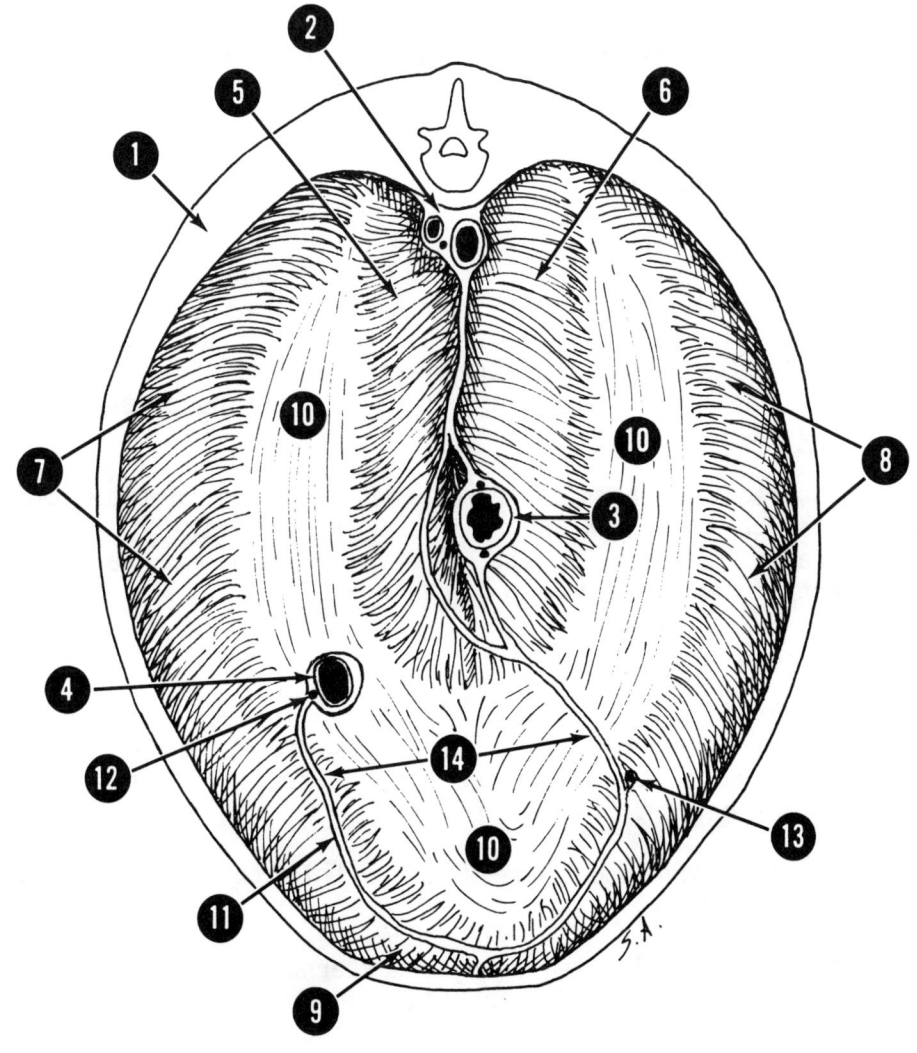

Figure 12-6

The Diaphragm of a Dog (cranial aspect)

1. Body wall
2. Aorta, azygos vein, and thoracic duct in the aortic hiatus
3. Esophagus and dorsal and ventral vagal nerve trunks in the esophageal hiatus
4. Caudal vena cava in the vena caval foramen
5. Right crus of lumbar part
6. Left crus of lumbar part
7. Right costal part
8. Left costal part
9. Sternal part
10. Central tendon
11. Plica vena cava
12. Right phrenic nerve
13. Left phrenic nerve
14. Mediastinal recess

After Nickel, Schummer, Seiferle, and Sack, 1973 [5]

species are done intercostally (see Chapter 11, Abdomen). This cranial convexity usually extends to the heart and explains the traumatic pericarditis often seen in hardware disease in cattle.

3. The apparent radiographic density of the diaphragm is due to the fluid density of the liver caudal to it, contrasted against the gas density of the lung field. On lateral radiographic perspectives of the thorax, either crus of the diaphragm can appear to be cranial to the other one. Usually the "down" crus (the one nearest to the table) will be pushed further forward by the weight of the abdominal viscera. The one most closely associated with the gastric air bubble is usually the left one. The right crus is associated with the portion of the central tendon penetrated by the caudal vena cava.

4. Diaphragmatic hernias are common sequelae to traumatic accidents. Although they can occur in any part of the diaphragm, they are usually located in the fleshy portions and rarely involve the central tendon or natural openings [16].

V. MISCELLANEOUS THORACIC STRUCTURES

A. The thymus is well developed in young individuals and difficult or impossible to find in adults. It has important immunological functions. In the ruminants, thymic tissue often extends to the cranial aspect of the cervical region.

B. A number of lymph nodes are found within the thorax. Among the more important are these:

1. Sternal nodes located along the sternum.
2. Tracheobronchial nodes located near the bifurcation of the trachea. These may enlarge and become radiographically detectable in some infectious diseases.
3. Caudal mediastinal nodes in the mediastinum caudal to the heart. In the ox, a single, large node is present at this location. Its enlargement can put pressure on the esophagus, causing problems with deglutition and/or eructation.

C. The esophagus is positioned dorsal to the trachea. It crosses the base of the heart and continues on to pass through the esophageal hiatus of the diaphragm. Three places along its course where it commonly suffers clinical blockage or stricture from either luminal foreign bodies or external pressure are:

1. thoracic inlet (choke)
2. base of the heart (vascular ring disease)
3. esophageal hiatus of diaphragm

(Further consideration of the esophagus is found in Head and Neck, Chapter 19.)

D. A number of important nerve trunks are found in the thorax.

1. The left and right phrenic nerves are derived from the ventral

branches of some of the caudal cervical spinal nerves. They pass through the thoracic inlet, course caudally across the pericardium, and enter the diaphragm. Heart surgeons should preserve them, although it has been shown that bilateral phrenicotomy does not paralyze the diaphragm [17].

2. The left and right sympathetic trunks course caudally along the dorsal aspects of the thoracic wall. In the cervical region, before they enter the thoracic inlet, they are still combined with the vagus nerves as the vagosympathetic trunks. Near the thoracic inlet (middle cervical ganglion), the sympathetic trunk and vagus nerve on each side split away from one another. The sympathetic trunks course dorsally and continue caudally along the dorsal aspect of the thoracic cavity, receiving rami communicantes from the spinal nerves. The ganglia along their course are called sympathetic trunk ganglia except for the initial thoracic one on each side which is larger than the rest and is termed the cervico-thoracic (stellate) ganglion. A number of branches to the thoracic organs are present. At the caudal aspect of the thoracic cavity the sympathetic trunks course over the diaphragm to enter the abdomen and continue caudally.

3. The left and right vagal nerves split away from the sympathetic trunks at the middle cervical ganglia. They course caudally across either side of the base of the heart and each one splits into a dorsal branch and a ventral branch. The left and right dorsal branches recombine on the dorsal aspect of the esophagus to form the dorsal vagal trunk. Likewise, the left and right ventral branches recombine on the ventral aspect of the esophagus to form the ventral vagal trunk. These follow the esophagus through the diaphragm and innervate the organs of the digestive system as far caudally as the colon.

At the level of the middle cervical ganglia, the vagal nerves give rise to the recurrent laryngeal nerves which course cranially around the aorta (left side) or right subclavian artery (right side) to innervate structures in the neck as far cranially as the larynx. The cranial extent of each recurrent laryngeal nerve is the caudal laryngeal nerve, and it innervates most of the intrinsic muscles of the larynx except for the cricothyroideus m. This nerve (or its recurrent laryngeal parent nerve) is involved in equine laryngeal hemiplegia (commonly called roaring). The cause of the nerve damage remains unknown, but about 90% occur on the left side. Denervation of the intrinsic laryngeal muscles produces the characteristic noise on forced respiration because the glottis is partially obstructed from the relaxed and adducted vocal fold. A number of surgical corrections have been described involving a ventral laryngotomy [18].

E. The thoracic duct is the major channel returning lymph to the circulatory system from the abdomen, pelvis, and pelvic limbs. It is on the right side near the aorta caudally, and usually crosses to the left side near or just caudal to the heart. It empties into the venous system near the left external jugular vein. The exact locus varies with species and individual. It is not uncommon for the thoracic duct to be double.

Rupture of the duct results in chylothorax, which is sometimes surgically corrected by ligation. The presence of multiple channels and the difficulty in finding the duct often makes this surgery less than satisfactory. Its location during surgery may be facilitated by feeding the patient a fatty meal beforehand [3]. If a break is actually found, the duct should be ligated on both sides of it. (See Chapter 13.)

References

1. International Committee on Veterinary Gross Anatomical Nomenclature. 1983. Nomina Anatomica Veterinaria, third ed. Published by the Committee, Ithaca, New York.

2. Habel, R. E. 1981. Applied Veterinary Anatomy, second ed. Published by the author, Ithaca, New York.

3. Archibald, J. ed. 1974. Canine Surgery, second ed. American Veterinary Publications, Santa Barbara, California.

4. Shively, M. J. 1982. Twenty more veterinary anatomic lies, half truths, and misleading statements. Jour. Vet. Med. Ed. 9(1):20-21.

5. Nickel, R., A. Schummer, E. Seiferle, and W. Sack. 1973. The Viscera of the Domestic Mammals. Verlag Paul Parey, Berlin.

6. Ettinger, S. J. 1983. Textbook of Veterinary Internal Medicine, second ed. W. B. Saunders, Philadelphia.

7. Kealy, J. K. 1979. Diagnostic Radiology of the Dog and Cat. W. B. Saunders, Philadelphia.

8. Schummer, A. H., H. Wilkens, B. Vollmerhaus, and K. H. Habermehl. 1981. The Circulatory System, the Skin, and the Cutaneous Organs of the Domestic Mammals. Translated by W. Siller and A. Wright. Verlag Paul Parey, Berlin.

9. Knauer, K. 1982. Personal communication.

10. Tilley, L. P. 1977. Symposium on feline cardiology. Vet. Clin. N. Am. 7:2.

11. Ettinger, S. J., and P. F. Suter. 1970. Canine Cardiology. W. B. Saunders, Philadelphia.

12. Buchanan, J. W., and R. P. Botts. 1972. Clinical effects of repeated cardiac punctures in dogs. JAVMA 16(17):814-818.

13. Owens, J. M., and D. N. Biery. 1982. Radiographic Interpretation for the Small Animal Clinician. Ralston Purina Company, Saint Louis, Missouri.

14. Ott, B. S., B. A. Raymond, R. L. North, and G. E. Pickens. 1964. Diagnosis and surgical repair of congenital pulmonary stenosis in the dog. JAVMA 144(8):851-856.

15. Weirich, W. E., C. R. Smith, F. P. Incropera, and I. Mandelbaum. 1973. Hypothermia for cardiac arrest surgery in the dog. JAAHA 9(6):540-547.

16. Wilson, G. P., C. D. Newton, and J. K. Burt. 1971. A review of 116 diaphragmatic hernias in dogs and cats. JAVMA 159:1142-1146.

17. Evans, H. E., and G. C. Christensen. 1979. Miller's Anatomy of the Dog, second ed. W. B. Saunders, Philadelphia.

18. Mansmann, R. A., E. S. McAllister, and P. W. Pratt, eds. 1982. Equine Medicine and Surgery. American Veterinary Publications, Santa Barbara, California.

13

CENTRAL ANGIOLOGY AND LYMPHATIC SYSTEM

I. BRANCHES OF THE AORTA

The aorta is the parent vessel of all of the systemic arteries. It begins at the aortic valve of the left ventricle and terminates near the lumbosacral junction. The aorta is divided into three segments: the ascending aorta, aortic arch, and descending aorta [1].

A. Ascending aorta--courses cranially from the left ventricle and supplies two branches in all domestic species

1. Left coronary artery
   a. paraconal interventricular branch
   b. circumflex branch
2. Right coronary artery

In the dog and ruminants, a subsinuosal interventricular branch arises from the circumflex branch of the left coronary artery. This branch supplies much of the interventricular septum. This pattern, in which the whole left ventricular wall is supplied by the left coronary artery, results in an unequal size of the two coronary arteries and is called a left coronary type of supply [2]. In the pig and horse, the subsinuosal interventricular branch arises from the right coronary artery and the resulting pattern is known as a bilateral coronary type of supply [2]. The coronary arteries in these animals are more closely matched in size, and the left coronary artery supplies only part of the interventricular septum. In cats, the pattern is variable, but it is most commonly of the left coronary type [2].

B. Aortic arch--curves $180°$ dorsally and caudally. It has one branch in the horse and ruminants (brachiocephalic trunk). In the carnivores and pig, it has two branches (brachiocephalic trunk and left subclavian a.).

1. Brachiocephalic trunk (present in all domestic mammals)

   a. Left and right subclavian aa. (These vessels are distributed primarily to the limbs. In the carnivores and pig, the left subclavian artery arises as a separate branch of the aortic arch.)
   b. Bicarotid trunk (ungulates)
   or
   Separate left and right common carotid aa. (carnivores)

2. Left subclavian artery (arises directly from the aortic arch in the carnivores and pig--Fig. 13-1/A)

From this it can be seen that the major differences in the arborization of the brachiocephalic trunks of the various domestic species are the common (ungulates) or separate (carnivores) origins of the common carotid aa. and the locus of origin of the left

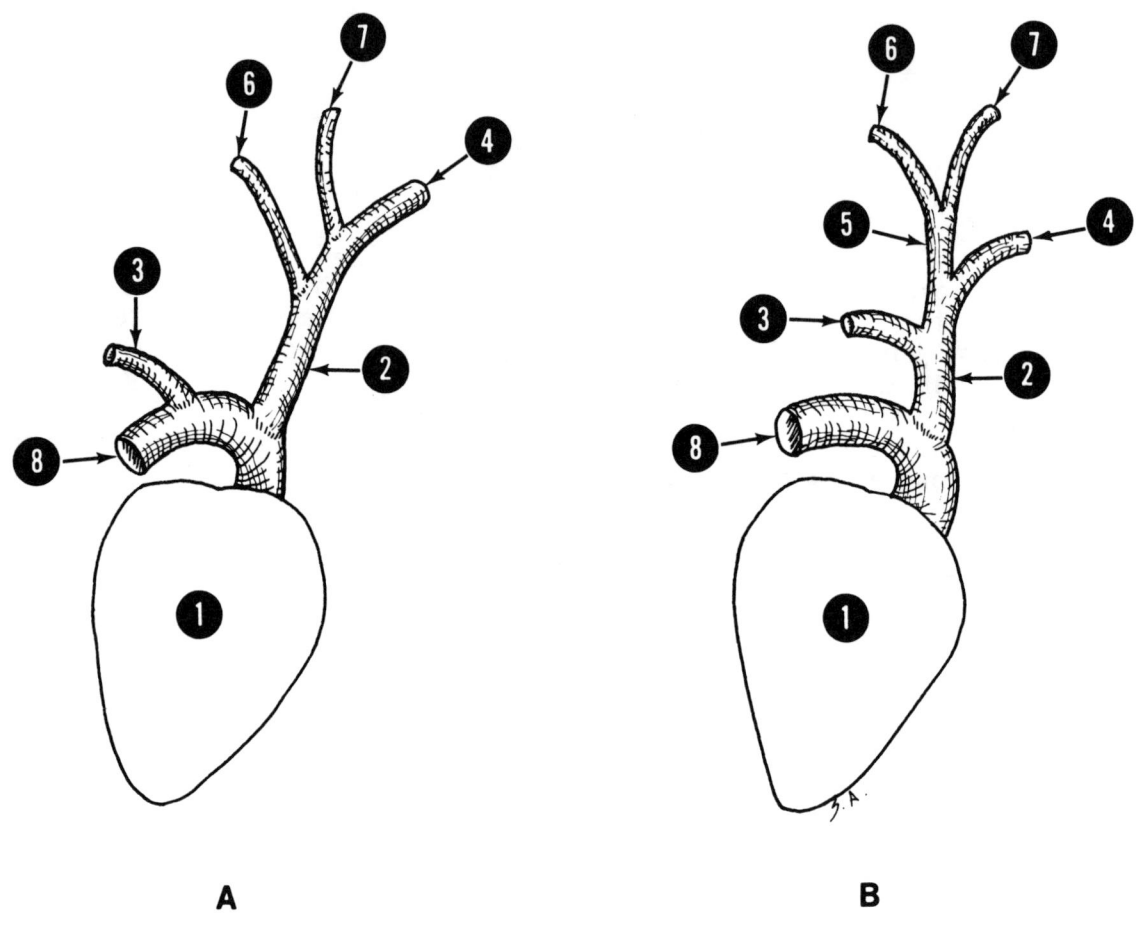

Figure 13-1

Branches of the Aortic Arch in the Carnivores (A)
and in the Horse and Ruminants (B) (dorsal aspect)

1. Heart
2. Brachiocephalic trunk
3. Left subclavian artery
4. Right subclavian artery
5. Bicarotid trunk (ungulates only)
6. Left common carotid artery
7. Right common carotid artery
8. Continuation of the aorta

The pattern in the pig resembles the one present in the horse and ruminants (B) except that the left subclavian a. (3) originates directly from the aortic arch as it does in the carnivores (A).

subclavian a. from the brachiocephalic trunk (ruminants and horse) or from the aortic arch (carnivores and pig).

Each subclavian artery supplies several branches either directly or indirectly (Fig. 13-2).
a. vertebral a.--courses through the transverse foramina of the cervical vertebrae supplying branches to the spinal cord and surrounding structures.
b. deep cervical artery--courses cranially in the deep muscles of the neck.
c. dorsal scapular a.--courses dorsally to supply the muscles near the dorsal border of the scapula.
d. supreme intercostal a.--courses caudally just ventral to the necks of the ribs and supplies some of the cranial aspects of the thoracic wall (intercostal spaces).*
e. costocervical trunk--a common trunk for two (horse and pit), three (carnivores, or all four (ruminants) of the above branches.
f. internal thoracic a.--courses parallel to the sternum just off the midline to supply the ventral ends of the dorsal intercostal arteries. It is of concern in midsternal thoracotomies if one strays too far from the midline and in intercostal thoracotomies if one extends the incision too far ventrally.
g. superficial cervical a.--courses cranially to supply branches to the shoulder region and superficial branches to the neck.

To summarize the variations in the origins of these vessels, in all domestic animals the internal thoracic a. and the superficial cervical a. originate as separate entities near the thoracic inlet. The remaining vessels (a-f above) arise together as the costocervical trunk or independently as follows:

(1) In the ruminants, all of the remaining arteries noted above (a-f) arise together and further proximally as the costocervical trunk. Therefore, each subclavian artery has only three branches in these species (Fig. 13-2/B).
(2) In the carnivores, there are four branches of each subclavian artery because the vertebral a. arises independently rather than from the costocervical trunk (Fig. 13-2/C).
(3) Horses have the carnivore pattern (four branches) on the right side, but on the left there are five branches because the deep cervical artery arises independently (Fig. 13-2/A). Also in the horse, the right subclavian a. arises much further cranially than its counterpart. Consequently, its two initial branches (costocervical

---

*In the dog, the parent trunk of the first few dorsal intercostal aa. courses dorsal to the necks of the ribs instead of ventral to them as it does in all other domestic mammals (including the cat). Consequently, in the dog this vessel is termed thoracic vertebral a. instead of supreme intercostal a. [1,2].

Figure 13-2

Schematic Representation of the Branches of the Left Subclavian Artery in the Horse (A), Ox (B), and Dog (C)

1. Subclavian a.

2. Costocervical trunk

3. Supreme intercostal a. (called thoracic vertebral a. in the dog because it courses dorsal to the necks of the ribs)

4. Dorsal scapular a.

5. Deep cervical a.

6. Vertebral a.

7. Superficial cervical a.

8. Internal thoracic a.

9. Continuation of the subclavian a. which becomes the axillary a. as it leaves the thoracic cavity by coursing around the first rib

The right subclavian artery in most species has a similar pattern of distribution. In the horse, however, the right side resembles the pattern in the dog with the deep cervical artery (5) originating from the costocervical trunk.

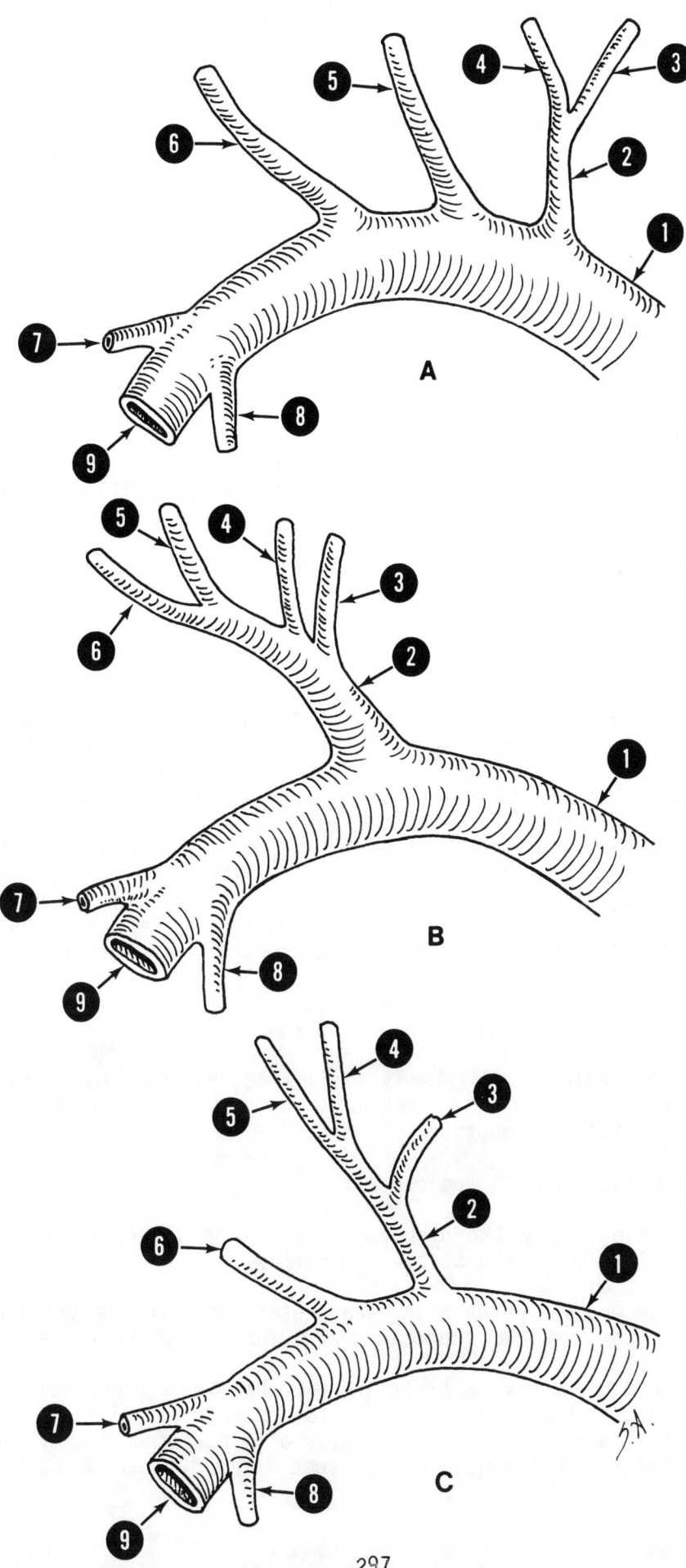

trunk and vertebral a.) may actually arise from the brachiocephalic trunk [2], but for simplicity they are still classified as branches of the subclavian a.
- (4) The pattern in the pig resembles that in the horse by having asymmetric branching on left and right sides, but the difference is related to the origin of the vertebral a. rather than to the origin of the deep cervical a.

C. Descending aorta--divided regionally into the thoracic aorta (branches 1 through 4 below) and the abdominal aorta (branches 6 through 16) (Fig. 13-3)

1. Bronchoesophageal a.

   This vessel may be paired or single. Its bronchial and esophageal branches may arise independently. Finally, it may arise from one of the dorsal intercostal aa. rather than from the aorta.

2. Miscellaneous small branches to the esophagus, pericardium, and mediastinum may be identifiable in some species or individuals.

3. Dorsal intercostal aa.

   The first few dorsal intercostal aa. on each side arise directly or indirectly from the costocervical trunk. The aorta supplies the rest of them directly. Toward their ventral ends, they divide to send a branch along the cranial border of each rib. Both branches (the one along the cranial border and the one remaining on the caudal aspect) anastomose with the internal thoracic artery near the sternum. Since they receive arterial input both dorsally and ventrally, surgical disruption of intercostal vessels during a thoracotomy will require attention to both cut ends for hemostasis. In addition, since the dorsal intercostal aa. are positioned near the caudal aspect of a rib, an intercostal incision should be made in the middle of an intercostal space [3].

4. Dorsal costoabdominal aa.

   This pair of vessels is similar to the intercostal aa. but is located caudal to the last pair of ribs and therefore is not "intercostal" in location.

5. Phrenic aa. (cranial and caudal)

   These supply the diaphragm. For those interested in details, they differ among the species as follows:

   a. The cranial phrenic aa. are present only in the horse and they arise from the thoracic aorta instead of from the abdominal aorta.
   b. In the carnivores, the caudal phrenic and cranial abdominal aa. arise as a common trunk (phrenicoabdominal a.).
   c. The caudal phrenic aa. usually originate from the celiac a. in the pig and ruminants. In some individual animals, the right

Figure 13-3

Major Branches of the Aorta
(ventral aspect)

1. Ascending aorta
2. Aortic arch
3. Brachiocephalic trunk
4. Left subclavian (in ungulates this artery originates from the brachiocephalic trunk - see Fig. 13-1)
5. Thoracic aorta (supplies cranial part of the descending aorta)
6. Diaphragm
7. Abdominal aorta (supplies caudal part of the descending aorta)
8. Celiac a. (supplies left gastric, splenic, and hepatic aa. in all species)
9. Cranial mesenteric a. (primarily distributed to the intestines)
10. Paired branches to the diaphragm (these have a number of species differences in regard to name, location, and what they supply - see text)
11. Paired renal aa.
12. Paired gonadal (testicular or ovarian) aa. (these arise from the terminal part of the aorta in the ruminants)
13. Caudal mesenteric a. (supplies descending colon)
14. Paired deep circumflex iliac aa. (in ungulates these arise from the external iliac aa.)
15. Paired external iliac aa. (the major blood supply to the pelvic limbs)
16. Paired internal iliac aa. (the major blood supply to the pelvic viscera)
17. Median sacral a. (supplies the tail)

Segmental branches including the dorsal intercostal aa., dorsal costoabdominal aa., and lumbar aa. are not shown.

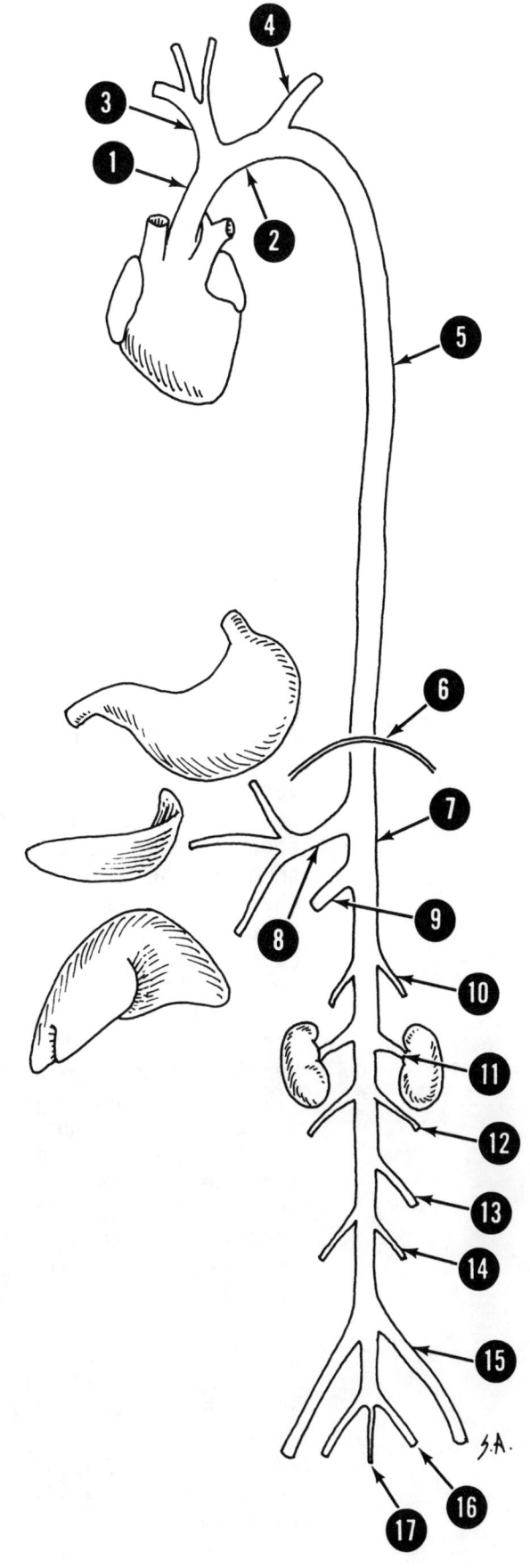

and left vessels may originate together and sometimes the origin is from the aorta rather than from the celiac a.

6. Cranial abdominal aa.

These vessels, distributed to the lateral abdominal wall, are present only in the carnivores and the pig [2]. In carnivores, they arise in common with the caudal phrenic aa. as the phrenicoabdominal trunks. These vessels course across the suprarenal glands of carnivores, supply some vessels to them, and require manipulation during suprarenalectomies (adrenalectomies). Several other small vessels supply the adrenal gland. With some species variations, these may arise from the caudal phrenic aa., celiac a., cranial mesenteric a., lumbar aa., renal aa., cranial abdominal aa., and/or the aorta.

7. Celiac a.

The celiac artery has three major branches:

a. Left gastric artery - courses toward the lesser curvature of the stomach near the esophagus.
b. Splenic artery - primarily supplies the spleen and, in most species, some pancreatic branches. The small vessels which continue on to the greater curvature of the stomach in non-ruminants are termed short gastric arteries. When they reach the stomach, they contribute to the left gastroepiploic artery along the greater curvature. The presence of these vessels prevents hemostasis during splenectomies in carnivores by the simple method of ligating the main splenic artery and then removing the spleen. (Retrograde hemorrhage will occur through the short gastric arteries which will be disrupted when the spleen is removed.) In ruminants, the splenic artery usually supplies the right and left ruminal arteries which course along the right and left longitudinal grooves of the rumen (Fig. 13-4). The ruminal arteries arise directly from the celiac a. in some individuals and the left one may arise from the left gastric a. [2].
c. Hepatic artery - supplies several hepatic branches to the liver parenchyma as well as a cystic artery to the gallbladder (except in the horse). The hepatic artery also supplies the right gastric artery to the lesser curvature of the stomach and the gastroduodenal artery. This latter vessel terminates by dividing into the right gastroepiploic artery (along the greater curvature of the stomach or abomasum) and the cranial pancreaticoduodenal artery (along the descending duodenum caudally).

8. Cranial mesenteric a.

The cranial mesenteric artery supplies most of the intestine and there are a number of unimportant species variations in its branches. Regardless of species, it gives rise to a caudal pancreaticoduodenal artery, an ileocolic artery, and a series of jejunal arteries. The ileocolic artery is distributed to the ileum, cecum, and it often supplies the right colic artery to the ascending colon. The middle colic artery is the branch of the cranial mesenteric vasculature most closely associated with the transverse colon. In the horse, the cranial mesenteric a. is a common site for the aneurysms caused by Strongylus vulgaris. Blockage of some of its branches by Strongylus species may cause colic (Fig. 13-5).

9. Caudal mesenteric a.

   The caudal mesenteric artery is the smallest of the three major unpaired branches of the abdominal aorta. It supplies the descending colon and divides within the mesocolon into two major branches: the left colic artery (directed cranially) and the cranial rectal artery (directed caudally).

10. Renal aa.

    Although these vessels are usually singular to each kidney, surgeons should watch for double or triple renal arteries during nephrectomies [4]. They often supply small twigs to the suprarenal glands and may also supply one of the gonadal aa. in some individuals.

11. Gonadal aa. (testicular or ovarian aa.)

    The testicular or ovarian arteries arise just caudal to the renal arteries in most species, but, they arise from the terminal aorta or even from the external iliac vessels in ruminants. It is clinically significant when doing ovariohysterectomies in carnivores that the ovarian vessels are not closely associated with the suspensory ligament. (See Chapter 16.) Tiny vessels which may course along the ligament are usually inconsequential.

12. Lumbar aa.

    This series of paired vessels, homologous to the dorsal intercostal vasculature, supplies the lumbar area. In some loci, a given pair may arise as a common trunk and the total number of pairs corresponds to the lumbar vertebral number. The last pair originates from the median sacral a. (in the carnivores, small ruminant, and pig) or from the iliolumbar aa. (ox). In the horse, the last two pair originate from the external iliac aa. [2].

13. Deep circumflex iliac aa.

    These vessels originate from the aorta only in the carnivores. In other species they are branches of the external iliac aa. They course laterally to supply the lateral abdominal wall and surrounding structures.

14. External iliac aa.

    The external iliac arteries are the major vessels which supply the pelvic limbs. After supplying the deep femoral artery, each one

Figure 13-4

Major Branches of the Celiac Artery of the Ox

    A. Visceral (right) aspect of stomach
    B. Parietal (left) aspect of stomach

1. Abdominal aorta

    2. Cranial mesenteric a.

    3. Celiac a.

        4. Left gastric a.

            5. Left gastroepiploic a.

            6. Accessory reticular a.

        7. Hepatic a.

            8. Right gastric a.

            9. Gastroduodenal a.

                10. Cranial pancreaticoduodenal a.

                11. Right gastroepiploic a.

    12. Splenic a.

        13. Left ruminal a. (may originate from left gastric a.)

        14. Reticular a.

    15. Right ruminal a.

        Used with permission of Dr. J. E. Smallwood

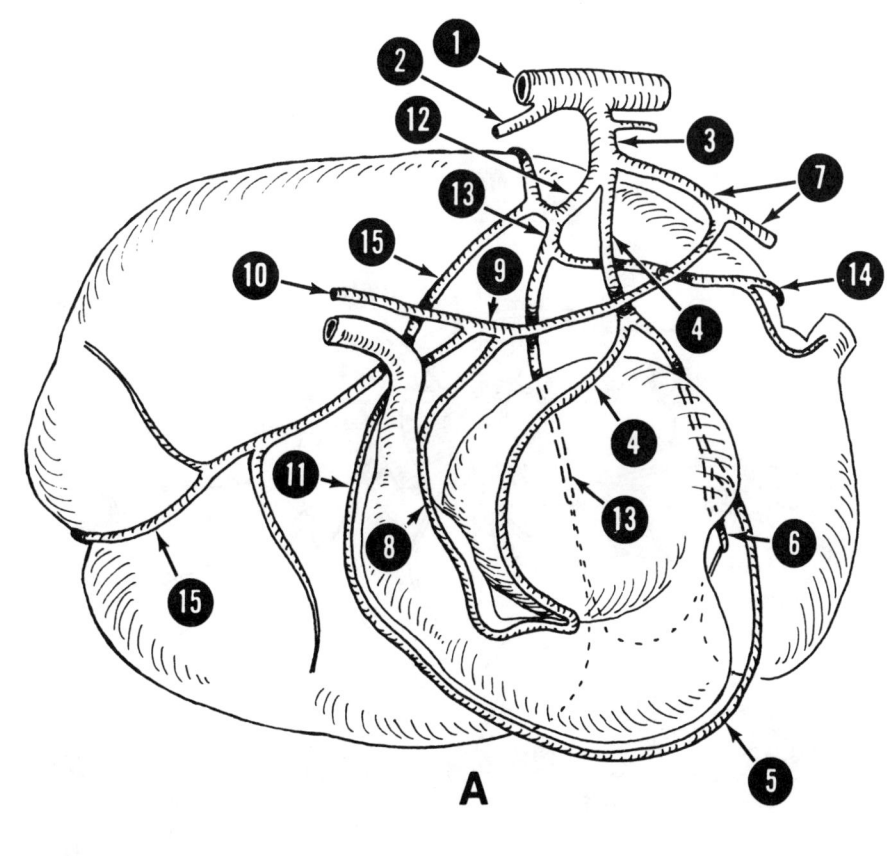

A

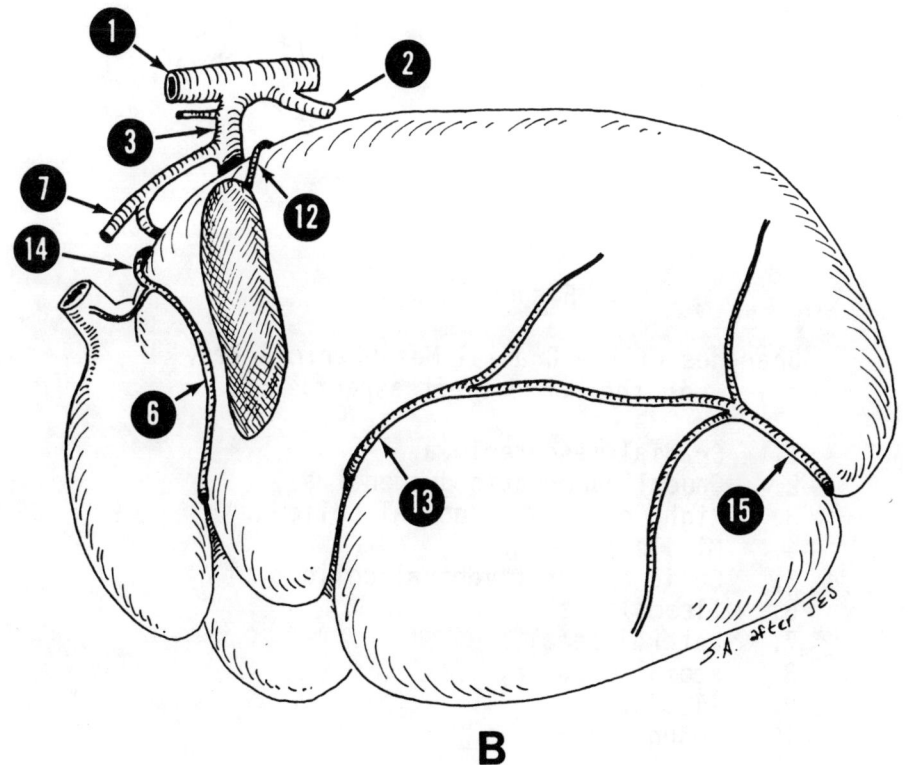

B

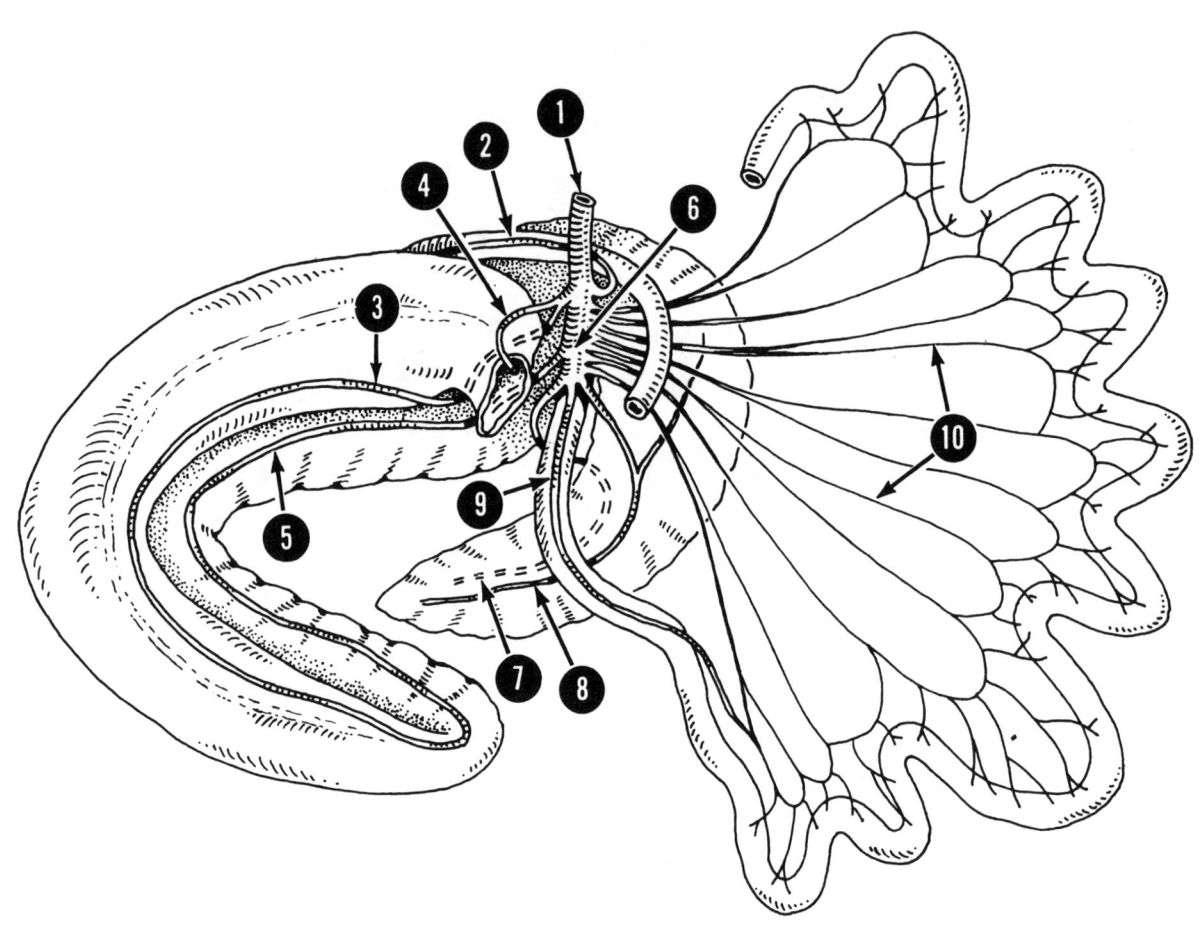

Figure 13-5

Branches of the Cranial Mesenteric Artery
in the Horse (left aspect)

1. Cranial mesenteric a.
2. Caudal pancreaticoduodenal a.
3. Right colic a. ("dorsal colic a.")
4. Middle colic a.
5. Colic branch ("ventral colic a.")
6. Ileocolic a.
7. Lateral cecal a.
8. Medial cecal a.
9. Ileal a.
10. Jejunal aa.

The order of origin of 3, 5, 6, and 7 may vary.

After Schummer et al., 1981 [2]

penetrates the abdominal wall through the vascular lacuna and continues on down its respective limb as the femoral artery. Saddle thrombi in the caudal aorta of cats may block the external iliacs causing lameness or paralysis as well as regional hypothermia. Five "P's" may be observed on physical examination of affected cats: pulselessness, pain, pallor (cyanosis) of footpads, polar (cool) pelvic limbs, and paresis [5]. Thrombus formation in the caudal aorta, external iliac aa., or femoral aa. due to Strongylus vulgaris sometimes causes lameness in horses [6]. The only branch of the external iliac a. present in all species is the deep femoral a. The deep femoral a. has the following branches:

a. Pudendoepigastric trunk--this short vessel may originate from the external iliac a. in horses. It has two major branches:
   (1) Caudal epigastric a.--courses cranially on the deep surface of the rectus abdominis m.
   (2) External pudendal a.--courses through the inguinal canal and divides into two major branches:

   (a) Superficial caudal epigastric a.--courses cranially along the superficial aspect of the cranial abdominal wall. In mares and female ruminants, this vessel is also known as the cranial mammary a. In cattle, its satellite vein (superficial caudal epigastric v. as well as its cranial anastomotic continuation, the superficial cranial epigastric v.) is the so-called "milk vein" or "superficial abdominal vein" [1].
   (b) Ventral scrotal a. or ventral labial a.--In mares and female ruminants, the ventral labial a. is also known as the caudal mammary a. [1].

   In horses, the external pudendal a. also supplies the cranial a. of the penis which is one of three sources of blood to the equine penis. The others are the middle a. of the penis (from the obturator a.) and the dorsal a. of the penis (from the internal pudendal a.).

b. Medial circumflex femoral a.--a counterpart to the lateral circumflex femoral a. (which arises from the femoral a.). The medial circumflex femoral a. supplies a number of named branches in the various species (obturator branch, deep branch, ascending branch, transverse branch, and acetabular branch). In the horse, the middle a. of the penis arises from the obturator branch of this vessel. The horse also has an iliacofemoral a. which arises from the obturator a. and substitutes for the ascending and transverse branches of the medial circumflex femoral a.

The external iliac arteries supply the following small, species specific branches (these arteries are typically present in the other species but they have origins from other sources).

   (1) deep circumflex iliac aa. in ungulates (See item 13 in this chapter.)
   (2) cremasteric and uterine aa. in horses as well as the last 2 pairs of lumbar aa.

(3) caudal abdominal aa. in carnivores, sheep, and cattle (supplies abdominal wall)

15. Internal iliac aa.

The internal iliac aa. are distributed to the pelvic viscera and to the hip and thigh. They supply several branches (directly or indirectly) including the umbilical aa. (round ligg. of the urinary bladder) and the cranial gluteal, prostatic (or vaginal), and iliolumbar aa.* The cranial gluteal a. courses across the cranial part of the greater ischiatic notch to enter and ramify in the gluteal musculature. It and branches of the iliolumbar a., which courses ventral to the cranial ilium, may bleed profusely when the gluteals are elevated for pelvic fracture repair. The prostatic artery was formerly known as the "urogenital a." and it is homologous to the vaginal a. of the female. There is considerable species variation in the pattern of origin of these vessels. In all species, the internal iliac arteries terminated by dividing into:

a. Internal pudendal a.--distributed primarily to the pelvic viscera. In some species, it supplies some of the branches listed above (umbilical a. in the horse, prostatic or vaginal aa. in the carnivores and horse), and it terminates by dividing into the ventral perineal a. and the a. of the penis or clitoris.
b. Caudal gluteal a.--distributed primarily to the hip and thigh.

The length of the internal iliac aa. varies from quite short (horse) to very long (ruminants) depending on the osition of the terminal division into internal pudendal and caudal gluteal aa. The goat is unusual in that its internal and external iliac aa. on each side arise together as a common iliac a.

16. Median sacral a.

This artery to the tail may actually arise cranial to the origins of the internal iliac aa. Its caudal continuation which remains on the ventral aspect of the tail is termed the middle caudal a., and it or its satellite vein may be used to "tail bleed" cattle. In the horse, the median sacral a. is poorly developed or absent, but the middle caudal a. is nonetheless present and arises from the caudal gluteal a. [2].

II. MAJOR SYSTEMIC VEINS

A. Cranial vena cava

---

*The prostatic a. (vaginal a. in the female) was formerly known as the urogenital a. The uterine a. is a branch of this vessel in carnivores, but in the horse the uterine a. originates from the external iliac a., and in the ruminants it is an initial branch of the umbilical a.

This short vessel returns blood to the heart from the head and thoracic limbs. In the carnivores and pig, it is formed by convergence of the two (left and right) brachiocephalic vv., each of which is formed by the convergence of an ipsilateral external jugular v. and subclavian v. In the ruminants and horse, there are no brachiocephalic veins because the external jugular v. and subclavian v. on each side enter the cranial vena cava separately.

B. Azygos vein (left and/or right)

The azygos vein(s) returns blood to the heart from the dorsal and lateral thoracic wall. Of primarily academic interest is the fact that left azygos veins occur only in swine and ruminants, but right azygos veins occur in the carnivores, ruminants, horse, and sometimes in the pig [1]. Right azygos veins typically empty into the cranial vena cava although they may join the right atrium directly. Left azygos veins usually join the great cardiac vein. Hemiazygos veins may supplement or substitute for the azygos vein. They cross to the other side of the vertebral column and continue caudally along it. Right hemiazygos veins may occur in pigs and ruminants, and left ones may occur in carnivores and horses [2].

C. Caudal vena cava

The caudal vena cava returns blood to the heart from the abdomen, pelvis, and pelvic limbs. It is formed by the convergence of the left and right common iliac veins. Its major tributaries include the hepatic, renal, gonadal, and the lumbar vv. It also receives cranial and caudal phrenic vv. (phrenicoabdominal v. in the carnivores) and the deep circumflex iliac v. in all domestic mammals except the pig. Some other small branches are present in the various species.

D. Portal vein

Essentially all of the blood leaving the aorta through the celiac, cranial mesenteric, and caudal mesenteric arteries is carried to the liver by the portal vein. The relatively short portal vein is formed by the convergence of the relatively large cranial mesenteric vein and the small caudal mesenteric vein. After its formation, the major tributaries which join the portal vein are the gastroduodenal v. and the splenic v.

III. PULMONARY CIRCULATION

The single vessel leaving the right ventricle is the pulmonary trunk. Domestic mammals have one pulmonary trunk. It divides into two (left and right) pulmonary arteries. ("Main pulmonary artery (segment)," which is often used to designate the pulmonary trunk, is an unwieldly and inefficient term.) Each pulmonary artery divides into individual branches to the various lobes of the lung. The pulmonary trunk (and the right ventricle) are common places for adult heartworms (Dirofilaria immitis) to reside.

A number of pulmonary veins are present to return oxygenated blood to the left atrium. Some of these may converge before entering the atrium. It is sometimes of value radiographically that the images of the branches of the pulmonary veins are ventral and caudal to those of the pulmonary arteries.

Radiologists often use the terms "ventral" and "central" to refer to the fact that the pulmonary veins are ventral to their arterial counterparts in lateral perspectives and central (closer to the median plan) in V-D or D-V perspectives. Arterial and venous differentiation is significant radiographically because pulmonary over-circulation or vascular hypertrophy may result in arteries which are larger in diameter than their corresponding veins. Causes include PDA, dirofilariasis, left-right shunts (atrial and ventricular septal defects), and congestive heart failure [7].

IV. FETAL CIRCULATION (Figs. 13-6, 13-7)

    A. There are two peculiarities in fetal biology which require differences in the circulatory pattern [8]:

        1. The lungs are shrunken, nonfunctional, and present a large resistance to blood flow.

        2. Oxygenation (and other nutrient-waste exchange) in fetal blood occurs at the placenta, which is physically distinct from the fetus.

    B. There are specific anatomical structures present because of the biological peculiarities:

        1. A pair (left and right) of umbilical arteries originate from the internal iliac arteries and carry fetal blood out through the umbilical cord to the placenta for nutrient-waste exchange.

        2. A single definitive umbilical vein returns fetal blood from the placenta to the fetus. It courses from the umbilical cord to the liver and continues through the liver as a channel, the ductus venosus.

        3. An interatrial septal passageway, the foramen ovale, allows some of the blood to bypass the lungs by flowing directly from the right atrium to the left atrium.

        4. A vascular connection between the pulmonary trunk and aorta, the ductus arteriosus, allows most of the blood which enters the right ventricle to bypass the lungs by shunting it directly into the aorta.

    C. The circulatory pattern in the fetus (Fig. 13-6)

Oxygenated blood returning to the fetus through the umbilical vein is shunted through the liver in the ductus venosus. As it enters the hepatic veins, it is joined and diluted by the blood in the liver from the hepatic artery and portal vein. It then flows into the caudal vena cava where it is further diluted by blood returning toward the heart from the pelvic limbs and caudal abdomen. At the right atrium, the blood is diluted once again by blood returning to the heart from the head, thorax, and thoracic limbs (cranial vena cava and azygos vein). Some of the blood in the right atrium flows directly into the left atrium through the foramen ovale, and the rest enters the right ventricle as in the adult. From the right ventricle, this blood enters the pulmonary trunk enroute to the lungs. However, a large percentage of it bypasses the lungs by flowing directly into the aorta through the ductus arteriosus. The left atrium receives the blood which entered it from the foramen ovale as well as the small amount returning from the lungs. This blood is pumped into the left ventricle and on into the aorta just as it is in the adult.

D. The changes that occur at birth (or shortly thereafter)

1. The initiation of respiration expands the lungs and reduces their resistance to blood flow. This in turn allows more blood to flow through them, and the increased venous return to the left atrium is believed to cause functional closure of the foramen ovale. This closure occurs because the increased pressure in the left atrium physically holds a thin flap of endocardium (the valve of the foramen ovale) tightly against the left atrial opening of the foramen ovale.

2. Functional respiration by the neonate also increases the partial pressure of oxygen in the neonate blood. This is believed to cause contraction of smooth muscle in the wall of each of the following, resulting in their functional closure:

    a. umbilical arteries
    b. umbilical vein and ductus venosus
    c. ductus arteriosus

E. Changes with time (Fig. 13-7)

The various fetal circulatory structures that have no adult function are gradually replaced with connective tissue and become vestigial:

1. The pre-bladder portions of the umbilical arteries typically regress to become the round ligaments of the urinary bladder, but occasionally they remain patent and carry part of the blood supply to the bladder. They are surrounded by folds of peritoneum termed the lateral ligaments of the bladder. The post-bladder portions of the umbilical arteries (between the bladder and umbilicus) usually regress beyond recognition.

2. The umbilical vein becomes the round ligament of the liver--a fibrous cord surrounded by the falciform ligament which courses from the umbilicus to the liver.

3. Within the liver the ductus venosus becomes a fibrous cord termed the ligamentum venosum.

4. The ductus arteriosus becomes the ligamentum arteriosum. Occasionally it fails to regress properly and remains clinically as a patent ductus arteriosus. This condition usually requires surgical correction by ligation because of the circulatory disturbances which it causes.

Figure 13-6

Circulatory Scheme in the Fetus

1. Umbilicus
2. Umbilical vein
3. Ductus venosus
4. Hepatic vein
5. Caudal vena cava
6. Right atrium
7. Cranial vena cava
8. Right lung
9. Right pulmonary vein(s)
10. Right pulmonary artery
11. Brachiocephalic trunk
12. Left subclavian artery
13. Ductus arteriosus
14. Left pulmonary artery
15. Left pulmonary vein(s)
16. Left lung
17. Left atrium
18. Left ventricle
19. Right ventricle
20. Foramen ovale
21. Ascending aorta
22. Pulmonary trunk
23. Descending aorta
24. Celiac artery
25. Left gastric artery
26. Splenic artery
27. Hepatic artery
28. Cranial mesenteric artery
29. Caudal mesenteric artery
30. External iliac artery (left)
31. Internal iliac artery (left)
32. Umbilical arteries (left and right)
33. Common iliac veins (left and right)
34. Portal vein
35. Urinary bladder

Many branches of the aorta and caudal vena cava were intentionally omitted, and no attempt was made to illustrate the azygos vein.

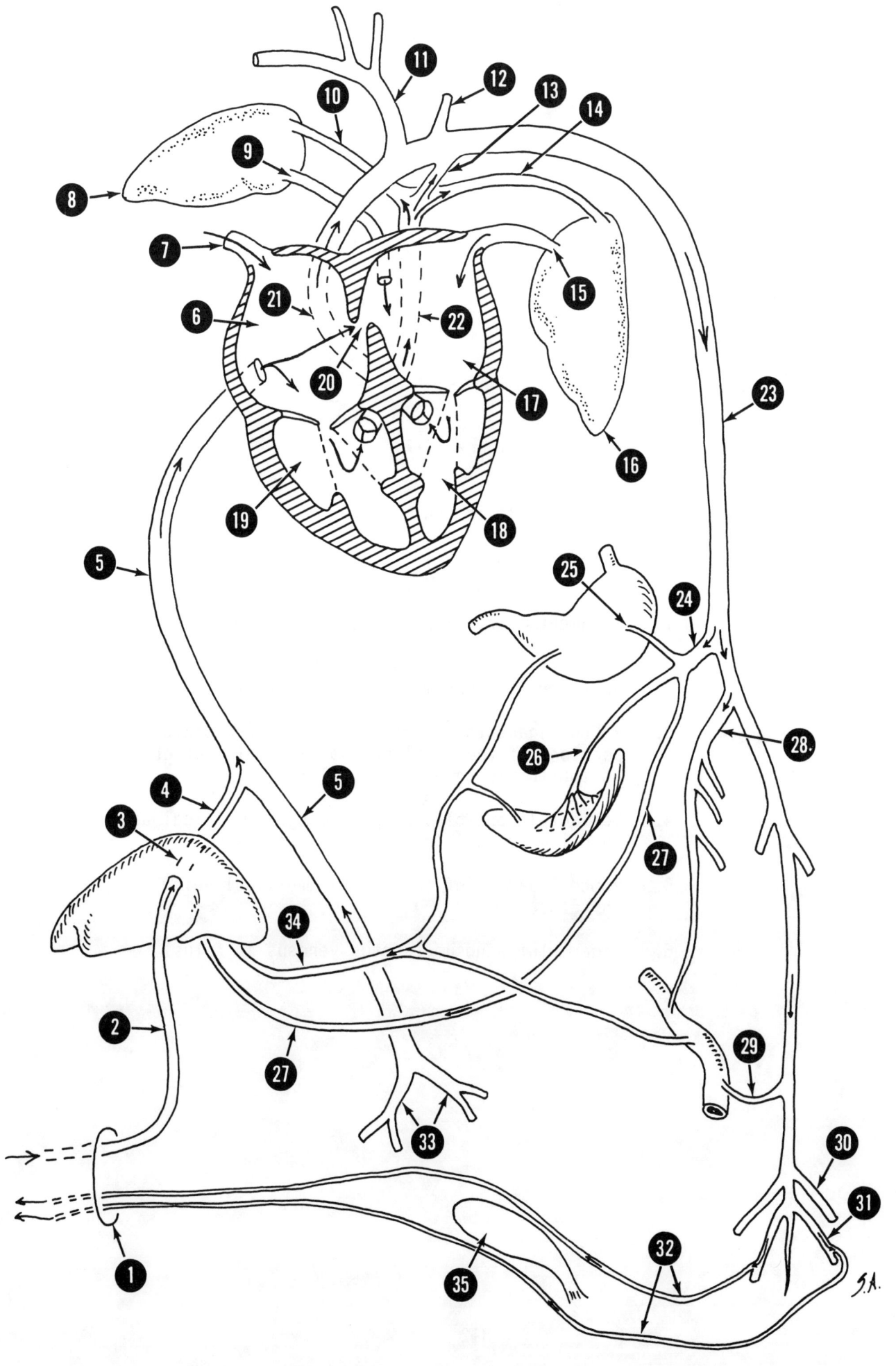

Figure 13-7

Circulatory Scheme in the Neonate and Adult
(Only those structures which undergo
changes at birth are labeled; compare
to Fig. 13-6.)

1. Ligamentum arteriosum (Ductus arteriosus in fetus)

2. Fossa ovalis (foramen ovale in fetus)

3. Round ligaments of urinary bladder (Prebladder portions of the umbilical aa. - remain patent postpartum in some individuals)

4. Vestigial post-bladder portions of umbilical aa. (usually impossible to find in adults)

5. Round ligament of the liver (umbilical vein in fetus)

6. Ligamentum venosum (ductus venosus in fetus)

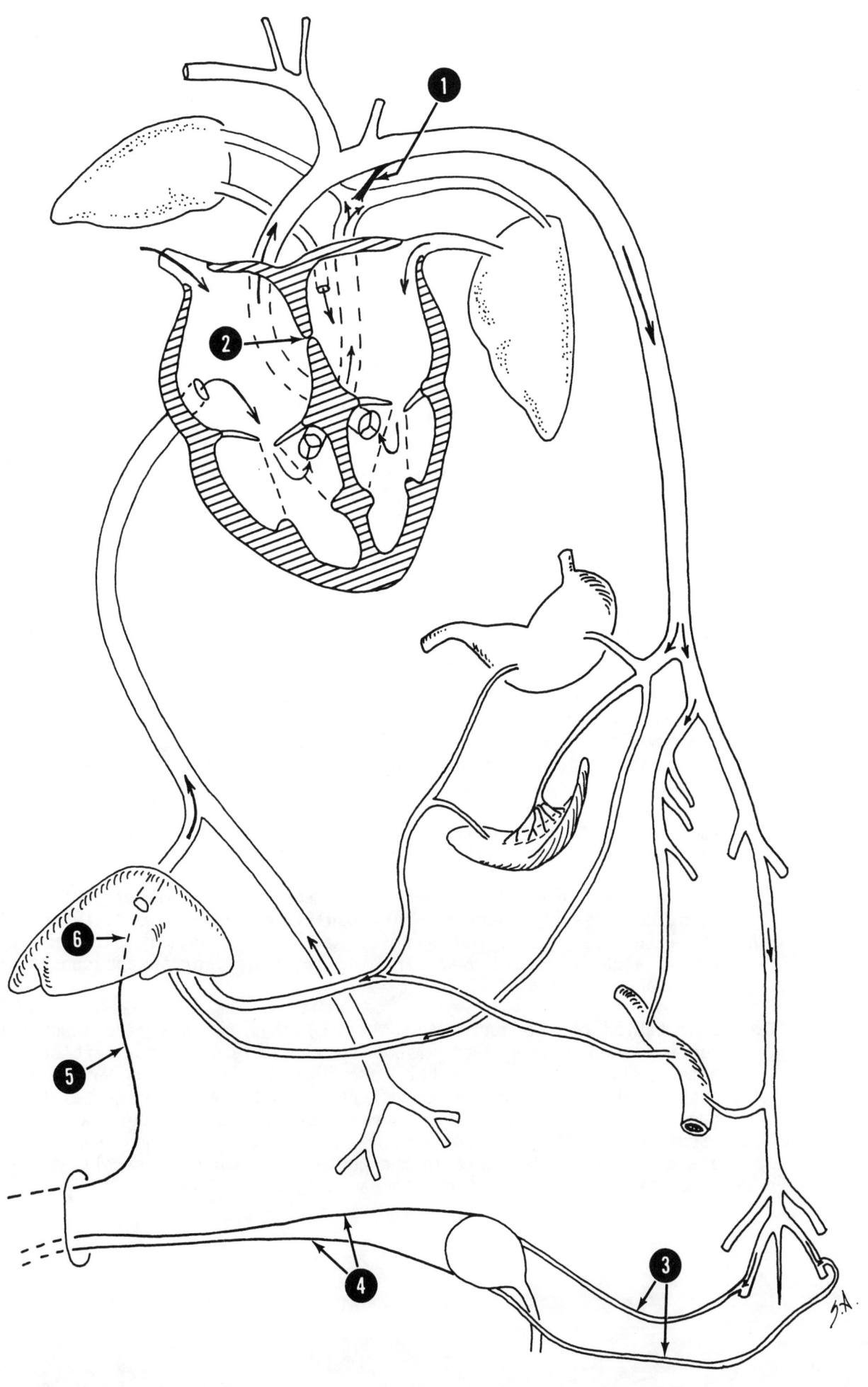

5. The foramen ovale normally fibroses to become the fossa ovalis. It may not seal off in some individuals (probe patency), but this usually is not pathological because the intra-atrial pressure on the left side keeps it physically closed.

V. ANOMALIES OF THE GREAT VESSELS (Fig. 13-8)

Embryologically the dorsal aorta is paired and receives six pairs of aortic arches. Although not all are present at the same time, some of these persist and some regress in forming parts of the great vessels near the heart.

A number of developmental anomalies of the large vessels occur. These typically require angiography or exploratory surgery for diagnosis. In addition to patent ductus arteriosus, which has already been discussed, these anomalies include transposition of the great vessels and persistent truncus arteriosus [8] as well as the following:

A. Persistent right aortic arch (Fig. 13-8/D). This is the most frequently encountered vascular ring anomaly in the dog, and accounts for about 95% of the cases involving esophageal constriction.[5] In this condition, the right fourth aortic arch and right dorsal aorta persist as the aorta instead of the left ones. If the ductus arteriosus also forms from the right side (right sixth aortic arch), no problem usually occurs. However, if the ductus forms from the left primordium as is the usual case, it may entrap the esophagus in a vascular ring and cause dysphagia [8,9].

B. Abnormal origin of the right subclavian artery (Fig. 13-8/B). Variations in the origin of the subclavian vessels are often observed in the anatomy laboratory, but only rarely do they cause clinical signs. In those that do, the right subclavian artery usually develops from a primordium attached to the left aspect of the aortic arch. As it crosses back to the right side for distribution to the right thoracic limb, it must cross the dorsal aspect of the esophagus and may constrict it. The clinical signs are usually associated with the constriction [8,10].

C. Double aortic arch (Fig. 13-8/C). In this rare condition, the embryonic right dorsal aorta (part of which usually regresses) persists as well as the left dorsal aorta (which normally remains). This results in a double aortic arch forming a vascular ring which may entrap and constrict the trachea and esophagus [8,11].

D. Coarctation of the aorta (Fig. 13-8/E) [8]. In this rare condition the aortic lumen is narrowed distal to the origin of the left subclavian artery. It may be preductal (proximal to the ductus arteriosus) or postductal (distal to the ductus arteriosus). In the preductal type, the ductus arteriosus is usually persistent, but in the postductal form it usually is vestigial. Collateral circulation between the proximal and distal parts of the aorta in the post-ductal form is established through the intercostal and internal thoracic arteries.

E. Interrupted aortic arch (Fig. 13-8/F) [8]. In this rare condition the fourth arch on the left side fails to develop into the definitive aortic arch and, as a result, the aorta may supply the head, and the pulmonary trunk (via a patent ductus arteriosus) supplies the rest of the body.

F. Double caudal vena cava [8]. In this condition the left member of paired primordial vessels persists as well as the right one. No clinical signs are usually present.

G. Absence of caudal vena cava [8,12,13]. In this condition the primordium for the caudal vena cava fails to persist and, as a result, blood from the caudal part of the body returns to the heart in the azygos vein. This is sometimes called an azygos continuation of the caudal vena cava and no clinical signs are usually present.

H. Double cranial vena cava. This condition results from a failure of a common channel to form and usually has no clinical significance [8]. Double cranial vena cava is normal in rabbits [14]. In dogs, the left primordium sometimes remains without the right one and empties into the caudal aspect of the left atrium (as does the left one of the two present in rabbits). No clinical signs are usually attributable to the vena cava, but coexisting anomalies are often present [14].

I. Portocaval shunt. In this clinically significant condition, all or some of the blood in the portal vein usually bypasses the liver and empties directly into the caudal vena cava [15]. In a rarer form, the ductus venosus may persist as a patent channel. The spectrum of disease produced by these anomalies is very diverse [5].

J. Anomalous pulmonary veins. In this condition, some or all of the pulmonary veins drain into the right atrium or the cranial vena cava. The clinical significance depends on the number of anomalous vessels [16].

VI. LYMPHATIC SYSTEM

The lymphatic system includes the lymphatic tissue and the lymphatic vessels. Lymphatic tissue comprises the parenchyma of a number of gross organs and is also diffusely scattered throughout the tubular portions of parts of the visceral body systems. Lymphatic vessels include the lymph capillaries and lymph vessels which anastomose with venous channels. The lymphatic vessels differ functionally from venous channels by having a special resorptive property at their terminal ends and in their innate motor ability.

A. Lymphatic tissue and organs

Lymphatic tissue functions in body defense. It is one of the specialized connective tissues and has fixed cells (reticular cells) as well as mobile cells (lymphocytes, plasma cells, macrophages).

1. Diffuse lymphatic tissue occurs in the mucous membranes of the visceral body systems. In the intestine, these are called "Peyer's

Figure 13-8

Selected Anomalies of the Great Vessels
(ventral aspect)

A. Patent ductus arteriosus
B. Abnormal origin of the right subclavian a.
C. Double aortic arch
D. Persistent right aortic arch
E. Coarctation of the aorta (preductal type)
F. Interrupted aortic arch

1. Aorta (ascending)
2. Brachiocephalic trunk (not present in B)
3. Right subclavian artery
4. Left subclavian artery
5. Right and left common carotid aa.
6. Pulmonary trunk (A,D,E,F)
7. Right pulmonary artery (A,D,E,F)
8. Left pulmonary artery (A,D,E,F)
9. Ductus arteriosus (A,E,F)
10. Trachea (B,C)
11. Esophagus (B,C)

After Langman, 1981 [8]

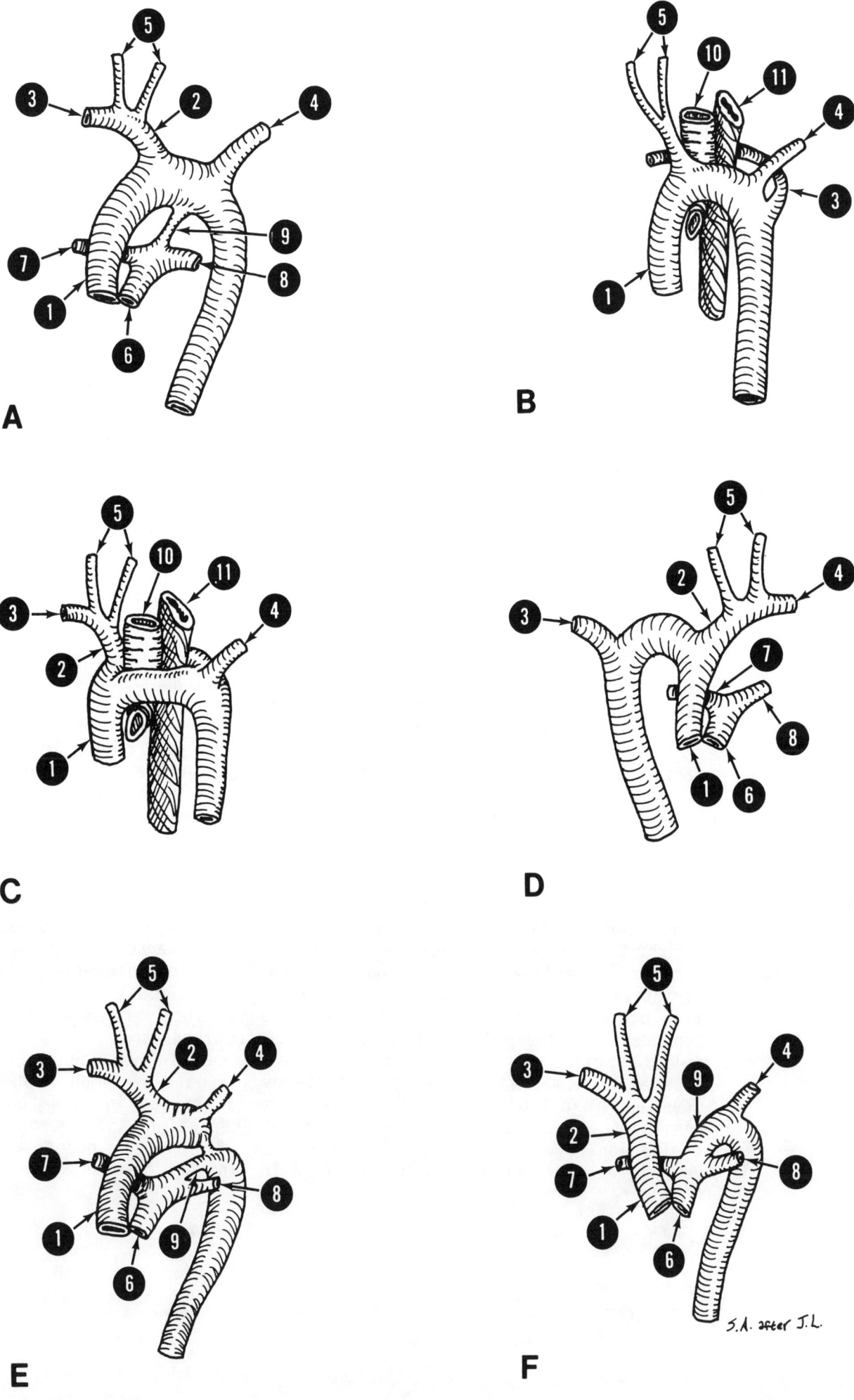

Patches". Similar accumulations occur in the greater omentum ("milk spots") and in the pia mater ("arachnoid cell accumulations").

2. Tonsils are subepithelial accumulations of lymphatic tissue in the pharynx. The major ones form a ring at the entrance to the esophagus and larynx where they contact potential pathogens. A comparison of the specific tonsils found in the various domestic species is presented in Chapter 19, Head.

3. Lymph nodes are encapsulated collections of lymphatic tissue located along the course of lymphatic vessels. Several afferent lymphatic vessels enter the convex margin of the node and one or two efferent vessels leave a depressed hilus. Within the lymph nodes of most domestic mammals the lymphatic nodules are concentrated peripherally in the cortex, but in the pig, they are centrally located. Lymph flow is also reversed in the lymph nodes of pigs (the afferent vessels enter at the hilus and the efferent vessels leave through the other parts of the capsule).

Lymph nodes occur singly or in groups of several thousand (colic lymph nodes of the horse). In the carnivores and ruminants, there are usually only one or two lymph nodes at each site, whereas the pig and horse typically have a group of many small nodes. The total number of lymph nodes present in various species have been estimated at 8000 in the horse, 300 in the ox, and 60 in the dog [2].

Lymph nodes are named according to their location, and these loci are relatively constant among the different domestic species. Functionally, analogous groups of lymph nodes (i.e., those which receive afferent vessels from approximately the same region in the various species) are termed lymphocenters [1]. There are 19 lymphocenters in the body: 5 in the head and neck, 5 in the thorax and thoracic limb, 4 in the abdomen, and 5 in the pelvis and pelvic limb (Table 13-1).

Lymph nodes are clinically important for several reasons. Because of their significant enlargement in response to some pathogens, lymph nodes are important indicators of infection. The "normal size" of a lymph node, however, is a difficult diagnostic problem because there is no absolute norm. There can be considerable size variation between individual nodes at a given locus. Variations even occur between the two sides of the same animal. It is also of considerable medical importance that infectious and neoplastic cells carried away in the lymph may be trapped in more centrally located nodes and initiate metastases. Finally, lymph nodes involved in pathogenic processes may undergo changes in color and consistency that are important in meat inspection and necropsy evaluations. Needle or surgical biopsies of involved nodes may provide valuable diagnostic information in a number of diseases.

Table 13-1

Lymph Nodes of Domestic Mammals

Key: 0 - Absent   2 - Present and normally palpable
     1 - Present but not normally palpable   3 - Inconstantly present

	Cat	Dog	Pig	Sheep	Goat	Ox	Horse
Parotid lymphocenter							
parotid lnn.*	1	2	1	1	1	2	1
Mandibular lymphocenter							
mandibular lnn.	1	2	1	1	1	2	2
accessory mandibular lnn.	3	0	1	0	0	0	0
pterygoid ln.	0	0	0	0	0	3	0
Retropharyngeal lymphocenter							
medial retropharyngeal lnn.	1	1	1	1	1	1	1
lateral retropharyngeal lnn.	1	3	1	1	1	2	1
rostral hyoid ln.	0	0	0	0	0	3	0
caudal hyoid ln.	0	0	0	0	0	3	0
Superficial cervical lymphocenter							
(dorsal) superficial cervical lnn.	1	2	1	1	1	2	2
middle superficial cervical lnn.	0	0	1	0	0	0	0
ventral superficial cervical lnn.	1	0	1	0	0	0	0
accessory superficial cervical lnn.	0	0	0	3	0	1	0
Deep cervical lymphocenter							
cranial deep cervical lnn.	0	3	1	3	3	3	1
middle deep cervical lnn.	3	3	3	3	3	1	1
caudal deep cervical lnn.	1	3	1	1	1	1	1
costocervical ln.	0	0	0	3	3	1	0
subrhomboid	0	0	0	0	0	3	0
Axillary lymphocenter							
(proper) axillary lnn.	1	2	0	1	1	1	1
axillary ln. of the first rib	3	0	1	1	1	1	0
accessory axillary ln.	1	3	0	2	0	3	0
cubital lnn.	0	0	0	3	0	0	2
infraspinous ln.	0	0	0	0	0	3	0
Dorsal thoracic lymphocenter							
thoracic aortic lnn.	3	0	1	1	1	1	1
intercostal lnn.	3	3	0	1	1	1	1
Ventral thoracic lymphocenter							
cranial sternal lnn.	1	1	1	1	1	1	3
caudal sternal lnn.	3	0	0	3	0	1	3
cranial epigastric ln.	3	0	0	0	0	0	0
Mediastinal lymphocenter							
cranial mediastinal lnn.	1	1	1	1	1	1	1
nuchal ln.	0	0	0	0	0	0	3

*NAV lists dorsal and ventral parotid lymph nodes [1]

Table 13-1 (Continued)

Key: 0 - Absent 2 - Present and normally palpable
1 - Present but not normally palpable 3 - Inconstantly present

	Cat	Dog	Pig	Sheep	Goat	Ox	Horse
medial mediastinal lnn.	0	0	0	1	1	1	1
caudal mediastinal lnn.	0	0	1	1	1	1	3
phrenic lnn.	3	0	0	0	0	3	0
Bronchial lymphocenter							
left tracheobronchial lnn.	1	1	1	1	1	1	1
right tracheobronchial lnn.	1	1	1	0	3	3	1
middle tracheobronchial lnn.	1	1	1	0	3	3	1
cranial tracheobronchial lnn.	0	0	1	1	1	1	0
pulmonary lnn.	3	3	0	0	3	3	3
Lumbar lymphocenter							
lumbar aortic lnn.	1	1	1	1	1	1	1
lumbar proper lnn.	0	0	0	0	0	3	0
renal lnn.	0	0	1	1	1	1	1
ovarian ln.	0	0	0	0	0	0	3
testicular ln.	0	0	3	0	0	0	0
phrenicoabdominal ln.	0	0	3	0	0	0	0
Celiac lymphocenter							
celiac ln. (non ruminants)	0	0	1	-	-	-	1
celiac & cranial mesenteric lnn.	-	-	-	3	3	1	0
splenic lnn.	3	1	1	1	1	1	1
gastric lnn. (non ruminants)	3	3	1	-	-	-	1
right ruminal lnn.	-	-	-	1	3	1	-
left ruminal lnn.	-	-	-	3	0	3	-
cranial ruminal lnn.	-	-	-	3	3	1	-
reticular lnn.	-	-	-	3	3	3	-
omasal lnn.	-	-	-	3	3	1	-
ruminoabomasal lnn.	-	-	-	3	0	1	-
reticuloabomasal	-	-	-	3	3	1	-
dorsal abomasal lnn.	-	-	-	1	1	1	-
ventral abomasal lnn.	-	-	-	3	3	3	-
hepatic (portal) lnn.	1	1	1	1	1	1	1
accessory hepatic lnn.	0	0	0	0	0	1	0
pancreaticoduodenal lnn.	1	3	1	1	3	1	1
omental lnn.	0	0	0	0	0	0	1
Cranial mesenteric lymphocenter							
cranial mesenteric lnn. (nonruminants)	0	0	3	0	0	0	1
jejunal lnn.	1	1	1	1	1	1	1
cecal lnn.	1	0	0	1	0	1	1
ileocolic lnn.	0	0	1	0	1	0	0
colic lnn.	1	1	1	1	1	1	1
Caudal mesenteric lymphocenter							
Caudal mesenteric lnn.	1	1	1	3	3	1	1
vesicular ln.	0	0	0	0	0	0	3

Table 13-1 (Continued)

Key: 0 - Absent 2 - Present and normally palpable
1 - Present but not normally palpable 3 - Inconstantly present

	Cat	Dog	Pig	Sheep	Goat	Ox	Horse
Iliosacral lymphocenter							
medial iliac lnn.	1	1	1	1	1	1	1
lateral iliac lnn.	0	0	1	3	0	3	1
sacral lnn.	1	1	1	1	1	1	1
anorectal lnn.	0	0	3	1	1	1	1
uterine lnn.	0	0	3	0	0	0	3
obturator ln.	0	0	0	0	0	0	3
Deep inguinal lymphocenter							
iliofemoral lnn.	3	3	1	3	0	1	0
deep inguinal lnn.	0	0	0	0	3	0	1
femoral ln.	3	3	0	0	0	0	0
epigastric ln.	0	0	0	0	0	3	0
Superficial inguinal lymphocenter							
superficial inguinal lnn.	1	2	1	2	2	2	2
caudal epigastric ln.	1	0	0	0	0	0	0
subiliac lnn.	3	0	1	2	2	2	2
coxal ln.	0	0	0	3	0	3	3
accessory coxal ln.	0	0	0	0	0	3	0
ln. of paralumbar fossa	0	0	0	0	0	3	0
Ischiatic lymphocenter							
ischiatic lnn.	1	0	1	1	3	1	1
gluteal ln.	0	0	1	0	0	3	0
tuberal ln.	0	0	0	3	3	3	0
Popliteal lymphocenter							
deep popliteal lnn.	0	0	3	1	1	1	1
superficial popliteal lnn.	1	2	3	0	0	0	0

4. Hemal nodes ("hemolymph nodes") differ from regular lymph nodes in that they filter blood instead of lymph. In fact, they are connected to the blood vascular system rather than to lymphatic channels. Among the domestic mammals they are found only in the ruminants. Hemal nodes are found mainly in the cephalic and cervical regions as well as in the thoracic, abdominal, and pelvic cavities. They are often found near regular lymph nodes. They are easily distinguished from the latter, however, by their reddish-brown (vs. blue-gray) color. Hemal nodes should be distinguished from lymph nodes which have taken up erythrocytes after local hemorrhage in their collecting area.

5. Spleen. The spleen has been discussed in Chapter 11, Abdomen.

6. Thymus. The thymus develops from the ventral diverticulae of the third pharyngeal pouches. In early development, these diverticuli elongate into a tube-like structure which contacts the pericardium caudally. Various parts of these primordia remain, regress, and/or fuse in the various species until the thymus reaches its maximal development at birth. At birth, the fully developed, generalized thymus consists of cervical lobes (left and right), an intermediate lobe, and a thoracic lobe. In the carnivores and horse, only the thoracic lobe is developed. The cervical lobes are prominent in ruminants and the pig, and these are connected to the thoracic lobe by an unpaired intermediate lobe. Developmentally, the pig and ox also have cranial parts of the thymus, but they persist only until the end of intrauterine development [2].

B. Lymphatic vessels

Lymphatic vessels are found throughout the entire body. They supplement the venous side of the circulatory system. The fluid which they carry is termed lymph, and it varies in composition according to the activity of the animal and the part of the body from which it originates. The lymphatic channels include the lymph capillaries and lymph vessels. The larger lymphatic channels fuse into lymph collecting ducts and trunks which ultimately terminate in the so-called "venous angle" on each side. (The left and right "venous angles" are the points of confluence of the venous drainage from the head and the ipsilateral thoracic Limb.) The larger lymphatic channels include the following:

1. Left and right jugular trunks ("tracheal ducts") course parallel to the trachea. They sometimes terminate directly in their respective venous angles. Alternatively, the right one may unite with the axillary lymphatic channels to form the right lymphatic duct. The left jugular trunk may unite directly with the thoracic duct near the venous angle.

2. The thoracic duct is the large lymphatic channel which conveys lymph from the cysterna chyli to the left venous angle. Its origin from the cysterna chyli is single in ruminants and pigs, but in dogs and horses it is double (sometimes even triple in dogs). The thoracic duct traverses the diaphragm through the aortic hiatus in all species except the ruminants where it courses independently through the musculature of the lumbar part of the diaphragm. Although it begins on the right of the midline, the thoracic duct subsequently courses to the left, at the level of the fifth or sixth thoracic vertebra. Even in those cases where there is a single origin, the thoracic duct may divide so that it is double or triple over part of its length. Anastomoses between these parallel channels may form "ladder-like" connections which are partially responsible for the difficulty in surgical correction of chylothorax by ligation of the thoracic duct [2]. The thoracic duct terminates at the left venous angle near the level of the first rib.

3. The cysterna chyli lies on the right, dorsal side of the aorta, between the origins of the diaphragmatic crura. It extends from the second lumbar vertebra to the last thoracic vertebra. It is poorly visualized without special anatomic preparation and is often taken on faith by veterinary students. The cysterna chyli receives the following lymphatic channels (the regions that they drain can be deduced from their names).

   a. lumbar trunks (left and right)
   b. celiac trunk
   c. intestinal trunk
   d. colic trunk
   e. jejunal trunk
   f. gastric trunk
   g. hepatic trunk

   In all domestic mammals except the horse, the celiac trunk and intestinal trunk unite to form the single visceral trunk and enter the cysterna chyli as a single lymphatic channel.

References

1. International Committee on Veterinary Gross Anatomical Nomenclature. 1983. Nomina Anatomica Veterinaria, third ed. Published by the Committee, Ithaca, New York.

2. Schummer, A. H., H. Wilkens, B. Vollmerhaus, and K. H. Habermehl. 1981. The Circulatory System, The Skin, and the Cutaneous Organs of the Domestic Mammals. Translated by W. Siller and A. Wight. Paul Parey, Berlin.

3. Shively, M. J. 1982. Twenty more veterinary anatomic lies, half truths, and misleading statements. Jour. Vet. Med. Ed. 9(1):20-21.

4. Shively, M. J. 1978. Origin and branching of renal arteries in the dog. JAVMA 173(8):986-989.

5. Ettinger, S. J. 1983. Textbook of Veterinary Internal Medicine, second ed. W. B. Saunders, Philadelphia.

6. Adams, O. R. 1974. Lameness in Horses, third ed. Lea and Febiger, Philadelphia.

7. Owens, J. M., and D. N. Biery. 1982. Radiographic Interpretation for the Small Animal Clinician. Ralston Purina Company, Saint Louis, Missouri.

8. Langman, J. 1981. Medical Embryology, fourth ed. Williams and Wilkens, Baltimore.

9. Buchanan, J. W. 1968. Thoracic surgery in the dog and cat--III Patent ductus arteriosus and persistent right aortic arch surgery in dogs. J. Small Anim. Pract. 9:409-428.

10. Ettinger, S. J. and P. F. Suter. 1970. Canine Cardiology. W. B. Saunders, Philadelphia.

11. Klotz, A. P. and N. R. Brewer. 1952. Double aortic arch in a dog. North Am. Vet. 33(12):867-869.

12. Hickman, J., J. E. Edwards, and F. C. Mann. 1949. Venous anomalies in a dog. Anat. Rec. 104:137-146.

13. Wallace, C. R. 1960. Absence of posterior vena cava in a dog. JAVMA 136: 27-28.

14. Buchanan, J. W. 1963. Persistent left cranial vena cava in dogs; angiocardiography, significance, and coexisting anomalies. J. Am. Vet. Radiol. Soc. 4:1-8.

15. Suter, P. F. 1975. Portal vein anomalies in the dog: Their angiographic diagnosis. J. Am. Vet. Radiol. Soc. 16:84-97.

16. Shively, M. J. 1978. Anomalous pulmonary venous connection in a dog. JAVMA 166:1102-1103.

URINARY SYSTEM

The urinary system is the subdivision of the urogenital system which functions in the formation, transport, storage, and excretion of urine. The major organs comprising this system are the kidneys, ureters, urinary bladder, and urethra.

I. KIDNEY

   The kidneys are paired excretory organs which receive about 20-25% of the cardiac output and convert about 0.1% (1/1000) of this to urine through the processes of filtration, secretion, and selective reabsorption.

   A. Basic features [1,2]

   dorsal and ventral surfaces
   lateral and medial borders
   cranial and caudal extremities ("poles")
   cortex--the outer portion of the kidney which contains most of the glomeruli
   medulla--the inner part of the kidney made up primarily of tubules
   lobe--a unit of the kidney consisting of both cortex and medulla. (These are not externally obvious among domestic mammals except in the ox.)
       renal pyramid--the medullary component of a lobe
           base--the portion of a pyramid adjacent to the cortex
           renal papilla--the apex of a pyramid which projects toward the hilus
   renal hilus--the indentation which receives the ureter and renal vessels
   renal pelvis--the expanded initial portion of the ureter within the kidney
   renal sinus--the space occupied by the renal pelvis and renal vessels
   renal crest--the longitudinal ridge of medulla formed by fusion of the renal papillae that projects into the renal pelvis of carnivores, small ruminants, and horses

   B. Comparative features

   1. The shapes of the kidneys vary considerably among the species (Fig. 14-1). The kidneys of the carnivores, small ruminants, and the pig are bean-shaped. Those of pigs are distinctly flattened. In horses, the left one is bean-shaped but the right one is distinctly heart-shaped. In fact, the right kidney of horses is unique among the domestic animals in being the only kidney which is physically wider (transverse axis) than it is long (cranial-caudal axis). In the ox, the kidneys are lobated ovoids with the left one somewhat pointed on its cranial aspect.

   2. The kidneys are located in the lumbar area with their dorsal surface adjacent to the diaphragmatic crura. Generally, they are located just to each side of the midline, are retroperitoneal, and

are held in place by perirenal fat and fascia. However, the left kidney of the cat is somewhat pendulous and mobile. In both dogs and cats, it may be displaced further caudally by a full stomach. The left kidney of ruminants is displaced by the rumen to the right of the median plane and lies caudal to the right one. Specific locations of the kidneys in the various species are shown in Table 14-1.

Table 14-1

Specific Locations of the Kidneys

	Right Kidney	Left Kidney
dog	T12-13 to L1-2	about one vertebra further caudally
cat[a]	L2-3	the same level (or just slightly caudal)
ruminant	T13-L3	2 vertebrae further caudally
horse[b]	T15-17	T17-L3
pig[c]	L1-4	L1-4

Notes:
a. The kidneys of cats are located further caudally than those of dogs.
b. The left kidney of the horse is physically longer than the right one and thus extends over one more vertebra.
c. The kidneys of the pig are almost symmetrically placed, and either one may be located slightly cranial to the other one. The pig is the only domestic mammal in which the right kidney does not contact the liver [2].

3. The kidneys of dogs, sheep, and goats are so similar that they are difficult to distinguish grossly.

4. Feline kidneys have distinct capsular veins (Fig 14-1/B). These are not present in any of the other domestic mammals and should be recognized as normal.

5. The kidney of the ox has external lobation (18-20 lobes) and has no renal pelvis or crest. Instead of expanding on entering at the hilus, the ureter forms two primary branches and each of these redivides to form a total of 18-22 calices (funnel shaped "mini-pelvises") which invest the renal papillae. Since the renal papillae remain unfused (some fusions of 2-5 units occur) and drain into the individual calices, a renal crest by definition is not present (Fig. 14-2). (Kidneys which have calices do not have a renal crest and vice versa.)

6. Porcine kidneys have a renal pelvis, but individual calices do project from it and invest the bases of both single and groups of 2-5 fused papillae. No renal crest is present.

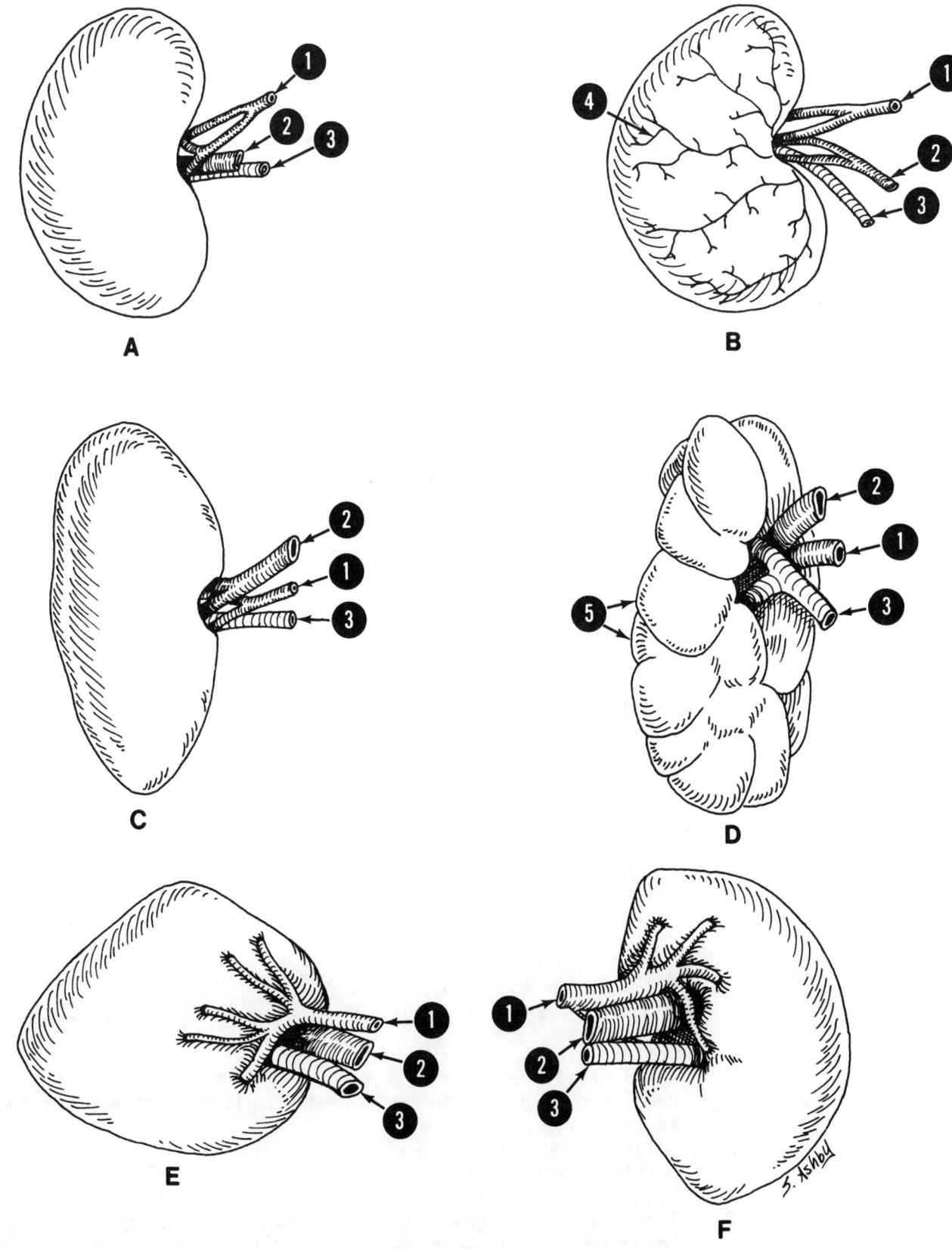

Figure 14-1

Ventral Aspects of the Kidneys of the Dog (A), Cat (B), Pig (C), Ox (D), and Horse (E and F) (right kidneys A-E, left kidney F)

1. renal artery
2. renal vein
3. ureter
4. capsular veins (cat only)
5. externally obvious lobes (ox only)

7. Equine kidneys have a small renal pelvis which is extended toward each extremity by a terminal recess. These recesses are several centimeters long (Fig. 14-2/C7). The pelvis contains a yellowish mucus that is secreted by glands in its wall. These glands also extend into the initial parts of the ureters [2]. The mucus gives equine urine a turbid appearance.

8. In some mammals (whales), each kidney is represented by a number of separate units, each consisting of a cortex and a medullary portion that drains into a calyx. In the ox, partial fusion of these have occurred, but the separate lobes represent the original development of the kidney as separate units. In the pig, the fusion is more complete so that external lobation is not present, but internally the divisions can still be seen as they drain into separate calices. In the other domestic species, the fusion is essentially complete [2].

C. Medical and Surgical Significance

1. Although paracostal approaches are convenient for unilateral nephrectomies, midline approaches are often used for nephrectomies in carnivores [3]. Even though the kidneys are not readily accessible through the ventral midline, bilateral evaluation can be done through the single midline incision. In addition, some surgeons prefer to ligate the ureter near the bladder to prevent possible reflux of urine into the otherwise long ureteral stump. This can be done through a midline incision but not through a paracostal one. Partial nephrectomies may be performed if a lesion is confined to one extremity [3]. Bilateral nephrectomies are not done in veterinary practice since the cost of dialysis is prohibitive.

2. The retroperitoneal location of the kidneys makes it theorectically possible to perform a nephrectomy without invading the peritoneal cavity. In veterinary medicine this fact is mainly an academic curiosity with little clinical significance.

Figure 14-2

Kidneys of the Dog (A), Ox (B), and Horse (C)
Sectioned Longitudinally in the Dorsal Plane

1. Ureter
2. Renal pelvis--not present in the ox
3. Renal crest--absent in the ox (and pig); present but not shown in the horse
4. Calices--present in the ox and pig only
5. Cranial branch of ureter--present in the ox only
6. Caudal branch of ureter--present in the ox only
7. Terminal recess--present in the horse only - it is difficult to grossly section a kidney in a plane which includes the whole length of the terminal recess.
8. Opening of terminal recess in renal pelvis--present in the horse only
9. Renal artery--shown on the horse only

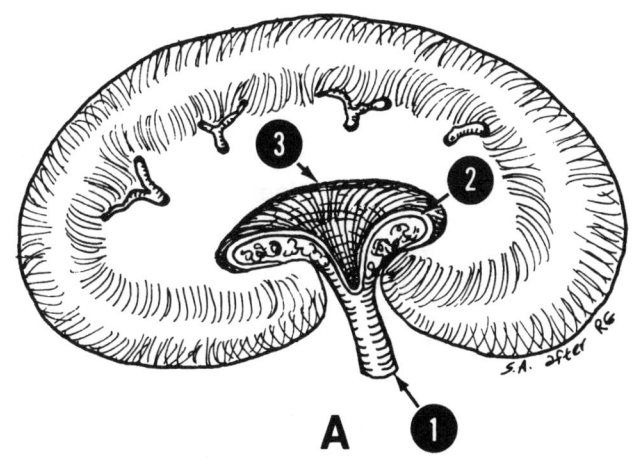

A

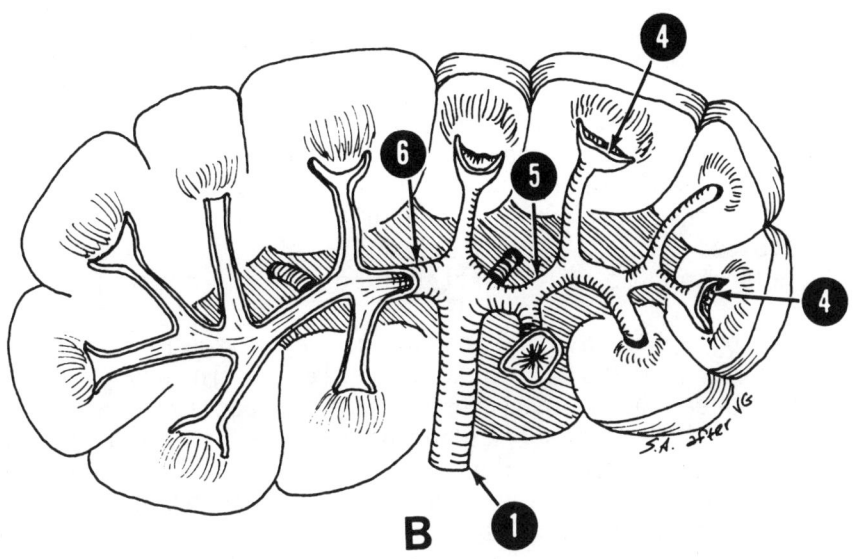

B

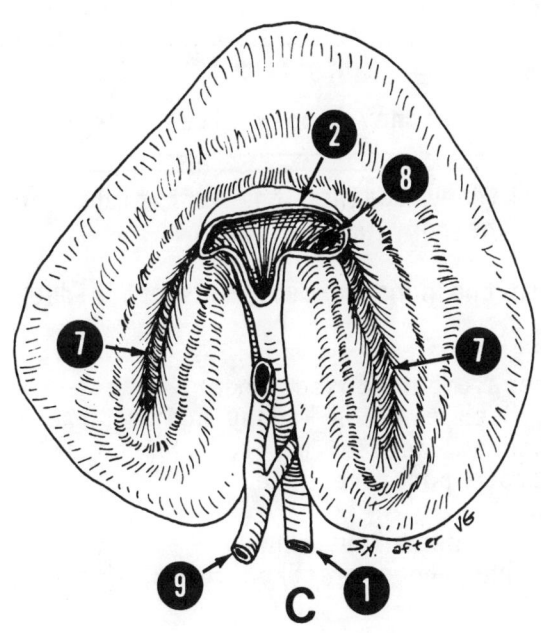

C

3. Before performing unilateral nephrectomies (because of traumatic injury, hydronephrosis, etc.), a surgeon should always evaluate the status of the other kidney since severe disease or nonfunction in it might contraindicate removal of the first one. During the surgery, one should watch for multiple renal arteries. As many as 3 have been reported in the dog (5 in man) [4]. Even single renal vessels normally bifurcate before they enter the kidney. In some animals, this split occurs close to the aorta giving a false appearance of multiple renal vessels. In the horse, one or more small "polar" branches typically enter the kidney near its extremities in addition to the major renal artery which enters at the pelvis.

4. Nephrotomies are sometimes indicated in cases of renal ("staghorn") calculi. The kidney is typically opened by "bivalving" it (longitudinally splitting it along its lateral border). Reconstruction may be effected by sutures [3,5] or by gentle pressure for a few minutes to allow the halves to "clot" together [6]. The latter technique avoids the renal destruction caused by sutures.

5. Renal biopsies are occasionally indicated for histopathological examination, and several techniques for biopsy are available [7]. Some common procedures are illustrated in Table 14-2. To prevent iatrogenic hemorrage, the hilar region of the kidney should be avoided [5,8]. Some surgeons prefer to biopsy the kidney during laparotomy to allow better exposure and control.

6. Radiographic evaluation of kidney size is often of value clinically. Kidneys are usually enlarged in any acute renal disease, hydronephrosis, pyelonephrosis, or neoplasia. They are smaller than normal in end-stage kidney disease and in renal hypoplasia. Because the right kidney is usually visualized too poorly for measurements on plain films, and even the left one is often difficult to see, intravenous nephrography is typically used to estimate kidney size. In dogs, studies have shown that the radiographic length ratio between the kidneys and the second lumbar vertebra is about 3:1 (the vertebral measurement to include only the body and not the

Table 14-2

Kidney Biopsy Sites

Horse	Push the left kidney against the left flank (per rectum) and pass the needle through the body wall.
Ox	Performed as in the horse except the left kidney is pushed against the <u>right</u> body wall.
Dog	Incise the paralumbar fossa under sedation and local anesthesia. Insert a finger to fix the kidney against the lateral abdominal wall. Direct the biopsy needle toward the caudal aspect of the kidney through a separate puncture site.
Cat	The kidneys are pendulous enough to hold for biopsy without an incision. They have been mistaken for tumors and fetuses.

From Habel, 1981 [8]

intervertebral discs). If the renal length is less than 2.5 times or more than 3.5 times the length of L2, the kidney should be considered to be abnormally small or large, respectively [9].

7. The giant kidney worm <u>Dioctophyma renale</u> affects many species of carnivores, mustelids, and the pig. In the definitive host, the parasite is most often found in the peritoneal cavity and may be clinically quiescent, even if one kidney is parasitized and destroyed. Clinically, urinary signs usually occur if both kidneys are involved or in unilateral cases with other renal disease. Surgical removal of the worm is the only known treatment [9].

8. A number of congenital and heritable diseases affect the kidneys including aplasia, hypoplasia, and polycystosis. Familial renal disease occurs in Norwegian Elkhounds and Lhasa Apso dogs [9].

II. URETER

Each ureter courses from the renal hilus to the urinary bladder and penetrates the dorsal wall of the bladder at an oblique angle near its neck (Fig. 14-3).

A. Basic features

abdominal part
pelvic part
layers of wall:
    outer serosal layer
    middle muscular layer
    inner mucosal lining

B. Clinical features

1. The ureters may be obstructed internally by urinary calculi, neoplasms, or blood clots. They may also be occluded by external pressure from abdominal neoplasms or displacement of the urinary bladder. Accidental surgical ligation has also occurred. The condition is usually unilateral and results in a hydronephrotic syndrome. Bilateral obstruction causes a uremic crisis.

2. Ectopic ureters may end blindly and cause hydronephrosis, or they may terminate in the uterus, vagina, or urethra, causing urinary incontinence. Except for one reported case in a male dog, urinary incontinence in dogs as a result of ectopic ureters has been found only in females [9]. Toy breeds are more commonly affected than larger dogs.

3. In males, the ductus deferens on each side loops around the ipsilateral ureter and some cases of ureteral dislodgement have been reported by those using the "pull" method of tomcat castration (Fig. 14-3; also see Chapter 15, Male Reproductive System).

4. The oblique angle at which the ureter enters the urinary bladder helps to prevent reflux of urine [10]. This angle should be duplicated by surgeons treating ectopic ureters via reimplantation in order to prevent possible post-surgical, vesico-ureteral reflux. Reflux, which has also been reported in association with other

urinary diseases, can perpetuate a cystitis and expand its involvement to include the kidneys [9].

5. In cattle, diseased ureters may be palpated per rectum. They are enlarged and firm in cases of pyelonephritis and enlarged but fluctuant in cases of ureteral calculi [8].

III. URINARY BLADDER

The urinary bladder is an organ of considerable distensibility and mobility. When empty, the bladder is located almost entirely within the pelvic cavity, and its wall is relatively thick. When full, however, the bladder wall is thin and the bladder extends cranially for a considerable distance through the cranial pelvic opening and onto the abdominal floor.

A. Basic features (Fig. 14-3) [1]

dorsal and ventral surfaces
apex [vertex] of the bladder--the cranial, free end
body--the central, main part
neck--the constricted portion which joins the urethra
median lig.--the unpaired, ventral fold of peritoneum which is the caudal counterpart of the falciform lig.
lateral ligg.--the paired peritoneal folds which support the bladder laterally and envelop the round ligg.
   round ligg.--the vestigial, prebladder remnants of the left and right umbilical aa.
urachus--the vestigial connection of the apex of the bladder to the umbilicus
ureteral ostium (left and right)--the opening of each ureter into the bladder near the neck
internal urethral ostium--the opening of the initial part of the urethra into the bladder
trigone--the triangular area between the two ureteral ostia and the internal urethral ostium

B. Comparative and clinical features

1. Several conditions can alter the normal position of the urinary bladder [9].

    a. In males, it may be displaced cranially by prostatic enlargement (from hyperplasia, neoplasia, cysts, or abscesses).

    b. In females, it may be pulled into the pelvic cavity by uterine or vaginal prolapse, and it may also prolapse through the urethra.

    c. It may be fixed in an abnormal position by adhesions or held there by adjacent tumors.

    d. It may rotate around its long axis (torsion) to cause partial or complete obstruction.

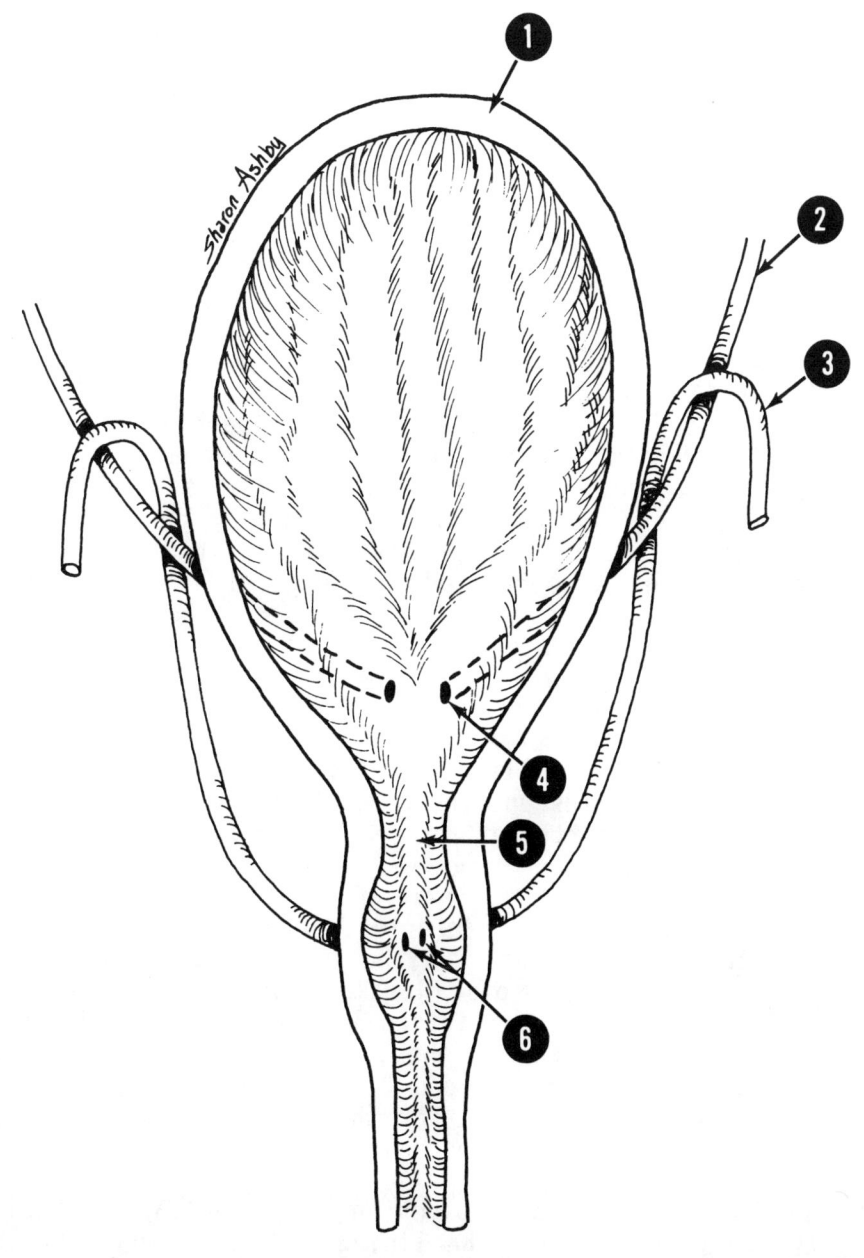

Figure 14-3

Ventral View of Sectioned Urinary Bladder of a Male

1. Bladder wall at the apex (vertex)
2. Left ureter
3. Ductus deferens
4. Ureteral ostium
5. Beginning of the urethra (internal urethral ostium)
6. Openings of deferential ducts on colliculus seminalis

e. It may be found in a perineal, inguinal, or ventral abdominal hernia.

2. Urinary calculi occasionally collect (and increase in size) in the urinary bladder. Those composed primarily of phosphates or oxalates (the most common ones) are usually radiopaque, while those composed primarily of urate or cystine are typically radiolucent.* They may be removed by a routine cystotomy. Some can be prevented through diet and medication.

3. The urachus usually degenerates after birth and is difficult or impossible to identify in the adult. Occasionally, it remains open as a patent urachus or it may be partially patent and develop cysts. Patent urachus may be diagnosed in neonates by the observation of urine dripping from the umbilicus. Intravenous urography or retrograde cystography may be needed to confirm the diagnosis. Secondary omphalitis and cystitis may be present. The problem can be corrected by surgical resection of the urachal stalk.

4. The median ligament of the bladder attaches to the ventral body wall from the umbilicus to the pelvis in the fetus, and serves as the caudal counterpart of the falciform ligament. It surrounds and supports the post-bladder (bladder-to-umbilicus) portions of the umbilical arteries and the urachus. Much of it degenerates with the urachus after birth.

5. The left and right umbilical arteries originate as initial branches of the internal iliac arteries. They course to the bladder within the lateral ligaments of the bladder and then continue to the umbilicus in the median ligament of the bladder. The prebladder portions (between the internal iliac aa. and the bladder), which become the round ligaments, may remain patent after birth and continue to supply blood to the bladder in the adult. The post-bladder portions of the arteries (bladder-to-umbilicus) usually regress beyond recognition.

6. The bladder wall consists of an outer serosa, a muscular layer, and an inner mucosa [1]. The lining mucosa is very friable and becomes hemorrhagic even with very gentle manipulation. The muscle layer is formed of smooth muscle, but near the internal urethral ostium there are skeletal muscle fascicles which form a functional, but not grossly identifiable, sphincter.

7. The bladder may be emptied by cystocentesis with a small gauge needle. This procedure may be necessary to prevent rupture of the bladder in tomcats with urethral obstructions. The site should be prepared for surgery and the abdominal puncture should be made on the midline just cranial to the pelvic symphysis, since the bladder

---

*A memory aid for the radiopaque calculi is that "op" in radiopaque can be matched with oxalate and phosphate. In a similar manner, radiolucent calculi include those composed of urate and cystine.

will shrink back into the pelvic cavity as it empties. It is also helpful in this regard to direct the needle dorsocaudally at about a $45°$ angle. Occasionally, when doing laparotomies, the surgeon will encounter a full bladder, which is bothersome. It may be emptied with a sterile syringe and needle or expressed. When penetrating the bladder wall with a needle, the angle of entry should be markedly oblique to reduce the possibility of subsequent leakage. After cystocentesis, a bladder should not be subjected to digital pressure for several hours [9].

8. Radiographic visualization of the urinary bladder may assist diagnosis of bladder displacement, cystic calculi, or neoplasia. Negative contrast (using air, CO_2, or N_2), positive contrast, or double contrast techniques may be used. The bladder should be emptied and survey (plain) films taken prior to introduction of the contrast medium. Blood clots and air bubbles may produce identifiable and confusing shadows.

9. Urinary incontinence (inability to urinate when and/or where desired) may be caused by congenital malformations, primary bladder disease, or iatrogenic vesico-urethral damage. Incontinence may be classified as neurogenic, nonneurogenic, or paradoxical [9].

   a. Neurogenic incontinence results from damage to the bladder's nerve supply. This may be caused by direct damage to the sacral nerves which supply the bladder (vertebral lesions, etc.) resulting in a "paralytic bladder", or it may result from a lesion of the C.N.S. between the brain and sacral part of the cord ("cord bladder").

   b. Nonneurogenic incontinence results from ectopic ureters, congenital problems of the urethra and/or its sphincters, patent urachus, or endocrine imbalances after ovariohysterectomies.

   c. Paradoxical incontinence results from partial obstruction of the urethra due to calculi, strictures, or neoplasms.

   These types of incontinence may be differentiated as follows:

Type of Incontinence	Normal Micturition	Distended Bladder	Easily Catheterized
Neurogenic	-	+	+
Nonneurogenic	+	-	+
Paradoxical	-	+	-

10. Human cystoscopes may be used to examine the interior of the urinary bladder in medium to large bitches, but the anatomy of the canine urethra makes the procedure impossible in male dogs [8].

IV. URETHRA

The urethra functions to eliminate urine that is stored in the urinary bladder. It is a musculomembranous tube joining the neck of the bladder to the body surface. The wall of the urethra has the same basic layers as that of the urinary bladder. In addition, it contains the striated urethralis muscle which allows some voluntary control of urination.

A. Basic features

   Male urethra

   pelvic part--the portion between the bladder and penis
       pre-prostatic part--the short initial segment
       prostatic part--the portion surrounded by the prostate gland
           urethral crest--the longitudinal ridge of mucosa projecting
               from the dorsum of the urethra
           colliculus seminalis--the area on the urethral crest on which
               the genital ducts open
           ejaculatory ostium--the combined opening of the ductus
               deferens and vesicular gland in the horse and ruminants
   spongy part--the portion of the urethra within the penis
   external urethral ostium--the urethral opening at the tip of the penis
   mucosal layer--the urethral lining
   stratum spongiosum--the vascular layer which surrounds the mucosa
   muscular layer--the external layer consisting of smooth muscle and, in
       the pelvic part, the urethral (striated) muscle

   Female urethra

   urethral crest--as in the male
   external urethral ostium--opens into the vaginal vestibule
   layers of wall
       mucosal layer
       muscular layer
       adventitial layer

B. Comparative features

   1. The mucosa of the urethra in the ox normally contains lymphatic nodules.
   2. There are urethral glands associated with the mucosa in the pig and the horse.
   3. In the horse and small ruminants, the urethra projects beyond the glans penis via the urethral process (see Chapter 15, Male Reproductive System).
   4. The cow and sow have a blind diverticulum of the vaginal vestibule, the suburethral diverticulum, located ventral (caudal) to the urethra. The suburethral diverticulum joins the vestibule adjacent to the external urethral ostium (see Chapter 16, Female Reproductive System).

C. Clinical features

   1. Congenital anomalies of the urethra include its absence, duplication, hypospadia and epispadia (opening of the urethra on the ventral or dorsal surface of the penis or perineum), abnormal diverticula, and accessory meatus [9].

2. A cystitis-urethral obstruction complex occurs primarily in male cats (feline urolithiasis, feline urological syndrome, or plugged-tomcat syndrome). Queens often have the cystitis with its accompanying dysuria and hematuria, but rarely do they suffer the urethral obstruction. The obstructants include cells, crystals, mucoid materials, and various combinations of them. Dry cat foods, alkaline urine, and diets high in mineral content may be predisposing factors. Vitamin A and/or castration are not considered to be factors in obstructive urolithiasis in cats. The etiology may be viral. Indwelling catheters may be preferred over repeated catheterizations since iatrogenic truma can result in strictures. Cystocentesis may be required in severe cases. Urinary acidifiers and antibiotics are indicated. Recurring cases may require urethrostomies (perineal, preputial, antepubic) [9].

3. The urethra can be easily catheterized in most species. In male ruminants and pigs, this procedure is facilitated by administration of an ataractic drug to straighten the sigmoid flexure. In female ruminants and pigs, the suburethral diverticulum may tend to catch the tip of the catheter tube (which should be directed over it). Bulls can often be induced to urinate by washing the prepuce with warm water. Cows often urinate in response to gentle stroking of the ventral perineal area (the so-called "escutcheon").

4. Trauma to the urethra may result from automobile accidents, bite wounds, urethral calculi, or iatrogenically from catheterizations.

5. Calculi can block the urethra at any point, but in male dogs the most common locus is just proximal to the os penis. The high incidence of blockage at this point is apparently related to the non-expansibility of the urethra as it courses through the groove in the ventrum of the os penis [8]. Tomcats also have an os penis, but it does not surround the urethra and is not responsible for the obstructions which occur. In bulls and steers, calculi often lodge in the distal part of the sigmoid flexure, and in rams and bucks, the most usual place is in the urethral process. Obstructing calculi are more common in steers than in bulls (even though both groups form calculi at about the same rate) because bulls can pass calculi more easily due to a larger urethral lumen (see Chapter 15, Male Reproductive System) [11]. In female mammals, the shorter and relatively more expansible urethra makes obstructive urolithiasis relatively rare, but the production of calculi occurs with equal frequency in both sexes [11].

References

1. International Committee on Veterinary Gross Anatomical Nomenclature. 1983. Nomina Anatomica Veterinaria, third ed. Published by the Committee, Ithaca, New York.

2. Nickel, R., A. Schummer, E. Seiferle, and W. Sack. 1973. The Viscera of the Domestic Mammals. Paul Parey, Berlin.

3. Archibald, J., ed. 1974. Canine Surgery, second ed. American Veterinary Publications, Santa Barbara, California.

4. Shively, M. J. 1978. Origin and branching of renal arteries in the dog. JAVMA 173(8):986-989.

5. Bojrab, M. J. ed. 1975. Current Techniques in Small Animal Surgery. Lea and Febiger, Philadelphia.

6. Gorley, I. M. 1975. Nephrectomy and nephrolithotomy. Vet. Clin. North Am. 5(3):401-413.

7. Osborn, C. A. 1971. Clinical evaluation of needle biopsy of the kidney and its complications in the dog and cat. JAVMA 158(7):1213-1228.

8. Habel, R. E. 1981. Applied Veterinary Anatomy, second ed. Published by the author, Ithaca. New York.

9. Osborne, C. A., D. G. Low, and D. R. Finco. 1972. Canine and Feline Urology. W. B. Saunders, Philadelphia.

10. Feeney, D. A., C. A. Osborne, and G. R. Johnston. 1983. Vesicoureteral reflux induced by manual compression of the urinary bladder of dogs and cats. JAVMA 182(8):795-797.

11. Blood, D. C., J. A. Henderson, and O.M. Radostits. 1979. Veterinary Medicine, fifth ed. Lea and Febiger, Philadelphia.

MALE REPRODUCTIVE SYSTEM

The major parts of the male reproductive system include the testes, the epididymis and ductus deferens associated with each testis, the distal part of the urethra, the penis, the scrotum, and the accessory sex glands. Major species differences are related to which accessory sex glands are present and the structure of the penis (Fig. 15-1).

I. TESTIS

Each testis functions to produce spermatozoa and the male sex hormone testosterone. The spermatozoa are produced within the microscopic seminiferous tubules, and the interstitial cells between the tubules produce the hormone. The sperm mature in the epididymis, and nourishing and extending fluids are added by the accessory sex glands at ejaculation to produce semen.

A. General features (Fig. 15-2) [1]

capital extremity--the end associated with the head of the epididymis
caudal extremity--the end associated with the tail of the epididymis
medial and lateral surfaces
epididymal and free borders
tunica albuginea--the dense connective tissue which encapsulates the testicular parenchyma
mediastinum testis--the central connective tissue core which contains the rete testis
septula of the testis--trabeculae of connective tissue which divide the testicular parenchyma into lobules
seminiferous tubules--the sperm producing portions of the parenchyma
rete testis--a collection of small tubules in the mediastinum which carry sperm from the seminiferous tubules to the capital extremity
efferential ducts--the channels which perforate the tunica albuginea to connect the rete testis to the head of the epididymis

B. Comparative features

1. The testes of the ram, buck, and boar are relatively large while those of carnivores and horses are relatively small. There is no seasonal change in testicular size in domestic mammals [2].

2. The orientation of the testis within the scrotum varies among the species. In the horse, the capital-caudal axis is nearly horizontal. In the dog, cat, and pig, it is tipped down by various degrees so that the capital extremity is lower than the caudal extremity. In the ox, the capital extremity is tipped up so far that the testicular axis is almost vertical (Fig. 15-2) [2].

3. The mediastinum testis of the stallion is confined to the capital extremity [2] and is considered to be absent by some authors [3].

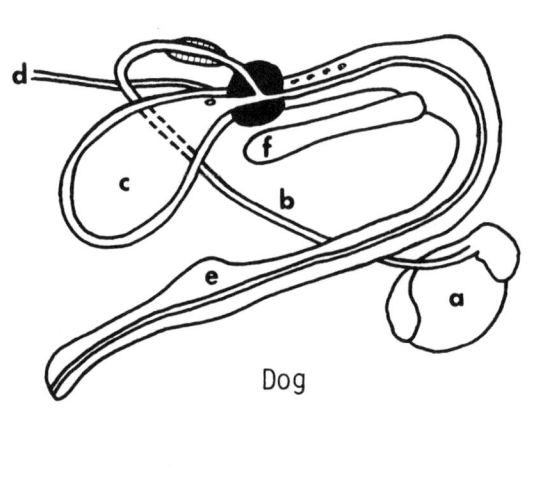
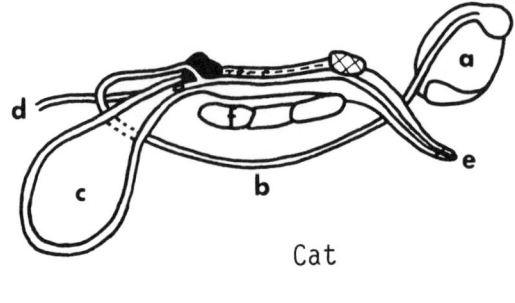
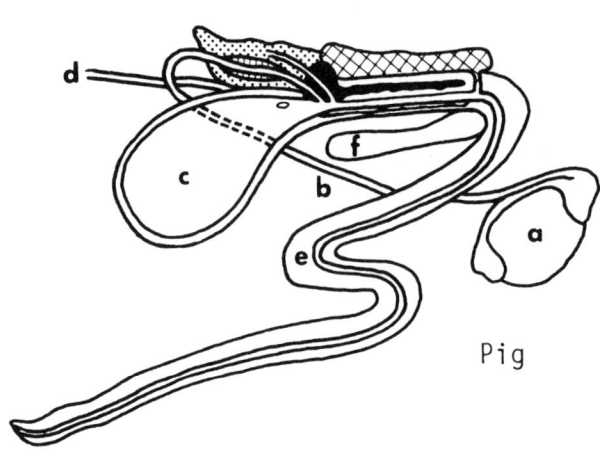
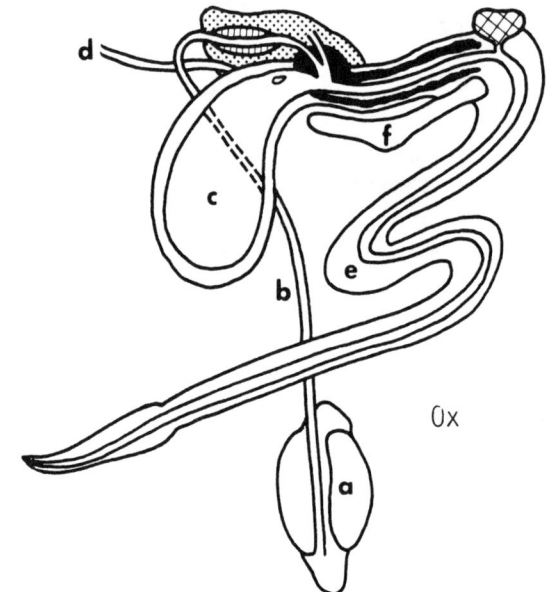
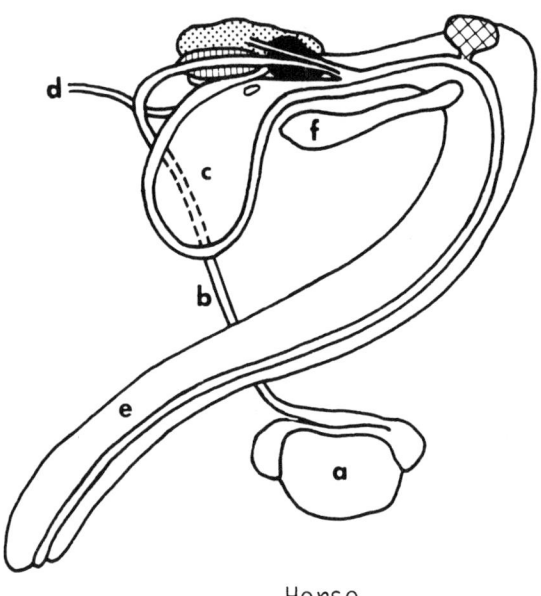

Figure 15-1

Male Genital Organs

- ▨ ampulla*
- ■ prostate gland
- ▦ vesicular gland**
- ▩ bulbourethral gland

a. right testis and epididymis
b. ductus deferens
c. urinary bladder
d. ureter
e. penis and extrapelvic urethra
f. pelvic symphysis

*glandular part of ductus deferens in pig
** seminal vesicle in horse

After Nickel, Schummer, Seiferle, and Sack, 1973 [2]

C. Clinical considerations

1. Castration and cryptorchidism will be discussed in some of the following sections.

2. Testicular neoplasia has a relatively low incidence in domestic animals, except in the dog, and occurs more commonly in undescended testes than in scrotal ones. Primary tumors involve the interstitial cells, sustentacular (Sertoli) cells, or germinal epithelium [4].

3. Testes may degenerate because of circulatory disturbances, age, heat, irradiation, localized or systemic diseases, or hormonal changes. Testicular inflammation usually precedes degeneration and testicular fibrosis usually follows it [4].

4. Testicular hypoplasia is more commonly observed in ungulates than in carnivores and may occur unilaterally [4].

II. EPIDIDYMIS

The epididymis is an elongated organ which lies adjacent to the testis and continuously receives immature sperm, which enter it through the efferent ducts. These ducts join the single, tortuous duct of the epididymis, where sperm complete their maturation. At ejaculation, peristaltic contractions force sperm into the ductus deferens, which is continuous with the tail of the epididymis.

A. General features [2]

head--the end where the efferential ducts enter
body--the central portion
tail--the portion which is continuous with the ductus deferens
duct of the epididymis--the single continuous channel within the epididymis
lobules of the epididymis--the wedge-shaped masses formed by the efferential ductules before they unite to form the duct of the epididymis
paradidymis--vestigial remnants of the mesonephric ducts

B. Comparative features

1. The number of efferential ducts which unite to form the duct of the epididymis varies from 13-23 among individuals and species [2].

2. The total length of the duct of the epididymis varies from about 2 meters (cat) to 75 meters (horse) [2].

C. Clinical considerations

1. The epididymis and initial part of the ductus deferens of some species have secretory cells which may produce some male sex hormones and this may explain the phenomenon of "proud cut" horses (castrated males that retain their male sexual behavior). The validity of this theory remains undocumented and has been seriously questioned by some recent investigations.

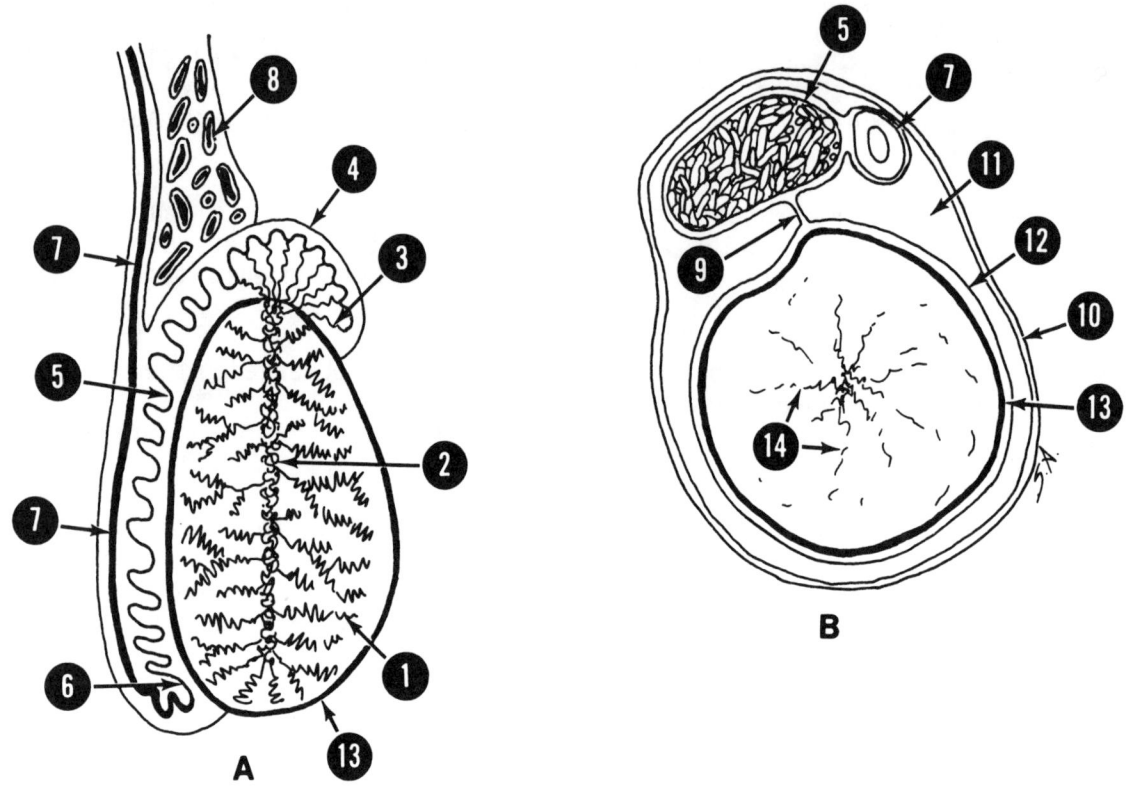

Figure 15-2

Schematic Sectional Views of the Testis of a Bull

    A. Longitudinal section
    B. Transverse section

1. seminiferous tubules
2. rete testis (within the mediastinum testis)
3. efferential ducts
4. head of epididymis
5. duct of epididymis in the body of the epididymis
6. duct of epididymis at the tail of the epididymis
7. ductus deferens
8. pampiniform plexus
9. mesorchium
10. parietal vaginal tunic and spermatic fascia
11. vaginal cavity
12. visceral vaginal tunic
13. tunica albuginea
14. septula of testis

After Nickel, Schummer, Seiferle, and Sack, 1973 [2]

2. The most common clinical syndrome of the epididymis is inflammation resulting from bacterial infection (especially <u>Brucella, Corynebacterium,</u> and <u>Actinobacillus</u> spp.)

III. SCROTUM

In a normal mature male the testes and epididymides are located in the scrotum. The thermoregulatory function of the scrotum necessary for spermatogenesis is a well-accepted phenomenon which birds and some mammals (such as elephants and whales) defy. Seasonal ascent and descent of the testes associated with rut (periodic sexual behavior) is not seen in domestic mammals.

A. Major features [1]

skin of the scrotum--integument which forms the external wall of the scrotum
    raphe--the line formed by the junction of the right and left halves of the scrotal skin
tunica dartos--the inner layer of the scrotal wall formed by connective tissue and bundles of smooth muscle (dartos m.)
    septum of the scrotum--the partition which divides the scrotal cavity into two compartments

B. Comparative features

1. The scrota of pigs and cats are located directly ventral to the anus and are not pendulous.

2. In the horse, dog, and ruminants, there is a varying amount of intervening perineum between the anus and scrotum. These animals have pendulous scrota.

3. The scrota of dogs, stallions, bulls, and boars are relatively glabrous, while those of small ruminants and cats are hairy [4].

C. Clinical considerations

1. Castration in companion animals is often done to control sexual behavior. In food animals, it is done for economic reasons. Many techniques are available and the one selected is often determined by personal preference. Common techniques include the following:

a. Pigs, cats, and horses are usually castrated through two scrotal incisions. In pigs, no anesthesia is used and the spermatic cords are pulled or cut without ligating them. In cats, the cords may be pulled, ligated and cut, or cut and then tied on each side by separating the ductus deferens from the ipsilateral spermatic vessels and tying these two components in a knot [5]. In horses, the cords are cut and crushed with an emasculator. Part of the scrotal septum may be removed to prevent premature closure of the incision sites and associated complications [6].

b. Dogs are usually castrated through a single incision just cranial to the scrotum. The whole spermatic cord and its tunics are ligated (closed technique) or the parietal vaginal tunic may be opened and the spermatic cord components may be ligated more directly (open technique). See part VII. [7].

c. Ruminants may be castrated through separate scrotal incisions or by cutting off the bottom third of the scrotum and pulling each testis out. In very young animals, the cords may be broken by tension. In larger animals, they are usually severed, or crushed and severed with an emasculator [8].

2. Failure of testicular descent into the scrotum on one or both sides results in cryptorchidism. Horses with this condition are often called "ridglings," "rigs," or "originals" [8]. Undescended testicles produce hormones but usually no sperm, and they have a higher incidence of neoplasia. It is considered unprofessional to castrate a unilateral cryptorchid, unless you also intend to attempt to remove the undescended testis.

3. The scrotal skin is very sensitive and subject by its location to frostbite, insect bites, photosensitization, and ectoparasitism. The extreme irritability of this area in dogs is one reason why castration is usually done through an incision just cranial to the scrotum rather than through the scrotum itself [7].

IV. DUCTUS DEFERENS

The ductus deferens transports spermatozoa from the tail of the epididymis to the urethra. Its initial part is tortuous and closely associated with the epididymis. It then courses proximally with the testicular vessels and nerves to form the part of the spermatic cord which passes through the inguinal canal. Inside the abdominal cavity, the testicular vessels and nerves course toward the kidneys (where the testes originally developed), and each ductus deferens turns toward the pelvic inlet and courses toward the neck of the urinary bladder. Near the bladder the ductus deferens thickens to form the ampulla in some species. Glands in the ampulla add a viscous, mucoid secretion to the seminal fluid. The ductus deferens terminates by joining the pelvic urethra on the colliculus seminalis.

A. Comparative features

1. The ampulla is very well developed in the horse and less so in the dog and ruminants. The cat and pig have no ampulla as such, but they do have some glands in the wall of the distal part of the ductus deferens [2].

2. In the horse and ruminants, and often in the pig, the ductus deferens unites near its termination with the excretory duct of the ipsilateral vesicular gland. These form a common ejaculatory duct which then enters the pelvic urethra at the colliculus seminalis [2].

3. A remnant of the paramesonephric ducts (uterus masculinus) is usually present between the ampullae of the horse. It may often be identified in bulls as well [2].

B. Clinical considerations

1. It is of clinical significance that each ductus deferens loops around the ipsilateral ureter, since tension on the ductus during a "pull" type castration puts tension on the ipsilateral ureter. The anatomic possibility of dislodging a ureter by this technique has led to criticism of its use in cats. This author believes that an empty bladder removes the danger of dislodging the ureter, since the empty bladder is mobile and free to turn as tension is applied to the ductus deferens. This movement may relieve direct tension on the ureter. When distended, however, the bladder is lodged at the pelvic inlet and is unable to turn. In addition, the position of entry of the ureters is further cranial in a full bladder. The problem probably occurs in toms brought in one day and castrated the next day (many are reluctant to urinate in a strange environment, so they have full bladders at the time of surgery).

V. INGUINAL CANAL (Fig. 15-3)

The inguinal canal is a passageway in the abdominal wall. In males, it transmits the spermatic cord, genitofemoral nerve, external pudendal vasculature, and the efferent lymphatic vessels from the superficial inguinal lymph nodes. In females, it transmits only the latter three structures.* Its superficial opening is the superficial ("external") inguinal ring, and its deep opening is the deep ("internal") inguinal ring. The actual canal is not a hollow cylinder but is collapsed because of its oblique passage through the abdominal wall. It is therefore somewhat difficult to conceptualize. The superficial inguinal ring is a slit in the aponeurosis of the external abdominal oblique muscle. It is easily located and visualized by following the spermatic cord through it. The deep inguinal ring, however, is not well defined anatomically. It is a long, slender triangle, bounded cranially by the caudal edge of the internal abdominal oblique muscle, caudally by the inguinal ligament (the caudal free border of the aponeurosis of the external abdominal oblique m.), and medially by the attachment of the rectus abdominis m. (prepubic tendon). All of the spermatic cord components course through at least part of the inguinal canal. It is a matter of semantic debate whether the cremaster muscle, which is derived as a slip from the internal abdominal oblique, passes all the way through the canal or "sneaks" in from the side.

Inguinal hernias are very common in horses and pigs and have been shown to be hereditary in these two species [4]. Inguinal hernias occur in the other domestic mammals, but with a lower frequency. Affected animals should be castrated or not used for breeding [4]. Inguinal hernias may progress to scrotal hernias.

---

*In bitches, a vaginal process of peritoneum courses through the inguinal canal. It surrounds the round ligament of the uterus and some fat.

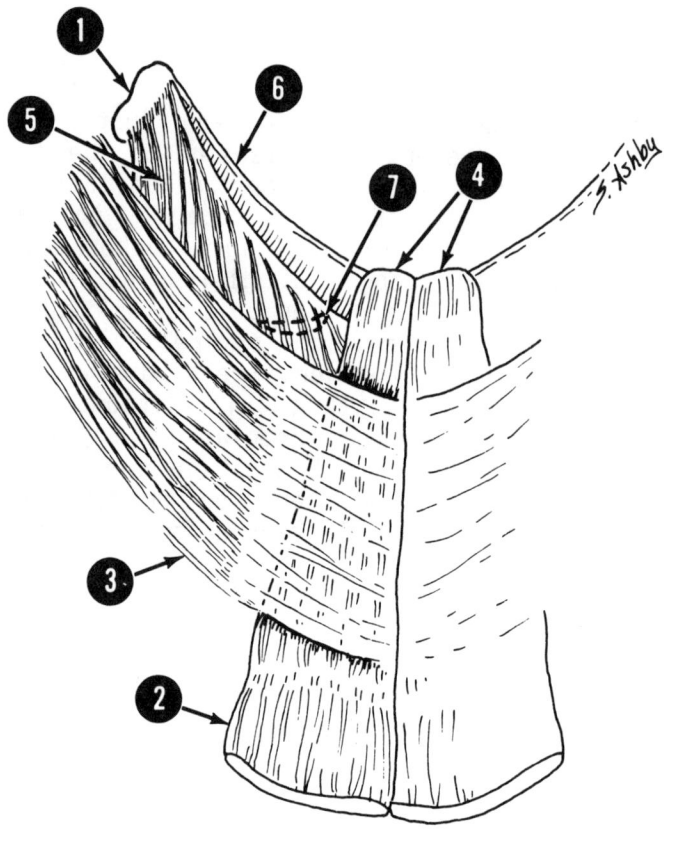

Figure 15-3

Pelvic Inlet from an Intra-Abdominal Perspective

1. tuber coxae

2. rectus abdominis m.

3. transversus abdominis m.

4. prepubic tendon

5. internal abdominal oblique m.

6. inguinal ligament (caudal free border of external abdominal oblique m.)

7. dotted lines indicate the superficial inguinal ring--a slit in the aponeurosis of the external abdominal oblique m.

   The deep inguinal ring is the slitlike triangle formed by 4, 5, and 6.

VI. DESCENT OF THE TESTES (INTO THE SCROTUM)

The testes begin development within the abdominal cavity near the kidneys. A connective tissue cord, the gubernaculum, extends from the caudal aspect of each embryonic testis into the inguinal canal. During development, the testis moves caudally, following the gubernaculum into and eventually through the inguinal canal. The forces involved in this migration are not understood, and although a number of possible factors have been mentioned, the ultimate explanation remains undetermined. It is particularly peculiar that no connections between the gubernaculum and the scrotal wall have been demonstrated during development; thus, simple tension from shrinkage of the gubernaculum ("rubber-band" theory) does not explain testicular descent. It has been shown that the gubernaculum enlarges to dilate the inguinal canal sufficiently to allow the testis to pass through. After the descent of each testis, its gubernaculum persists as connective tissue joining the tail of the epididymis to the scrotal wall (ligament of the tail of the epididymis) and also joining the tail of the epididymis to the testis (proper ligament of the testis).

In ruminants, testicular descent is complete at about 3-4 months fetal age. In the pig, completion of the descent occurs just before birth and, in carnivores, shortly after birth. In horses, it may occur several days before or after birth [2].

VII. SPERMATIC CORD AND VAGINAL TUNIC (Fig. 15-4)

The spermatic cord is the group of structures which extends from the caudal extremity of the testis through the inguinal canal. Included are the ductus deferens and its tiny vessels as well as the testicular artery, vein, lymphatics, and nerves. Some authors include the cremaster muscle, others do not.

As each testis, epididymis, and ductus deferens descend through the inguinal canal, they carry with them the visceral peritoneum which originally invested their surfaces. This serous layer, attached directly to them, is the visceral vaginal tunic (Fig. 15-4/6). The parietal layer of peritoneum which precedes each testis through the inguinal canal to the scrotal cavity is the parietal vaginal tunic. (The term vaginal process is synonymous with vaginal tunic and refers collectively to the parietal and visceral portions.) The "vaginal ring" is the circular structure formed by the parietal peritoneum as it passes through the deep inguinal ring to become the parietal vaginal tunic. The parietal vaginal tunic is adherent to the spermatic fascia, lining the scrotum and extending through the inguinal canal. The potential space between the parietal and visceral vaginal tunics is the vaginal cavity, which is continuous with the peritoneal cavity. The portion of the vaginal cavity between the testis and epididymis is the testicular bursa (homologous to the ovarian bursa of the female).

Supporting folds of parietal vaginal tunic are given special names:

mesorchium--the peritoneum which suspends the testis and surrounds the testicular artery, vein, nerve, and lymphatics. The relationship between the testis and mesorchium is identical to that between the jejunum and the mesentery.

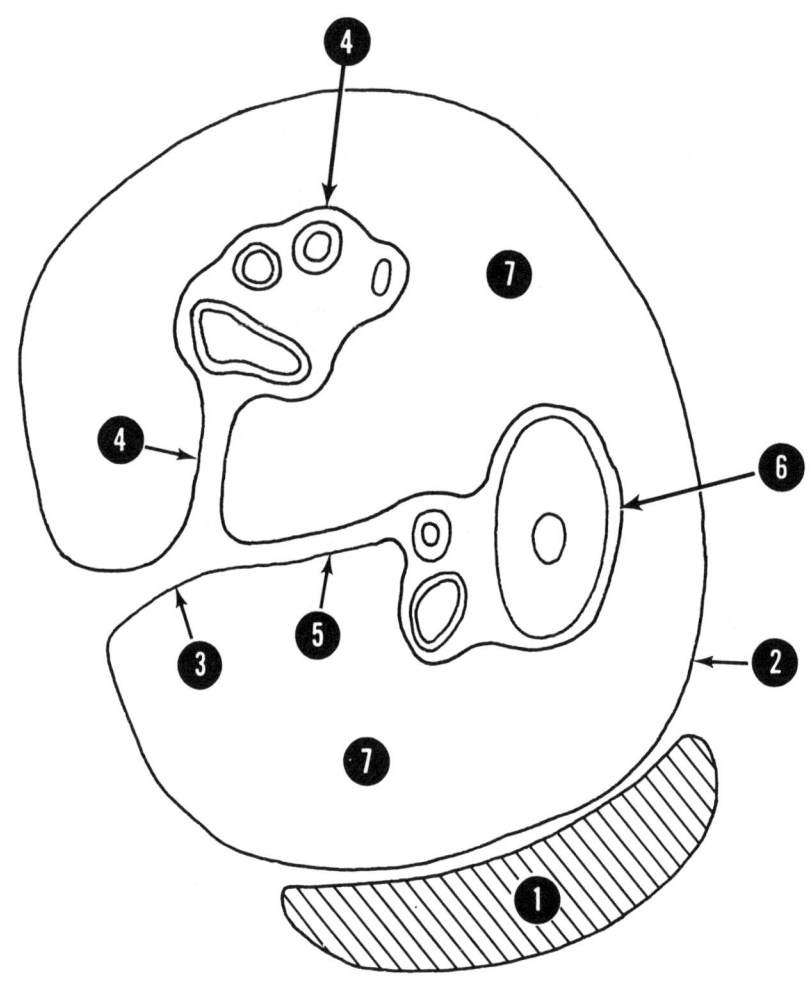

Figure 15-4

Schematic View of Spermatic Cord (transverse section)

1. cremaster muscle
2. parietal vaginal tunic
3. mesofuniculus--a double layer of vaginal tunic homologous to the mesentery
4. mesorchium--a special part of the parietal vaginal tunic which surrounds the testicular artery, vein, nerve, and lymphatic. It is continuous distally with the visceral vaginal tunic covering the testis.
5. mesoductus deferens--a special part of the parietal vaginal tunic which suspends the ductus deferens and deferential vessels. It is continuous with the visceral vaginal tunic surrounding the ductus deferens.
6. visceral vaginal tunic
7. vaginal cavity

mesofuniculus--the portion of the mesorchium between the origin of the mesoductus deferens and the outer part of the parietal vaginal tunic around the cord

mesoductus deferens--the suspending fold of peritoneum which supports the ductus deferens

mesoepididymis--the suspending fold of peritoneum which supports the epididymis

"Open" and "closed," as applied to castration techniques, refer to whether the vaginal cavity has (open) or has not (closed) been exposed by the procedure. For example, in castrating a dog, the surgeon may isolate the whole cord external to the parietal vaginal tunic without invading the vaginal cavity. If he then ligates the whole cord and severs it distal to the ligation, the procedure was "closed." However, if he incises the parietal vaginal tunic to place a ligature directly around the visceral vaginal tunic surrounding the component structures, the procedure is "open" because the vaginal cavity was invaded. Most castrations in most species are performed open (see Part III.C.).

VIII. ACCESSORY SEX GLANDS (Fig. 15-5)

The accessory sex glands are very closely associated with the pelvic urethra and differ among the various species. They include the prostate, vesicular, and bulbourethral glands (Table 15-1). Some authors consider the ampullae to be accessory sex glands, too, but technically they are parts of the deferential ducts. The accessory sex glands add volume, nutrients, buffers, and lubricants to the ejaculate.

Table 15-1

The Accessory Sex Glands

	Prostate Gland	Vesicular Gland	Bulbourethral Gland
dog	+	-	-
cat	+	-	+
pig	+	+	+
ruminants	+	+	+
horse	+	+	+

A. Prostate gland

The prostate gland is present in all domestic mammals and consists of a body (visible on the outside of the urethra) and a disseminate part (forming a glandular layer in the urethral wall). Some species have only a body (horse), some have only a disseminate part (small ruminants), and the others have both [2].

1. The body in the carnivores is divided into right and left lobes which completely surround the urethra in the dog but do not meet ventrally in the cat. The disseminate part in these species consists of a few scattered lobules in the urethral wall.

Figure 15-5

Accessory Sex Glands

A. Stallion (dorsal aspect)
B. Bull (left aspect)

1. ureter
2. ductus deferens and ampulla
3. uterus masculinus (shown in horse only)
4. seminal vesicle (A), vesicular gland (B)
5. prostate gland (body)
6. pelvic urethra surrounded by urethralis m
7. bulbourethral gland
8. spongy urethra and bulb of penis surrounded by bulbospongiosus m.
9. retractor penis m.
10. ischiocavernosus m.
11. sigmoid flexure (bull only)
12. urinary bladder (shown in bull only)

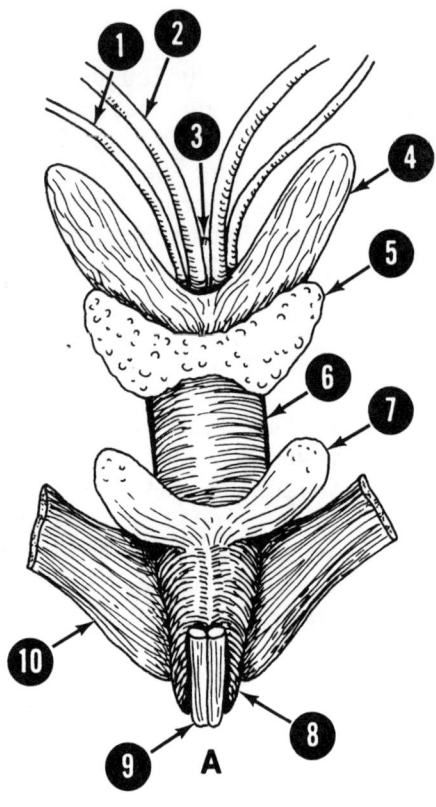

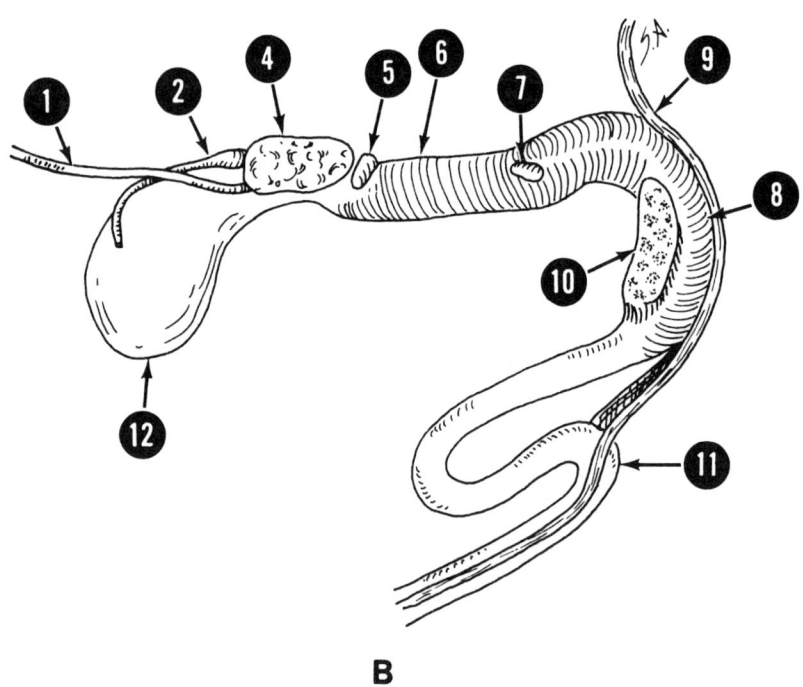

After Nickel, Schummer, Seiferle, and Sack, 1973 [2]

2. In the ox and pig, the body is a small mass on the dorsal aspect of the urethra and the disseminate part is covered by the urethralis muscle.

3. The small ruminants have only the disseminate part (no body).

4. The horse has no disseminate part and the body consists of right and left lobes which lie on the dorsal aspect of the urethra and are connected by an isthmus.

The prostate suffers clinical problems, mainly in the dog, and these are usually hyperplasia or inflammation. The common clinical signs of prostatitis include constipation, preputial discharge, and pain on rectal palpation. Castration and estrogens are used to treat hyperplasia and antibiotics are of value in prostatitis. Removal of the prostate may be indicated by neoplasia. It may be accomplished by transecting the urethra on both sides and then anastomosing the urethra [7]. Scottish terriers have very large prostate glands.

B. Vesicular gland

The vesicular gland is paired and is positioned on the dorsolateral aspect of the neck of the urinary bladder. The vesicular gland is absent in carnivores. In the horse and ruminants, the excretory duct of the vesicular gland joins the terminal part of the ductus deferens to form an ejaculatory duct. This same arrangement may also occur in the pig, but usually the procine excretory duct and ductus deferens open independently into the urethra. In the horse, as in man, the vesicular gland is termed the seminal vesicle because it is hollow. The vesicular gland does not store sperm [2].

C. Bulbourethral ("Cowper's") gland

The paired bulbourethral gland is present in all domestic mammalian species except the dog. It lies on the dorsal aspect of the caudal part of the pelvic urethra near the bulb of the penis. In the pig, the gland consists of two large cylindrically shaped structures which are covered by the bulboglandularis muscle. In the other domestic mammals, the bulbourethral glands are nearly spherical. The right and left glands each have one excretory duct which joins the urethra (except in the horse where each gland has several ducts) [2].

IX. PENIS

The penis of domestic mammals is a highly specialized and complex organ. It attaches to the ischia and extends to the glans at the distal, free end. It surrounds the terminal part of the urethra and functions in both the reproductive and urinary systems.

A. General features [1]

root--the attachment to the left and right ischia
crura--the initial portions (left and right) which fuse to form the body. These are covered by the ischiocavernosus mm.

body--the main part of the penile shaft formed by the corpora cavernosa, corpus spongiosum, and the urethra
urethral surface--the surface nearest to the urethra
dorsal surface--the surface furthest from the urethra
free part of the penis--the portion distal to the point of attachment of the prepuce
glans penis--the distal part on which the urethra opens
prepuce--the cutaneous sheath which surrounds the glans and free part of the penis
    external lamina--the outer layer which is continuous with the skin of the abdominal wall
    internal lamina--the inner layer which is continuous with the skin on the free part of the penis

    preputial orifice--the opening where the internal and external laminae meet
    preputial cavity--the space around the free part of the penis when it is retracted into the prepuce
cranial and caudal preputial muscles--poorly developed muscles which are responsible for pulling the prepuce cranially to cover the penis, or caudally to expose the penis
corpus cavernosum penis--the paired erectile bodies which lie dorsal and lateral to the urethra
corpus spongiosum penis--the unpaired erectile body which surrounds the spongy ("external" or "penile") part of the urethra
bulb of the penis--the proximal, expanded erectile body, a caudal evagination of the corpus spongiosum penis, which is surrounded by the bulbospongiosus muscle
corpus spongiosum glandis--the erectile tissue of the glans which is continuous with the corpus spongiosum penis
tunica albuginea--the dense connective tissue which surrounds the erectile tissue of the penis. It is divided into parts which surround the corpora cavernosa and a portion which surrounds the corpus spongiosum

B. Comparative and physiological considerations

1. Although the two corpora cavernosa are developmentally paired and separate proximally to form the crura, they fuse distally with only a septum between them. In the carnivores, this septum remains intact, but in the other species, it is so perforated by openings that a single functional erectile body is formed from both corpora (Figs. 15-6A/1, 15-6B/1) [2].

2. The erectile tissue in the corpora cavernosa, corpus spongiosum penis, corpus spongiosum glandis, and bulb of the penis consists of numerous cavernous spaces separated by connective tissue trabeculae. Depending on the relative amount of connective tissue present, penises of various species may be classified as fibroelastic (pig and ruminants) or musculocavernous (carnivores and horse). Fibroelastic penises, because of their connective tissue content, tend to be firm even when they are not erect [2].

Figure 15-6

Transverse Sections of the Penis in Various Males

A. Stallion, near cranial aspect of scrotum

B. Bull, near caudal aspect of body of penis

C. Dog, through pars longa glandis and prepuce

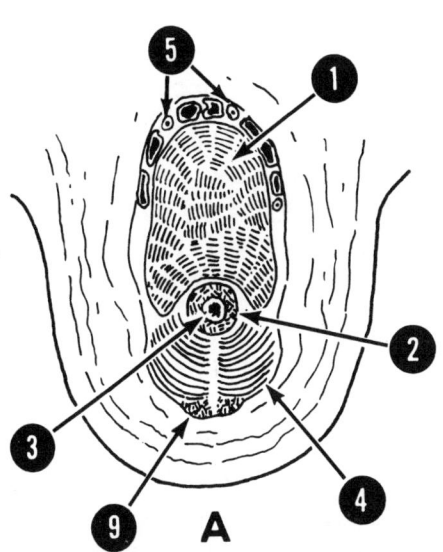

1. corpus cavernosum penis
2. corpus spongiosum penis
3. urethral lumen
4. bulbospongiosus m. (horse)*
5. dorsal arteries of penis (horse, ox)**
6. deep arteries of penis (ox)**
7. os penis (dog)
8. corpus spongiosum glandis (dog)**
9. retractor penis muscle (horse)**

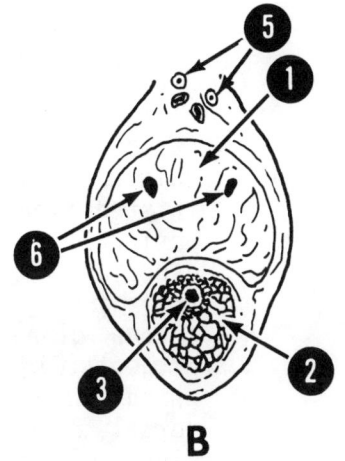

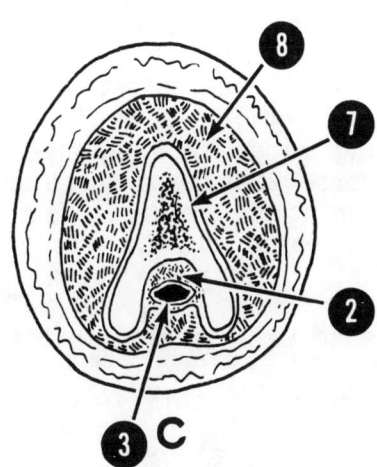

* Extends distally to the glans only in the horse

** Present in all species but not illustrated on all of them because of the different planes of section.

After Nickel, Schummer, Seiferle, and Sack, 1973 [2]

3. The principal physiological cause of erection is an engorgement of the cavernous bodies, caused by an increased blood supply to them and a decreased drainage from them. The hydrostatic pressure in the cavernous bodies is elevated markedly above arterial systolic pressure by a mechanism not fully understood. In the bull, the mean peak pressure has been shown to be about 14,000 mm Hg. [10].

4. The pig and ruminants have sigmoid flexures in the bodies of their penises. Most of the elongation during erection in these species occurs because the sigmoid flexure is straightened. The sigmoid flexure configuration is regained at detumescence by elastic connective tissue ligaments at the flexure [2].

5. In all species except the cat, the penis is directed cranioventrally from its point of attachment on the ischia. In the cat, the penis is directed caudoventrally and the urethral surface remains on the dorsal (caudodorsal) aspect.

6. Carnivores have an os penis located between the urethra and the dorsal surface of the penis. In dogs, the os penis is deeply grooved on its ventral aspect for passage of the urethra. In tomcats, the small os penis is not grooved.

7. The glans penis differs markedly among the domestic mammals (Fig. 15-7). In the cat, it is covered with cornified, epithelial, proximally-projecting spines which may explain why a queen often screams as the tom withdraws. The dog's glans penis is divided into a pars longa glandis distally and a bulbus glandis. The bulbus glandis engorges to a great extent at erection and is responsible, along with the vestibular bulbs of the bitch, for the physical "tie" between the sexes at coitus. In the pig, the glans penis is twisted into a "corkscrew" configuration. The ruminants also have a twisted glans and, in addition, they have a free extension of the urethra, termed the urethral process. The urethral process is especially well-developed in small ruminants. The glans penis of the horse has a constriction (collum glandis) just behind the corona glandis, an encircling ridge from which conical papillae project (Fig. 15-8/14). The horse also has a short urethral process which is surrounded by an indentation known as the fossa glandis. A dorsal diverticulum from the fossa glandis called the urethral sinus collects smegma and debris to form the "bean" (Fig. 15-8/12).

8. The prepuce of the horse is so well-developed that an additional portion called the preputial fold originates from the base of the internal lamina. The cranial edge of this fold is the preputial ring (Fig. 15-8/6) [2].

9. In the boar, there is an opening in the dorsal wall of the prepuce which leads to a blind preputial diverticulum. The diverticulum is partially divided into left and right parts by a septum (Fig. 21-9). Decomposing urine and epithelial debris in this pouch (100+ ml) are responsible for the boar's characteristic odor [2].

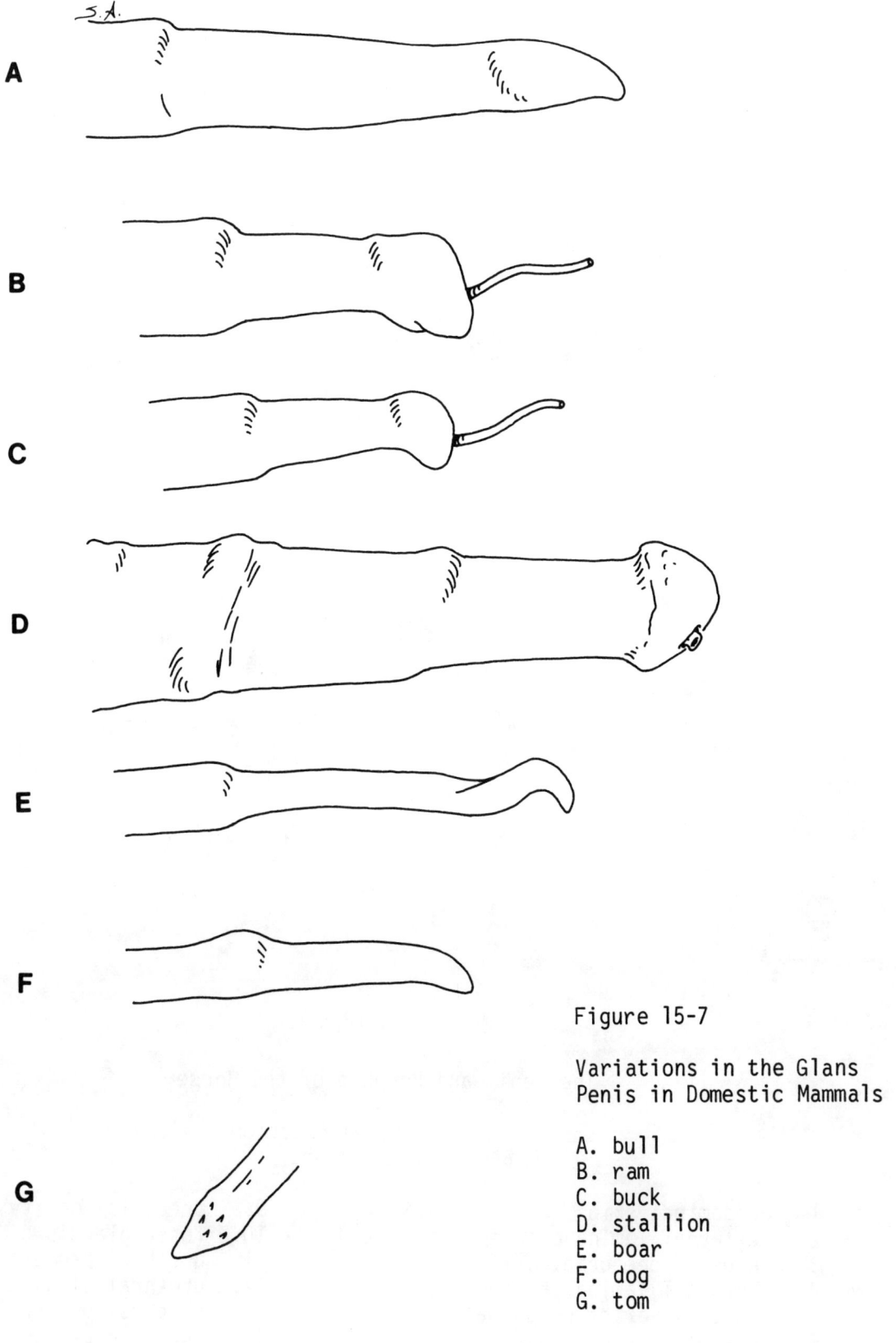

Figure 15-7

Variations in the Glans Penis in Domestic Mammals

A. bull
B. ram
C. buck
D. stallion
E. boar
F. dog
G. tom

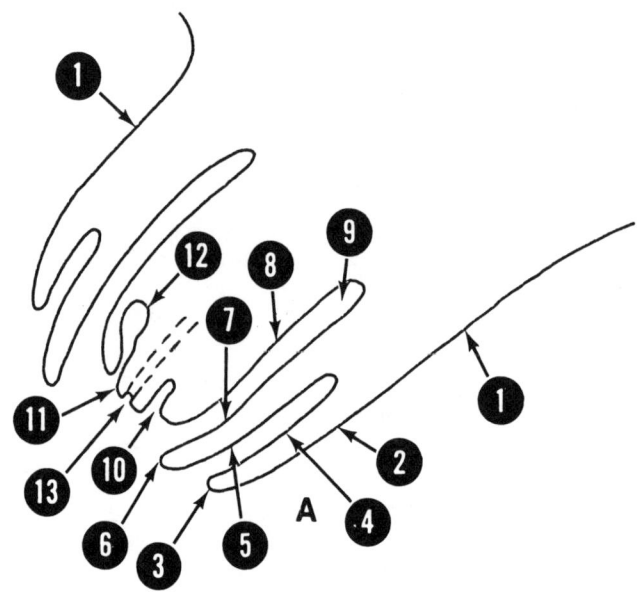

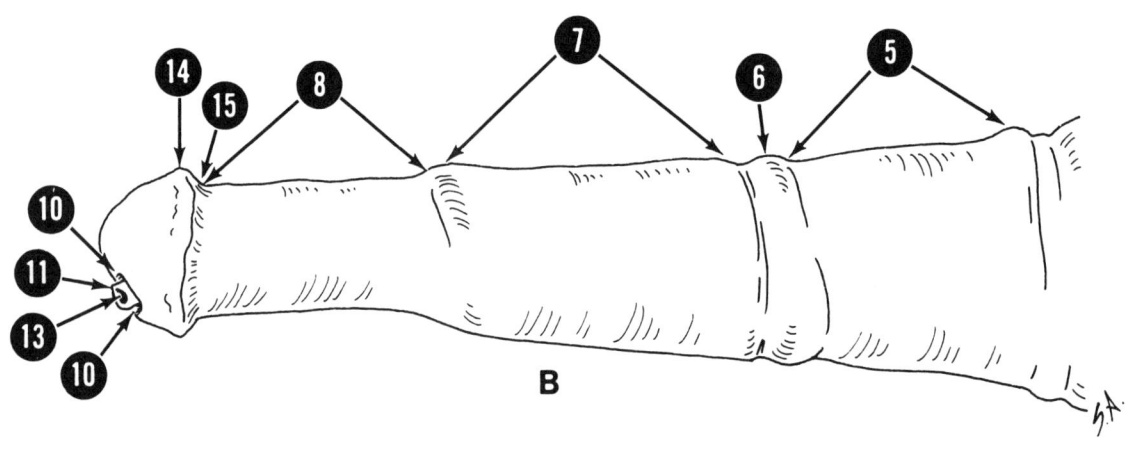

Figure 15-8

The Penis and Prepuce of the Horse

    A.   Retracted (sectional view)
    B.   Extended

1. abdominal skin
2. external lamina of prepuce
3. edge of preputial orifice
4. internal lamina of prepuce
5. outer layer of preputial fold
6. preputial ring
7. inner layer of preputial fold
8. skin on free part of penis
9. preputial cavity
10. fossa glandis
11. urethral process
12. urethral sinus
13. external urethral orifice
14. corona glandis
15. collum glandis

10. The horse lacks preputial muscles. The caudal ones are absent in the carnivores and are sometimes absent in the pig [2]. Absence or incomplete development of the caudal preputial muscles occurs in bulls of <u>Bos indicus</u> derivation.

11. The muscles directly associated with the penis include:

    a. bulbospongiosus m.--surrounds the bulb of the penis and the urethra at the root of the penis. It is continuous with the .rethralis muscle which surrounds the pelvic urethra. In the horse, it continues distally to the glans and covers the urethra ventrally and laterally. Contraction of this muscle causes increased pressure in the urethra which may expel the semen at ejaculation [4].

    b. ischiocavernosus m.--originates from the ischiatic arch and ischiatic tuberosity. This paired muscle envelops the crura and supports the erect penis. In the bull, a pumping action involving this muscle may explain the extremely high pressures attained in the cavernous spaces during erection [10].

    c. retractor penis m.--originates on the ventral aspect of the first few caudal vertebrae. The proximal part of this paired smooth muscle supports the rectum. The distal part is attached to the urethral surface of the penis. Several unimportant variations in this muscle occur among the domestic species.

12. The innervation of the male reproductive organs is derived from a number of sources. The scrotum and part of the prepuce are innervated by the iliohypogastric, ilioinguinal, and genitofemoral nerves. The genitofemoral nerve also innervates the vaginal tunic and cremaster muscle. The pudendal nerve supplies the penis and part of the prepuce, and the perineal (as well as branches of the caudal rectal) nerves supply the bulbospongiosus, ischiocavernosus, and retractor penis muscles.

13. The blood supply to the male reproductive tract is derived from several sources. The penis is supplied primarily by terminal branches of the internal pudendal aa. (dorsal aa. of the penis). In the horse, branches of the external pudendal aa. are also involved (cranial aa. of the penis) as well as branches of the obturator aa. (middle aa. of the penis). The testis, epididymis, and ductus deferens on each side are supplied by the ipsilateral testicular a. The accessory sex glands and pelvic urethra are supplied primarily by branches of the internal pudendal aa.

C. Clinical considerations

1. Urethral calculi affect several species and cause obstructions that may be fatal if not corrected. In cattle, they usually lodge at the distal part of the sigmoid flexure. In sheep, they may occur at the sigmoid flexure or at the urethral process [11]. In dogs, the usual locus is just proximal to the os penis [12]. The popular theory held for several years that early castration of male cats increased

the incidence of the disease is no longer considered to be valid [13]. Urethral calculi may be treated conservatively by backflushing and/or surgically by a number of urethrostomy procedures.

2. Semen collection for evaluation and/or artificial insemination is frequently performed. It may be done electrically in dogs, pigs, and ruminants. In dogs, ejaculation may be induced by manually grasping the penis behind the bulbus glandis. A manual technique is also effective in boars. Artificial vaginas are often used in horses and cattle [4].

3. Inability to protrude the penis from the prepuce (i.e., "extend the penis") can result from a number of causes. Sometimes it occurs because of phimosis, a stricture of the preputial orifice. It should be emphasized, however, that phimosis only implies a narrowed preputial orifice and it may or may not result in an inability to protrude the penis from the prepuce. In addition to a narrowed preputial orifice, inability to extend the penis can also be caused by adhesions, tumors, and hematomas. In dogs, boars, and bulls, the condition has been reported in association with an anomalous fibrous band, "persistent frenulum," which joins the prepuce to the glans [4]. Transection of the band relieves the problem. In bulls, adhesions sometimes occur between penis and prepuce which result in phimosis or deviation of the erect penis. Lack of penile protrusion may also occur because of a congenitally short penis or retractor penis muscles. Finally, the condition can be caused by prolapse of the prepuce, and circumcision may be necessary [4].

4. Inability to retract the penis into the prepuce (paralysis of the penis) can result from several causes. In bulls, uncomplicated cases may be treated by resecting and shortening the retractor penis muscles. In bulls and horses, a reefing operation may be performed by removing a sleeve of preputial skin several centimeters long. The cut edges are then anastomosed. If the cause was related to protrusion of the penis through a stenotic preputial orifice (paraphimosis), appropriate corrective surgery may be required. Several cases of penile paralysis have been reported in horses following use of some types of tranquilizers [4].

5. Catheterization of the urinary bladder through the male urethra is a relatively simple procedure. In the horse, several feet of catheter are needed. In the cat, a straight metal catheter may be used, but its use may be justifiably criticized, since trauma may cause fibrosing constrictions. In male ruminants and boars, the sigmoid flexure must be straightened. In bulls, a fold of mucosa projecting over the opening of the excretory duct of each bulbourethral gland prevents a catheter from entering the pelvic urethra.

6. Before collecting semen from stallions, the penis may be washed and a "bean", if present, may be removed. Some collection protocols do not involve washing the penis. Strong soaps should not be used because they may permit overgrowth of opportunistic microbes.

7. In boars used for artificial insemination, the preputial diverticulum may be surgically removed to improve semen quality. This prevents the contents (decomposing urine and epithelial debris) from mixing with the semen and lowering sperm motility. The diverticulum may also be removed to prevent "balling up" (a masturbation process, considered a vice, in which the boar ejaculates into the diverticulum). For removal, an incision is made on the lateral side of the prepuce about 5 cm caudal to the preputial orifice and then the diverticulum is dissected free [14].

8. Preputial lacerations and prolapses are relatively common in bulls and usually result from trauma. Prolapses are especially common in bulls of Bos indicus derivation. The condition in these animals may be aggravated by absence or incomplete development of the caudal preputial muscles [15].

9. Bulls occasionally (and stallions rarely) suffer hematomas of the penis from trauma during service ("broken penis"). Conceptually, these consist of a "blow-out" of the corpus cavernosum through the tunica albuginea. These are surgically treated 7-10 days after the injury and the tunica albuginea is carefully reapposed following removal of the clotted hematoma. Sometimes repair is complicated by development of a shunt between the corpus cavernosum and dorsal veins of the penis [15]. This can be radiographically assessed by corpus cavernography.

10. A number of surgical techniques involving the penis have been used to produce "teaser" (marker) bulls. These include penectomy, penotomy, penopexy, and translocation of the penis including the sheath. Other surgical procedures for teaser bulls include transection or resection of the epididymis or ductus deferens, and preputial manipulations including iatrogenic phimosis and preputial deviation procedures [15]. Techniques involving the epididymis or ductus deferens are less likely to lower libido than procedures involving the penis and prepuce. However, if the penis can be protruded normally, venereal disease can be easily spread.

11. The pudendal nerves of the ox can be blocked on the medial aspect of the broad sacrotuberous ligament. The left and right nerves are first located by rectal palpation. Each nerve courses ventrocaudally from its lumbosacral origin and passes through the ipsilateral lesser sciatic foramen, the cranial border of which is palpable. Just before the nerve passes through the foramen, it is positioned just dorsal to the palpable internal iliac artery. A five inch needle is passed medial to the sacrosciatic ligament and anesthetic is deposited around the nerve. Continued injection as the needle is withdrawn will block the caudal rectal nerves. This procedure will block the perineal and anal regions as well as the penis in bulls (causing protrusion of the penis).

12. Perineal anesthesia in the horse can be affected by blocking the perineal nerves with an injection on each side 2 cm dorsal to the ischiatic arch and 2 cm lateral to the anus. Anesthetic should be deposited both subcutaneously and 0.5 cm deeper to insure that both

of the larger perineal nerve branches are blocked. The pudendal nerve branches to the penis (dorsal nerves of the penis) can be blocked from one of the perineal nerve injection sites by advancing the needle until it strikes the ischial arch on the midline.

References

1. International Committee on Veterinary Gross Anatomical Nomenclature. 1983. Nomina Anatomica Veterinaria, third ed. Published by the Committee, Ithaca, New York.

2. Nickel, R., A. Schummer, E. Seiferle, and W. Sack. 1973. The Viscera of the Domestic Mammals. Paul Parey, Berlin.

3. Getty, R. 1975. Sisson and Grossman's The Anatomy of the Domestic Animals, fifth ed. W. B. Saunders, Philadelphia.

4. Roberts, S. J. 1971. Veterinary Obstetrics and Genital Diseases (Theriogenology), second ed. Published by the author, Ithaca, New York.

5. Catcott, E.J. ed. 1975. Feline Medicine and Surgery. American Veterinary Publications, Santa Barbara, California.

6. Mansmann, R. A., E. S. McAllister, and P. W. Pratt, eds. 1982. Equine Medicine and Surgery. American Veterinary Publications, Santa Barbara, California.

7. Archibald, J. ed. 1974. Canine Surgery, second ed. American Veterinary Publications, Santa Barbara, California.

8. Frank. E. R. 1964. Veterinary Surgery, seventh ed. Burgess Publishing Co., Minneapolis, Minnesota.

9. Beckett, S. D., D. F. Walker, R. S. Hudson, T. M. Reynolds, and R. I. Vachon. 1974. Corpus cavernosum penis pressure and penile muscle activity in the bull during coitus. J. Vet. Res. 35(6):761-764.

10. Watson, J. W. 1964. Mechanism of erection and ejaculation in the bull and ram. Nature 204 (4953):95-96.

11. Blood, D. C., J. A. Henderson, and O. M. Radostits. 1979. Veterinary Medicine fifth ed. Lea and Febiger, Philadelphia.

12. Osborn, C. A., D. G. Low, and D. R. Finco. 1972. Canine and Feline Urology. W. B. Saunders, Philadelphia.

13. Herron, M. A. 1972. The effects of prepubertal castration on the penile urethra of the cat. JAVMA 160(2):208-211.

14. Aamdal, J., I. Hogset, and O. Filseth. 1958. Extirpation of the preputial diverticulum of boars used in artificial insemination. JAVMA 132(12):522-524.

15. Amstutz, H. E., ed. 1980. Bovine Medicine and Surgery, second ed. American Veterinary Publications, Santa Barbara, California.

16. Habel, R. E. 1981. Applied Veterinary Anatomy, second ed. Published by the author, Ithaca, New York.

FEMALE REPRODUCTIVE SYSTEM

The female reproductive system includes the ovaries, uterine tubes, uterus, vagina, vestibule, vulva, and clitoris. These develop from the same primordia as the organs of the male reproductive tract (Table 16-1).

I. OVARIES

The ovaries, which are homologous to the testes of the male, produce ova and the female sex hormones, estrogen and progesterone.

A. Major features [1]

hilus--the indentation where the vessels and nerves enter the ovary
tunica albuginea--the dense connective tissue capsule around the ovary
corpus luteum--the post ovulation body formed by follicular cells
corpus albicans--the fibrous remnant of a corpus luteum
proper ligament--the dense connective tissue between the ovary and uterine horn (Fig. 16-1), a remnant of the female gubernaculum (cranial part)
mesovarian border--the edge where the mesovarium attaches
free border--the area opposite the mesovarian border

B. Comparative features

1. The ovaries of the carnivores and cow are elongated ovoids. Those of the small ruminants are flattened spheroids. In the sow, the ovary has a tuberculate appearance because of the numerous large follicles. The ovary in mares is bean-shaped with a particularly well-developed hilus [2].

2. The ovary of the mare has a distinct ovulation fossa at the hilus where most follicles mature.

3. In the pig and ruminants, the ovaries are located near the cranial pelvic opening ("pelvic inlet"), but in the other domestic mammals they are near the caudal poles of the kidneys in the sublumbar area.

C. Clinical considerations

1. Removal of the ovaries alone (ovariectomy, oophorectomy) is rarely done in domestic animals. In mares and cows, oophorectomies may be done through either an abdominal incision or a vaginal incision (colpotomy) [3]. In carnivores, oophorectomies are contraindicated without simultaneous removal of the uterus (ovariohysterectomy) because of a high incidence of postoperative pyometra [4].

2. Rectal palpation of the ovaries in the mare and cow is an important clinical procedure in evaluation of the reproductive tract. Maturing follicles may be larger than the main part of the

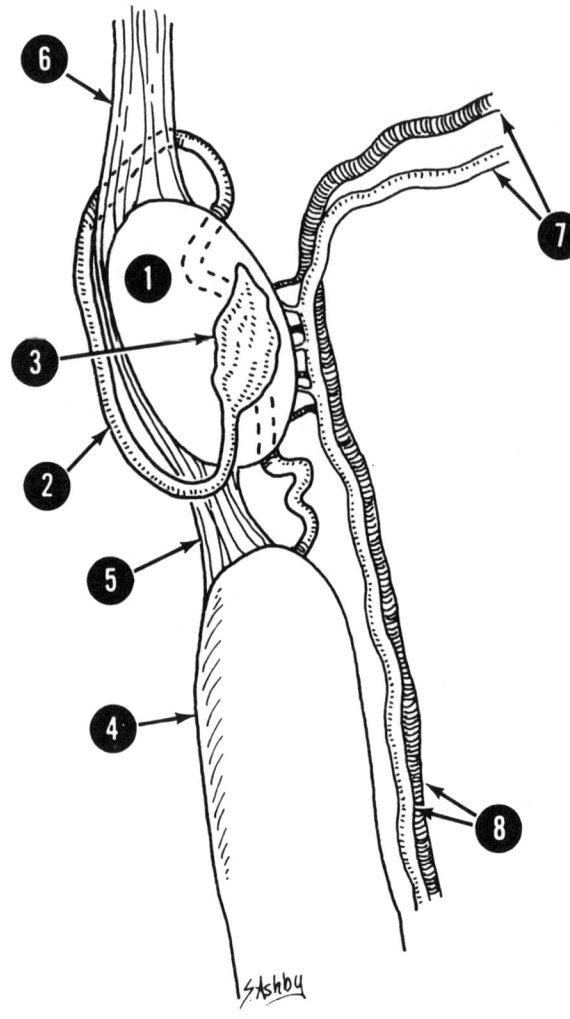

Figure 16-1

Schematic View of an Ovary, Uterine Tube, and Uterine Horn

1. ovary
2. uterine tube
3. infundibulum
4. uterine horn
5. proper ligament of the ovary
6. suspensory ligament
7. ovarian a. and v.
8. uterine a. and v.

Table 16-1

Homologies of the Reproductive Organs in Male and Female Mammals

Male	Female
Testis	Ovary
Mesorchium	Mesovarium
Mesepididymis	Mesosalpinx
Testicular bursa	Ovarian bursa
Proper lig. of testis	Proper lig. of ovary
Lig. of tail of epididymis	Round lig. of uterus
Prostatic urethra	Urethra
Penis	Clitoris
Corpus spongiosum penis	Vestibular bulbs
Corpus cavernosum penis	Corpus cavernosum of clitoris
Scrotum	Labia
Scrotal raphe	Dorsal commissure of labia
Prepuce	Prepuce of clitoris

ovary itself. In cows, the blister-like developing follicles can be palpated (with experience) and distinguished from the easily identified, firmer corpora lutea which are elevated with depressed centers. In mares, ovarian follicles can be palpated, but it is virtually impossible to distinguish corpora lutea--partly because they are located in the ovulation fossa and partly because the thick tunica albuginea keeps them from projecting above the ovarian surface [5].

3. The ovarian arteries are usually direct branches of the aorta and they course to the ovary in the mesovarium. After supplying branches to the ovary, they continue along the left and right uterine horns and anastomose with the uterine arteries. The ovarian arteries (and veins) and the uterine arteries (and veins) are the major hemostatic concerns during ovariohysterectomies (see Broad Ligament, Part VIII).

4. The ovaries are subject to a number of diseases and abnormalities. They may be hypoplastic, cystic, neoplastic, or congenitally absent. One may also descend through the inguinal canal.

5. The relationship of the ovary to the ovarian bursa is shown in Figure 16-2. Although most ovulated eggs are "captured" by the infundibulum, some occasionally manage to "sneak out" through the opening of the ovarian bursa and become lost in the peritoneal cavity [6]. If fertilized, these may (rarely) establish an abdominal pregnancy.

II. UTERINE TUBE ("OVIDUCT")

The uterine tubes are located between the two fused layers of peritoneum comprising the mesosalpinx which form the lateral wall of the ovarian bursa (Fig. 16-2). They "capture" and transport ovulated eggs to the uterus and serve as the normal locus for fertilization.

A. Major features [1]

infundibulum--the funnel-shaped, expanded, ovarian end of the uterine tube
abdominal ostium--the opening of the uterine tube in the ovarian bursa
fimbria--the irregular processes of the infundibulum
ampulla--the wide initial segment of the uterine tube
isthmus--the narrow distal segment of the uterine tube
uterine ostium--the opening into the uterine horn

B. Comparative and clinical considerations

1. Inflammatory processes and blockages of the uterine tubes occur in domestic mammals, but they are rarely diagnosed or treated.

2. The simultaneous transport of ova distally and sperm proximally is a remarkable feat. The small size of the sperm is a more important factor in this movement than the motility of the spermatozoa, which is haphazard at best.

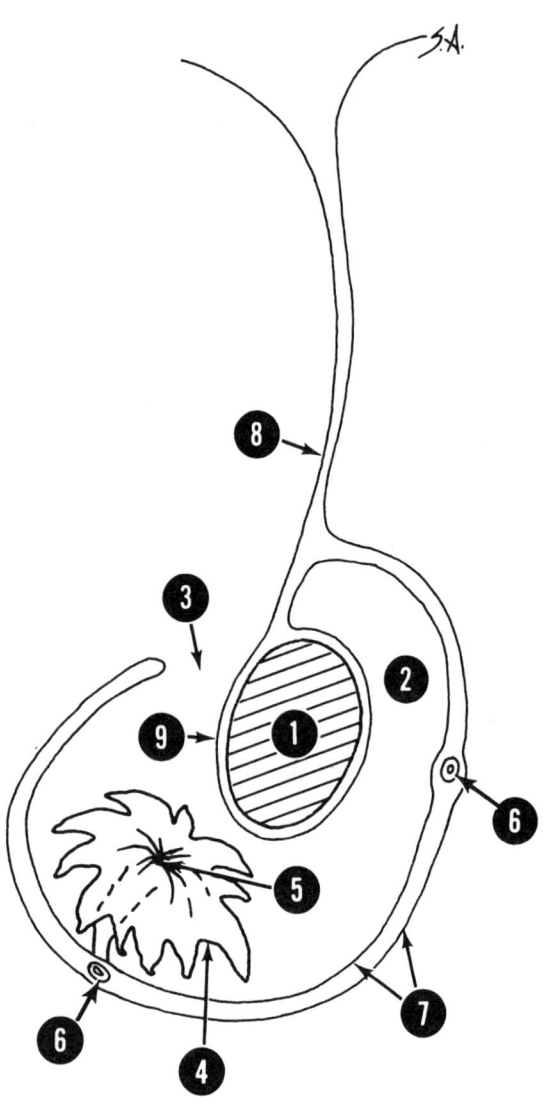

Figure 16-2A

Schematic Section through an Ovary and Ovarian Bursa

1. ovary
2. ovarian bursa
3. opening of ovarian bursa
4. infundibulum
5. abdominal ostium of uterine tube
6. transverse section of uterine tube
7. double layer of peritoneum (mesosalpinx) forming the wall of the ovarian bursa
8. mesovarium
9. visceral peritoneum on surface of ovary

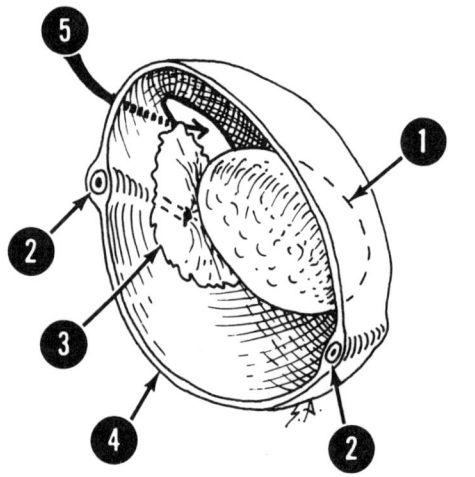

Figure 16-2B

Semi-schematic Section through an Ovary and Ovarian Bursa

1. ovary
2. uterine tube
3. infundibulum
4. mesosalpinx
5. opening of ovarian bursa

3. Tubal ligation can be used to sterilize an animal, but it does not eliminate estrus (which may be a major concern).

4. The paroophoron and epoophoron are vestigial remnants of the mesonephros and mesonephric (Wolffian) duct which may be identifiable in the mesosalpinx as blind, flexuous tubules. They are most evident in young adults and tend to disappear with age. Terminal hydatids (hydatids of Morgagni) are remnants of the epoophoron, which consist of pedunculated cysts of the fimbria [5,7].

III. UTERUS

The uterus receives the fertilized ovum, nourishes and houses the developing embryo, and expels the mature fetus through the birth canal.

A. Major features [1]

    uterine horns--the two cranial extensions from the uterine body
        mesometrial border
        free border
    body of uterus--the single part of the uterus caudal to the horns
    left and right borders
    cervix-the constricted caudal part of the uterus
    cervical canal--the lumen within the cervix
        longitudinal folds
        cervical glands
    internal uterine ostium--the uterine opening of the cervical canal
    external uterine ostium--the vaginal opening of the cervical canal
    round lig. of the uterus--a fibrous remnant of the female gubernaculum (caudal part) in a fold of the broad lig. (Fig. 16-3).

B. Comparative features

1. The uterine mucosa of the ruminants has focal elevations called caruncles which form the maternal component of the placentomes. The fetal component of each placentome in ruminants is called a cotyledon. Assessment of the size of the placentomes is one criterion for aging a pregnancy.

2. In the carnivores and artiodactyles, the medial walls of the uterine horns fuse near the uterine body to form an internal partition termed the uterine velum (Fig. 16-4/5) [2].

3. The cranial end of the body of the uterus of the mare is termed the uterine fundus [1].

4. There is considerable species variation in the morphology of the cervical canal. In carnivores, it is very short. In mares, it has a number of well-developed, longitudinal folds. In sows, the cervical canal is very long and the longitudinal folds have

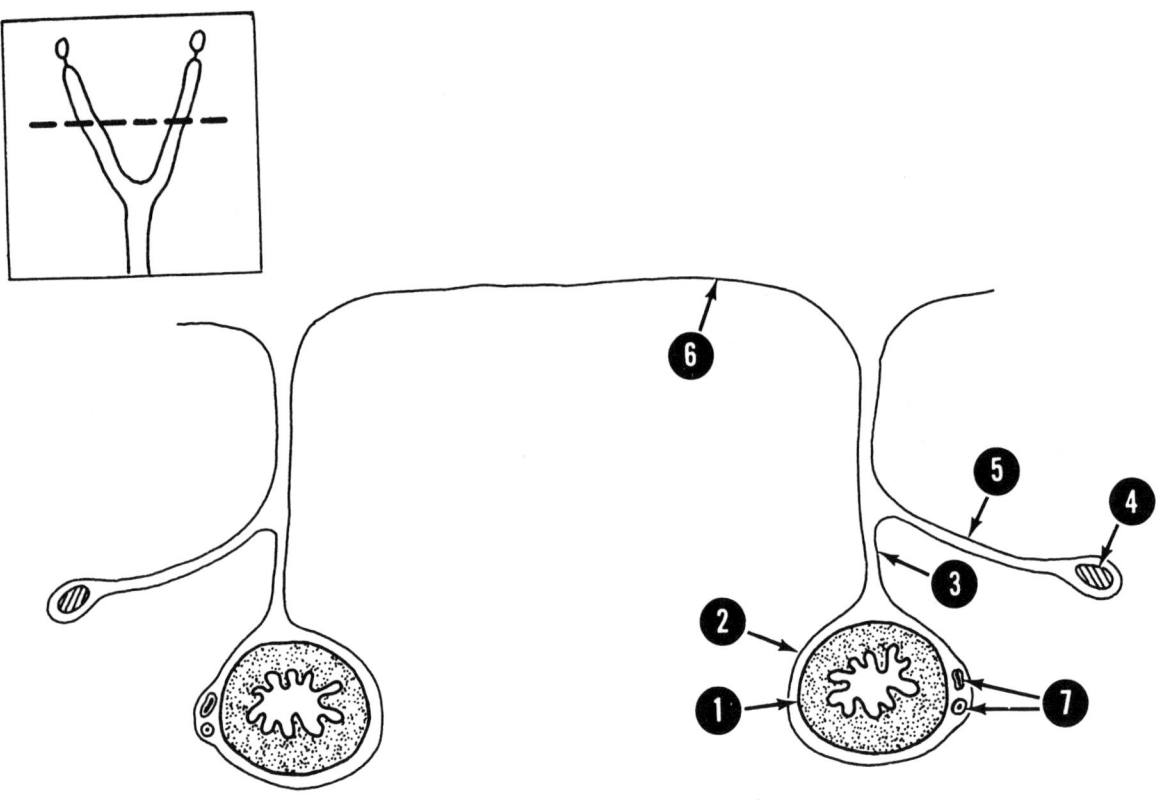

Figure 16-3

Schematic Transverse Section through the Uterine Horns
(cranial to the uterine body)

1. uterine horn
2. visceral peritoneum
3. mesometrium
4. round ligament of uterus
5. fold of mesometrium which surrounds round lig. of uterus
6. parietal peritoneum
7. uterine a. and v.

rounded prominences on them (cervical pulvini). In ruminants, the cervical mucosa has circular (transverse) folds as well as longitudinal ones [2].

5. In the bitch, the round ligament of the uterus (surrounded by peritoneum) extends through the inguinal canal and ends blindly, surrounded by the peritoneal vaginal process.

6. Folds of peritoneum termed dorsal and ventral intercornual ligaments connect the caudal aspects of the uterine horns of ruminants.

7. The uterine horns of sows are very long and tortuous, while those of mares are short and poorly developed.

C. Clinical considerations

1. Removal of the ovaries, oviducts, and uterus to render the animal sterile is one of the most common elective surgical procedures in carnivores. The mechanics of the procedure are discussed under Broad Ligament (Part VIII) since all of the portions of the female reproductive system involved are suspended within it. Pregnancy or estrus may complicate the otherwise simple surgery because of the markedly increased blood supply [4].

2. Cesarean section (usually indicated by dystocia) is frequently performed in most domestic species but rarely in mares. Local analgesia is often induced to avoid the depressant effects of general anesthesia on the fetuses. In dogs, a midline abdominal incision is usually used, in pigs a midline or flank incision, and in cattle a midline, paramedian, or flank incision (either side) is used. In all species, the uterus is incised in a relatively avascular area and is closed with an inverting suture pattern. In mares, the severed edges of the uterus should be oversewn to reduce hemorrhage.

3. Uterine torsion occasionally occurs in the cow and mare. It may be diagnosed per rectum as increased tension as well as malposition of the left and right mesometria (one side goes under the uterus and one side over it, depending on the direction of the torsion) [5]. Uterine torsion may also be diagnosed via vaginal examination.

4. Uterine prolapse may occur in several species. It may often be corrected manually and held in place with various specialized suture patterns. Amputation may be done when replacement is impossible or contraindicated because of a severely damaged uterus [5].

5. The placenta is composed of two parts. The fetus contributes the chorioallantois and the dam contributes her endometrium. Grossly, four types exist based on the shape of the area of contact between the chorioallantois and the uterus.

    a. Diffuse (horse and pig)--the entire surface of the

chorioallantois is covered with villi and microvilli that evaginate into the endometrium.

    b. Zonary (carnivores)--contact between the uterus and chorioallantois is limited to a band, 2-8 cm wide around the circumference of the fetal membranes.

    c. Cotyledonary (ruminants)--focal contacts occur (75-120 in cow and 80-90 in ewe).

    d. Discoid (primates and rodents)--a single focal contact occurs.

In the generalized placenta, there are 6 layers which separate maternal and fetal blood. The maternal endometrium has three layers (endothelium, connective tissue, and lining epithelium) and the chorioallantois has 3 layers (surface epithelium, connective tissue, and endothelium). All 6 of these layers are present in the mare, sow, and ruminants. The term epitheliochorial is applied to these placentae (maternal epithelium is in contact with the chorioallantois). In the placentae of carnivores, the uterine epithelium and connective tissue are not present and so these are termed endotheliochorial (endothelium of uterus is in contact with chorioallantois). In humans and rodents, all 3 uterine layers are absent (hemochorial placentation). Although some classification schemes have included other categories (endothelioendothelia and hemoendothelia), electron microscopic studies have denied their existence [5].

Placentae are classified as deciduate if part of the maternal tissues are shed at parturition (man, rodents, carnivores). In adeciduate (indeciduate) placentae (ungulates), the maternal layers are left intact (except for parts of the caruncles of ruminants) [5].

6. The most widely accepted technique of pregnancy diagnosis in cattle is rectal palpation. The first anatomic change is increase in size of the gravid horn due to accumulation of fluid. This may be detectable as early as 4 weeks. The non-gravid horn also fills, but not until 40-45 days. If the horns are symmetrical and fluid filled, twins should be suspected. (Unicornual twins are rare and difficult to diagnose.) If the uterus is fluid-filled, one of the following four positive signs of pregnancy should be sought. If the uterus is not in the pelvic cavity, it should be retracted for this examination and the horns should be straightened and examined throughout their length. The intercornual ligaments serve as a convenient locus to place a hooked finger for this retraction [8]. The ventral ligament is better developed than the dorsal one.

    a. Palpation of the chorioallantoic (CA) membrane. This is called the "fetal membrane slip". The CA feels like a cord within the uterine lumen and is first palpable at 30-35 days. (The "times" associated herein with various aspects of pregnancy diagnosis may vary by several days according to the experience of the palpator.)

    b. Palpation of the amnionic vesicle (AV). It is located at the greatest diameter of the gravid horn. It is first palpable at 30-35 days.

    c. Palpation of the placentomes. These can first be detected at about 70 days and enlarge as the pregnancy progresses.

    d. Palpation of the fetus (first palpable at 65-70 days).

7. Pregnancy diagnosis in the mare can be based on several anatomic changes [5]:

    a. Thickness of the uterine wall--increases in both pregnant and nonpregnant mares to day 16. From day 16 to day 21 it increases 3 times in thickeness in pregnant mares, and in nonpregnant mares it becomes thinner again. Uterine tone follows a similar pattern.

    b. Palpation of the amnionic vesicle--may be detected between 20 and 30 days as a ventral bulging of the uterus near the divergence of the horns. Dorsal bulging may occur at 40 days but is not marked. (Caution should be used during palpation because rupture of the amnionic vesicle or fetal heart sac will induce abortion.)

    c. Enlargement of the uterine horn containing the fetus-- increase from about 5 cm in diameter to 15 cm between 30 and 90 days.

    d. Palpation of the fetus--can usually be done between 90 and 120 days. The "membrane slip" technique, of value in early pregnancy detection in the cow, is contraindicated in mares because abortion may be induced [9]. (The diffuse placentation doesn't lend itself to a "slip"). The Ascheim-Zondek (A.Z. or "rat") test may be used to determine serum levels of gonadotropin hormones. Other serum tests are also used such as the mare immuno-pregnancy test (MIP). The MIP remains positive for some time after abortion or fetal death [9]. A urine estrogen test may also be used between 120 and 150 days.

8. Ultrasound devices are now being used with increasing frequency for pregnancy detection (especially in mares and sows).

9. Several lesions on rectal palpation of the bovine uterus and ovary may resemble a gravid uterus. These include pyometra, hydrometra, fetal maceration or mummification, ovarian tumors, uterine lymphoma, and adhesive perimetritis. Errors can also be made by mistaking the urinary bladder for the uterus; the ovaries for placentomes; or the rumen, a kidney, a perivaginal abscess, or a hematoma for the fetus [8].

10. Retained fetal membranes (RFM) is a major reproductive problem in cattle which affects dairy animals more significantly than beef breeds [5]. Although RFM may be removed manually, this procedure is usually contraindicated because it may induce endotoxic shock. It may be advisable to wait for natural expulsion. If conservative treatment is used (instillation of antibacterial agents), RFM are usually naturally expelled within two weeks.

IV. VAGINA

The vagina is the female copulatory organ which also serves as an important part of the birth canal.

A. General features [1]

fornix--the annular recess which encircles the protrusion of the cervix into the vagina
hymen--the transverse fold, identifiable in the young, which separates the vagina from the vestibule
ostium--the opening of the vagina into the vestibule

B. Comparative and clinical considerations

1. A common rectovaginal opening may be produced because of lacerations which occur during parturition, especially in mares. These may also involve the vestibule and vulva. If left unrepaired, vaginitis and metritis often occur.

2. Vaginal smears are sometimes used in carnivores to evaluate the stage of the estrous cycle.

3. Perivaginal hematomas in cows may be single or multiple and typically result from dystocia in first calf heifers. They have no clinical significance and recede within a few weeks, but they should not be mistaken for lymph nodes or neoplasms.

4. Perivaginal abscesses may result from perforation of the vaginal wall at parturition. If troublesome, these may be surgically drained.

5. Imperforate hymen is a congenital anomaly occasionally observed in heifers. It may cause accumulation of postestral blood and mucus and result in straining and a fetid discharge. In some heifers, a band of tissue may be present in the vagina near the cervix which may cause dystocia unless it is transected.

6. Pneumovagina in cows and mares ("windsuckers") may result from a conformational defect in the perineum. Animals with especially high placed ischiatic tuberosities may have deeply placed vulvae in which the lips do not close properly. Uncomplicated cases may have no clinical significance, but if feces enter the vagina, vaginitis and/or metritis may result. Corrective surgeries for this condition have been described [5].

V. VESTIBULE

The vestibule is the caudal part of the tubular portion of the female reproductive tract and is common to both the urinary and reproductive systems.

A. General features

external urethral ostium--the opening of the urethra commonly used to separate the vestibule from the vagina
minor vestibular glands--glands in the vestibular wall that
major vestibular glands--produce a lubricating mucus

B. Comparative and clinical considerations

1. The urethra in the bitch opens on a papilla termed the urethral tubercle. This should be distinguished from the clitoris.

2. The sow and cow have a suburethral diverticulum which is a blind pouch in the floor of the vestibule adjacent to the external urethral orifice. It may "catch" the catheter during catheterization.

3. The wall of the vestibule contains erectile venous plexuses which are organized into vestibular bulbs (left and right) in the mare and bitch. Erection of the vestibular bulbs of the bitch are responsible for the "tie" during copulation in dogs. They force the vestibular wall tight against the penis just behind the enlarged bulbus glandis.

4. Remnants of the mesonephric ducts ("canals of Gartner") may be present in the vestibular wall on each side of the urethral orifice and, especially in the cow, may open at two small orifices (Fig. 16-4) [2].

5. Major vestibular glands ("glands of Bartholin") are found only in the cow, queen, and sometimes in the ewe. They are compact masses (one on each side) which open on the floor of the vestibule, caudal and lateral to the urethral orifice through two ducts (left and right) [2]. Occasionally, these become cystic and in cows they may be incised and drained.

6. Minor vestibular glands are present in the bitch, sow, ewe, and mare. They open through numerous individual ducts along the ventral or lateral aspect of the vestibule. Mucoid secretions from both major and minor vestibular glands lubricate the reproductive organs at copulation and parturition. These secretions may contain pheromones [2].

VI. VULVA (FEMALE PUDENDA)

The vulva is the external part of the female reproductive system.

Figure 16-4

Reproductive Organs of a Cow
(dorsal aspect with uterus, vagina,
vestibule, and vulva opened)

1. ovary
2. proper lig. of ovary
3. uterine tube
4. uterine horn (right)
5. uterine velum
6. uterine body
7. caruncles
8. cervix
9. cervical canal
10. vagina
11. external urethral ostium
12. openings of mesonephric ducts
13. openings of major vestibular glands
14. labium (right)
15. depression for clitoris
16. ventral commissure of labia
17. vestibule

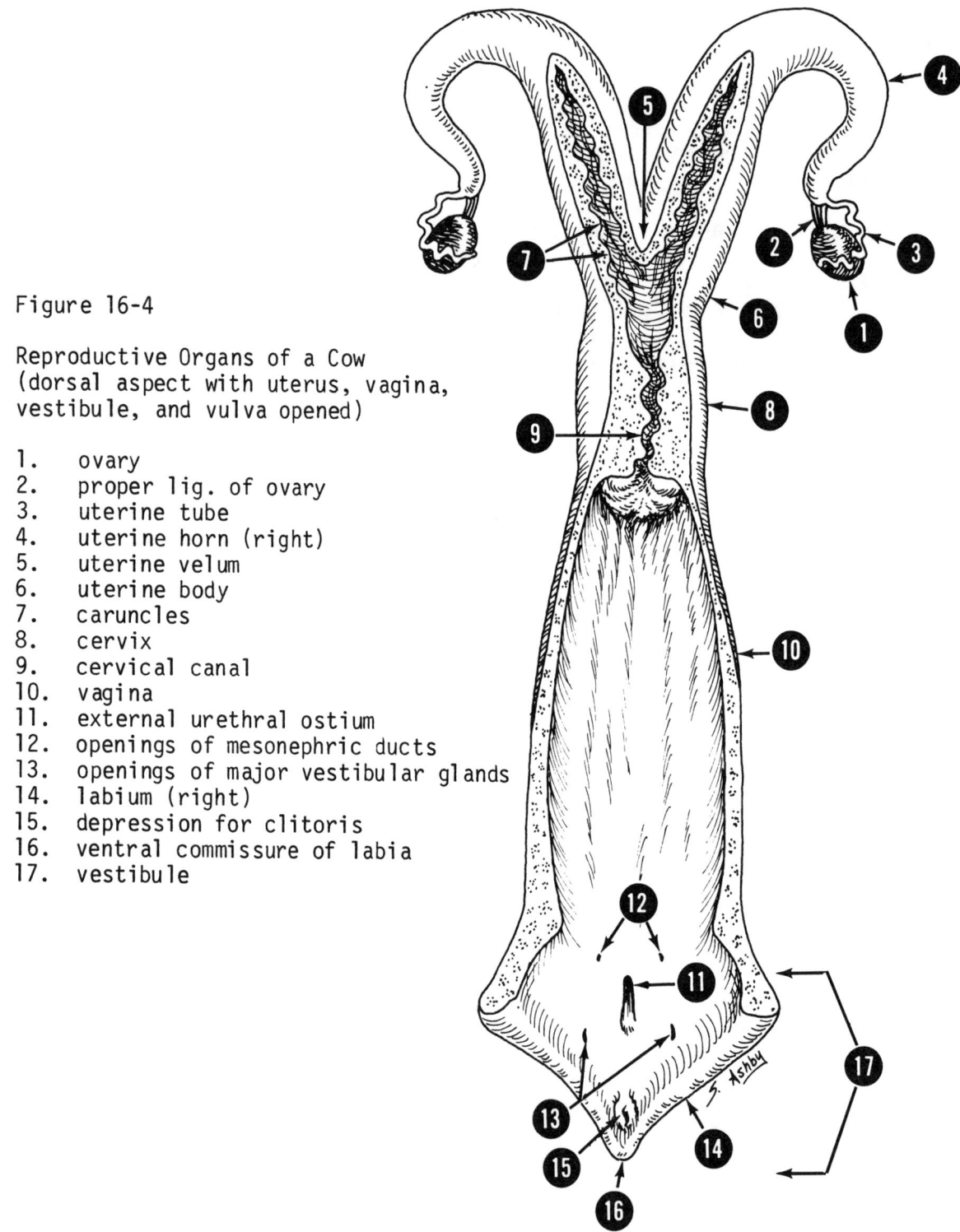

A. General features

   labium pudendi (vulvae)--the right and left lips

   ventral commissure--the pointed ventral junction of the labia
   dorsal commissure--the rounded dorsal junction of the labia
   rima pudendi--the vulvar cleft

VII. CLITORIS

The clitoris is the female counterpart of the penis and is located within the ventral commissure of the vulva.

A. General features [1]

   left and right crura--the two roots which attach to the ischiatic arch
   body--the shaft formed by the junction of the crura
   glans--the only exposed part of the clitoris
   clitoral prepuce--the connective tissue surrounding the glans
       clitoral fossa--the depression from which the glans protrudes
   corpus cavernosum of the clitoris--the erectile tissue within the clitoris

B. Comparative features

   1. In the bitch, the glans is well developed, but in the queen it is comparatively small.

   2. In the cow, the glans is located in a shallow depression rather than in a true fossa.

   3. In the mare, the clitoris can usually be seen in the ventral aspect of the vulvar cleft. The clitoral fossa in mares serves as a residing locus for the contagious equine metritis (CEM) organism. Surgical obliteration of this fossa may lower the incidence of the disease.

   4. An os clitoridis, homologous to the os penis, is present in some bitches and may be observed radiographically.

VIII. BROAD LIGAMENT

The broad ligament is the peritoneum which supports the female reproductive system, and its three major parts have already been considered (see Chapter 11, Abdomen). The mesometrium, which suspends the uterus, also reflects around the round ligament of the uterus (Fig. 16-3). The mesosalpinx primarily forms the lateral wall of the ovarian bursa and the uterine tube is suspended between its two layers of peritoneum. The ovarian bursa enclosed by the mesosalpinx is more extensive in some species than in others and it has two openings: the opening of the ovarian bursa (into the main part of the peritoneal cavity) and the abdominal ostium of the uterine tube (in the middle of the infundibulum). The mesovarium continues cranially after suspending the ovary, and the fold of it which attaches to the caudal rib near the diaphragm is the suspensory ligament of the ovary. The suspensory ligament is well developed in carnivores, but more difficult to delineate in ungulates.

The ovariohysterectomy ("spay") is one of the most common elective surgical procedures performed in carnivores. The ovaries, uterine tubes, and uterus are removed through a midline or paramedian incision. To get better exposure of the ovarian vessels for ligation, the suspensory ligaments are cut or torn, allowing the ovaries to be pulled caudally. Although inexperienced surgeons are often fearful of disrupting the ovarian vessels by this manipulation, close examination of the area will show that the vessels are enveloped by the mesovarium medial to the ovaries, whereas the suspensory ligaments are formed by the mesovarium cranial to the ovaries.* Surgeons occasionally report small bleeder vessels within the suspensory ligament, but these can usually be ignored. Ligatures are usually placed on the ovarian vessels, and then the broad ligament and round ligament are broken down by blunt disruption (tearing). Finally, the uterine (or cervical or vaginal) stump is clamped, ligated, and severed, including the left and right uterine vessels that parallel it. These vessels are derived from the internal iliac vasculature and course parallel to each other on each side of the uterus. They anastomose cranially with branches of the ovarian vasculature. In small dogs and cats, the uterine vessels may be ligated with the vaginal stump in a single ligature. In larger animals, surgeons may ligate the left and right vessels separately, and then place a third transfixing ligature around the whole stump.

References

1. International Committee on Veterinary Gross Anatomical Nomenclature. 1983. Nomina Anatomica Veterinaria, third ed. Published by the Committee, Ithaca, New York.

2. Nickel, R., A. Schummer, E. Seiferle, and W. Sack. 1973. The Viscera of the Domestic Mammals. Paul Parey, Berlin.

3. Frank, E. R. 1964. Veterinary Surgery, seventh ed. Burgess Publishing Co., Minneapolis, Minnesota.

4. Archibald, J., ed. 1974. Canine Surgery, second ed. American Veterinary Publications, Santa Barbara, California.

5. Roberts, S. J. 1971. Veterinary Obstetrics and Genital Diseases. Published by the author, Ithaca, New York.

---

*The often noted fact that the left ovarian vein of carnivores typically empties into the left renal vein rather than directly into the caudal vena cava is academic and has no practical significance.

6. Shively, M. J. 1979. Twenty-four anatomic fibs, half-truths, and misleading statements. J. Vet. Med. Ed. 6(3):182-187.

7. Sisson, S., and J. Grossman. 1953. The Anatomy of the Domestic Animals, fourth ed. W. B. Saunders, Philadelphia.

8. Callahan, C. J. 1980. In Bovine Medicine and Surgery, second ed. edited by H. E. Amstutz. American Veterinary Publications, Santa Barbara, California.

9. Ramge, J. C. 1982. Personal communication.

17

ODONTOLOGY

I. GENERAL FEATURES

The teeth of domestic animals are arranged in two dental arches (superior and inferior) and are the principal organs of mastication. They also aid in prehension and, in some species, they serve as formidable weapons. A typical domestic animal tooth consists grossly of a visible crown, one or more embedded roots, and a slightly constricted neck. Individual protrusions from the crown are termed cusps. Teeth with a distinct neck between the crown and root(s) are termed brachyodontic or low-crowned teeth. In contrast, the canine teeth of pigs, the "cheek teeth"* of ruminants, and all teeth of horses have no distinct neck and are termed hypsodontic or high-crowned teeth. Most hypsodontic teeth continue to erupt throughout life.**

Mammalian teeth are composed of three substances: dentine, enamel, and cement. Dentine constitutes the bulk of a tooth and surrounds the dental cavity. The dental cavity contains the dental pulp, which is a mass of connective tissue, vessels, and nerves. In hypsodontic teeth, enamel surrounds the dentine, and cement, a substance similar to bone, surrounds the enamel. In brachyodontic teeth, the enamel coating is limited to the crown and cement covers the root(s) only.

The roots of the teeth are embedded into bony sockets termed alveoli. Each alveolus is lined by a thin shell of dense bone termed the lamina dura. The radiodense lamina dura is separated from the tooth root by a thin, radiolucent periodontal membrane. A generalized loss of distinct laminae durae is an early radiographic indication of a demineralization syndrome (hyperparathyroidism). If the process is localized, it may have resulted from periodontal disease.

The teeth of mammals are divided into four types according to location and function. The incisors are embedded in the incisive bones and in the incisive part of the mandible. These are followed caudally by the canines, premolars, and molars which are embedded in the maxillae and the mandible. As already noted, the premolars and molars are often grouped under the heading cheek teeth. The superior teeth collectively form the superior dental arch and the inferior teeth form the inferior dental arch.*** Each arch contains spaces or gaps (diastemata, singular = diastema) between the contact surfaces

---

*"Cheek teeth" is an unofficial but useful term referring collectively to the premolars and molars. It has no official counterpart.
**The canine teeth of horses lack a neck, but are not considered to erupt throughout life.
***Superior and inferior are the correct directional terms to use in reference to teeth (versus dorsal and ventral) [1]. Upper and lower are more popular.

of the teeth (especially between the incisors and the cheek teeth). The superior arch is innervated by the maxillary nerve and the inferior arch is innervated by the mandibular alveolar nerve.

A given tooth has four surfaces: occlusal, vestibular, lingual, and contact [1]. The occlusal surface faces the opposite dental arch and is the principal mastication surface. Animals are said to be isognathous (equal-jawed) when the whole occlusal surface of the superior (upper) arch makes contact with the whole occlusal surface of the inferior (lower) arch on centric occlusion. This requires the arches to be the same width and is true in the pig. All other domestic mammals are anisognathous with the inferior arch narrower than the superior arch. The vestibular surface lies adjacent to the lips or cheeks and may be classified as labial or buccal, depending on which of these structures a given tooth faces. The lingual surface is opposite to the vestibular surface and lies adjacent to the tongue. The contact surface faces adjacent teeth in the same arch and all teeth except the last cheek teeth have two contact surfaces: mesial and distal. On the first incisor, the mesial surface is the contact surface adjacent to the median plane. On other teeth, the mesial surface is the contact surface directed toward the first incisor. The contact surface opposite the mesial surface is termed the distal surface (further away from the median plane).

In some laboratory species, only one set of teeth develops (monophyodontic dentition), but in all domestic mammals, two sets develop (diphyodontic dentition). The first set (deciduous teeth) appears early in life and consists of fewer and smaller teeth than the permanent dentition which gradually replaces it. The deciduous dentition contains no molars or first premolars and provides the young mammal with a fully functional set of teeth that can be accommodated by its smaller jaws. Replacement by the permanent teeth is gradual and follows a definite sequence that is useful in the estimation of age.

In addition to being classified as diphyodontic and as brachyodontic or hypsodontic, the different tooth types present in domestic species qualify them as heterodontic (vs. homodontic species such as sharks and odontocetes in which all teeth are alike). Finally, since their teeth are embedded in alveoli, domestic mammals are termed thecodontic. In contrast, the teeth of some lower vertebrates are classified as acrodontic because the teeth rest on the bone rather than being embedded in alveoli. Other species have pleurodontic dentition in which the teeth are attached to the side (inside edge) of the bone [2].The proper name for a dental implantation (joint) is gomphosis.

II. DENTAL FORMULAE

Dental formulae are used as a shorthand method of designating the particular dental complement of a given species. Because of bilateral symmetry, the parenthetical portion of a formula is used to describe only one-half (left or right) of the arches, and the whole expression is multiplied by two to arrive at the correct total number. Within the parentheses, letters are used for the four tooth types and "fractions"

Table 17-1

Dental Formulae of Domestic Mammals

	Permanent	Deciduous
Pig	$2(I\frac{3}{3}\ C\frac{1}{1}\ P\frac{4}{4}\ M\frac{3}{3}) = 44$	$2(I\frac{3}{3}\ C\frac{1}{1}\ P\frac{3}{3}) = 28$
Horse	$2(I\frac{3}{3}\ C\frac{1}{1}\ P\frac{3(4)}{3}\ M\frac{3}{3}) = 40\text{ or }42$	$2(I\frac{3}{3}\ C\frac{1}{1}\ P\frac{3}{3}) = 28$ (See 5 below)
Dog	$2(I\frac{3}{3}\ C\frac{1}{1}\ P\frac{4}{4}\ M\frac{2}{3}) = 42$	$2(I\frac{3}{3}\ C\frac{1}{1}\ P\frac{3}{3}) = 28$
Cat	$2(I\frac{3}{3}\ C\frac{1}{1}\ P\frac{3}{2}\ M\frac{1}{1}) = 30$	$2(I\frac{3}{3}\ C\frac{1}{1}\ P\frac{3}{2}) = 26$
Ruminants	$2(I\frac{0}{4}\ C\frac{0}{0}\ P\frac{3}{3}\ M\frac{3}{3}) = 32$	$2(I\frac{0}{4}\ C\frac{0}{0}\ P\frac{3}{3}) = 20$

Notes:

1. Among the domestic species, only the pig has the full, generalized mammalian complement of 44 permanent teeth. In the other domesticated mammals, the dentition is reduced in one or more areas and with the exception of the ruminants, these reductions are limited to the premolars and/or molars.

2. In those animals in which a full complement of permanent premolars (4 in each position) is not present, the missing premolars are the most rostral ones [3]. To be more specific:

    a. In ruminants, the 3 permanent premolars are the second, third, and fourth premolars (P2, P3, and P4).
    b. In the cat, the 3 permanent superior premolars are P2, P3, and P4, and the 2 permanent inferior premolars are P3 and P4. (Superior P1's and inferior P1's and P2's are absent.)
    c. In the horse, the three fully developed premolars in each arch are P2, P3, and P4. The first superior premolars of the horse are vestigial and often absent. They are responsible for the parenthetical 4 in the premolar section of the equine dental formula and are known among horsemen as the wolf teeth (dentes lupi). Similar vestigial P1's, also known as wolf teeth, are present in the inferior arch, but they rarely erupt.

3. In species which do not have a full complement of permanent molars (3 in each position), those which are missing are the most caudal ones [3].

4. The deciduous dental formulae are identical to the permanent formulae except that the molars and first premolars (P1's) have no deciduous predecessors.

5. The deciduous canine teeth of horses do not erupt and are never functional. Consequently, the equine deciduous formula is often written to indicate no canine teeth and a total of 24 [4]. In mares, the permanent canine teeth are typically very small and may not erupt, reducing the total number of teeth to 36 or 38 [2].

indicate the number of each type present with the numerator representing the number of that type in the superior arch and the denominator representing the number present in the inferior arch. The dental formulae of the domestic mammals are presented in Table 17-1.

III. DENTITION OF CARNIVORES (Figs. 17-1, 17-2)

The teeth of carnivores are brachyodont and so anisognathous that the lingual surface of the superior teeth slide over the vestibular surface of the inferior teeth when the jaws are being closed. As a result, only dorsoventral movement of the mandible (centric occlusion) occurs at the temporomandibular joint (i.e., side-to-side motion does not occur). The dental complement of cats is relatively constant, but that of dogs is often reduced in the brachycephalic breeds. The upper canine teeth are positioned caudal to the lower canines when the mouth is closed. The premolars increase in size from the rostral ones to the caudal ones and the molars decrease in size from the rostral to caudal. The upper fourth premolars occlude with the lower first molars. These four teeth are the sectorial ("carnassial") teeth and are the largest teeth in the mouth. Most of the upper premolars make no contact with the lower premolars. Puppies and kittens are typically edentulous (lack erupted teeth) during the first few weeks of life. The deciduous dentition erupts from the third to the sixth week and by two months of age a full set is typically present and in wear. The permanent teeth gradually replace the deciduous ones beginning at about 2 months of age [5]. Replacement is usually complete by 7 months of age.

Determination of age by dentition is of questionable value in carnivores because there is wide variation in dental data, both individually and with the various breeds. Husbandry and oral conformation also influence the appearance of the dentition. The chance of judging an animal's age correctly by its teeth is considered to be accurate by some authors [6] and inaccurate by others [7]. (Table 17-2). In young dogs, the criteria used are based primarily on wear data involving the cusps of the incisors. Each incisor has a large cusp and at least one small cusp (superior I1's and I2's have two small cusps). In Table 17-2, "cusp worn off" refers to the large cusp. Small dogs and those with brachygnathic or prognathic conformation are the ones most likely to deviate from these data [3].

Because it is of value when performing extractions, knowledge of the number of roots in the various permanent teeth of carnivores may be useful:

	Dog	Cat
teeth with 1 root	All I,C,P1, and inferior M3	All I,C, and superior P2
teeth with 3 roots	Superior P4, superior molars (last 3 upper teeth)	Superior P4
teeth with 2 roots	All except those noted above	

A useful memory aid for the number of roots of canine cheek teeth is 122333 for superior teeth and 1222221 for inferior teeth. In the cat, these numbers are 1232 and 222, respectively.

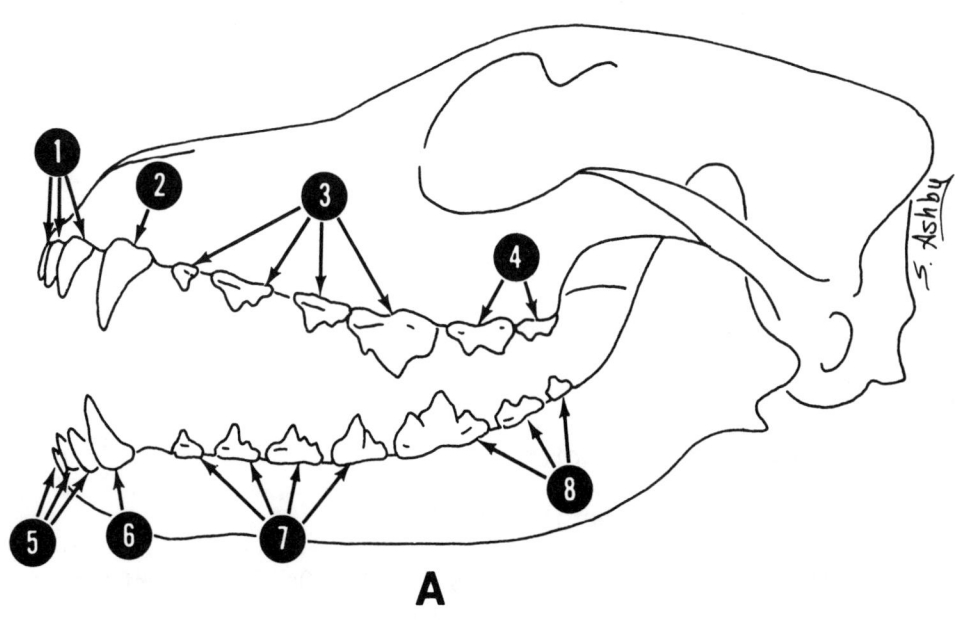

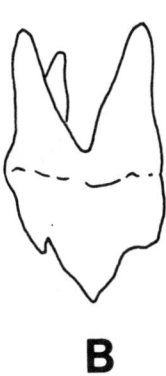

Figure 17-1

Permanent Dentition of the Dog

A. Teeth in situ (left aspect)
B. Isolated superior fourth premolar

1. Superior incisors (I1, I2, I3)
2. Superior canine
3. Superior premolars (P1, P2, P3, P4)
4. Superior molars (M1, M2)
5. Inferior incisors (I1, I2, I3)
6. Inferior canine
7. Inferior premolars (P1, P2, P3, P4)
8. Inferior molars (M1, M2, M3)

Table 17-2

Dental Aging Criteria for Dogs

5 mo.	Permanent incisors have erupted. I3 not yet in wear
6 mo.	Permanent canines erupted
1½ yr.	Cusp worn off inferior I1
2½ yr.	Cusp worn off inferior I2
3½ yr.	Cusp worn off superior I1
4½ yr.	Cusp worn off superior I2
5 yr.	Cusp of inferior I3 worn slightly. Occlusal surface of inferior I1 and I2 rectangular; Slight wear of canines
6 yr.	Cusp worn off superior and inferior I3; Canines worn blunt; Inferior canine shows impression of superior I3
7 yr.	Inferior I1 worn down to root so that occlusal surface is elongated in the labiolingual direction
8 yr.	Occlusal surface of inferior I1 is beveled in front
10 yr.	Inferior I2 and superior I1 have occlusal surfaces elongated labiolingually
12 yr.	I1's begin to fall out
16 yr.	Incisors gone
20 yr.	Loss of canines

From Habel, 1981 [3]

The teeth of carnivores are well adapted to their natural, functional role of grasping and holding their prey, tearing pieces from it, and crushing large pieces in preparation for swallowing. Their dentition is not designed for efficient grinding, which is found in other domesticated mammals.

As noted in the discussion of dental formulae, cats are missing the first upper premolars and the first two lower premolars. Brachycephalic dogs typically have reduced dentition (particularly in the cheek teeth of the lower arcade), and the teeth which are present are often crowded so much that they are rotated with the long axis positioned transversely [5]. Prognathia (elongated mandible--"overshot") is often present in these animals as well.

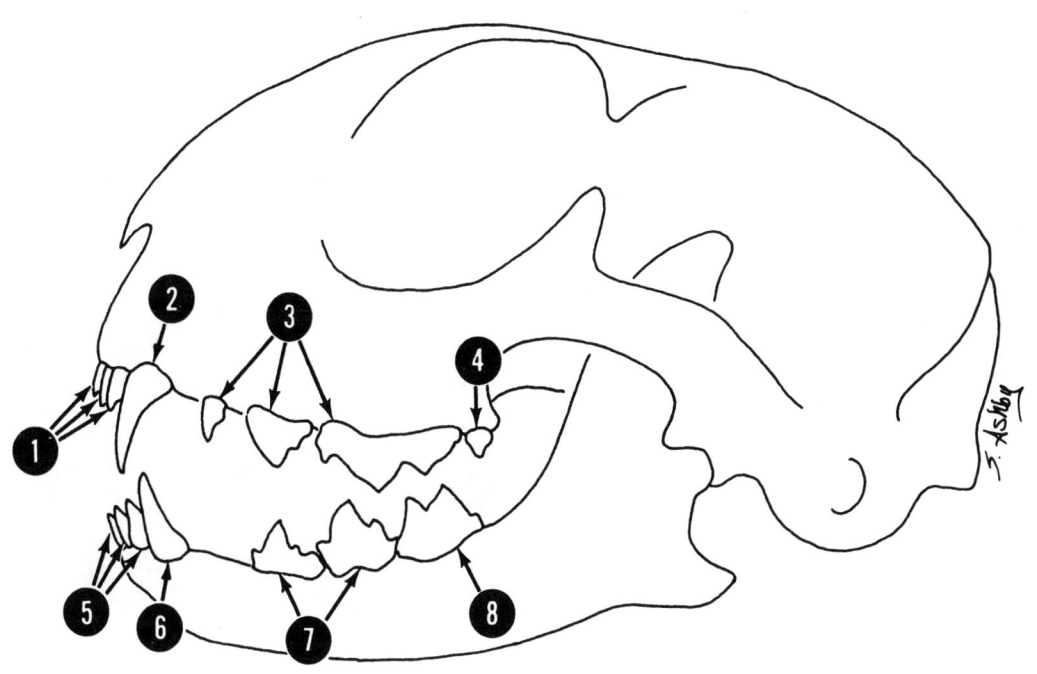

Figure 17-2

Permanent Dentition of a Cat (left aspect)

1. Superior incisors (I1,I2,I3)
2. Superior canine
3. Superior premolars (P2,P3,P4)
4. Superior molar
5. Inferior incisors (I1,I2,I3)
6. Inferior canine
7. Inferior premolars (P3,P4)
8. Inferior molar

Brachygnathia (shortened mandible - "undershot") is less frequently observed in carnivores. ("Overshot" and "undershot" are sometimes used with reversed (opposite) meanings. Prognathia and brachygnathia are not subject to the alternative interpretations.)

Dogs and cats are occasionally presented with one or more supernumerary teeth. Extra incisors and premolars are most common. This often results from a failure to shed deciduous teeth, but in some instances these represent additional (duplicate) teeth. Because of the owners' concern and the fact that the chance of dental problems is increased (periodontal disease, etc.), supernumerary teeth (particularly retained deciduous ones) are often extracted. However, if they cause no crowding and are not awkwardly positioned, they may be left in situ. Other developmental problems include:

> anodontia--failure of a tooth (usually a permanent tooth) to develop. Its deciduous predecessor often remains 3 to 5 years in such cases before it is shed.

> gemination--twinning of a tooth due to a splitting of the tooth bud. The two parts usually remain attached to each other and rarely cause clinical problems.

> dens in dente--improper development of a tooth bud resulting in an extra enamel cap outside of the major part of the tooth. These teeth often deteriorate because cracks in the outer enamel allow bacterial invasion.

The upper sectorial teeth sometimes abscess with the presenting sign being an external swelling or draining tract ventral to the orbit. In cats, these abscesses may rupture into the orbit and drain from the eye. Extraction is indicated and may necessitate splitting the tooth into rostral (2 roots) and caudal (1 root) parts and separately removing each part. (Since the three roots diverge as they enter the maxilla, attempts to extract the whole tooth intact may result in broken roots which are difficult to remove and may serve as a nidus for infection if left in situ.)

The basic principle of tooth extraction in carnivores involves forcing a dental elevator into the alveolus which in turn forces the root out. In normal teeth, this is very difficult and may require a gingival incision and an osteotomy of the alveolar wall. Endontic, periodontic, and orthodontic techniques are occasionally applied to carnivores. A dentist is often involved on a consulting basis.

IV. PORCINE DENTITION (Fig. 21-1)

The teeth of pigs are brachyodont with the exception of the hypsodont canines. They are also isognathous. The canine teeth of the pig are very large and are known as tusks. The lower tusk may reach a total length of 18 cm (in a boar) and the lateral and medial edges of the exposed parts are kept sharp by constant contact with the mesial contact surface of the smaller upper tusk. Sows' tusks are much smaller than those of a boar. Premolars and molars increase in size from rostral to caudal. The deciduous I3's and C's ("needle teeth") are erupted in newborn piglets, and are often clipped to prevent injury and/or discomfort to the sow during suckling. The other deciduous teeth erupt during the first few weeks of life with the deciduous second incisors typically being last to erupt at 2 to 3 months [8]. Replacement by permanent teeth begins at about 8 months of age and is complete by about 18 months of age. The first, second, and third molars erupt at about 5, 10, and 20 months of age, respectively. Root numbers in pigs have little, if any, clinical significance [8]:

1 root - Incisors and canines

2 roots - P1, lower P2

3 roots - Upper P2 and upper P3, lower P4

4 roots - Lower M1 and lower M2

6 roots - Lower M3 and all upper molars

Lower P3 has 2 or 3 roots and upper P4 has 4 or 5 roots

Selective breeding has resulted in marked changes in the skull shapes in some porcine breeds, and this has influenced the eruption, position, and shape of the teeth. As a result, determination of age by the teeth is approximate at best [8]. As in the carnivores, the mandibles move mainly in a dorsoventral direction during mastication, but some lateral motion is possible. The lower incisors serve as shovellike extensions of the mandible and are useful in exposing edibles in the ground ("rooting").

V. RUMINANT DENTITION (Figs. 17-3, 17-4)

The incisors of ruminants are brachyodont and the cheek teeth are hypsodont. Incisors and canines are absent in the upper arcade* and are replaced by a dental pad. This pad is covered by a heavy, cornified epithelium and acts as an antagonist to the lower incisors. The lower canine teeth have functionally evolved as incisors and are so designated (I4). In addition to their formal numerical designations, the incisors of ruminants are commonly known as central (I1), first intermediate (I2), second intermediate (I3), and corner (I4) incisors. They have distinct necks. The lingual borders of the occlusal surfaces of the incisors have ridges separated by notches. When wear has reduced a tooth sufficiently to remove these features, a tooth is said to be level [3]. The cheek teeth increase in size from rostral to caudal and they continue to grow for some time after eruption. Thereafter, they slowly advance from their sockets. Considerable lateral movement of the jaw occurs during mastication.

The number of roots possessed by the various teeth are [8]:

teeth with 1 root--all incisors

teeth with 2 roots--all lower cheek teeth

teeth with 3 roots--all upper cheek teeth

---

*Primordia for these teeth have been demonstrated in embryos but disappear before birth.

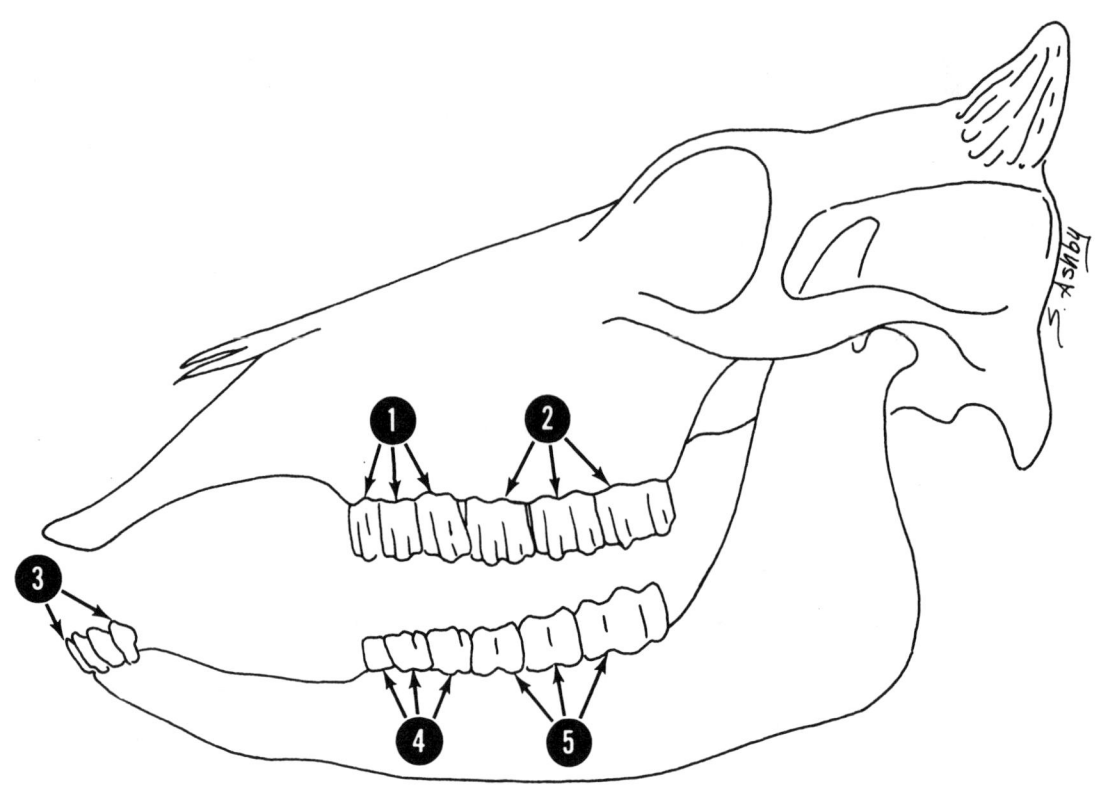

Figure 17-3

Permanent Dentition of an Ox (left aspect)

1. Superior premolars (P2, P3, P4)
2. Superior molars (M1, M2, M3)
3. Inferior incisors (I1, I2, I3, I4)
4. Inferior premolars (P2, P3, P4)
5. Inferior molars (M1, M2, M3)

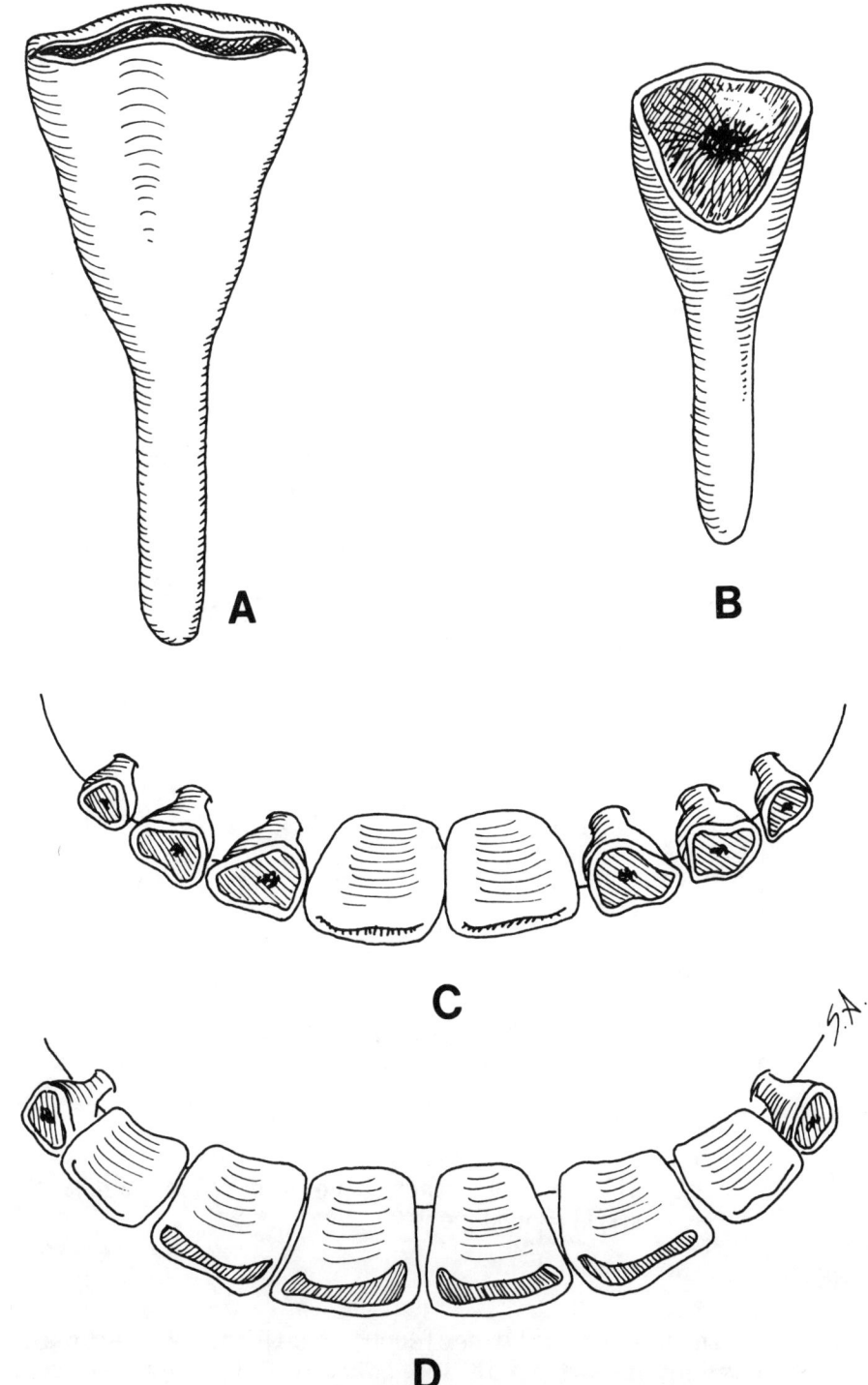

Figure 17-4

Aging Features in Bovine Incisors

A. Bovine incisor just coming into wear (lingual aspect)

B. "Level" bovine incisor (lingual aspect)

C. Two-year-old ox showing permanent central incisors and well worn deciduous I2, I3, and I4

D. Three-year-old ox with impending replacement of deciduous corner incisor

After Habel, 1981 [3].

Eruption and important aging dates for ruminant teeth vary according to the species:

A. Ox

1. All deciduous teeth may be present at birth. However, the third incisors and all teeth caudal to them may not erupt for several more (up to 21) days [8]. It may also be of value in aging to note the following[3]:

    a. By 2 weeks of age, the gum has receded to the neck of I1.
    b. By 3-4 weeks of age, the gum has receded to the necks of all incisors.

2. The permanent teeth erupt according to the following schedule: ($\pm$ a few months) [8]

    The numbers to remember for aging are:

    I 0/1--14-25 months   1½ years
    I 0/2--17-33 months   2 years
    I 0/3--22-40 months   2½ years
    I 0/4--32-42 months   3 years

    P 2/2--24-28 months
    P 3/3--24-30 months   Eruption of these teeth is
    P 4/4--28-34 months   less variable than the
    M 1/1--5-6 months   incisors but is seldom
    M 2/2--15-16 months   considered in aging [3].
    M 3/3--24-28 months

3. The following data may also be of value in aging oxen [3]:

    5 years--all incisors are in wear
    6 years--I1 is level and neck is visible (Fig. 17-4/B)
    7 years--I2 is level and neck is visible
    8 years--I3 is level and neck is visible
    9 years--I4 is level and neck is visible
    15 years--all incisors that have not fallen out are reduced to small round pegs

B. Sheep

1. As in the ox, all deciduous teeth may be erupted at birth. However, the central and corner incisors often do not appear for up to 8 days and the premolars may not erupt for up to 4 weeks [8].

2. The permanent teeth erupt according to the following schedule [8].

    A useful memory aid:

    I 0/1--12-18 months   1 year

```
          I 0/2--21-24 months        ⎛ 2 years
          I 0/3--27-36 months        ⎨ 3 years
          I 0/4--36-48 months        ⎝ 4 years

          P 2/2--21-24 months
          P 3/3--21-24 months
          P 4/4--21-24 months
          M 1/1--3 months
          M 2/2--9 months
          M 3/3--18 months
```

C. Goat [8]

1. The first three deciduous incisors are present at birth and the corner incisor erupts at 1 to 3 weeks of age. The deciduous premolars erupt at 3 months of age.

2. The permanent incisors erupt at 15, 21, 27, and 36 months of age for I1, I2, I3, and I4, respectively. The permanent premolars erupt at 17 to 20 months of age and the molars erupt at 5 to 6, 8 to 10, and 18 to 24 months for M1, M2, and M3.

VI. EQUINE DENTITION (Figs. 17-5, 17-6, 17-7)

The teeth of horses are hypsodont, anisognathous and, with the exception of canine teeth, they continue to erupt throughout life. The first, second, and third incisors are often termed central, intermediate, and corner incisors, respectively. They are several (6 to 7) centimeters long and are curved with the concavity on the lingual aspect. The curvature is most pronounced in the exposed part of the crown in a young horse so that the crowns of the incisors in young animals meet their antagonists almost vertically. As the horse ages, the teeth wear and the embedded, straighter portions erupt, making the occlusal angle more acute as viewed from the lateral aspect. The shape of the occlusal surface of the incisors changes with age (because of eruption, wear, and the cross-sectional shape of the incisor) from oval (transversely), to rounded, to triangular, and finally back to oval (rostrocaudally) in an old horse. Knowledge of this is of some value in aging horses, although eruption data and the disappearance of the infundibula are used more frequently. The infundibulum is a centrally-placed depression in the occlusal surface of the incisor which is commonly known as the "cup." Although present on both deciduous and permanent incisors, infundibula are used for aging only in adults. They are about 12 mm deep on upper incisors and 6 mm deep on lower incisors. As the tooth wears, (at about 2 mm/year) the cup becomes shallower and ultimately disappears. The enamel forming the bottom of the cup remains for several years as the enamel spot. As the cup disappears, the dental star appears nearby on the vestibular aspect of the occlusal surface. The dental star is the secondary, darker dentine which fills in the pulp cavity as wear causes the occlusal surface to approach it. The dental star first appears on I1 at 8 years as a transverse line. It becomes oval and moves toward the center of the occlusal surface as the enamel spot disappears. By 13 years, it is centered in all incisors and by 15 years all stars are round.

The canine teeth lack infundibula and are located in the diastemata, a little closer to the corner incisors than to the cheek teeth. They usually develop in stallions but are often absent in mares.

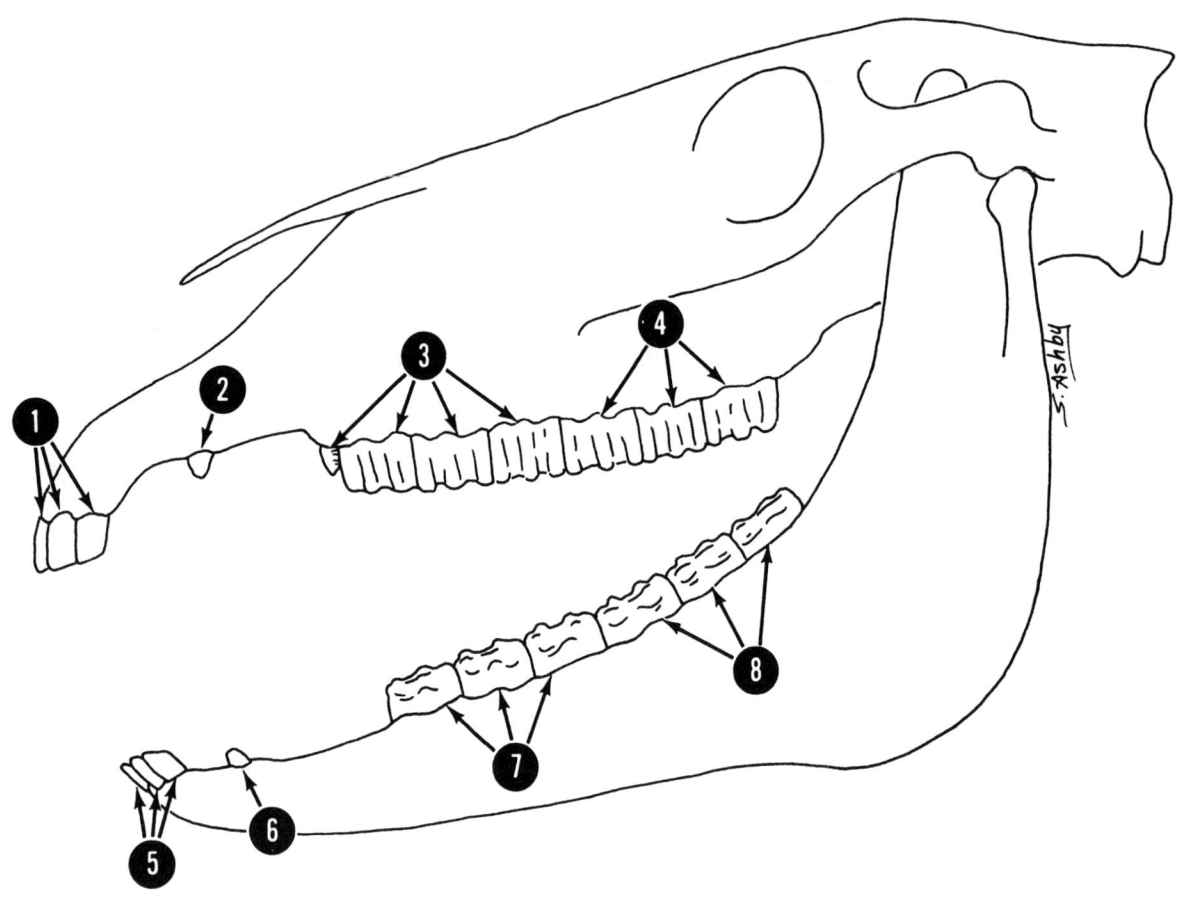

Figure 17-5

Permanent Dentition of a Horse (left aspect)

1. Superior incisors (I1, I2, I3)
2. Superior canine
3. Superior premolars (P1="wolf tooth", P2, P3, P4)
4. Superior molars (M1, M2, M3)
5. Inferior incisors (I1, I2, I3)
6. Inferior canine
7. Inferior premolars (P2, P3, P4)
8. Inferior molars (M1, M2, M3)

There are typically six upper and six lower cheek teeth on each side (P2, P3, P4, M1, M2, M3). Occasionally, rudimentary P1's ("wolf teeth") are present as noted in the dental formulae section. They are incorrectly blamed for a number of maladies. Horsemen may request their removal since they may cause problems with certain types of bits. The upper cheek teeth are nearly square in cross section and the lower ones are narrower transversely and elongated in a rostral-caudal direction. The cheek teeth complete their growth at 6-7 years,* and at that time they are 8-10 cm long and project 1.5-2 cm above the gums. The cheek teeth are structurally complex with many folds and ridges. They have infundibula, but the depressions are filled up with cement so that no "cups" occur.

Because of the anisognathism, only about the lingual third of the occlusal surface of the upper arch is in contact with the vestibular half of the lower arch at centric occlusion [8]. As the mandible moves to one side during mastication, all contact between upper and lower arches on the opposite side is lost. Also, as a result of the anisognathism, the vestibular side of the lower arch wears more rapidly than the lingual aspect. In the upper cheek teeth, the lingual aspect wears more rapidly for the same reason. "Floating" is a clinical procedure to file off the resulting sharp edges ("points") on the lingual border of the lower arch and the vestibular border of the upper arch. Unless removed, these edges may lacerate the tongue and cheeks. Large projections resulting from abnormal wear may have to be removed with molar cutters.

Successful estimation of age in horses by examination of the teeth may be necessary to establish or maintain credibility with some clients. The features used include eruption data (which are relatively accurate) and several wear-related features of the incisors including cup disappearance, the shape of the occlusal surface, and dental star appearance (as well as the seven-year-hook, Galvayne's groove, and others).

Dates of eruption, "in wear," and leveling are more significant in aging than disappearance of cups and other wear-related data. Wear data is influenced by several factors including diet and the amount of sand in the pasture soil. Consequently, the appearance of an animal's teeth may not match its chronological age. In addition, disappearance of the cups is not an accurate aging criterion because it depends upon the depth of the enamel infundibulum and on the amount of cement in the bottom (both of which are variable). Consequently, cup data are disregarded if they do not agree with eruption data [3].

Only inferior teeth are normally used to estimate age, and most observations are limited to the incisors. Superior teeth are examined by some individuals, but they lag behind the lower teeth and examination of them has not been shown to increase the accuracy of the age estimation [3].

---

*They continue to erupt, however, throughout life [9]. Eruption refers to extrusion from the alveolus. Growth refers to an increase in the size (primarily length) of the tooth.

Figure 17-6

Aging Features in Equine Incisors
(sagittal section of unworn second inferior incisor with occlusal
surfaces shown at various ages)

- A. 4 years--in wear
- B. 5 years--level
- C. 7 years--cup gone
- D. 10 years--enamel spot remains, dental star present, round shape
- E. 17 years--enamel spot gone, dental star present, triangular shape

    1. cement--not shown in C, D, or E because it wears off by those ages
    2. enamel
    3. dentine
    4. infundibulum
    5. dental cavity--fills in with secondary dentine to form the dental "star" before ages shown in D and E.
    6. enamel spot
    7. dental star

When the dental star appears on the occlusal surface, it is on the vestibular aspect of the enamel spot (D and E).

After Habel, 1981 [3]

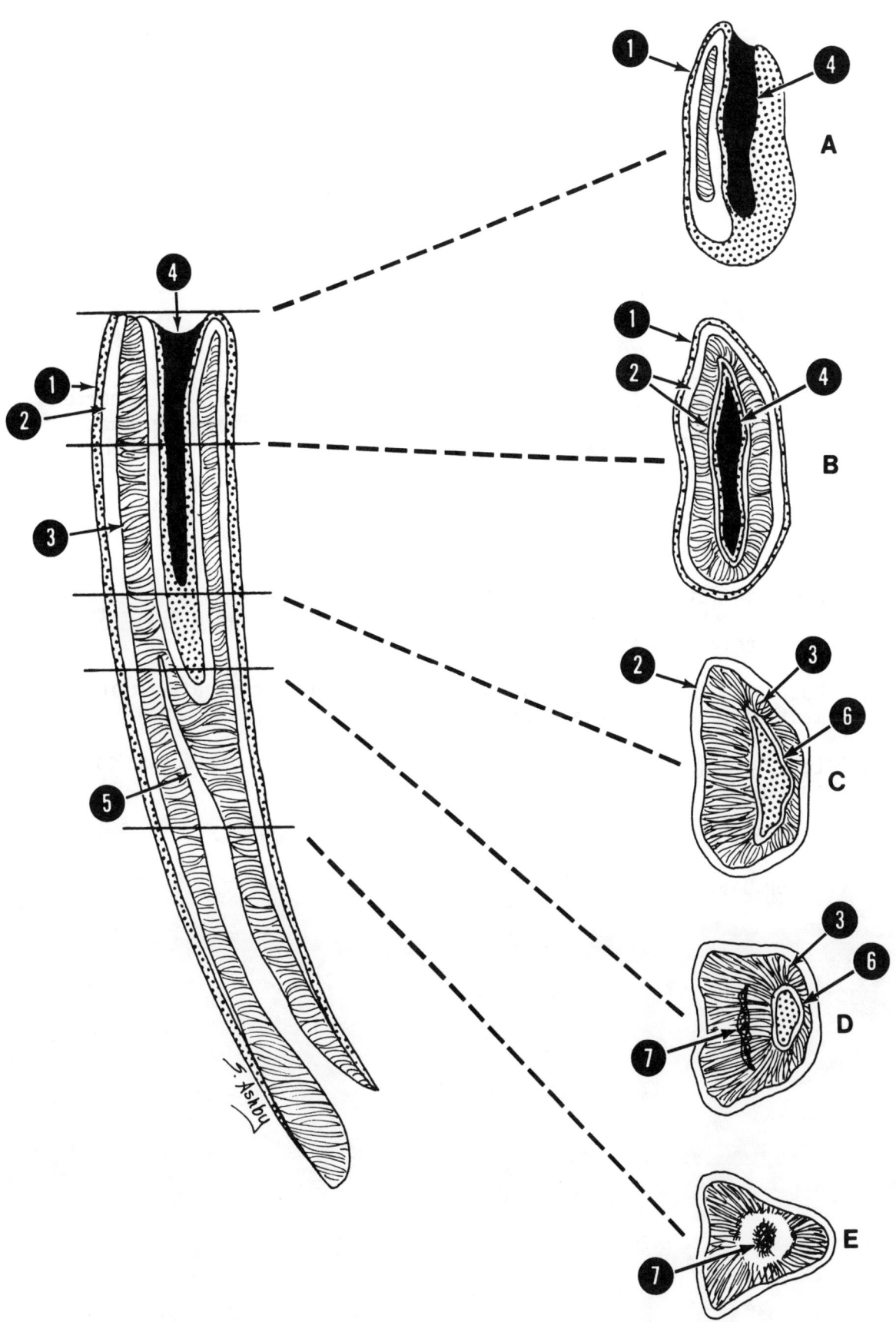

Figure 17-7

Typical Appearance of Equine Incisors at 2 years (A, B, C)
and 4 years (D, E, F)

A. Rostral aspect of a 2-year-old. The deciduous incisors have shorter crowns than the permanent ones and they also lack the shallow groove on the labial surface. A common mistake in aging is to assume deciduous incisors to be permanent ones.

B. Left aspect of a 2-year-old.

C. Occlusal surfaces of inferior incisors of a 2-year-old. The presence of infundibula in deciduous teeth has caused some significant aging errors. Horses 2-2½ years of age are sometimes mistakenly aged at 6-8 years.

D. Rostral aspect of a 4-year-old. The permanent central and intermediate incisors are erupted and in wear.

E. Left aspect of a 4-year-old. Note the small deciduous corner incisors.

F. Occlusal aspect of inferior incisors of a 4-year-old.

After Davis, 1966, [11]

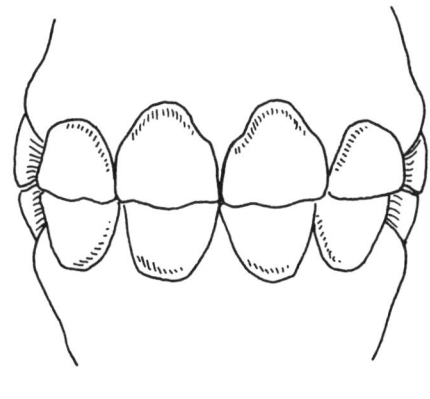

A

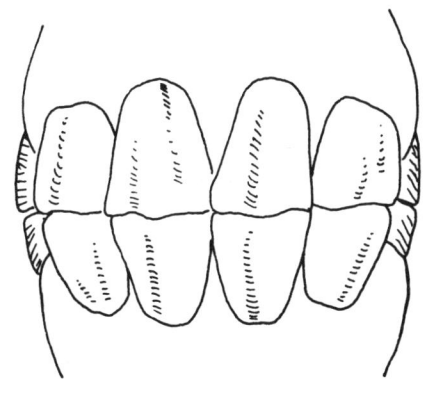

D

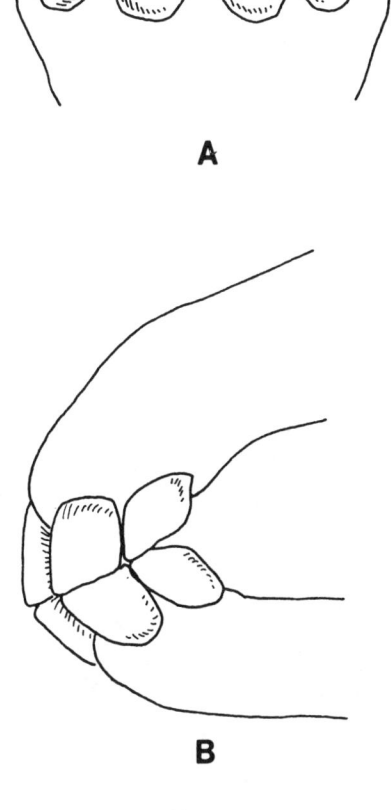

B

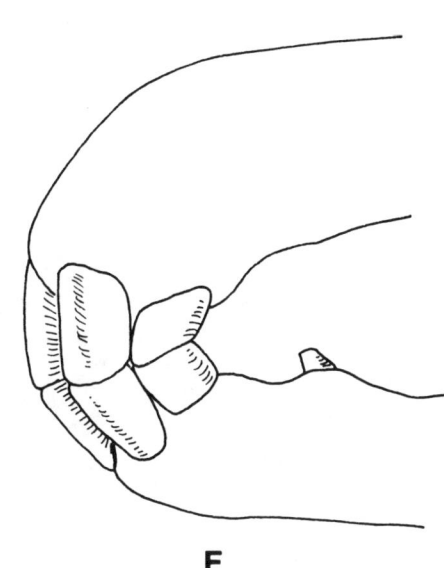

E

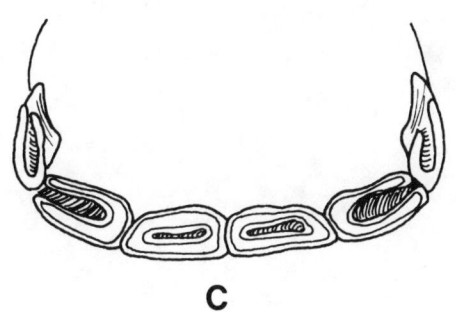

C

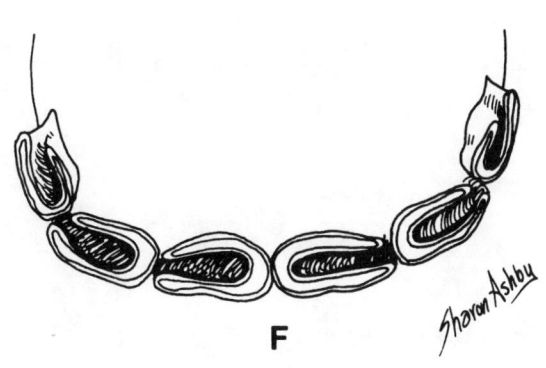

F

Figure 17-8

Typical Appearance of Equine Incisors
at 7 years (A, B, C) and 15 years (D, E, F)

A. Rostral aspect of a 7-year-old.

B. Left aspect of a 7-year-old. The inconstant "seven-year-hook" can be observed on the superior corner incisor. The well-erupted canine teeth age this animal at 5 plus years even before the occlusal surfaces of the inferior incisors are examined.

C. Occlusal surfaces of inferior incisors of a 7-year-old. The cups are gone from the central and intermediate incisors but enamel spots remain.

D. Rostral aspect of a 15-year-old.

E. Left aspect of a 15-year-old. Galvayne's groove is about halfway down to the occlusal surface of the superior corner incisor.

F. Occlusal surfaces of inferior incisors of a 15-year-old. All incisors lack enamel spots and all have dental stars.

After Davis, 1966 [11].

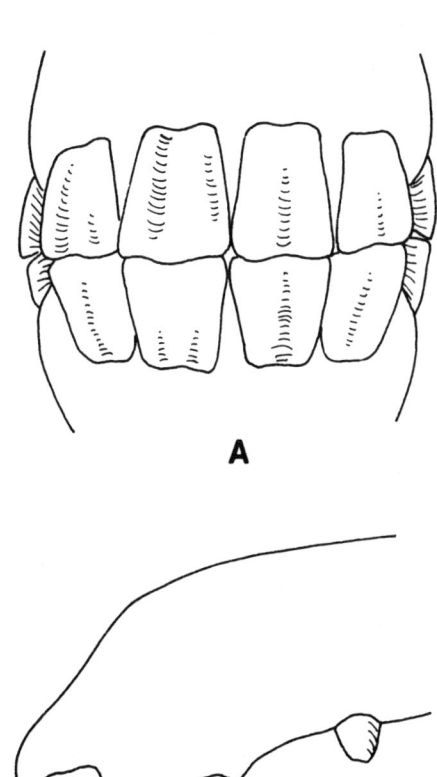
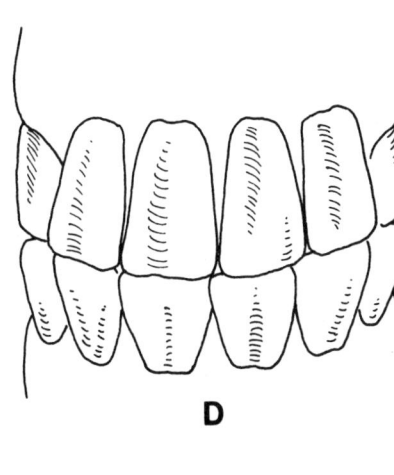
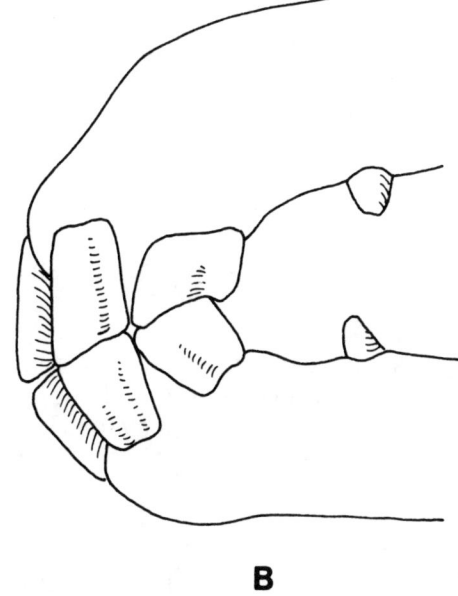
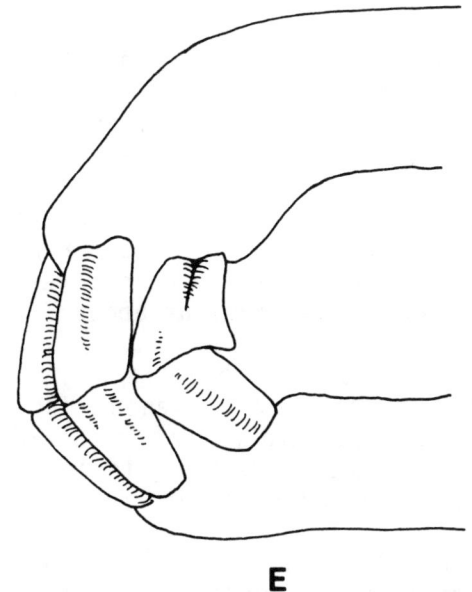
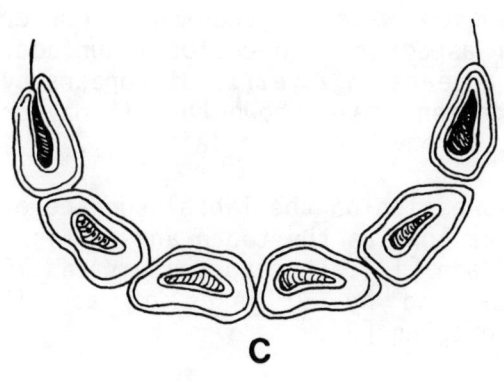
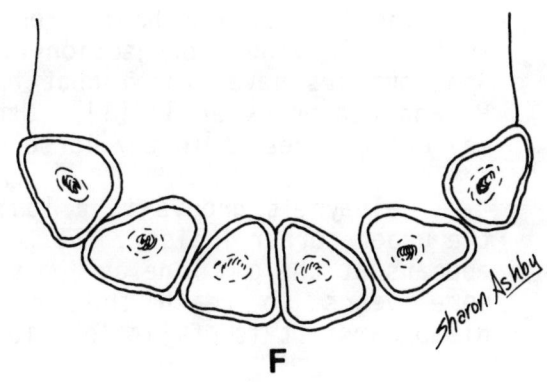

399

Eruption data for equine teeth are given below. These data from Nickel et al, 1973 [8] may vary by a few months from other sources.

TEETH	Age at Deciduous Eruption	Age at Permanent Eruption
I 1/1	Before or near birth	$2\frac{1}{2}$--3 years
I 2/2	3 to 8 weeks	$3\frac{1}{2}$--4 years
I 3/3	5 to 9 months	$4\frac{1}{2}$--5 years
C 1/1	Rarely erupt	4--5 years
P 2/2	Before birth	$2\frac{1}{2}$ years
P 3/3	or during	$2\frac{1}{2}$ years
P 4/4	first week	$3\frac{1}{2}$ years
M 1/1		1 year $\pm$ a few months
M 2/2		2--$2\frac{1}{2}$ years
M 3/3		$3\frac{1}{2}$--$4\frac{1}{2}$ years

Of value in aging is to remember 7 days, 7 weeks, 7 months (or 8-8-8--both are just memory aids and neither is exactly right, see chart above) for the eruption of deciduous I1, I2, and I3; and $2\frac{1}{2}$, $3\frac{1}{2}$, $4\frac{1}{2}$ years for the eruption of the permanent incisors. Eruption dates of other teeth (except canine teeth) are seldom used in aging. After eruption, an incisor requires about six months to erupt far enough to begin wear. Once the whole occlusal surface is in wear, an incisor is said to be "level." All deciduous incisors are level at about 2 years. Permanent I1 and I2 are level at 5 years, and permanent I3 is level at about 7 years [3].

The most reliable "wear" data used in aging is the disappearance of the cups in the lower permanent incisors. This requires an average of about 3 years of wear and occurs at 6-7-8 years for I1, I2, I3. As noted previously, however, these data are disregarded if they do not agree with eruption, "in wear," or leveling data.

Conflicting data for aging are available concerning retention of the bottom of the infundibulum as the enamel spot [3]. Although most authors have stated that it disappears from all lower incisors by 13 years of age, a well documented investigation has shown it to be present in a majority of horses through 16 years of age [10]. Specific data regarding enamel spots, dental stars, and shapes of the occlusal surfaces are published in the Official Guide for Determining the Age of the Horse", edited by Davis [11].

The "seven-year-hook" results from uneven wear of the upper corner incisor, leaving a projection at the distal aspect of the occlusal surface. Some authors have stated that this feature appears at 7 years, disappears by 9, and reappears at 11 [11]. Other investigations have shown that it may or may not be present in any horse over 6 [10]. It may appear unilaterally.

Galvayne's groove is a longitudinal depression on the labial surface of the upper corner incisor. The groove is not as long as the tooth and it first appears at the gum line at about 10 years of age [11]. It supposedly takes 10 more years to reach the occlusal surface and by 30 years of age it disappears. It is of little value in accurate aging [3].

A common mistake in aging is to assume that deciduous incisors are permanent incisors. Deciduous incisors have shorter crowns, more distinct necks, and they usually lack the distinct longitudinal groove on the labial surface which is characteristic of permanent incisors. Deciduous incisors do, however, have infundibula. The deciduous third incisors are notably smaller than their intermediate and central counterparts. In estimating the age of a horse or any other animal by its dentition, the statement should be carefully worded to imply that the animal has the teeth of an X-year-old (i.e., avoid saying the animal is X years old) [3]. This will help maintain credibility in those cases where dental data do not match chronological age.

Selected definitions in regard to equine dentistry include:

bishoping--the unethical practice of altering the teeth of an older horse in an attempt to masquerade it as a younger animal. Techniques include drilling and staining false cups in the incisors.

cap--a deciduous cheek tooth which remains attached to the occlusal surface of its permanent replacement. Caps may have to be removed because they sometimes cause pain.

full mouth--a horse in which all permanent teeth have erupted (about 5 years of age and older).

in wear--refers to a tooth which has grown out to the occlusal level of the other teeth in its arch.

level--a term indicating that the entire occlusal surface is in wear.

parrot mouth--brachygnathia.

sow mouth--prognathia.

shear mouth--an excessively narrow lower arcade. This requires frequent floating.

scissor mouth--a mouth in which uneven wear in the incisors gives them oblique (to the left or right) occlusal surfaces rather than horizontal ones.

smooth mouth--an animal too old to age accurately.

step mouth--an uneven occlusal surface of a dental arch. Protrusion and lack of wear of a tooth because of a missing antagonist is the common cause. Such teeth may require frequent cutting. The term "wave mouth" is sometimes applied to horses in which the height difference of adjacent teeth is subtle or the transition in height is especially smooth.

Surgical procedures involving equine teeth usually involve floating, cutting, or extraction. To extract the lower cheek teeth, the mandible is trephined along its lateroventral border and the selected tooth is repelled with a hammer and punch. Upper cheek teeth are repelled through trephinations into the maxillary or conchofrontal sinus as noted in Chapter 19, Head.

References

1. International Committee on Veterinary Gross Anatomical Nomenclature. 1983. Nomina Anatomica Veterinaria, third ed. Published by the Committee, Ithaca, New York.

2. Getty, R. 1975. Sisson and Grossman's The Anatomy of the Domestic Animals. W. B. Saunders, Philadelphia.

3. Habel, R. E. 1981. Applied Veterinary Anatomy, second ed. Published by the author, Ithaca, New York.

4. Sisson, S., and J. Grossman. 1953. The Anatomy of the Domestic Animals, fourth ed. W. B. Saunders, Philadelphia.

5. Evans, H. E., and G. C. Christensen. 1979. Miller's Anatomy of the Dog, second ed. W. B. Saunders, Philadelphia.

6. Boenisch, F. 1913. Beitrag zur altersbestimmung des hundes mach schneidezahnen. Arch. Tierheilh. 39:289-327.

7. Meyer, L. 1942. Das gebib des deutschen schaferhundes mit besonderer berucksichtigung der zahnaltersbestimmung und der zahnanomalien. Dissertation, Zurich.

8. Nickel, R., A. Schummer, E. Seiferle, and W. Sach. 1973. The Viscera of the Domestic Mammals. Paul Parey, Berlin.

9. Shively, M. J. 1982. Twenty more veterinary anatomic lies, half-truths, and misleading statements. J. Vet. Med. Ed. 9(1):20-21.

10. Weekenstroo, H. J. 1918. Onderzoekingen betreffende de veranderingen aan de tanden van het paard op verschillende leeftijden en hun waarde voor de leeftijdsbepaling. P. Stokvis en Zoon, 'S-Hertogenbosch.

11. Davis, R. W. ed. 1966. Official guide for Determining the Age of the Horse. Am. Assoc. Equine Practitioners, Golden, Colorado.

18

RACHIOLOGY

The vertebral column connects cranial and caudal parts of the body and houses and protects the spinal cord. The individual vertebrae which form the column are divided into five groups according to regional similarities (cervical, thoracic, lumbar, sacral, and caudal vertebrae). Knowledge of the anatomy of the vertebral column is very important in small animal medicine and surgery because of the relatively high incidence of intervertebral disc disease as well as other vertebral diseases and injuries. Vertebral anatomy also has important applications in spinal and paravertebral anesthesia techniques and in special radiographic procedures.

I. EPAXIAL MUSCLES OF TRUNK

   A. The epaxial muscles are those which are located dorsal to the level of the transverse processes of the vertebrae. Most of them consist of overlapping fascicles, which attach to the vertebral processes and help to support the vertebral column. Bilateral contraction extends the vertebral column as a whole and unilateral contraction twists (bends) the vertebral column longitudinally to the right or left.

      1. Iliocostalis m.--extends from the ilium to the caudal cervical region. This muscle is the most laterally located muscle in the group, and is divided regionally into lumbar, thoracic, and cervical parts.

      2. Longissimus m.--extends from the ilium to the skull. This muscle is positioned just medial to the iliocostalis m. and is divided into a number of regional parts: lumbar, thoracic, cervical, atlantal, and capital.

      3. Transversospinalis m.--located near the midline from the sacrum to the cervical region. The transversospinalis m. has three major parts:

         a. semispinalis m. (thoracic, cervical, and capital). The semispinalis capitis m. is the most familiar one, and consists of the biventer cervicis m. (dorsally) and the complexus muscle (ventrally).

         b. multifidi mm.

         c. rotator mm.

      4. Other epaxial muscles of the trunk include the following:

         a. spinalis m.--this small muscle is grouped with the iliocostalis m. and longissimus m. under the general heading erector spinae [1].

         b. interspinalis mm.--these occur between spines of adjacent vertebrae.

403

c. intertransversarius mm.--these occur between transverse processes of adjacent vertebrae in the cervical, thoracic, and lumbar regions.

B. Clinical considerations

1. The transversospinalis m. is the muscle of primary concern in dorsal (hemi-) laminectomies. Although the names "multifidi" and "rotators" are frequently used in reference to these surgeries, these muscles are not usually specifically identified and dealt with in the actual manipulations. Instead, the muscles as a group are reflected laterally to expose the laminae of the selected vertebrae.

2. The epaxial muscles are used by some veterinarians for intramuscular injections. Their use is criticized by others who maintain that the heavy fascia around them does not allow good drainage in case of iatrogenic abscessation. In addition, some clients feel uneasy when they witness injections given in the back.

II. MORPHOLOGY OF VERTEBRAE

A. General features (Fig. 18-1)

cranial extremity (head)
caudal extremity (vertebral fossa)
body--the dense portion ventral to the spinal cord
ventral crest--the longitudinal ridge along the ventral aspect of the body
arch--the dorsal part which surrounds the spinal cord
    pedicle--the basilar parts of the arch on each side
    lamina--the left or right half of the dorsal part of the arch
spinous process--the single prominence projecting dorsally from the arch
transverse processes--the left and right prominences at the junctions of the pedicles with the body
articular processes (zygapophyses)--the paired cranial and caudal processes located at the junction of the laminae and pedicles
vertebral foramen--the foramen enclosed by the vertebral arch (collectively these form the vertebral canal)
cranial and caudal intervertebral notches--indentations on each side of the arches which, when articulated, form intervertebral foramina for the emergence of spinal nerves. Some spinal nerves emerge from lateral vertebral foramina which are passageways wholly within the arches of individual vertebrae (Fig. 18-2/3).

B. Regional and species specific features

There are 5 regional groups of vertebrae:

1. Cervical vertebrae

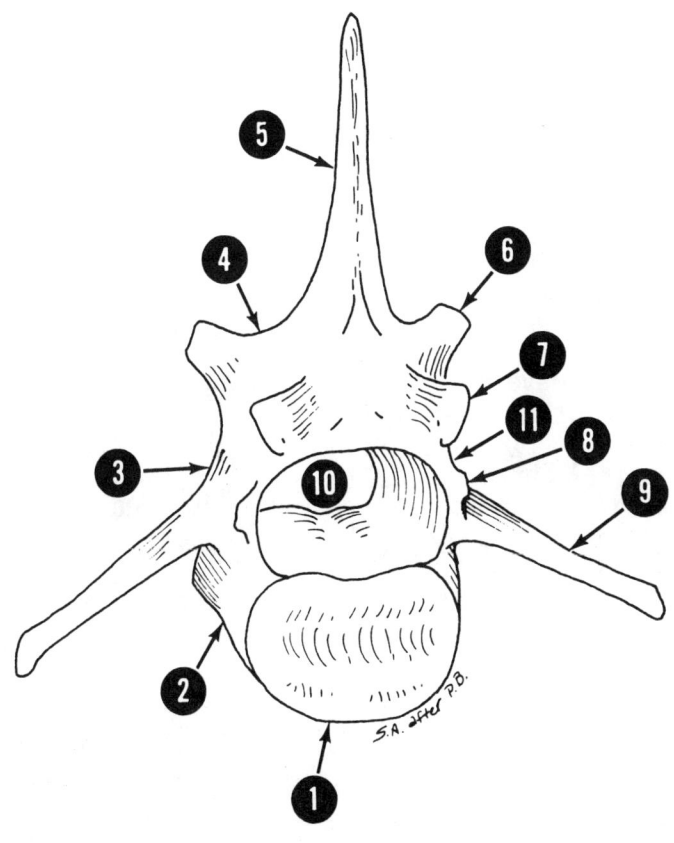

Figure 18-1

Features of a Vertebra
(caudal aspect of a canine lumbar vertebra)

1. caudal extremity
2. body
3. pedicle of arch
4. lamina of arch
5. spinous process
6. cranial articular process
7. caudal articular process
8. accessory process
9. transverse process
10. vertebral foramen
11. caudal intervertebral notch

After Evans and Christensen, 1979 [2]

a. All domestic mammals have 7 cervical vertebrae (Table 18-1) that are characterized by short spinous processes and a transverse foramen in the base of each transverse process.

b. The first cervical vertebra (C1) is called the atlas and it is atypical in several ways (Fig. 18-2):

   1) The body is poorly developed and is officially termed the ventral arch.

   2) The spinous process is absent.

   3) The transverse processes are very well developed (wings).

   4) There is an alar foramen in ungulates which transmits the ventral branch of the first cervical nerve through the wing. In the carnivores, the foramen is incomplete and is represented only as the alar notch.

   5) The ox does not have a transverse foramen in the atlas and it may be absent in the pig.

c. The second cervical vertebra (C2) is called the axis and has a very well-developed spinous process. It has the following specific features:

   1) The body has a cranial projection called the dens which articulates with the atlas. Developmentally, the dens represents part of the body of the atlas.

   2) The axis is the longest vertebra.

d. In the third through the sixth cervical vertebrae, the transverse process has a cranial projection termed the costal process. This latter process is the cervical homologue of a rib.

e. The sixth cervical vertebra has an especially well developed part of the transverse process termed the ventral lamina.

f. The seventh cervical vertebra has costal fovea for the heads of the first pair of ribs on the caudal part of its body. It has no transverse foramina (except in the pig).

2. Thoracic vertebrae

   a. Thoracic vertebrae are characterized by short bodies, long spinous processes, short transverse processes, and each of them bears a pair of ribs. The heads of the ribs articulate with foveae on the bodies of the vertebrae and the tubercles articulate with foveae on the transverse processes.

   b. The spinous processes of most of the thoracic vertebrae are inclined caudally, but near the caudal aspect of the thoracic

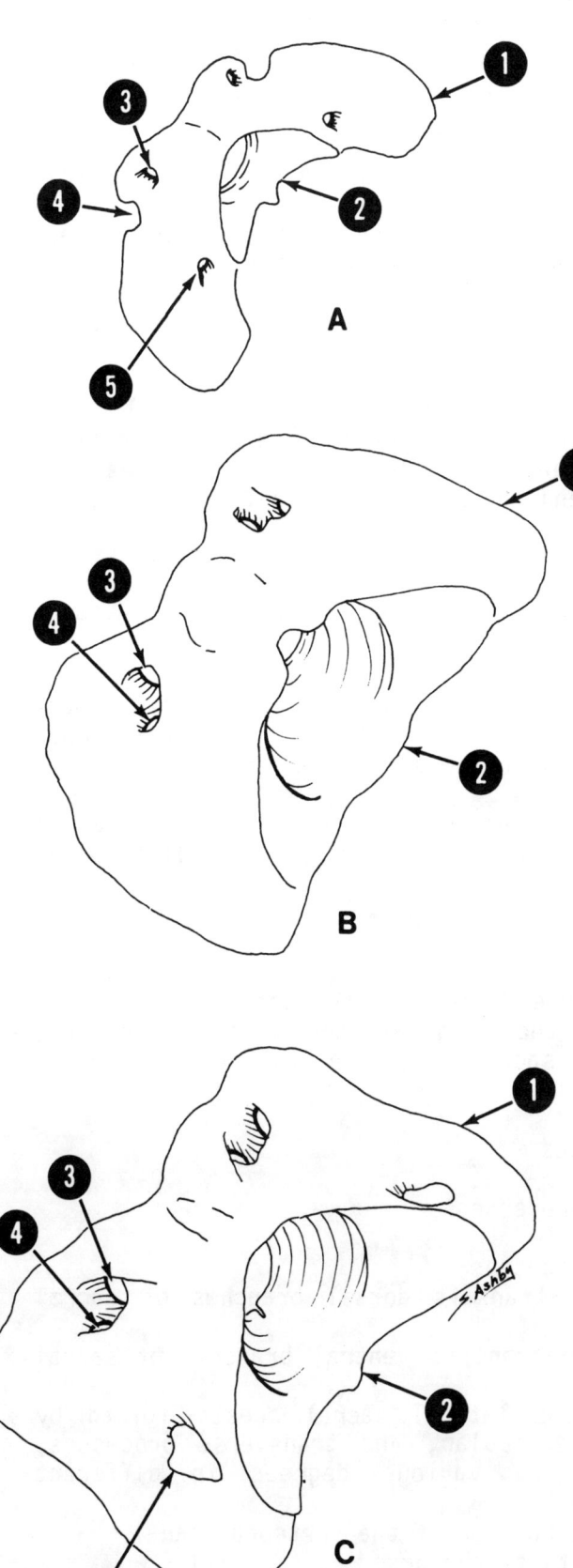

Figure 18-2

Features of the Atlas in the Dog (A), Ox (B), and Horse (C). (Caudodorsolateral aspect)

1. wing
2. ventral arch
3. lateral vertebral foramen
4. alar notch (dog); alar foramen (ox, horse)
5. transverse foramen (absent in ox)

region the inclination changes to a cranial orientation. The thoracic vertebrae with the most vertically oriented spine is termed the anticlinal vertebra and is usually T11 in dogs.

    c. Mammillary processes are small prominences for muscular attachment. They are present on all but the first few thoracic vertebrae and are also found on the lumbar, sacral, and caudal vertebrae. Initially, they occur on the transverse processes, but near the caudal aspect of the thoracic region they become associated with the cranial articular processes and remain in that position throughout the rest of the vertebral column.

    d. Accessory processes are small prominences on the caudal aspects of the pedicles in carnivores (Fig. 18-1/8). They occur from the middle (or caudal) thoracic region to the fifth or sixth lumbar vertebrae. They are best developed near the thoracolumbar junction and may be observed radiographically.

3. Lumbar vertebrae

    a. The lumbar vertebrae are characterized by long transverse processes which are directed cranially in carnivores.

    b. In the horse, the transverse processes of the last few lumbar vertebrae articulate with each other. Those of the last lumbar vertebra also articulate with the sacrum.

    c. Five lumbar vertebrae have been reported in several species of equidae (domestic horse, donkey, ass, mule, Przewalski horse) [3].

4. Sacral vertebrae

    a. The sacral vertebrae fuse into a single bony mass (sacrum) which articulates with the wings of the ilia to form the sacroiliac joint. The sacrum has the following specific features (Fig. 18-3) [1]:

        dorsal and pelvic surfaces
        base--cranial aspect
            cranial articular processes
        apex--caudal aspect
            caudal articular processes
        dorsal sacral foramina--transmit dorsal branches of sacral spinal nerves
        ventral sacral foramina--transmit ventral branches of sacral spinal nerves
        median, intermediate, and lateral sacral crests--formed by fusion of spinous, articular, and transverse processes, respectively (occur to various degrees in different species)
        sacral canal--the sacral portion of the vertebral canal
        wings--the lateral aspects of the base
        auricular surfaces - the surfaces which articulate with the ilia

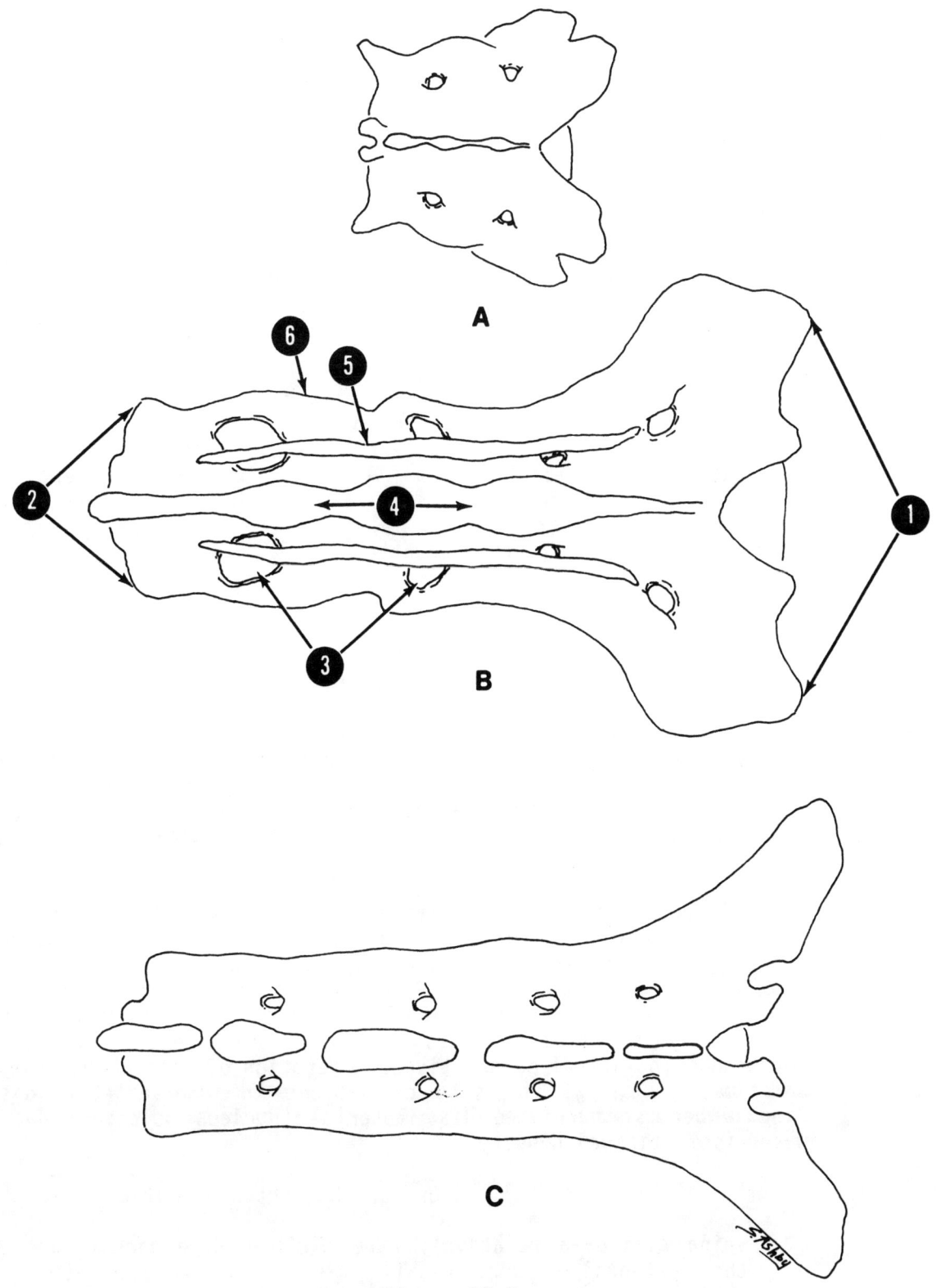

Figure 18-3

Sacrum of the Dog (A), Ox (B), and Horse (C) (dorsal surface)

1. base (cranial aspect)
2. apex (caudal aspect)
3. dorsal sacral foramina
4. median sacral crest (ox)
5. intermediate sacral crest
6. lateral sacral crest

5. Caudal vertebrae

   a. The caudal vertebrae get progressively smaller and lose their characteristic features.

   b. Hemal processes are paired ventral projections from the caudal vertebrae which can be identified in all species but are particularly prominent in cattle [1]. They form a channel which transmits the median sacral vessels. In cattle, a few of these (usually two of the Cd2-Cd5 series) are so well developed that they meet ventrally to form a complete hemal arch (Fig. 18-4). In the dog, separate (not fused to vertebrae) hemal arch bones are associated with one or more of the third to eighth caudal vertebrae (Fig. 18-4). Left and right bones often fuse to form a single V-shaped bone. Vertebrae further caudally have separate left and right hemal processes fused to the parent bone [2].

C. Clinical considerations

   1. In evaluating radiographs for signs of intervertebral disc disease, a narrowed or "wedged" space between adjacent vertebral bodies (disc space) is considered suspect. Because those spaces not in line with the central ray will always appear narrower than they really are, a space considered to be narrower than normal is judged to be so by comparing it with the adjacent ones cranially and caudally. Mineralized intervertebral discs may indicate old lesions and/or be age-related, and are usually considered to be incidental findings.

   2. The well-developed ventral laminae of the transverse processes of the sixth cervical vertebra in carnivores should not be mistaken for a foreign body in a lateral radiograph of the cervical region.

   3. The radiographic silhouettes of the intervertebral foramina in the lumbar region of carnivores have a radiolucent "horsehead" appearance in lateral perspectives. Alteration of this normal shape sometimes occurs at the site of lesions in intervertebral disc disease because herniated disc material (nucleus pulposus) has a water (soft tissue) density.

   4. A number of developmental lesions of the vertebral column occur:

      a. spina bifida--a relatively rare cleft in the dorsal part of the vertebral column, usually with a saclike protrusion of meninges (meningocele) over the defect [4].
      b. hemivertebra--a failure of proper ossification of a vertebral body, resulting in a misshapen (often wedge-shaped) vertebra. This may be insignificant clinically or present neurological signs [5].
      c. curvatures (bowing) of the vertebral column dorsally (kyphosis), laterally (scoliosis), or ventrally (lordosis). These

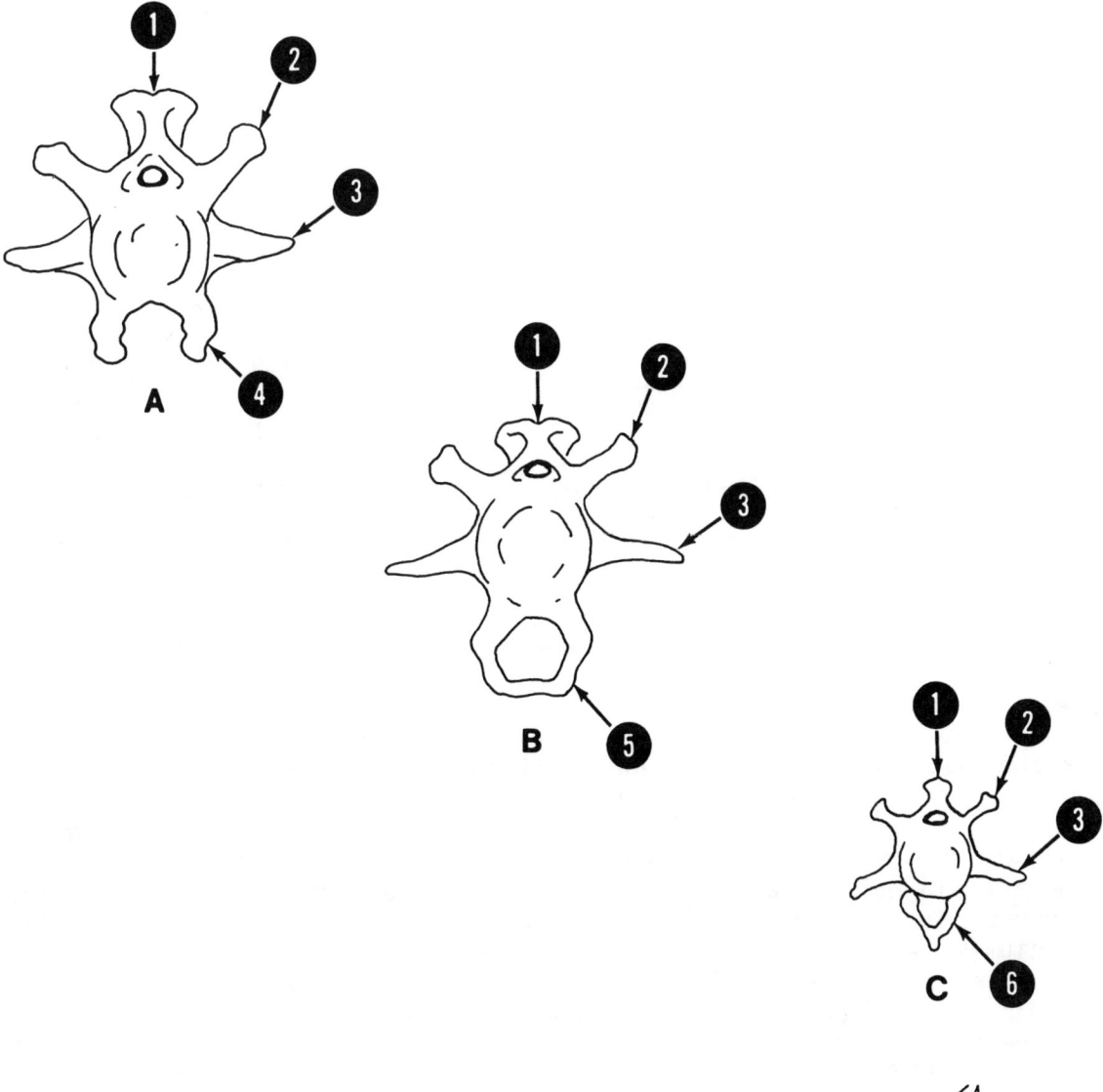

Figure 18-4

Hemal Processes and Hemal Arches
Associated with Caudal Vertebrae (cranial aspects)

        A.   Cd2 of ox
        B.   Cd4 of ox
        C.   Cd4 of dog

1. Spinous process
2. Cranial articular process
3. Transverse process
4. Hemal process
5. Hemal arch
6. Hemal arch bones (fused)

Table 18-1

Vertebral Formulae

Equus caballus	C7 T18 L6 S5 Cd15-21
Bos taurus (and *Bos indicus*)	C7 T13 L6 S5 Cd18-20
Ovis aries and *Capra hircus*	C7 T13 L6-7 S4 Cd16-18
Sus scrofa domestica	C7 T14-15 L6-7 S4 Cd20-23
Canis familiaris and *Felis catus*	C7 T13 L7 S3 Cd20-24

Notes:

1. All domestic mammals have the same number (7) of cervical vertebrae.

2. The "standard" number of thoracic vertebrae is 13, but pigs normally have at least 14, and some long bodied breeds often have 15 (as many as 17 have been recorded). The horse usually has 18 thoracic vertebrae.

3. The typical numbers of lumbar vertebrae (6 or 7) and sacral vertebrae (3 to 5) are often difficult to remember in the various species. An artificial memory aid which may be useful is to list the domestic species in order of decreasing size (as above) and then categorize them as large (horse and ox), medium-sized (sheep, goat, and pig) and small (dog and cat). The large animals have 6 lumbar vertebrae. The medium-sized animals have 6-7, and the small animals have 7 (L for lumbar and L for larger). In other words, the numbers of lumbar vertebrae get larger from the top to the bottom of the list. Similarly, the numbers of sacral vertebrae get smaller from the top to the bottom (S for sacral, S for smaller; the large animals have 5, the medium-sized animals have 4, and the small animals have 3).

4. The numbers of caudal vertebrae are quite variable. A useful number to remember for most species is 20. Sheep and goats have fewer as do some breeds of dogs and cats.

5. In many individual animals, variations in the vertebral formulae appear. In most cases, these are inconsequential clinically.

may require decompression and/or immobilization techniques [6].
- d. cervical vertebral instability (spondylolisthesis, wobblers) a subluxation of cervical vertebrae thought to be related to improper development and/or articulation of some of the articular processes. This condition affects dogs (especially Dobermans and Great Danes) and horses, and often has significant neurological signs [7]. The affected vertebrae (most often C3-C4 in horses and C5-C6 or C6-C7 in dogs) may be surgically fused [6]. In horses, a fusion procedure has been devised which involves insertion of a large plug of ilium into a hole drilled into the ventral aspect of the junction of the involved vertebral bodies [8].
- e. block vertebra--fusion of two or more vertebral bodies, often without clinical signs [6].
- f. transitional vertebrae--vertebrae adjacent to junctions of major regions of the vertebral column which have characteristics of the adjacent region. For example, the seventh cervical vertebra of some dogs has a cervical rib [4], and some animals have one less thoracic vertebra and one more lumbar vertebra than their typical counterparts. This condition may be termed "lumbarization" of the last thoracic vertebra. "Lumbarization" of T13 or S1, and "sacralization" of L7 have also been reported. "Sacralization" of Cd1 is very common in dogs [4].
- g. sacrococcygeal dysgenesis in Manx cats, which varies from spina bifida to complete agenesis, has been described. Locomotor disturbances and fecal/urinary incontinence may be present [9].
- h. atlantoaxial subluxation--most common in toy breeds of dogs. This condition may cause severe neurological signs and even death. Atlantoaxial subluxation is usually caused by congenital absence of the dens, but it may also occur as a result of a fractured dens or a ligamentous injury between the atlas and axis. It is corrected by wiring the atlas to the axis [6].

5. Acquired lesions of the vertebral column may result in spinal cord concussion (a traumatic injury with no radiographic signs that usually spontaneously resolves) or spinal cord contusion (damage characterized by edema, hemorrhage, and necrosis). Contusions may include hematorachis (hemorrhage into the subarachnoid or epidural space) and/or hematomyelia (hemorrhage into the spinal cord) [6]. The major types of acquired lesions include:

   a. fractures
   b. luxations and subluxations
   c. neoplasia
   d. degenerative lesions [6]

   1) intervertebral disc disease--a condition characterized by neurological deficits or signs resulting from compressed spinal cord or nerve injury from a ruptured intervertebral disc. These are often treated by decompression hemilaminectomies and/or fenestrations. (For a more thorough discussion, see Part III, Ligaments of the Vertebral Column).

2) spondylosis (deformans)--a lesion characterized by osteophytic spurs and/or bridges between adjacent vertebrae. The lesions usually involve the bodies of the vertebrae and are most common in the caudal thoracic and lumbar column.

3) spondylitis, spinal osteoarthritis--inflammation of the vertebral column resulting in destructive and proliferative lesions. If the intervertebral disc is involved, the lesion is termed discospondylitis.

4) dural ossification (ossifying pachymeningitis)--osseous metaplasia of the dura mater.

6. Regional anesthesia involving the spinal cord has considerable clinical use, particularly in large animals. The two general techniques are epidural injections and subarachnoid (spinal) injections. Epidural injections are made inside the vertebral canal but outside the dura mater. The anesthetic blocks the nerve trunks at the point of exit from the dura mater at the intervertebral foramina. Subarachnoid injections are made into the cerebrospinal fluid of the subarachnoid space (slightly deeper). This technique is not widely used in veterinary medicine for anesthesia, but is popular for the injection of contrast medium for myelography.

   a. Low (caudal) epidural. This block is usually made at Cd1-Cd2, but the sacrocaudal and other intercaudal junctions may also be used. The block does not affect motor control of the pelvic limbs, but does desensitize the tail, anus, vulva, perineum, caudal thighs, and part of the sacral region (i.e., "tail head" and surrounding area) [10]. If too much anesthetic is given, the motor nerves of the pelvic limbs may be affected as the anesthetic infiltrates cranially, and the animal may go down [11].

      1) Horse--inject Cd1-Cd2 about 10 cm cranial to the base of the tail. The needle should be angled ventrocranially about 10-30° from vertical [12].

      2) Ox--inject Cd1-Cd2 (at the most movable point when pumping the tail). The injection site is about 10 cm cranial to a line connecting the ischiatic tuberosities and the needle should be angled ventrocranially at about 45°.

      3) Sheep--inject 3-4 ml at S4-Cd1. The needle is held almost vertically. The procedure is used primarily in obstetrical cases.

      4) Dog--inject at S3-Cd1 or Cd1-Cd2 for surgeries involving the tail.

   b. High (cranial, lumbar) epidural. The lumbosacral junction is used for this block, and the general areas desensitized include the inguinal regions, flanks, prepuce and scrotum, inguinal mammary glands, and part of the lumbar region. High epidural blocks are more dangerous than low epidurals because uncompensated hypotension can result. They are primarily used for obstetrical and genital surgeries in the various species. The animal becomes ataxic caudally. If the dura is accidently penetrated (as noted by the appearance of CSF in the hub of the needle), only one-half of the dose should be given. A full epidural dose can be fatal if given subdurally. Intentional subarachnoid insertions can be used to withdraw samples of cerebrospinal fluid in ungulates, but in carnivores, the cisterna magna is a better site for CSF sampling [10].

1) Horse--the L-S junction is located 8-10 cm caudal to the level of the tuber coxae. A long (20 cm) needle with a stylet is recommended. Penetration of the yellow lig. can be felt at 10-12 cm. Some clinicians prefer not to use this block in horses because the animals occasionally become so ataxic that they injure themselves. (Horses rise from a prone position front legs first and may panic if their hind quarters remain immobile).

2) Ox--the palpable depression at the L-S junction is located at the same level as that in the horse.

3) Dog--the L-S junction is just caudal to the level of the iliac crests. The cord terminates at L6-L7, so there is little danger of penetrating the dura as is possible in the horse and ox.*

4) Pig and cat--the technique can be done, but there is greater danger of hypotension and circulatory collapse than with other species [10,13,14]

c. Lumbar epidural. This block may be used in cattle to obtain flank anesthesia without loss of motor control to the limbs. The L1-L2 junction is commonly injected (T13-L1 may be used). The needle is inserted just off the midline to avoid the thick supraspinous ligament. The injection is made at a level about 1-2 cm caudal to the cranial edge of the transverse process of L2 [11]. Pain is associated with penetration of the yellow ligament [10].

---

*The spinal cord is shorter than the vertebral canal in all species and is continued caudally after its termination by the cauda equina. The length differential occurs because the spinal cord segments in the lumbar and sacral portions of the cord are shorter than the corresponding vertebrae (the part of the cord which gives rise to the last pair of the lumbar spinal nerves, for example, is shorter than the last lumbar vertebra). "This apparent shortening of the spinal cord (medulla spinalis) is called the ascent of the cord (ascensus medullae)" [11].

7. Paravertebral lumbar anesthesia. This technique may be used in cattle to block the flank. Spinal nerves T13, L1, L2, and sometimes L3 are blocked 5 cm off the dorsal midline, and anesthetic is injected both above and below the transverse processes (to get the involved dorsal and the ventral branches of the nerves) in the following loci (Fig. 18-5):

> T13--along caudal border of the last rib
>
> L1, L2, and L3--along the caudal border of the transverse processes of L1, L2, and L3

This original technique of Farquharson [15] has the undesirable side effect of paralyzing the muscles of the back [11]. A modification of this technique, first described by Magda [16] and later by Cakala [17], is easier to perform. In the modified technique, anesthetic is injected at the ends of the transverse processes rather than 5 cm off the midline. The ends of the transverse processes of L1, L2, and L4 are used as markers to block spinal nerves T13, L1, and L2 respectively. Anesthetic is injected dorsal and ventral to the ends of the processes.

8. Line and inverted L blocks. Regional anesthesia may also be used to locally anesthetize the flank. The basis of the inverted L (also called 7 or reverse 7) is that the involved spinal nerves course caudally and ventrally as they innervate the abdominal wall.

III. LIGAMENTS OF THE VERTEBRAL COLUMN

The ligaments of the vertebral column stabilize the intervertebral articulations and are therefore important in maintaining integrity of the spinal cord.

A. General features [18]

Unofficially, there are two groups of ligaments based on their length:

1. "Long" ligaments

   supraspinous lig.--the dense connective tissue which courses along the tips of the spinous processes of the thoracic and lumbar vertebrae.
   nuchal lig.--the dense connective tissue extending from the cranial thoracic spines to the axis (dog) or skull (ungulates). It is often considered as a cranial continuation of the supraspinous ligament, but this concept is not quite valid, especially in the ox (see B-4 below).
   dorsal longitudinal lig.--the dense connective tissue which courses along the dorsal aspect of the vertebral bodies.
   ventral longitudinal lig.--the dense connective tissue which courses along the ventral aspect of the vertebral bodies. It is often quite thin and hard to identify.

2. "Short" ligaments

   intervertebral discs--these fibrocartilaginous joints occur between the bodies of the adjacent vertebrae (except C1-C2).

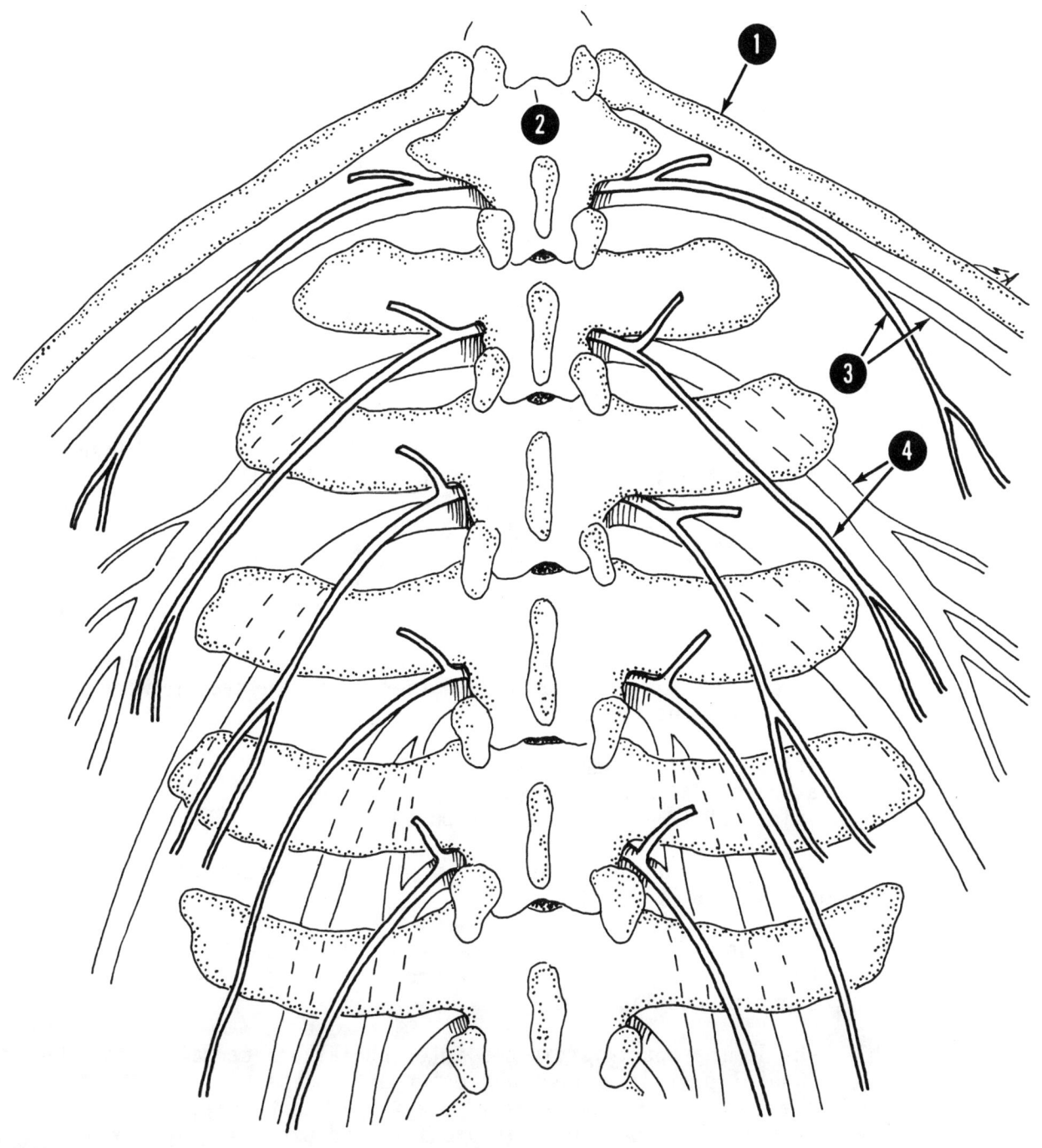

Figure 18-5

Relationship of Spinal Nerves T13-L4 to Their Respective Vertebrae in an Ox
(dorsal aspect)

1. Rib 13
2. Vertebra T13
3. Dorsal and ventral branches of spinal nerve T13
4. Dorsal and ventral branches of spinal nerve L1

After Habel, 1981 [11]

nucleus pulposus--the gelatinous inner part.
anulus fibrosus--the fibrocartilaginous peripheral part.
interspinous ligg.--these occur between spinous processes of adjacent vertebrae and are best developed in the thoracic region.
intertransverse ligg.--these occur between the transverse processes of the lumbar vertebrae.
yellow ligg. (ligg. flavum)--these join the arches of adjacent vertebrae.
intercapital ("conjugal") ligg. - these join the heads of a given pair of ribs passing transversely between the dorsal aspect of the anulus fibrosus and the dorsal longitudinal ligament (Fig. 18-6).

B. Comparative features

1. The cat has no nuchal ligament.

2. In the dog, the nuchal ligament is paired, cordlike, and attaches cranially to the spine of the axis (Fig. 18-7A) [2].

3. In the horse, the nuchal ligament has a single cordlike (funicular) part (formed by fusion of left and right primordia), and paired, sheetlike (laminar) parts (Fig. 18-7C). The funicular part extends cranially from the spinous processes at the withers (T2-T8) to attach to the occipital bone. The paired laminar parts extend ventrally from the funicular part (and from T2 and T3 spines) to attach to the spines of C2-C6. There are bursae between the funicular part and the [18]:

    atlas--cranial nuchal bursa
    axis--caudal nuchal bursa
    spines of T2-4--supraspinous bursa

4. In the ox, the nuchal ligament is similar to that of the horse except (Fig. 18-7B) [18]:

    a. the funicular part is paired and extends well back into the thoracic region. It is attached to each side of the supraspinous ligament.

    b. the laminar part is divided into cranial and caudal parts. The cranial part is paired and extends from the funicular part to the spines of the cranial cervical vertebrae (except the atlas). The caudal part is unpaired and extends from the spine of T1 to the spines of the caudal cervical vertebrae.

C. Clinical considerations

1. Inflammation of the cranial nuchal ("atlantal") bursa of horses may cause considerable pain. The condition is commonly called "poll evil," and resection of the ligamentum nuchae may be indicated for drainage [11].

2. Supraspinous bursitis in horses is commonly called "fistulous withers." It may require surgical exploration and drainage and particular precautions should be taken since Brucella spp. as well as other pathogens can be isolated from many cases.

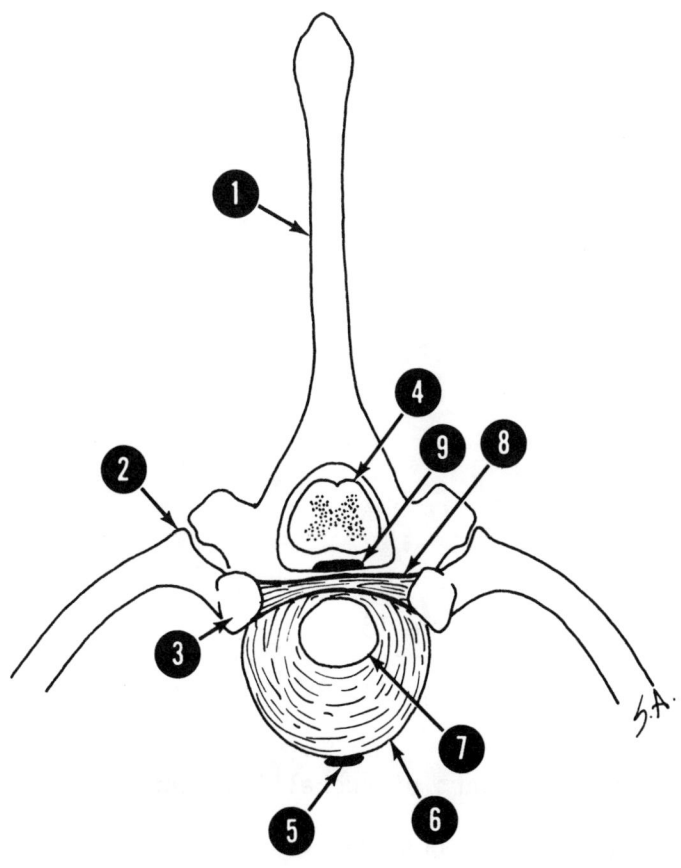

Figure 18-6

Selected Ligaments of the Vertebral Column
(transverse section of mid-thoracic region of a dog, cranial aspect)

1. spinous process of thoracic vertebra
2. tubercle of rib (articulating with transverse process of its parent vertebra)
3. head of rib (articulating with the cranial aspect of the body of its parent vertebra and with the caudal aspect of the next cranial vertebra)
4. spinal cord in vertebral canal
5. ventral longitudinal ligament (transverse section)
6. anulus fibrosus of intervertebral disc
7. nucleus pulposus of intervertebral disc
8. intercapital ligament
9. dorsal longitudinal ligament (transverse section)

Figure 18-7

Nuchal Ligament of the Dog (A), Ox (B), and Horse (C)

1. funicular part of nuchal ligament
2. supraspinous ligament
3. paired laminar part of nuchal ligament
4. unpaired laminar part of nuchal ligament (ox only)
5. cranial nuchal bursa (horse only)
6. caudal nuchal bursa (horse only)
7. supraspinous bursa (horse only)

After Nickel, Schummer, and Seiferle, 1954 [19]

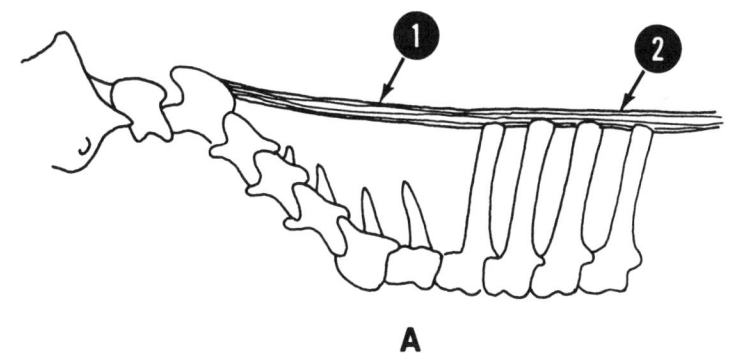

A

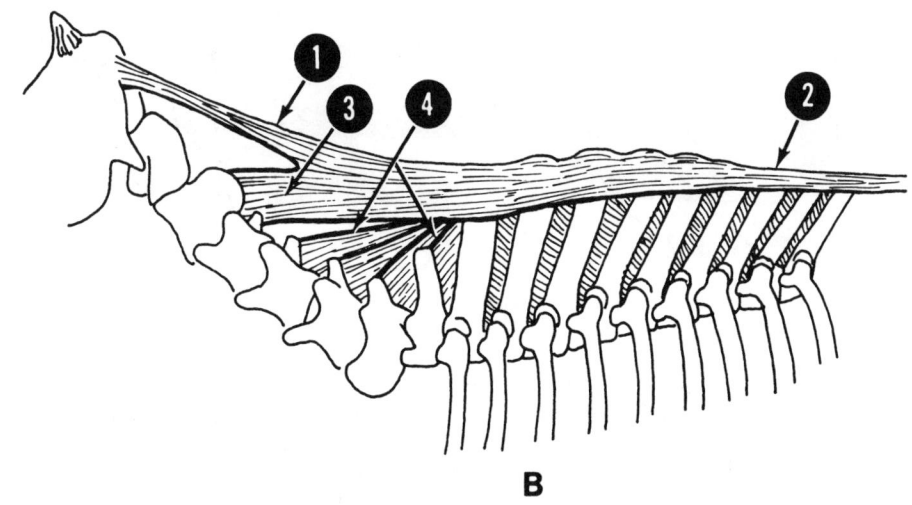

B

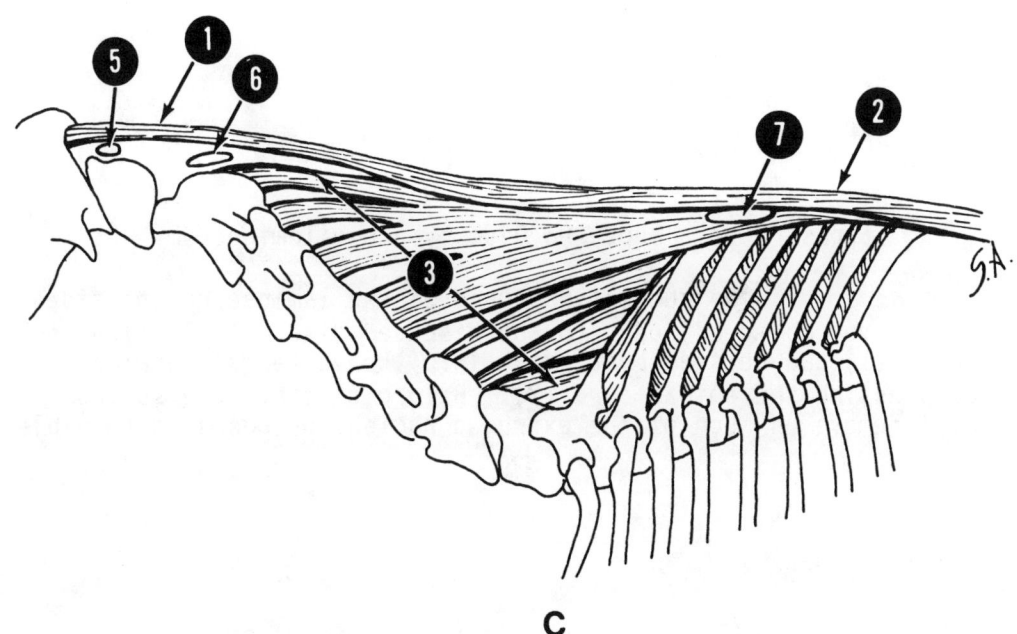

C

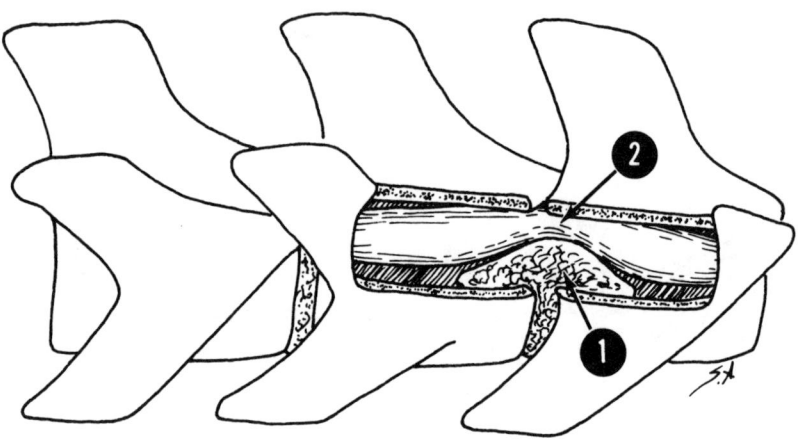

Figure 18-8

Exposure of a Ruptured Disc by a Hemilaminectomy

The surgeon has removed the laminae on one side of the vertebrae adjacent to the diseased disc. The nucleus pulposus (1) can be seen protruding into the vertebral canal and compressing the spinal cord (2). Before closing, the surgeon will remove as much of the extruded nucleus pulposus as possible.

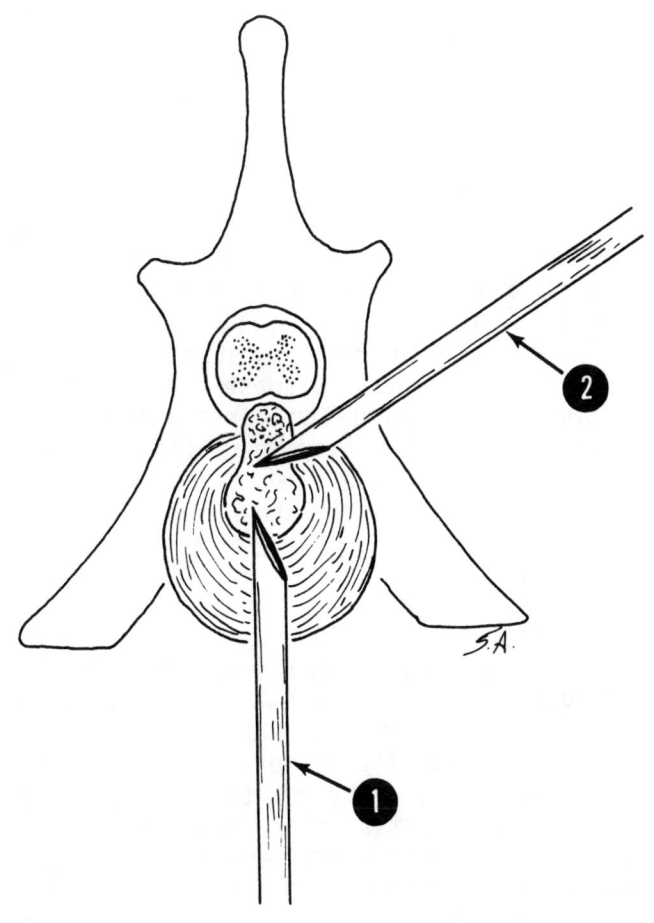

Figure 18-9

Surgical Fenestration of Anulus Fibrosus of a Diseased Disc
Ventrally (1) and Dorsolaterally (2)

As much of the nucleus pulposus as can be reached is removed.

3. Intervertebral disc disease in dogs usually results from dorsal or dorsolateral protrusion of the nucleus pulposus through the anulus fibrosus. Protrusions laterally or ventrally do not usually cause serious clinical signs because they exert no pressure on the spinal cord or spinal nerve roots. Unfortunately, the anulus fibrosus is thinnest dorsally and is more likely to rupture in that area. The highest incidence of i.v. disc disease occurs near the thoracolumbar junction (T11 to L1-L2) and in the cervical region. The main part of the thoracic region is rarely affected, and this is probably related to the presence of the intercapital ligaments which pass over and physically reinforce the dorsal part of the anulus fibrosus (intercapital ligaments are usually not present on the first 2 pair of ribs, nor on the last 2 pair). Dogs with mild neurological signs may respond to conservative treatment, but severe cases should be operated without delay. The surgical objective in i.v. disc disease is to eliminate pressure on the spinal cord by removing the dorsolateral aspects of the vertebral arches of the adjacent vertebrae (laminectomy or hemilaminectomy), and/or by removing the remaining nucleus pulposus through a surgical incision into the dorsolateral or ventral anulus fibrosus (fenestration). A large number of specific procedures have been developed [6].

   a. Hemilaminectomies (removal of the left or right half of the dorsal vertebral arch) are more popular than laminectomies because they accomplish the same purpose with fewer complications. After a dorsal midline (usually just off the midline) incision, the fibers of the transversospinalis muscle are separated just lateral to the spinous processes and then further blunt dissection is made to expose the dorsum of the vertebrae. The laminae and parts of the pedicles of the two vertebrae adjacent to the involved disc are removed, and often this osteotomy is extended cranially and caudally over the adjacent discs as well. The bone is usually removed with rongeurs and the initial entry may be facilitated by rongeuring off the articular processes and then trephining the arch at that point. This initial hole is then expanded. The vertebral venous sinuses on the ventral and ventrolateral aspects of the vertebral canal should be avoided if possible. The spinal cord may be touched, but no pressure should be applied (Fig. 18-8).

   b. Fenestrations are made in the anulus fibrosus. The objective of this surgery for ruptured discs is to remove any nucleus pulposus remaining within the anulus. Discs adjacent to herniated ones may be prophylactically fenestrated. In the cervical region, a ventral approach is often used--partly because the vertebral vessels coursing through the transverse foramina are bothersome. In other areas of the vertebral column, a dorsolateral approach is used and the procedure may be combined with a hemilaminectomy (Fig. 18-9). Because routine fenestrations may not be adequately decompressive, a number of variations have been developed. A currently popular one is the so called "ventral slot" procedure used in the cervical region. In this technique, a pneumatic drill is used to cut a longitudinal slot in the ventral aspects of the vertebral bodies. Disc material is removed through the opening this slot makes in the ventral aspect of the anulus fibrosus of the involved disc(s) [6].

4. In cases of cervical vertebral instability (c.v.i.) in horses (wobblers), a dorsal hemilaminectomy technique has been perfected by Wagner and Grant at Washington State University. They use the paired laminar parts of the nuchal ligament to advantage in their approach by passing between them--a relatively bloodless and "simple" procedure. To prevent hemorrhage into the exposed vertebral canal which may cause postoperative complications, they hang the animals by all four feet for a short time before recovery to effect better drainage [20].

5. Locating a spinal lesion in carnivores radiographically and then finding and operating the correct locus presents some special problems. The following facts may be helpful in this regard:

   a. The heads of most pairs of ribs articulate with facets on the cranial part of the body of their respective vertebra and with the caudal part of the body of the adjacent vertebra cranially. For example, the heads of the first ribs articulate with the cranial aspect of T1 as well as with the caudal aspect of C7; the heads of the second ribs articulate with T2 and with T1, etc. This same relationship is valid throughout most of the thorax. However, the last 2 or 3 pairs of ribs articulate further back on the bodies of their vertebrae and each is associated with only one vertebra.

   b. The palpable caudal border of the last rib is located at the same level as the caudal aspect of L2.

   c. The seventh lumbar vertebra is between the wings of the ilia, and the palpable spine just cranial to the ilial wings is L6.

   d. The cranial landmark for ventral cervical fenestrations can be found using the wing of the atlas. The ventral tubercle on the ventral arch of the atlas is located at the level of the caudal border of the wing of the atlas. The caudal extent of the ventral tubercle of the atlas marks the atlantoaxial joint (a synovial joint). Successive intervertebral junctions are marked by the subtle ventral tubercles located on the caudal aspects of the cervical vertebral bodies [6]. Cervical discs are oriented in oblique planes with the dorsal aspect of the disc further cranial than the ventral aspect.

References

1. International Committee on Veterinary Gross Anatomical Nomenclature. 1983. Nomina Anatomica Veterinaria, third ed. Published by the Committee, Ithaca, New York.

2. Evans, H. E., and G. C. Christensen. 1979. Miller's Anatomy of the Dog, second ed. W. B. Saunders, Philadelphia.

3. Stecher, R. M. 1961. Anatomical variations of the spine in the horse. J. Mammalogy 43:205-219.

4. Kealy, J. K. 1979. Diagnostic Radiology in the Dog and Cat. W. B. Saunders, Philadelphia.

5. Morgan, J. P. 1968. Congenital anomalies of the vertebral column of the dog: a study of the incidence and significance based on a radiographic and morphologic study. J. Am. Vet. Radiol. Soc. 9:21-29.

6. Hoerlein, B. F., ed. 1978. Canine Neurology, third ed. W. B. Saunders, Philadelphia.

7. Wright, F., J. Rest, and A. Palmer. 1973. Ataxia of the Great Dane caused by stenosis of the cervical vertebral canal: Comparison with similar conditions in the Basset Hound, Doberman Pinscher, Ridgeback, and the Thoroughbred horse. Vet. Rec. 92(1):1-5.

8. Wagner, P. C. 1979. Ilial bone plugs for cervical vertebral instability in horses. Paper presented at the Conference of the Veterinary Orthopedic Society, Vail, Colorado.

9. Leipold, H. W., K. Huston, B. Blauch, and M. Guffy. 1974. Congenital defects of the caudal vertebral column and spinal cord in Manx cats. JAVMA 164(5):520-523.

10. McFarland, L. Z. 1970. Veterinary Surgical Anatomy. Published by the author, Davis, California.

11. Habel, R. E. 1981. Applied Veterinary Anatomy, second ed. Published by the author, Ithaca, New York.

12. Heath, E. H., and V. S. Myers. 1972. Topographic anatomy for caudal anesthesia in the horse. VM/SAC 67:1237-1239.

13. Noordsy, J. L. 1978. Food Animal Surgery. Published by the author, Manhattan, Kansas.

14. Getty, R. 1963. Epidural anesthesia in the hog: Its technique and applications. Proc. AVMA:88-98.

15. Farquharson, J. 1940. Paravertebral lumbar anesthesia in the bovine species. JAVMA 97:54-57.

16. Magda, I. I. 1949. Prowodnikowaja anestiezija pri opieracijach na ziwotie krupnogo rogatogo skota. Vietierinarija 21:7.

17. Cakala, S. 1961. A technic for the paravertebral lumbar block in cattle. *Cornell Vet.* 51:64-67.

18. Getty, R. 1975. *Sisson and Grossman's The Anatomy of the Domestic Animals*, fifth ed. W. B. Saunders, Philadelphia.

19. Nickel, R., A. Schummer, and E. Seiferle. 1954. *Lehrbuch der Anatomic der Haustiere. Bewegungsapparat.* Paul Parey, Berlin.

20. Wagner, P. C. 1981. Dorsal cervical hemilaminectomy in the horse. Paper presented at the Conference of the Veterinary Orthopedic Society, Snowbird, Utah.

HEAD

The head is the most complex part of the body anatomically. It not only houses the brain and the organs for the special senses of vision, audition, olfaction, and gustation, but it also serves as the locus for the initial parts of the respiratory and digestive systems. In addition, it contains the greatest number and concentration of orifices, any one of which can serve as a portal of entry for potential pathogens.

I. SKULL

The skeletal framework of the head is composed of about 50 individual bones, many of which are complex in shape, are difficult to visualize in situ, and are generally unfamiliar when isolated from the rest of the skull. When articulated, their boundaries often appear to vanish because of ossification of the sutures which initially separated them, and they are perforated by a bewildering number of foramina, traversed in life by vessels and nerves. The skull has a cranial (neural) region which encloses the brain and the organs for sight, hearing, and equilibrium, and a facial region which houses the organs for smell and the teeth. The facial region varies considerably among the various breeds of dogs, but it is fairly uniform with each of the other domestic mammals. Most of the approximately 50 bones of the head are paired. The vomer, ethmoid, and occipital bones are unpaired.

A. Features of the skull as a whole (these involve more than one bone) [1,2]

cranial cavity--the space where the brain is located
rostral, middle, and caudal cranial fossae--the areas occupied by the olfactory lobes, main part of the brain, and cerebellum, respectively
temporal fossa--the area where the temporal muscle attaches
temporal line--the ridge of the frontal, parietal, and occipital bones which marks the dorsal aspect of the temporal fossa
zygomatic arch--the bony bridge formed by the zygomatic, temporal, and maxillary bones
jugular foramen ⎫
tympano-occipital fissure ⎬ all species have a jugular foramen through which cranial nerves 9, 10, and 11 leave the cranial cavity. In the carnivores and ruminants, its external opening is the tympano-occipital fissure
foramen lacerum--transmits the internal carotid a. (and the mandibular nerve in the pig and horse)
pterygopalatine fossa--the area which funnels down to form the maxillary foramen
osseous palate
    major palatine foramen--a vascular channel
        palatine fissure--the large paired osseous defect near the rostral aspect of the osseous palate
nasal cavity
    osseous nasal septum--the bony part of the nasal septum

Figure 19-1

Bones of the Skull

A. Cat
B. Dog
C. Pig
D. Sheep
E. Ox
F. Horse

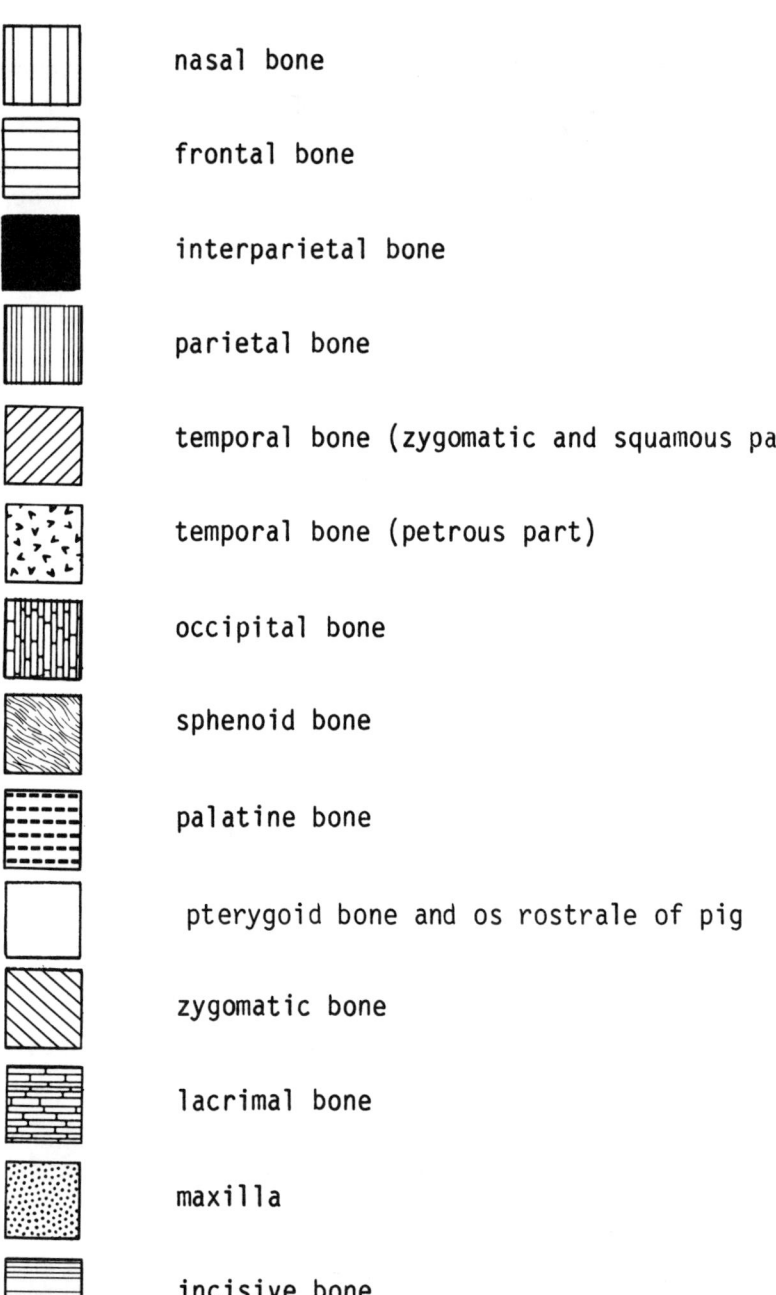

nasal bone

frontal bone

interparietal bone

parietal bone

temporal bone (zygomatic and squamous parts)

temporal bone (petrous part)

occipital bone

sphenoid bone

palatine bone

pterygoid bone and os rostrale of pig

zygomatic bone

lacrimal bone

maxilla

incisive bone

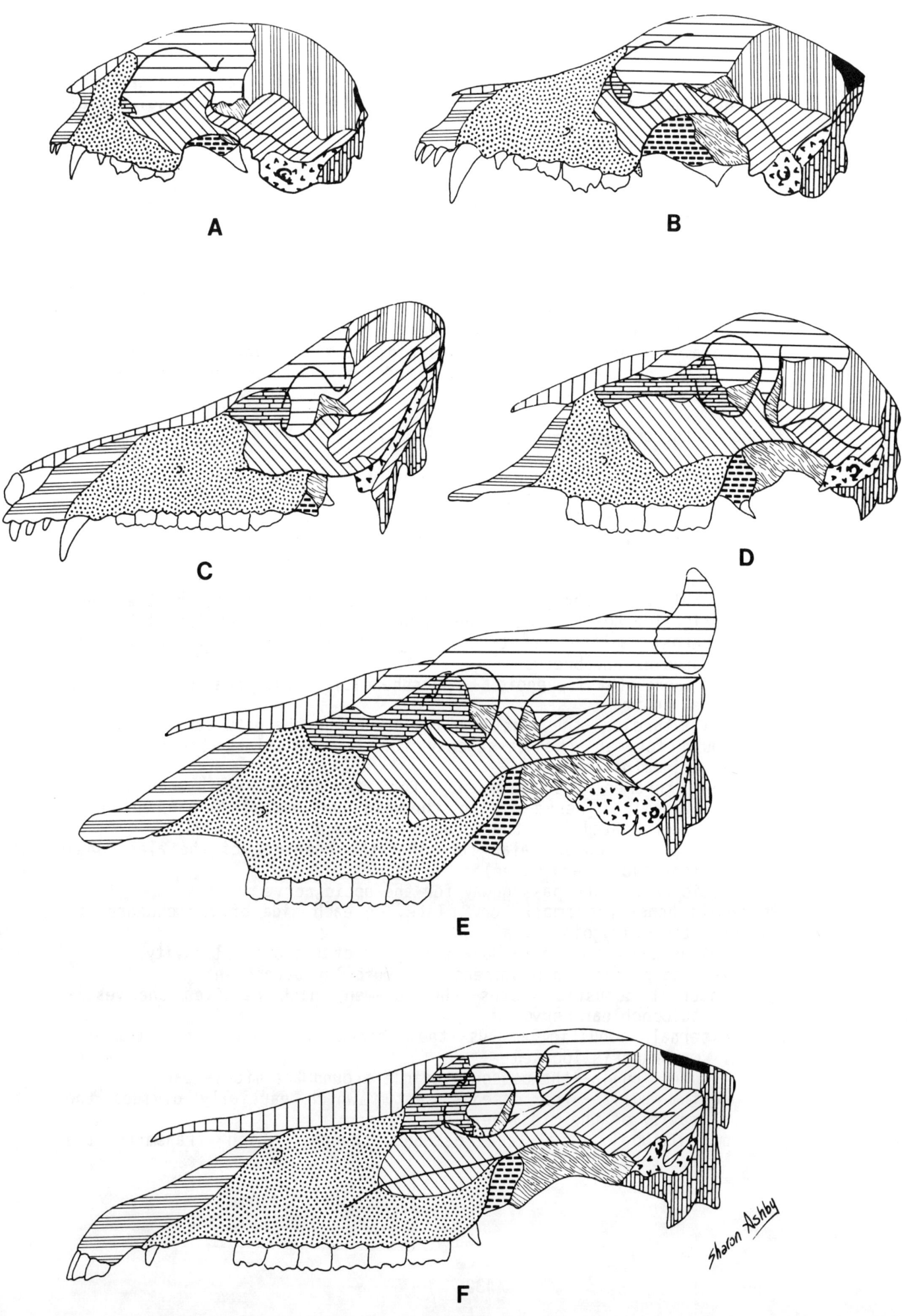

        dorsal, middle, ventral, and common nasal meatus--air passageways
        nasolacrimal canal--the bony canal that transmits the nasolacrimal duct
        choanae--the caudal nares
    orbit
        orbital lig. (carnivores and pig)--the band of connective tissue which completes the lateral rim of the orbit in the carnivores and pig. In the other domestic mammals, this structure is osseous and is formed by processes of the frontal bone as well as by parts of the zygomatic or temporal bones.
        orbital fissure (carnivores and horse)--the opening (just caudal to the optic canal) which transmits cranial nerves 3, 4, 5 (ophthalmic branch only), and 6
        foramen orbitorotundum (ox and pig)--a single orifice representing the combined orbital fissure and the round foramen (see sphenoid bone)

B.   Bones of the cranium (Figs. 19-1, 19-2) [1,2]

    Occipital bone--forms the caudal aspect of the cranial cavity
        foramen magnum--the opening which transmits the spinal cord
        occipital condyle--the portion which articulates with the atlas
        hypoglossal canal--the passageway for the hypoglossal nerve
        jugular process--the prominence for attachment of the digastricus m.
        nuchal crest--the prominent ridge on the caudal aspect of the bone
    Interparietal bone--the small bone just rostral to the occipital bone
        external sagittal crest--the ridge which develops with age in some species and breeds
    Sphenoid bone (basisphenoid + presphenoid)--forms the floor of the cranial cavity
        sella turcica--the portion which surrounds the pituitary gland
        round foramen--the passageway for the maxillary branch of the trigeminal nerve
        oval foramen--the passageway for the mandibular branch of the trigeminal nerve - (In the pig and horse, this opening is incorporated into the foramen lacerum.)
        rostral and caudal alar foramina--the openings of the alar canal (carnivores and horse)
        optic canal--the passageway for the optic nerve
    Pterygoid bone--the small bony plate, on each side of the choanae, to which the pterygoid mm. attach
    Temporal bone--forms the caudolateral part of the cranial cavity
        mastoid process--a prominence for muscular attachment
        internal acoustic meatus--the foramen which receives the vestibulocochlear nerve
        external acoustic meatus--the channel in which the tympanic membrane is located
        tympanic bulla--the osseous vesicle around the middle ear
        septum bullae--the osseous septum which partially divides the cavity of the middle ear
        musculotubal canal--the osseous channel which transmits the auditory tube

zygomatic process--the projection which forms the caudal part of the zygomatic arch
mandibular fossa--the depression which receives the head of the mandible
stylomastoid foramen--the hole which transmits the facial nerve
Parietal bone ⎰form the roof of the
Frontal bone ⎱cranial cavity
zygomatic process--the projection toward the zygomatic arch
cornual process--present only in some ruminants
Ethmoid bone--forms the rostral part of the cranial cavity
cribriform plate--perforated by numerous foramina for the olfactory nerves
ethmoid conchae ("turbinates")--the bony scrolls in the caudal aspect of the nasal cavity
dorsal nasal concha ("turbinate")--a rostral extension of one of the ethmoidal conchae
Vomer--forms part of the osseous nasal septum

C. Bones of the Face (Fig. 19-1, 19-2) [1,2]

Nasal bone--forms the osseous bridge of the nose
Lacrimal bone--forms the medial aspect of the orbit
lacrimal foramen and canal
fossa of the lacrimal sac
Maxilla--supports the superior cheek teeth and forms part of the osseous palate
infraorbital foramen--the opening which transmits the infraorbital nerve (rostral opening of the infraorbital canal)
alveolar juga--swellings around the roots of the teeth
maxillary foramen--the caudal opening of the infraorbital canal
lacrimal canal--the bony channel which transmits the nasolacrimal duct
zygomatic process--the bony process which forms the rostral extent of the zygomatic arch
Ventral nasal concha--the larger and better developed of the two major conchae ("turbinates")
Incisive bone--supports the superior incisors
Rostral bone--a bone which does not articulate with the rest of the skeleton. Found in the nose of pigs (os rostrale)
Palatine bone--the major osseous component of the hard palate
major and minor palatine foramina--vascular apertures in the osseous palate
Zygomatic bone--the major osseous component of the zygomatic arch
temporal process--the projection toward the temporal bone
frontal process--the projection toward the frontal bone
Mandible--the bone which supports all of the inferior teeth
body--the horizontal part
incisive part--the rostral part
molar part--the caudal part
mental foramina--passageways for the mental nerves
ramus--the vertical part
angle--the caudal border of the junction of the body and ramus

Figure 19-2

Major Features of the Canine Skull

    A.   Left aspect with zygomatic arch removed
    B.   Ventral aspect

1. Incisive bone
2. Masa bone
3. Infraorbital foramen (rostral opening of infraorbital canal)
4. Zygomatic process of frontal bone
5. Parietal bone
6. Interparietal bone
7. External occipital protuberance
8. Nuchal crest
9. Mastoid Foramen
10. Foramen magnum
11. Occipital condyle(s)
12. Jugular process
13. Stylomastoid foramen
14. External auditory meatus
15. Retroarticular process and foramen
16. Pterygoid bone
17. Zygomatic process of temporal bone (transected)
18. Rostral and caudal alar foramina
19. Orbital fissure
20. Optic canal
21. Ethmoid foramina
22. Sphenopalatine foramen
23. Caudal palatine foramen
24. Fossa for lacrimal sac
25. Zygomatic bone (transected)
26. Maxilla
27. Palatine bone
28. Major palatine foramen
29. Minor palatine foramen
30. Zygomatic arch
31. Tympanic bulla
32. Tympano-occiptal fissure
33. Hypoglossal canal
34. Foramen lacerum and musculotubal canal
35. Oval foramen

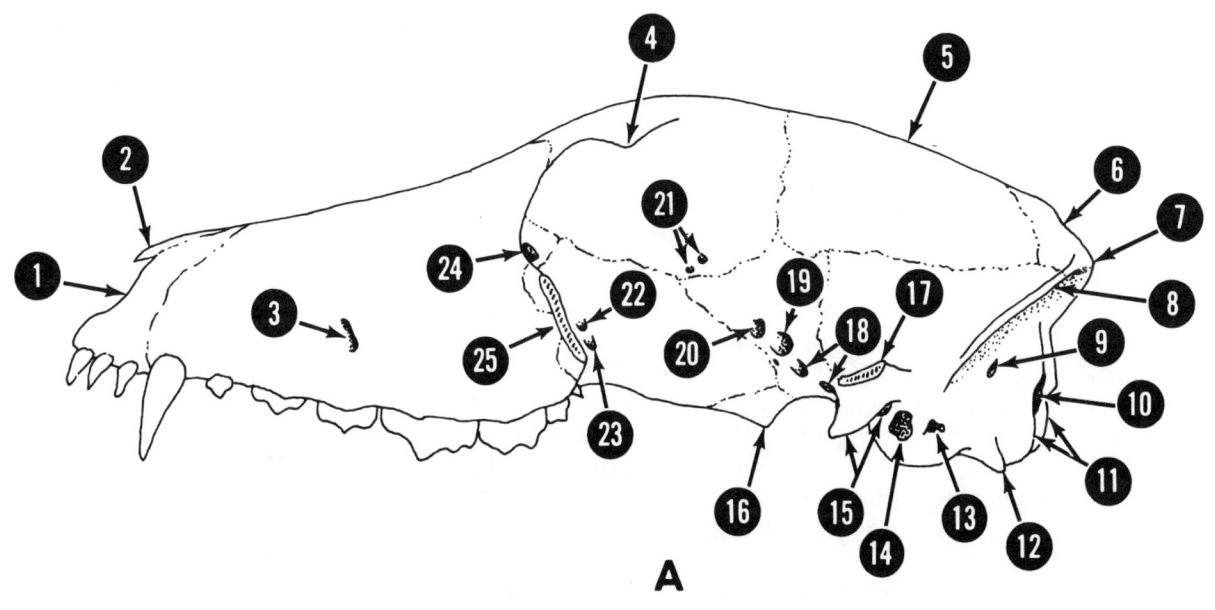
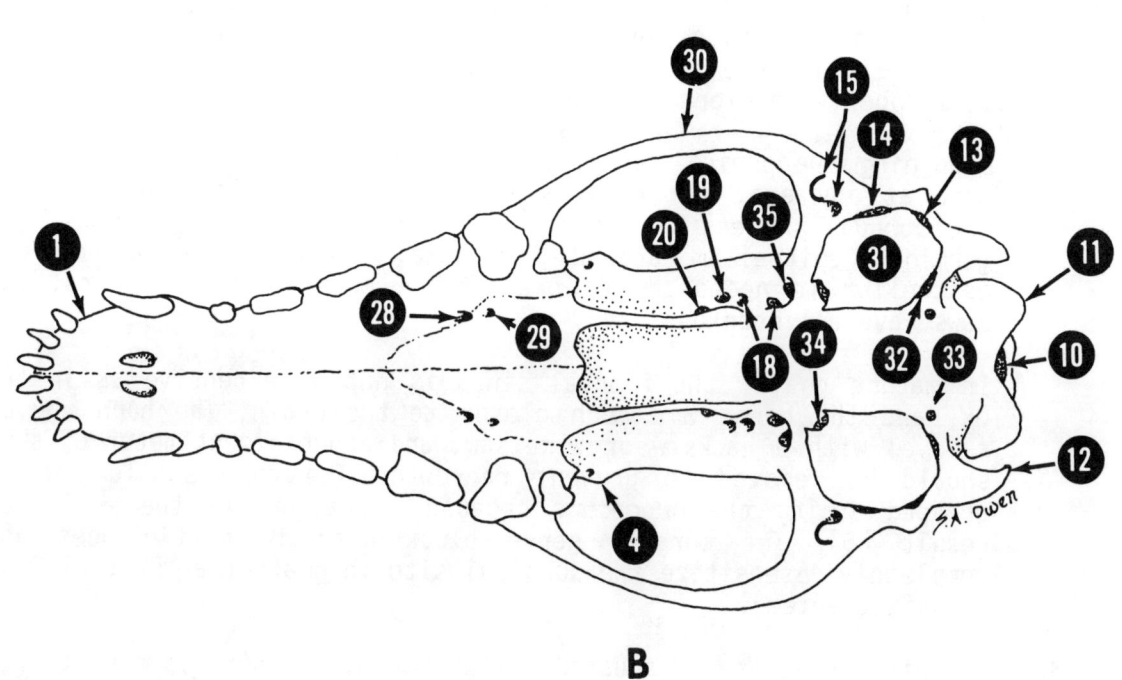

435

                    condyloid (condylar) process--the articular portion of the ramus
                        head and neck of mandible
                    coronoid process--the large prominence for muscular attachment
                    mandibular notch--the incisure between the condyloid and coronoid processes
                    mandibular foramen--the foramen which transmits the mandibular alveolar nerve
            Hyoid bones (Fig. 19-3)
                basihyoid bone--the only unpaired hyoid bone - connects left hyoid bones to right ones
                ceratohyoid bone--formerly spelled keratohyoid
                epihyoid bone--may be fractured in small dogs by "choke-chains"
                stylohyoid bone--divides the guttural pouch of horses into 2 parts
                tympanohyoid bone--may remain cartilaginous in carnivores
                thyrohyoid bone--the only hyoid bone which extends caudally from the basihyoid bone

    D. Medical and Surgical Procedures Involving the Skull

        1. Bullar osteotomy. The tympanic bulla is the most ventral part of the middle ear, and it may be entered to establish drainage in cases of otitis media in carnivores. It may be approached by 3 described techniques (oral, through the external auditory canal, or from the ventral aspect of the neck) [3]. In an oral approach, a Steinman pin works very well to open the bulla. In cats, the well developed septum bullae should be broken down or the bulla must be opened on both sides of the septum to insure good drainage. This septum divides the cavity of the middle ear unequally into 2 parts. It is poorly developed in dogs.

        2. Dehorning. Dehorning is easiest in very young animals but may be done at any age. The horn is an epidermal modification overlying the cornual process of the frontal bone. Since the horn grows from germinal epithelium around its base, adequate removal of the epithelium is necessary to prevent regrowth. Gouges, shears, and saws have all been used [4].

            In mature goats, the frontal sinus is not as extensive as in the ox, and the horns are much closer to the brain. The horn may be removed with a hacksaw or wire saw, and about a centimeter of skin should be removed to prevent regrowth. The horn should not be grasped during the procedure because a fracture of the skull may result [5]. The cornual nerve block used in cattle does not completely desensitize the surgical site in goats (see Part XI.B.4. in this Chapter).

        3. Trephinations are discussed with Paranasal Sinuses (Part VI, below).

II. MUSCLES OF THE HEAD

    Although the NAV [1] does not subdivide the muscles of the head into smaller groups, it may be helpful to do so since so few of them are clinically significant enough to warrant individual study.

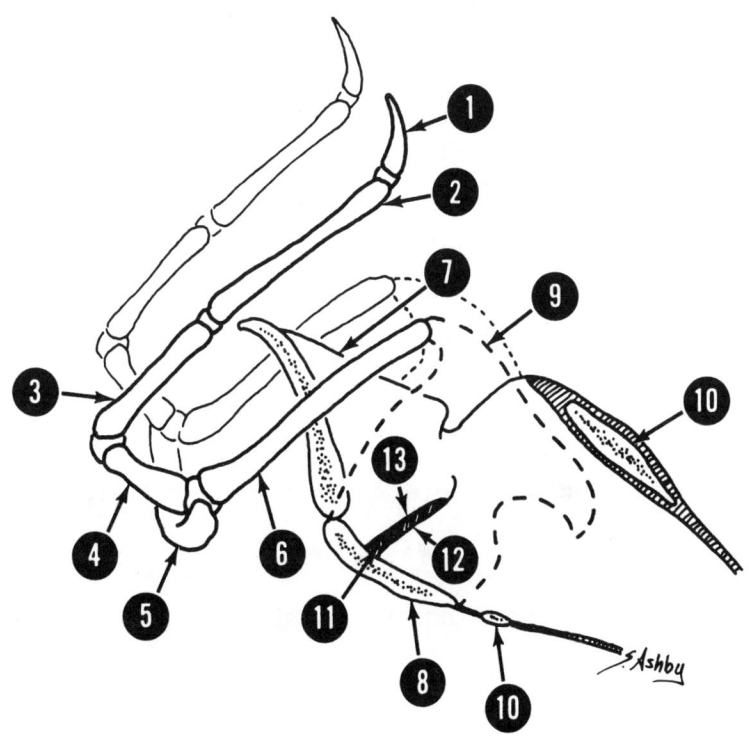

Figure 19-3

Larynx (Sectioned) and Hyoid Bones of a Dog

1. Tympanohyoid bone
2. Stylohyoid bone
3. Epihyoid bone
4. Ceratohyoid bone
5. Basihyoid bone
6. Thyrohyoid bone
7. Epiglottis
8. Thyroid cartilage (transected surface)
9. Thyroid cartilage (ghosted in from the side removed)
10. Cricoid cartilage
11. Lateral ventricle
12. Vocal fold
13. Vestibular fold

A. Facial muscles (innervated primarily by the facial nerve)

1. muscles of the cheeks and lips (including orbicularis oris, buccinator, etc.)
2. muscles of the forehead and dorsum of the nose (including orbicularis oculi, levator nasolabialis, etc.)
3. muscles of the external ear (including rostral, caudal, dorsal, and ventral groups)

B. Extrinsic muscles of the eye (innervated by the oculomotor, trochlear, and abducens nerves)*

ventral oblique m.
dorsal oblique m.
rectus mm. (dorsal, lateral, ventral, medial, located at 12, 3, 6, and 9 o'clock)
retractor bulbi mm. (4 fascicles at 1:30, 4:30, 7:30, and 10:30)

C. Muscles of mastication (innervated by mandibular branch of trigeminal n.)

masseter m. (masseteric myositis affects some small breeds of dogs)
temporal m.
pterygoid mm. (medial and lateral)
digastric m. (the caudal half is innervated by the facial nerve)

The digastricus m. opens the mouth and the others close it. Technically, the mandibular part of the sternocephalicus assists mastication as a synergist of the digastricus m. in the horse, ox, and goat, but it is not generally grouped with the muscles of mastication.

D. Muscles of the tongue (innervated by hypoglossal n.)

Included under this heading are the muscle fibers of the tongue itself (proper muscle of the tongue) as well as the three muscles which attach the tongue to the stylohyoid bone, other hyoid bones, and mandibular genu (styloglossus, hyoglossus, and genioglossus, respectively).

E. Muscles of the pharynx and soft palate (innervated primarily by the vagus and glossopharyngeal nn.)

This group includes all the "-pharyngeus" mm. and the small muscles (tensor veli palatini, levator veli palatini, etc.) of the palate.

---

*A memory aid formula for the innervation is $LR_6Do_4Rest_3$, where L = lateral rectus, R = retractor bulbi, Do = dorsal oblique, Rest = the rest of the extrinsic muscles of the eye, and 3, 4, and 6 are the numbers of the cranial nerves which supply them. In the cat, only the lateral two of the four fascicles of retractor bulbi muscle are supplied by the abducent nerve. The other two are supplied by the oculomotor nerve. This may be true in other domestic mammals, too, but it has not been investigated.

F. Muscles of the larynx and hyoid apparatus (innervated primarily by the vagus n.)

> These include the "-oideus" muscles. The cricothyroideus and cricoarytenoideus dorsalis muscles deserve individual recognition because of their actions of tensing and abducting the vocal folds, respectively.

III. SALIVARY GLANDS

There are three major pairs of salivary glands in domestic mammals: parotid, mandibular, and sublingual glands. In addition to these, there are several minor salivary glands, including those located in the lips, cheeks, and tongue (labial, buccal, and lingual glands, respectively). In the carnivores, the dorsal buccal glands are especially well developed. Since they are located medial to the zygomatic arch, the dorsal buccal glands are known as zygomatic salivary glands and their ducts open into the oral vestibule near the last upper cheek teeth.

A. Parotid gland

> The parotid gland is located in the retromandibular fossa which is the depression caudal to the ramus of the mandible and ventral to the wing of the atlas and base of the ear. In the carnivores, it is relatively small and triangular, but in the ungulates, it is large and its ventral extent overlaps the mandibular gland. The duct of the parotid gland empties into the oral vestibule adjacent to a superior cheek tooth (dog,* goat, horse, pig, third; sheep, fourth; ox, fifth) [7]. In the carnivores and usually in small ruminants, the parotid duct crosses the lateral surface of the masseter muscle. In the pig, ox, and horse, it courses first on the medial aspect of the mandible and then courses laterally under the mandible, accompanied by the facial artery and vein, to follow the border of the masseter muscle dorsally. These structures should be preserved during trephinations to repel the inferior cheek teeth in horses (particularly during approaches for the third and fourth ones) [9]. Translocation of the parotid duct into the lateral palpebral commissure ("canthus") of the eye has been used to surgically treat keratoconjunctivitis sicca in dogs [3]. At surgery, it may be differentiated from the dorsal and ventral buccal branches of the facial nerve by any or all of the following criteria:
>
> 1. The duct typically crosses the middle to ventral third of the masseter muscle with the nerves dorsal and ventral to it.
>
> 2. The duct is tightly bound to the epimysium of the masseter muscle, but the nerves are more loosely bound in the superficial fascia.

---

*Some authors state that the parotid duct opens adjacent to the fourth superior cheek tooth in the dog [10]. In reality, it is variable and is usually between the third and fourth ones.

3. The duct does not branch but the nerves do.

4. The duct is pinkish, translucent, or yellowbrown in color and the nerves are usually white.

B. Mandibular gland

The mandibular gland is located ventral and medial to the parotid gland which partially covers it. In the carnivores and pig it is oval. In the ruminants and horse, it extends rostrally into the intermandibular space. The mandibular duct courses rostrally to open on the sublingual caruncle of the floor of the oral cavity.

C. Sublingual glands

The sublingual glands are positioned ventral and caudal to the floor of the oral cavity. Two pairs of sublingual glands are present in domestic mammals. The monostomatic (one opening) sublingual gland (absent in the horse) has only one excretory duct, the major sublingual duct. In the ruminants, carnivores, and pig, it opens on the sublingual caruncle. The polystomatic (many openings) sublingual gland consists of a number of lobules, each of which secretes through its own minor sublingual duct. The polystomatic gland is rostral to the monostomatic gland in the carnivores and pig. In ruminants, it is dorsocaudal to the monostomatic gland. In carnivores, the caudal part of the monostomatic gland is attached to the cranial aspect of the mandibular gland. The cranial part of the monostomatic gland is slightly separated from the caudal part. The sublingual duct may open separately at the sublingual caruncle or in common with the mandibular duct. Blockage or rupture of the mandibular, sublingual, or combined duct produces the soft tissue swelling in the oral cavity termed salivary cyst (sialocele) or ranula. Swelling may also be noted in the pharyngeal and/or cervical regions. The mandibular and sublingual glands on the affected side are surgically removed [3].

IV. MOUTH AND ORAL CAVITY

A. Lips

The superior and inferior lips (labia) bound the oral cleft which opens into the oral cavity. The relatively mobile lips of horses and small ruminants are of considerable assistance in prehension, while the relatively stiffer lips of the ox and pig do not have much freedom of motion. The upper lip of carnivores and small ruminants is divided by an obvious median cleft, the philtrum [7]. In the pig and horse, the philtrum may be considered to be indistinct or absent.

B. Oral cavity

The oral cavity is bounded by the lips, cheeks, hard palate, a floor, and caudally it communicates with the pharynx. It is divided by the dentition into the oral cavity proper and the oral vestibule. The mucosa of the floor of the oral cavity has a central fold which attaches to the ventral aspect of the tongue (frenulum). The frenulum is double in the pig [7]. Two folds of mucosa on either side of the frenulum end rostrally as the sublingual caruncles on which the ducts of the mandibular and sublingual glands open. On the rostral aspect of the hard palate is the incisive papilla on which the two incisive ducts open. These ducts connect the oral cavity with the nasal cavity except in the horse where they end blindly under the epithelium of the oral cavity. The rostral portion of the hard palate in ruminants has a dental pad which substitutes functionally for the superior incisors. The soft palate is the caudal continuation of the hard palate.

C. Cheeks

Cheiloplasty may be indicated in some dogs with redundant cheeks to reduce hypersalivation [3]. Other individuals may require a similar procedure to remove infection-prone folds.

D. Tongue

The tongue is formed primarily by skeletal muscle. Its mucous membrane covering has numerous papillary projections named according to their shape. The filiform papillae (all species) and conical papillae* (ruminants) have mechanical functions. The fungiform (all species), vallate (all species), and foliate (usually absent in ruminants) papillae serve in a gustatory capacity. Five of the cranial nerve pairs have lingual functions including the hypoglossal nerve (motor to muscle); mandibular branch of the trigeminal nerve (tactile, pain, and temperature sensation); and the facial, glossopharyngeal, and vagus nerves (taste).

The major gross features of the tongue include the rostrally free apex, the body, and the root which attaches to the hyoid apparatus. In the dog, its dorsal surface is divided by a longitudinal median groove. In ruminants, the caudal aspect of the dorsal surface of the tongue is raised to form a prominence termed the torus linguae. In the ox, just rostral to the torus linguae, is a depression termed the fossa linguae. This area sometimes entraps burrs. The horse's tongue has a slender bar of cartilage in the median plane, and that of the dog has a similar structure, the lyssa, embedded in its apex [7].

The skeletal muscle forming the bulk of the tongue is the lingual muscle proper (intrinsic lingual muscle). The tongue is anchored to the mandible and hyoid apparatus by the extrinsic lingual muscles. These include the genioglossus (tongue to chin), hyoglossus (tongue to some of the hyoid bones), and styloglossus (tongue to stylohyoid bone). In addition, the "-hyoideus" muscles act to move the tongue since they attach to the hyoid apparatus. (These include mylohyoideus, geniohyoideus, stylohyoideus, occipitohyoideus, ceratohyoideus, hyoideus transversus, sternohyoideus and omohyoideus mm.).

---

*Conical papillae are essentially enlarged filiform papillae. Some authors limit them to the ruminants and some consider the carnivores to have them as well.

In toy breeds, too much tension on the tongue during tracheal intubation can result in fractures of the hyoid apparatus.

Self-sucking in cows may be corrected in some cases by surgically resecting either the left or right half of the tongue from the level of the frenulum to the apex [8].

V. NASAL CAVITY

    A. Nose

The nose is the portion of the face dorsal to the mouth which includes the nares. The nares lead into the nasal cavity which is connected to the paranasal sinuses and to the nasopharynx. The nasolacrimal ducts open at the junction of the skin and mucous membrane. In horses, this duct may be flushed retrograde to open blockages by cannulating the distal opening [9]. It can often be found by looking along the junction of pigmented and nonpigmented skin. The nose is supported by a number of cartilages and has several species variations:

1. In the carnivores and small ruminants, a definite cleft (philtrum) extends dorsally from the oral margin of the upper lip.

2. The nose of the pig contains a bone (os rostrale) supposedly advantageous to its "rooting" behavior.

3. In the horse, an alar fold projects laterally into the dorsal part of the nostril and divides the nostril into dorsal and ventral passages. The ventral passage is continuous with the nasal cavity, and the dorsal passage leads into a blind cutaneous pouch, the nasal diverticulum ("false nostril"). This may catch air during high speed running and keep the nostril flared.

    B. Nasal cavity

The nasal cavity is divided by a median septum formed by the vomer as well as by cartilage. Each side can be subdivided into rostral, middle, and caudal portions. The rostral, narrow portion leading from the nostrils, is the vestibule. The middle portion is the largest and contains the nasal conchae ("turbinates"). There are two principal nasal conchae, a smaller dorsal one and a larger ventral one. These scroll-like partitions consist of a thin plate of bone covered by a mucous membrane. They divide the nasal cavity into 3 major meatus (dorsal, middle, and ventral) which communicate along the nasal septum in a narrow space termed the common nasal meatus.* The ventral nasal meatus is the largest and is utilized for the passage of a stomach tube in large animals. The end of the tube is directed medially and ventrally to assure entering the ventral nasal meatus. This route may also be used in cats. The caudal part of the nasal cavity contains the numerous

---

*There are small ethmoidal conchae located in the caudal aspect of the nasal cavity, and the small nasal passageways located between them are called ethmoidal meatus.

ethmoidal conchae, and is continuous through the choanae with the nasopharynx. Striking the conchae with the end of the stomach tube during insertion or withdrawing it too rapidly can result in hemorrhage [9].

VI. PARANASAL SINUSES

The paranasal sinuses are bilaterally symmetrical, membrane lined, air-filled diverticula from the nasal cavity which invaginate the adjacent bones. They are not fully developed at birth and continue to grow in size as the animal matures. The sinuses are lined with a mucosa similar to that lining the nasal cavity, but variable in specific morphology from region to region. The true function of the sinuses remains obscure. Clinically, they have significance as infection-prone cavities, in equine dentistry, and in dehorning procedures. The orifices which join the paranasal sinuses to the nasal cavity proper are often difficult to find and are not important to identify. Sculptured skulls should be examined to determine the extent of the various sinuses and to identify them. The frontal and maxillary sinuses are best known, but several others are present in the various domestic animals [7]:

	Carnivores	Pig	Ruminants	Horse
Frontal sinus	+	+	+	+
Maxillary sinus	+	+	+	+
Sphenoid sinus	+ (cat only)	+	+ (ox only)	+
Palatine sinus	-	-	+	+
Lacrimal sinus	-	+	+	-
Conchal sinuses	-	+	+	+

A. Frontal sinus

Frontal sinuses are present in all domestic mammals. In the horse, small ruminants, and carnivores, they are located in the dorsal part of the skull between the nasal cavity, cranial cavity, and orbit. In the ox and pig, they extend caudally to invaginate the parietal, interparietal, occipital, and temporal bones. In horned ruminants, the cornual process of the frontal bone is also excavated by a diverticulum of the frontal sinus--an important consideration in dehorning procedures. The frontal sinuses communicate with the nasal cavity through openings into the meatus between ethmoidal conchae (frontal sinus apertures) except in the horse where they open into the maxillary sinuses through the fronto-maxillary aperture.* Species differences include the following [1,7]:

---

*In the horse, all paranasal sinuses communicate directly or indirectly with the middle nasal meatus. The rostral and caudal maxillary sinuses open directly into the nasal cavity (nasomaxillary aperture). The ventral conchal sinus communicates with the rostral maxillary sinus and the conchofrontal, middle conchal, and typically the sphenopalatine sinuses communicate with the caudal maxillary sinus. In the ox, the palatine and maxillary sinuses open directly into the nasal meatus through a common nasomaxillary aperture. The lacrimal sinus communicates with the maxillary sinus, and the frontal, sphenoid, and conchal sinuses open independently into ethmoidal meatus [7].

1. The horse and cat have undivided frontal sinuses. In the horse, the frontal sinus communicates with the dorsal conchal sinus to form the conchofrontal sinus. This may be trephined to repel the last upper cheek tooth (Fig. 19-4/1; see B.2. Maxillary sinus, below).

2. The dog has three frontal sinuses: rostral, medial, and lateral.

3. Three frontal sinuses are also present in the pig, but these are named medial rostral, lateral rostral, and caudal frontal sinuses. The latter is the largest.

4. The small ruminants have two frontal sinuses: a smaller medial one and a larger lateral one.

5. The ox has four frontal sinuses in each half of the skull including medial rostral, lateral rostral, intermediate rostral, and caudal frontal sinuses. The caudal frontal sinuses are by far the largest and include nuchal, postorbital, and (in some individuals) cornual diverticula. The cornual diverticulum is commonly opened by dehorning procedures in cattle (except those performed on young animals).

   Drainage of an infected frontal sinus in an ox may be established by trephination in one or more areas (Fig. 19-5) [8]:

   a. Into the nuchal diverticulum--halfway between the base of the horn and the dorsal midline
   b. Into the postorbital diverticulum at a point 3 cm caudal to the orbit and just medial to the orbit
   c. Into the rostral compartments--between the orbits and about 3 cm from the dorsal midline. The rostral compartments may also be trephined further rostrally, but the operator should move further laterally to stay within the sinus. To facilitate drainage, some of the bony trabeculae are broken down after the trephination.

B. Maxillary sinus

The maxillary sinus communicates with the nasal cavity through the nasomaxillary aperture. Species differences include the following:

1. The maxillary sinus of the carnivores is not considered to be a true sinus since it does not lie between the internal and external laminae of individual bones, but rather lies between the maxillary, lacrimal, and palatine bones. Its proper name in carnivores is maxillary recess [1,7].

2. The horse has two maxillary sinuses on each side: rostral and caudal, which are partially divided by a bony septum. Each has its own nasomaxillary aperture. The caudal maxillary sinus also communicates with the conchofrontal sinus through a frontomaxillary aperture (also called conchomaxillary aperture), and with the

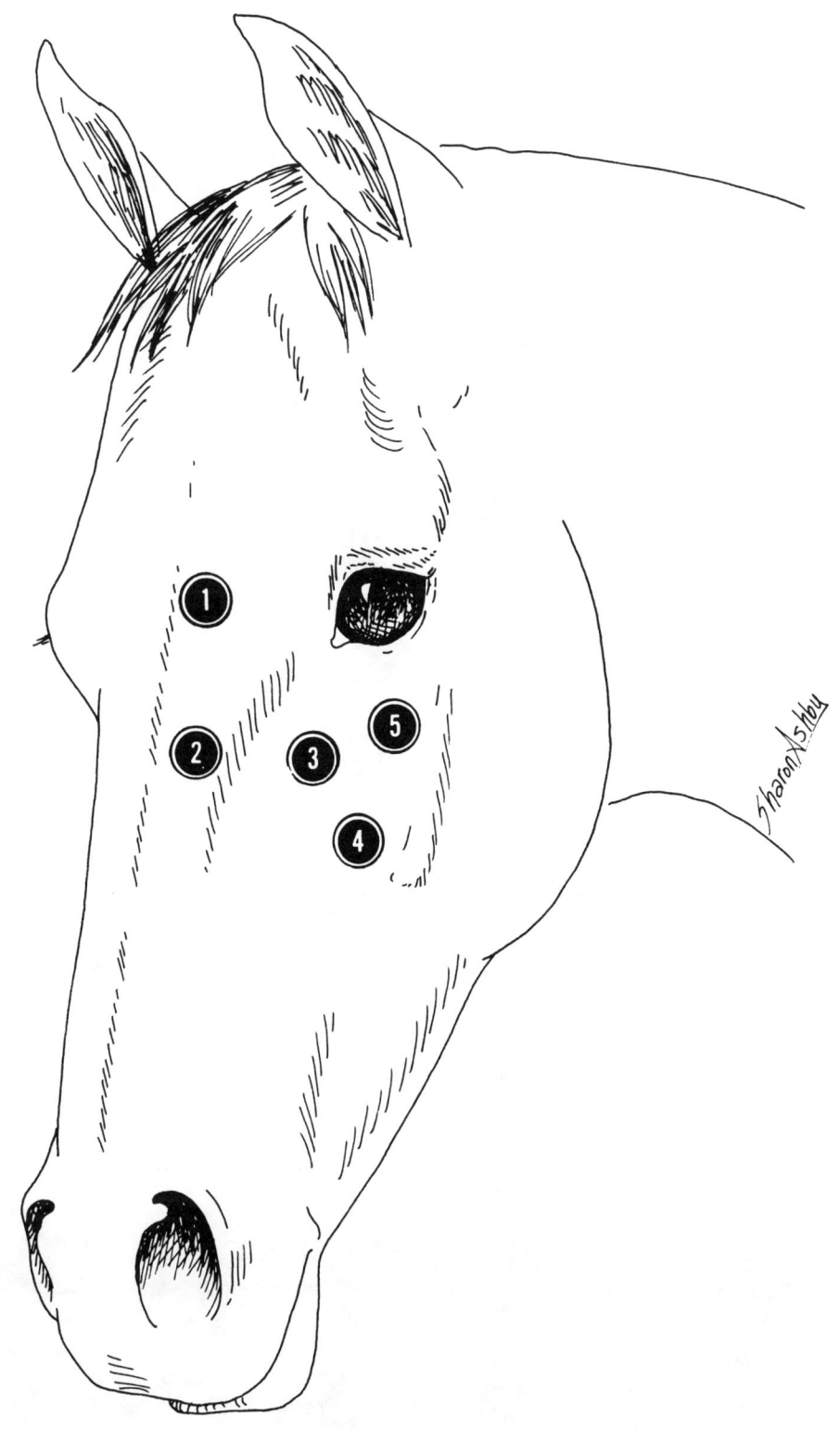

Figure 19-4

Trephination Sites in the Equine Head

1. Frontal (conchofrontal) sinus
2. Nasal cavity
3. Maxillary sinus
4. Rostral compartment of maxillary sinus
5. Caudal compartment of maxillary sinus

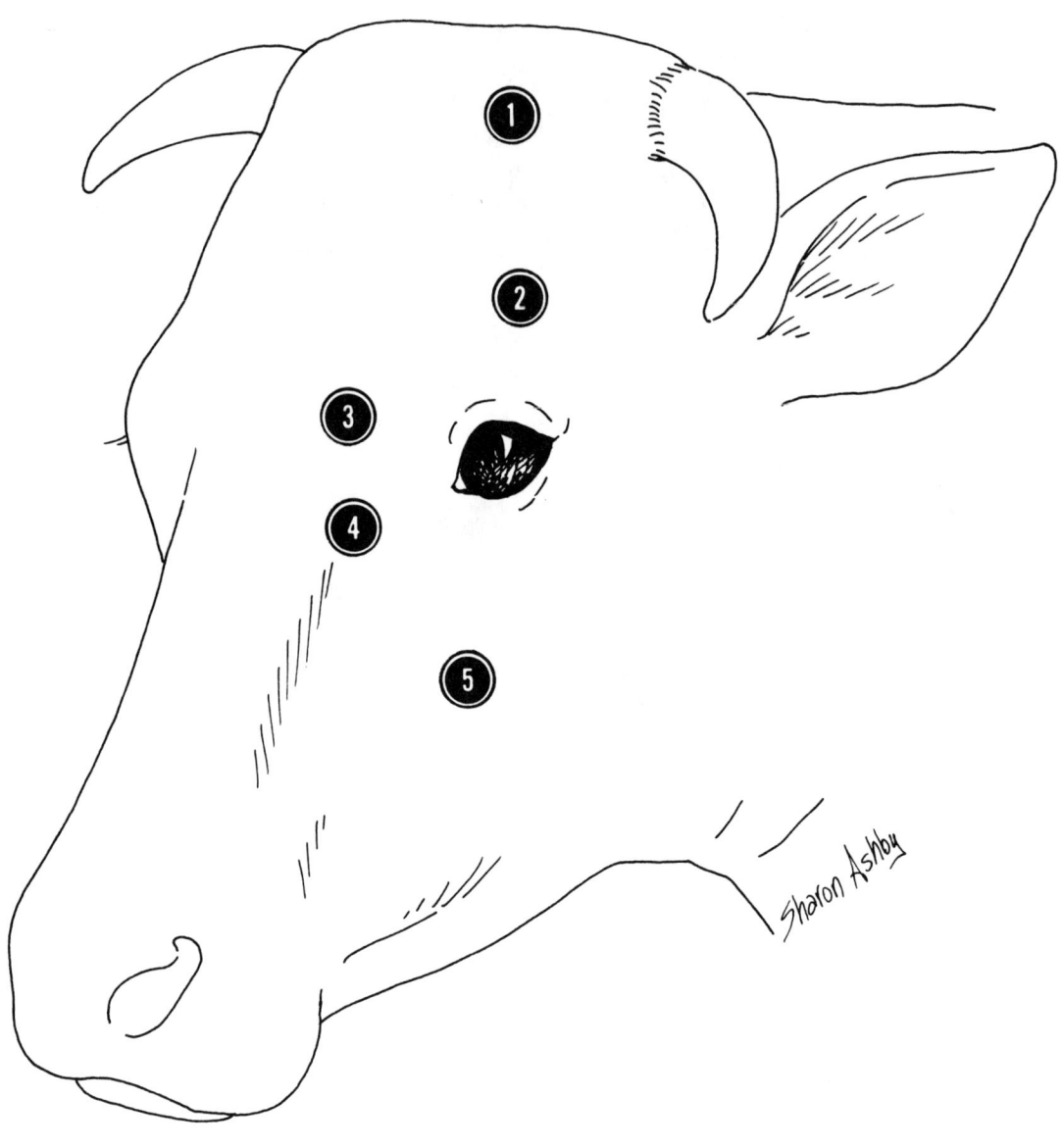

Figure 19-5

Trephination Sites in the Bovine Head

1. Frontal sinus (nuchal diverticulum)
2. Frontal sinus (postorbital diverticulum)
3. Frontal sinus (rostral compartments)
4. Conchal sinus
5. Maxillary sinus

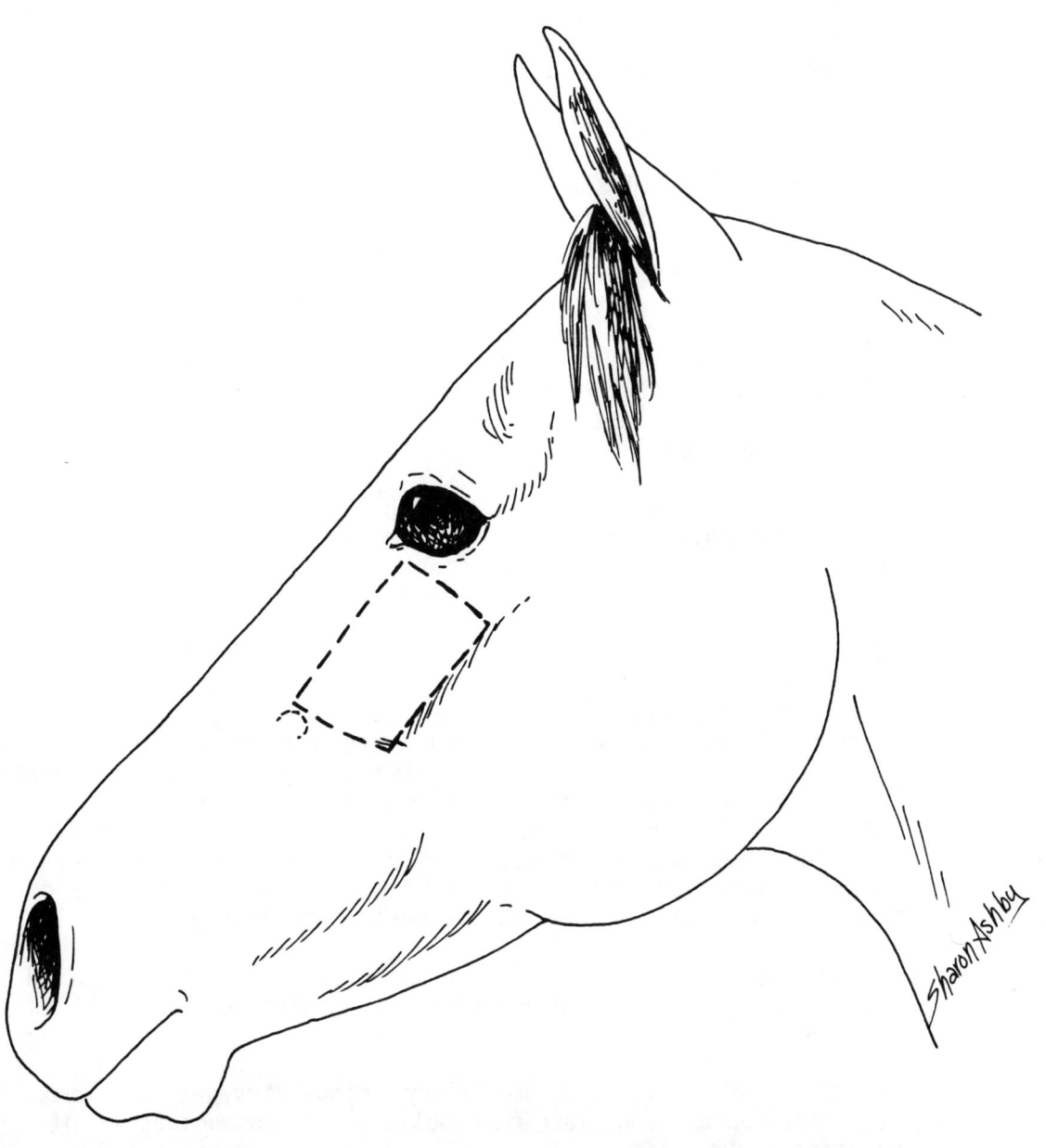

Figure 19-6

General Boundaries for Trephination of the
Maxillary Sinus in the Horse

The dorsal limit to avoid damaging the nasolacrimal duct is a line connecting the medial canthus of the eye and the infraorbital foramen (palpable). The ventral limit is the facial crest, an easily palpated ridge.

sphenopalatine sinus. The maxillary sinus is the only one which communicates directly with the nasal cavity in the horse [7]. The maxillary sinus is trephined to reach all of the superior cheek teeth for repulsion except the last one* (see A-1, above). The area entered is between two lines (Figs. 19-4 and 19-6):

    a. The dorsal limit (to avoid damage to the nasolacrimal duct) is a line between the infraorbital foramen and the medial palpebral commissure of the eye.

    b. The ventral limit (to stay above the roots of the teeth) is the facial crest.

The curvature of the teeth may be taken into account in selecting the exact rostral-caudal level for the trephination. The hole is made directly above the exposed part of the tooth for the first two cheek teeth, and just caudal to the tooth for the third, fourth, and fifth ones [9].

The last (sixth) superior cheek tooth may be repelled by trephining the conchofrontal sinus 3 cm off the midline, directly between the medial palpebral commissures ("canthi") of the eyes. A long punch is required and a curved one is often useful [8].

Mandibular teeth may be removed by repelling them through trephination sites in the ventrolateral aspect of the mandible. In young horses, the trephination site for the first cheek tooth is located immediately ventral to the tooth, and the site for the second through fifth cheek teeth is located just caudal to the level of the tooth. In older horses (over 9 years), the trephination sites shift rostrally on the second through fifth teeth until 12 years when they too are in direct line with the teeth. The last cheek tooth is repelled through a trephination site in the side of the mandible, and the masseter muscle must be reflected [9].

  3. In the pig, the single maxillary sinus is divided into rostral and caudal parts, and it excavates the zygomatic bone as well as the maxilla.

  4. In the ruminants, the maxillary sinus invades the maxilla, zygomatic bone, and lacrimal bulla, and communicates with the palatine sinus.

C. Sphenoid sinus

The sphenoid sinuses are relatively small and are absent in the dog and small ruminants. They open into the nasal cavity through the aperture of the sphenoid sinus. In the horse, the sphenoid sinus typically communicates with the palatine sinus to form the sphenopalatine sinus. However, it may open directly into the nasal cavity. The sphenoid sinus may be absent in both the ox and horse [7].

---

*In young horses, the sinus may not extend rostrally far enough to surround the first 2 cheek teeth.

D. Palatine sinus

The palatine sinus is not present in the carnivores and pig. In the ruminants, the palatine sinus communicates with the maxillary sinus through a wide maxillopalatine aperture and uses the same nasomaxillary aperture to communicate with the nasal cavity. In the horse, the palatine sinus opens rostrally into the caudal maxillary sinus and it is continuous caudally with the sphenoid sinus. The latter two are collectively termed the sphenopalatine sinus in the horse [7].

E. Lacrimal sinus

Lacrimal sinuses are found only in the pig and ruminants. They have several unimportant variations concerning their connections with the nasal cavity and with other sinuses [7].

F. Conchal sinuses

The conchal sinuses are formed by enclosure of the conchae in some species. Dorsal conchal sinuses (formed by the dorsal conchae) are present in the pig, ruminants, and horse. (In the horse, this joins the frontal sinus to form the conchofrontal sinus.) Ventral conchal sinuses (formed by the ventral conchae) are present in the pig, ox, and horse.

VII. PHARYNX

The pharynx is the passageway which connects the oral cavity with the esophagus, and the nasal cavity with the larynx.

A. The pharynx has three major divisions [1,7]:

1. The nasopharynx is part of the respiratory channel, and extends from the choanae to the intrapharyngeal opening. Its floor is formed by the soft palate, and the openings of the auditory tubes are in its lateral walls.

    In the horse, the auditory tubes have large dilations termed guttural pouches. The function of these is poorly understood, but each one is divided into a smaller lateral part and a larger medial part by the stylohyoid bones. Surgical drainage through the infamous "Viborg's triangle" is sometimes employed because of congestion [9]. The borders of this triangle are the tendon of the sternomandibularis m. (caudally), the ramus of the mandible (cranially) and the linguofacial vein (ventrally). A number of other approaches to the guttural pouches have also been used.

    Removal of the caudal free border of the soft palate (uvulectomy) may be indicated to reduce respiratory distress in some of the brachycephalic dogs. In addition, everted lateral ventricles may cause dyspnea in these animals and should be removed.

2. The oropharynx is part of the digestive tube extending from the palatoglossal arches to the base of the epiglottis. Its cranial

opening (bounded by the soft palate, palatoglossal arches, and root of the tongue) is the auditis pharyngeus.

    3. The laryngopharynx is common to both the respiratory and digestive channels. It is the caudal continuation of the oropharynx and extends from the base of the epiglottis to the level of the cricoid cartilage. Rostral parts of the larynx project up into the laryngopharynx. The wide, cranial part of the opening into the larynx is the auditis laryngis. It narrows caudally to form the glottis.

B. The openings into the pharynx include the:

1. paired choanae
2. paired pharyngeal openings of the auditory tubes
3. auditis pharyngeus
4. auditis laryngis which is closed by the epiglottis during swallowing
5. entrance into the esophagus

C. A number of pharyngeal muscles are present which primarily function in the swallowing reflex by constricting the pharynx. These include the various "-pharyngeus" muscles (pterygo-, palato-, stylo-, hyo-, thyro-, and crico-). Only one of these dilates the pharynx (stylopharyngeus caudalis). Sometimes the small muscles of the soft palate (the palatini's) are grouped with the pharyngeal muscles.

VIII. TONSILS

Tonsils are formed by lymph nodules and diffuse lymphatic tissue in the pharyngeal region. In some cases, they are distinct enough to be grossly obvious (palatine tonsil of carnivores), but in many cases, they are difficult to observe grossly except for the subtle mucosal invaginations (fossulae) which mark their location. Tonsils are named according to their position within the pharynx [7]:

A. Lingual tonsils are in the mucosa at the root of the tongue.
B. Palatine tonsils are on or in the lateral wall of the pharynx.
C. Tonsils of the soft palate are on the ventral surface of the soft palate.
D. Paraepiglottic tonsils are on or near the base of the epiglottis.
E. Pharyngeal tonsils are in the roof of the nasopharynx.
F. Tubal tonsils are in the lateral wall of the pharyngeal opening of the auditory tube.

Palatine tonsillectomies may be indicated in small animals. If a tonsillar snare is used, it should not be employed until dissection has produced an elongated pedicle. Otherwise, the whole tonsil will not be removed.

The following tonsils are present in the various domestic animals [7]:

	Carnivores	Pig	Ruminants	Horse
Lingual t.	*	*	+	+
Palatine t.	+	-	+	+
Tonsil of soft palate	*	+	*	+
Paraepiglottic t.	*	+	- ox + sheep, goat	-
Pharyngeal t.	+	+	+	+
Tubal t.	-	+	+	*

*Denotes diffuse tonsillar tissue not grossly identifiable.

IX. LARYNX

The larynx is the mucosa lined, cartilaginous tube joining the pharynx to the trachea. Its rostral opening (glottis) is passively closed during deglutition by the epiglottis and it contains the vocal organ.

A. Cartilages [1] (Fig. 19-3)

1. epiglottis (unpaired and rostral)
2. thyroid cartilage (unpaired and ventral and lateral)
3. arytenoid cartilages (paired and dorsal)
4. cricoid cartilage (unpaired and caudal)

A number of joints occur between the laryngeal cartilages. These have little clinical significance. The epiglottis passively closes over the glottis during deglutition to prevent aspiration of ingesta. The epiglottis is an important landmark in tracheal intubation. By pulling the tongue rostrally, the tube can usually be slipped over the epiglottis and on down the trachea. Cats are particularly prone to laryngospasm, and one should take care not to irritate the area or the intubation may be difficult. The thyroid cartilage articulates rostrally with the thyrohyoid bones. The arytenoid cartilages have vocal processes to which the vocal folds attach. The larynx of the horse may be surgically invaded through the cricothyroid ligament to correct laryngeal hemiplegia. The cricothyroid ligament is a heavy elastic membrane joining the ventral aspects of the cricoid and thyroid cartilages.

B. Lateral ventricles

The mucosal wall of the larynx in domesticated mammals (except the cat and ruminants) has evaginations on each side termed lateral ventricles [7]. The mucosal fold cranial to each lateral ventricle is the vestibular fold (absent grossly in the pig), and the mucosal fold caudal to the lateral ventricle is the vocal fold. Vocal folds are present in the cat and in ruminants even though they lack lateral ventricles. The vocal folds are transected and/or sutured down in devocalization procedures on carnivores [3]. Fluttering of the vocal fold and/or the laryngeal mucosa during forced respiration (inspiration) is believed to cause "roaring" in horses. This condition is also called laryngeal hemiplegia because it is typically unilateral (and usually affects the left side). It is believed to be related to dysfunction of the intrinsic muscles of the larynx due to paralysis of the recurrent laryngeal nerve. The condition may be corrected by a number of surgical procedures including excision of the mucosa of the lateral ventricle [9].

C. Muscles

The muscles of the larynx may be divided into an extrinsic group and an intrinsic group. The extrinsic muscles include those which connect the larynx with the hyoid bones, pharynx, and sternum. They are capable of moving the whole larynx (i.e., sternohyoideus, sternothyroideus, etc.) The intrinsic muscles include several named muscles, but only two will be singled out. The cricoarytenoideus dorsalis mm. attach to the dorsal surface of the larynx, joining the cartilages which the name indicates. Contraction of this paired muscle abducts the vocal folds by rotating the arytenoid cartilages (to which the folds attach) laterally. The cricothyroideus m. on the ventral aspect of the larynx tenses the vocal folds by buckling the cricothyroid articulation ventrally. All of the intrinsic muscles of the larynx are innervated by the caudal laryngeal nerve (terminal branch of the recurrent laryngeal nerve) except the cricothyroideus m. (cranial laryngeal n.). Both the cranial and caudal laryngeal nerves are branches of the vagus nerve.

X. BLOOD VESSELS OF THE HEAD (Fig. 19-7)

The cranial vessels form a complicated network with a considerable amount of detail far beyond the essence of value for a practitioner. In addition, there are just enough variations from one species to the next to add confusion. Only the major arterial channels will be considered:

A. Major arteries supplying the head

1. Common carotid artery

The paired common carotid arteries are the primary blood supply to the head. They originate from the brachiocephalic trunk, either as a single bicarotid trunk which then divides (ungulates), or as separate left and right common carotid arteries (carnivores). The only branches of the common carotid artery are thyroid and laryngeal aa. in the various species. The common carotid artery terminates by dividing into the internal and external carotid aa. In the cat and ruminants, the extracranial part of the internal carotid a. becomes vestigial (Fig. 19-7/4).

2. Internal carotid artery

The internal carotid artery has a variable enlargement, the carotid sinus, located near its origin from the common carotid artery. The internal carotid courses rostrally to supply blood to the cerebral arterial circle. In the ruminants and in adult cats,

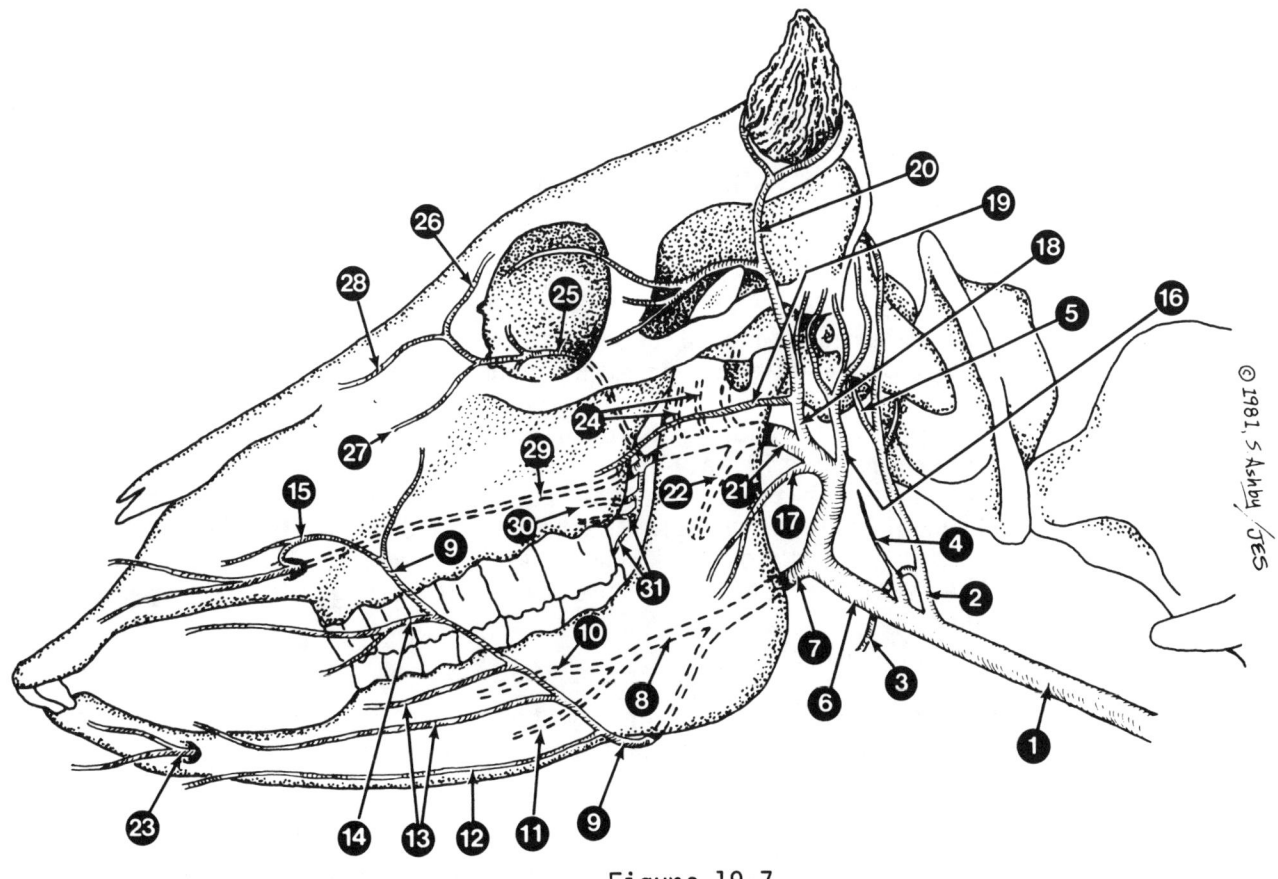

Figure 19-7

Branches of the Common Carotid Artery of the Ox

1. Left common carotid a.
2. Occipital a.
3. Ascending palatine a.
4. Internal carotid a. (extracranial segment degenerates postnatally)
5. Middle meningeal a.
6. External carotid a.
7. Linguofacial trunk
8. Lingual a.
9. Facial a.
10. Deep lingual a.
11. Sublingual a.
12. Submental a.
13. Inferior labial aa.
14. Superior labial a.
15. Rostral lateral nasal a.
16. Caudal auricular a.
17. Masseteric branch of external carotid a.
18. Superficial temporal a.
19. Transverse facial a.
20. Cornual a.
21. Maxillary a.
22. Inferior alveolar a.--to mandibular foramen
23. Mental a. from inferior alveolar a.
24. Rostral and caudal branches to rostral epidural rete mirabile
25. Malar a.
26. Angular a. of the eye
27. Caudal lateral nasal a.
28. Dorsal nasal a.
29. Infraorbital a.
30. Sphenopalatine a.
31. Major and minor palatine aa.

Used with permission of Dr. J. E. Smallwood

the portion of the internal carotid artery outside the cranial cavity degenerates. In the dog and pig, the artery courses through the carotid canal enroute to the cranial cavity.

    3. External carotid artery

The external carotid artery is the major rostral continuation of the common carotid a. Its major branches are:

- a. occipital a. (may also originate from the common carotid or internal carotid aa.)
- b. linguofacial trunk (in the ruminants and horse) or separate lingual and facial aa. (carnivores and pig). The facial a. is commonly used to check the pulse of horses. It courses under the ventral aspect of the mandible along with the parotid duct.
- c. caudal auricular a.

The external carotid artery terminates by dividing into the superficial temporal artery and the maxillary a.

B. Major veins draining the head

The venous channels of the head which have clinical importance are those involved in the formation of the cranial vena cava. These include the linguofacial and maxillary veins which join to form the ipsilateral external jugular vein. In the carnivores and pig, the external jugular vein and the subclavian vein on each side join to form a brachiocephalic vein. The two brachiocephalic veins (left and right) then unite to form the cranial vena cava. In the horse and ruminants, no brachiocephalic veins are present because the cranial vena cava is formed by a direct convergence of the left and right external jugular veins. The subclavian veins join the cranial vena cava directly in these species.

XI. CRANIAL NERVES (Fig. 19-8)

A. Basic information

A summary of factual information regarding the twelve pairs of cranial nerves is presented in Table 19-1. A working knowledge of this information is essential to a fundamental clinical background and to the application of nerve blocks and neurological diagnostic tests.

B. Medical and Surgical Applications

1. Maxillary nerve block (to anesthetize the superior arcade and lip of horses). The needle is inserted ventral to the facial crest or zygomatic arch at a level which is in line with the lateral palpebral commissure of the eye. The needle is then directed rostromedially to the maxillary foramen. A skull should be examined for landmarks and angles. This block will anesthetize all of the superior teeth, but is necessary only for the last 4. For the first 2 cheek teeth and the incisors, an infraorbital block may be used.

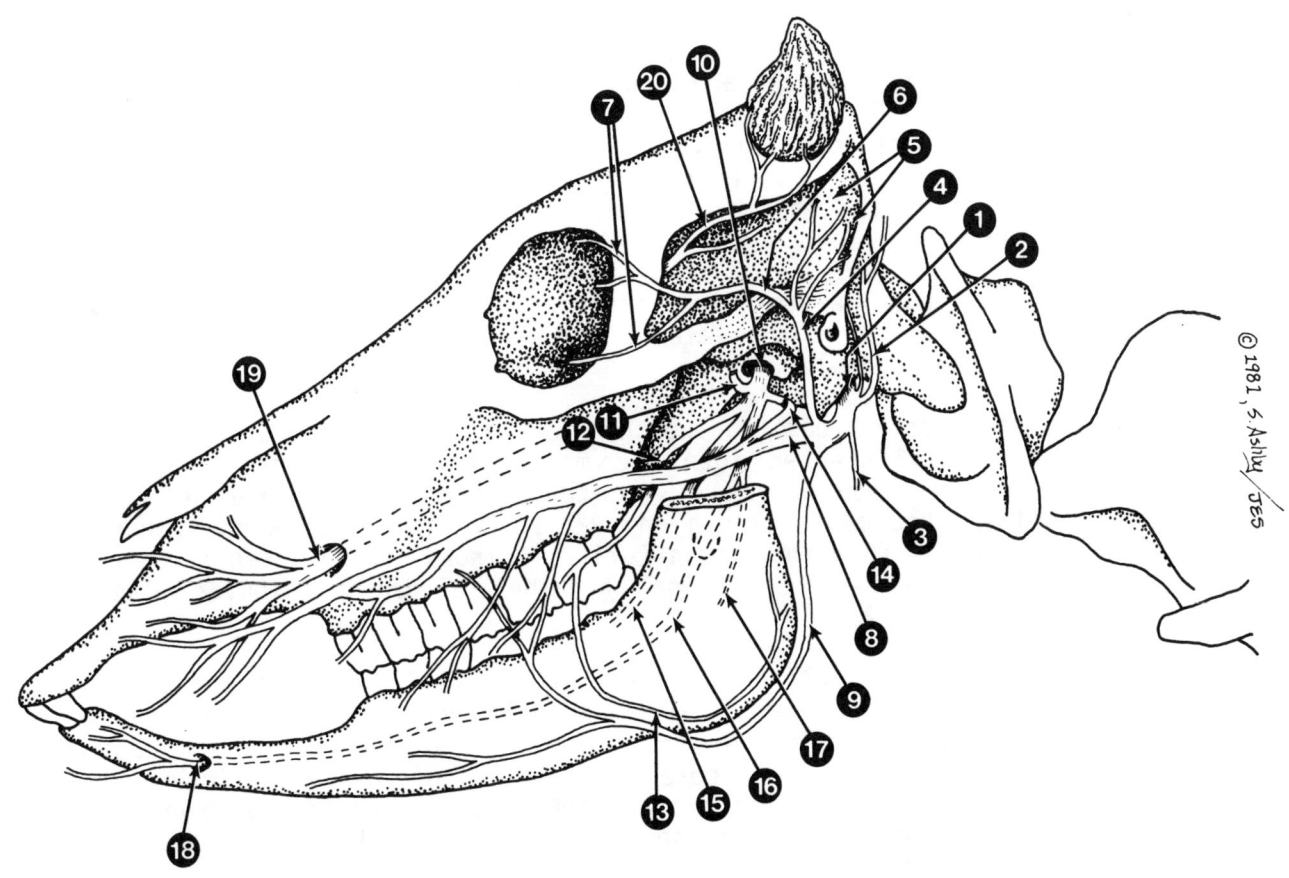

Figure 19-8

Selected Nerves of the Bovine Head

1. Facial n. (C.N. VII)--emerging from stylomastoid foramen
2. Caudal auricular n.
3. Branch of facial n. to digastric m.
4. Auriculopalpebral n.--can be "blocked" at arrow
5. Rostral auricular branches of auriculopalpebral n.
6. Zygomatic branch of auriculopalpebral n.
7. Palpebral branches of zygomatic branch of auriculopalpebral n.
8. Dorsal buccal branch of facial n.   {to muscles of the cheek,
9. Ventral buccal branch of facial n.   {lips, and nose
10. Mandibular n.--emerging from oval foramen
11. Stump of masticatory n.--to masseter and temporal mm.
12. Buccal n.--sensory to mucous membrane of oral cavity
13. Parotid branch of buccal n.
14. Auriculotemporal n.--joins dorsal buccal branch of facial n.
15. Lingual n.
16. Inferior alveolar n.
17. Mylohyoid n.
18. Mental n.--emerging from mental foramen
19. Infraorbital n.--emerging from infraorbital foramen
20. Cornual branch of the zygomaticotemporal branch of the zygomatic n. from maxillary n. (Some texts describe the zygomaticotemporal branch as a branch of the closely related lacrimal n. from the ophthalmic n.). The cornual branch can be blocked at the arrow (midway between eye and horn), where it lies just ventral to the palpable temporal line.

Used with permission of Dr. J. E. Smallwood

The needle is inserted into the infraorbital foramen located rostrodorsal to the end of the facial crest. This block will also anesthetize the nose and superior lip [11].

2. Inferior alveolar nerve block in horses (to anesthetize the inferior arcade and lip). The needle is inserted along the medial surface of the mandible to a point marked by the intersection of 2 lines:

   a. a caudal extension of the occlusal surface of the cheek teeth
   b. a line from the lateral palpebral commissure to the angle of the mandible

3. Mental nerve block (to anesthetize the inferior lip of horses). The needle is inserted into the mental foramina of the mandible to block the mental nerves as they emerge from the bone halfway between the canine tooth and P2. If the needle is deeply placed in the mental foramina, the inferior incisors can be desensitized. The mental nerves are terminal branches of the mandibular alveolar nerves.

4. Cornual nerve block (to anesthetize the horn for dehorning). In cattle, the needle is inserted halfway between the eye and the horn, just ventral to the temporal line. The cornual nerve is a branch of the zygomaticotemporal branch of the zygomatic branch of the maxillary nerve. (In some texts, it is described as a branch of the lacrimal branch of the ophthalmic nerve) [1]. About one-fourth of the cornual blocks in cattle fail to completely desensitize the horn. Failure can be attributed to an abnormal course of the cornual nerve (under the periosteum or in the bone); to a very long supraorbital or infratrochlear nerve; or to an abnormally long nerve of the frontal sinus. Dr. Habel points out that a ring block around the base of the horn will completely anesthetize it in the first two instances but not in the third one [11].

   In goats, the horn is supplied by the cornual branch of the infratrochlear nerve as well as by the cornual nerve. The cornual nerve may be blocked at a site similar to that in cattle, and the anesthesia completed with a block at the dorsomedial margin of the orbit [6].

5. Peterson's block is used for enucleation of the eye in the ox. It anesthetizes the third, fourth, and sixth cranial nerves as well as the ophthalmic and maxillary parts of the fifth. A 4 to 5 inch needle is inserted just caudal to the frontal process of the zygomatic bone. It is then directed rostromedially until it strikes the sphenoid bone near the foramen orbitorotundum. A similar block in horses can be made with a 5 inch needle introduced just caudal to the zygomatic process of the frontal bone. The needle is directed ventromedially about $40°$ from a horizontal axis until bone is struck near the orbital fissure. To operate on the eye, the auriculopalpebral n. to the orbicularis oculi m. must also be blocked. It can be palpated on the highest part of the zygomatic arch [11].

TABLE 19-1 CRANIAL NERVES

Number	Name	Function	Exit Foramen in Skull
I.	olfactory n.	olfaction	cribriform foramina
II.	optic n.	vision	optic canal
III.	oculomotor n.	motor to ventral oblique m.; dorsal, ventral, medial rectus mm. of eye, as well as levator palpebrae superioris m.; parasympathetic fibers to sphincter mm. of iris and to ciliary m.	*orbital fissure (Car, eq) or foramen orbitorotundum (Ru, su)
IV.	trochlear n.	motor to dorsal oblique muscle of eye	same as above
V.	trigeminal n. ophthalmic br.	sensory to and around eye	same as above
	maxillary br.	sensory to and around superior arcade and lip	*round foramen - rostral alar foramen (Car, eq) or foramen orbitorotundum (Ru, su)
	mandibular br.	sensory to and around inferior arcade, lip, and tongue; motor to muscles of mastication except caudal half of digastricus m.	oval foramen (Car, ru) foramen lacerum (eq, su)
VI.	abducens n.	motor to lateral rectus m. and retractor bulbi mm. of eye	*orbital fissure (Car, eq) or foramen orbitorotundum (Ru, su)
VII.	facial	motor to most muscles of facial expression and caudal half of digastricus m.; taste sensation from cranial two-thirds of tongue; parasympathetic fibers to lacrimal gl. and to mandibular and sublingual glands; sensory to soft palate and nasopharynx	stylomastoid foramen
VIII.	vestibulocochlear n.	balance and audition	does not emerge
IX.	glossopharyngeal n.	taste sensation from caudal one-third of tongue; parasympathetic fibers to parotid and zygomatic salivary glands; sensory to pharynx and carotid sinus; motor to stylopharyngeus m.	tympanooccipital fissure in Car and Ru and jugular foramen in eq and su
X.	vagus n.	motor to smooth m. and glands of respiratory and digestive systems and motor to heart; sensory to the respiratory and digestive systems; motor to muscles of pharynx and larynx; some taste fibers from pharynx, some sensory fibers from external auditory canal	same as above
XI.	accessory n.	motor to trapezius m. and partially to sternocephalicus, brachiocephalicus, and omotransversarius mm.	same as above
XII.	hypoglossal n.	motor to tongue	hypoglossal canal

*In the carnivores (Car) and horse (eq), the orbital fissure and round foramen are separate. In these species, cranial nerves 3, 4, and 6 emerge from the orbital fissure as well as the ophthalmic branch of cranial nerve 5. In the ruminants (Ru) and pig (su), the orbital fissure and round foramen are combined to form the foramen orbitorotundum which serves as a passageway for cranial nerves 3, 4, and 6, and both the ophthalmic and maxillary branches of cranial nerve 5.

6. Facial paralysis results from damage to the facial nerve. Initially, the face sags on the affected side and the nose may be drawn to the sound side.

7. A number of reflexes involving the cranial nerves may be used to assess their function as well as CNS integrity. Among the more widely used are the following:

   a. palpebral reflex--when the eyelids are touched, they close. The afferent limb of the reflex involves the ophthalmic branch of the trigeminal nerve and the efferent limb involves the facial nerve.

   b. corneal reflex--when the cornea is touched, the eyelids close. The pathways include the same ones as those of the palpebral reflex, but motor fibers to the retractor bulbi (CN6) should also cause retraction of the eyeball.

   c. pupillary light reflex--when increased light strikes the retina, the pupil decreases in size. Change in the size of the pupil in the stimulated eye is called the direct pupillary reaction, and change in the opposite pupil is called the indirect or consensual response. The constrictor pathway uses the optic nerve for the afferent limb of the arc and the oculomotor nerve for the efferent limb. The dilator pathway also uses the optic nerve for the afferent limb, but the efferent limb involves tracts down to the cranial thoracic part of the spinal cord and back up the sympathetic trunk.

XII. EYE (Figs. 19-9, 19-10, 19-11)

A. General features [1]

   anterior* and posterior poles--the central points anteriorly and posteriorly
   equator--the circumference halfway between the poles
   optic axis--the axis joining the poles which passes through the pupil
   fibrous tunic--the outermost of the 3 layers of the eyeball**
       sclera--the opaque "white" portion
       cornea--the transparent portion around the anterior pole
           limbus--the junction between the cornea and sclera
           layers:
               anterior epithelium--stratified and continuous with the conjunctival epithelium
               anterior limiting ("Bowman's) membrane
               substantia propria--connective tissue
               posterior limiting ("Descemet's") membrane

---

*The eye and ear are among the few areas where <u>anterior</u>, <u>posterior</u>, <u>superior</u>, and inferior are still considered to be proper nomenclature.
**"Tenon's capsule" refers to the fascial sheath (vagina bulbi) which surrounds the sclera.

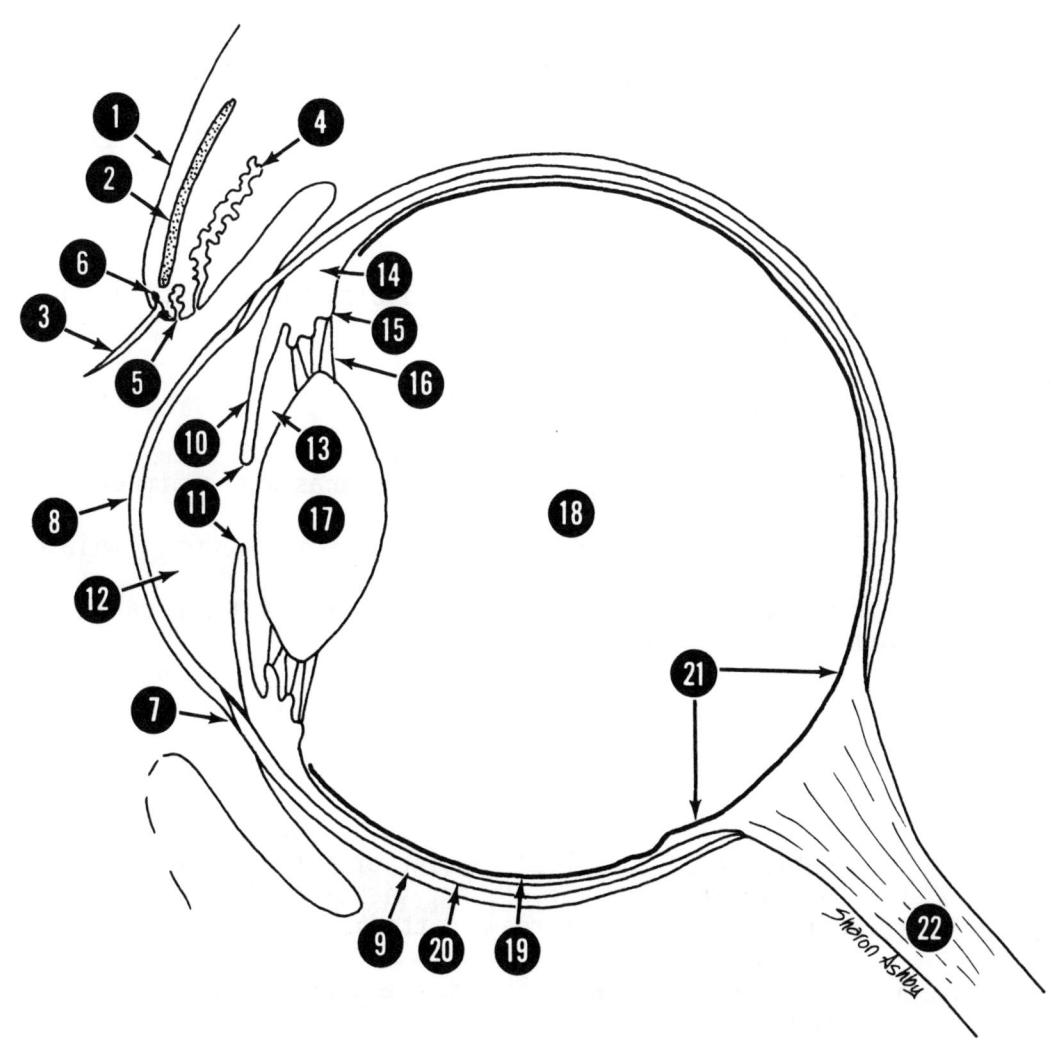

Figure 19-9

Parts of the Eye (sagittal section)

1. superior palpebra
2. tarsus
3. cilium
4. tarsal ("Meibomian") gland
5. ciliary gland (gland of "Moll")
6. sebaceous gland (gland of "Zeis")
7. limbus
8. cornea
9. sclera
10. iris
11. pupil
12. anterior chamber
13. posterior chamber
14. ciliary body
15. ciliary process
16. zonular fibers
17. lens
18. vitreous chamber
19. retina
20. choroid
21. area of optic disc
22. optic nerve

posterior epithelium--a single layer of epithelium (endothelium) which lines the anterior chamber
vascular tunic--the middle of the 3 layers of the eyeball ("uvea")
    choroid--the vascular layer between the retina and sclera
    ciliary body
        ciliary process--a ringlike projection which anchors the zonular fibers
        ciliary muscle--the smooth muscle which functions in accommodation
    iris
        pupillary and ciliary borders
        anterior and posterior surfaces
        pupil--the central aperture in the iris
            pupillary sphincter m.--parasympathomimetic, circular, smooth muscle
            pupillary dilator m.--sympathomimetic, radiate, smooth muscle
internal ("nervous") tunic--the innermost of the 3 layers of the eyeball
    retina
        optic part--the light sensitive part with the 10 classic layers
        blind part--the peripheral portion which lacks photoreceptors
            ciliary part--the part which extends onto the ciliary body
            iridial part--the part which extends onto the iris
        optic disc ("papilla")--point of entry of optic nerve
        macula--the area of highest visual acuity
    retinal vessels--the normal patterns are species specific (Fig. 19-11)
anterior chamber*--the space between the cornea and iris
    iridocorneal angle
posterior chamber*--the space between the iris and lens
vitreous chamber (compartment, posterior compartment)--the space posterior to the lens
    vitreous body--the viscoid body in the vitreous chamber
lens
    anterior and posterior poles   { homologous to the homonymous
    anterior and posterior surfaces { part of the eyeball
    axis and equator
    capsule--the transparent membrane which surrounds the lenticular epithelium
    epithelium of lens--the tissue which produces the lens
    cortex and nucleus--the outer and central parts of the lens, respectively
zonular fibers--attach the ciliary process to the equator of the lens
accessory organs of the eye
    extrinsic eye muscles--innervation formula is $LR_6 Do_4 Rest_3$
    orbital fascia--the irregular connective tissue around the eye
        periorbita--the cone-shaped connective tissue sheath around the muscles, vessels, and nerves of the eye

---

*Collectively, the anterior chamber and posterior chamber have previously been termed anterior compartment. They contain aqueous humor.

eyelids (superior and inferior palpebrae)
    anterior and posterior surfaces
    palpebral border
    tarsus--a fibrous connective tissue support (stiffener)
    medial and lateral commissures--points where the palpebrae meet ("canthi")
    medial and lateral angles of the eye--areas near the commissures
    cilia ("eyelashes")--prominent on the superior lid
    sebaceous glands (glands of "Zeis")--located around the bases of the cilia
    ciliary glands (glands of "Moll")--apocrine sweat glands
    tarsal ("Meibomian") glands--large sebaceous glands
conjunctival tunic
    third eyelid [semilunar conjunctival fold]--"nictitating membrane"
        cartilage
        superficial and deep glands
    lacrimal caruncle--the fleshy structure in the medial canthus
    bulbar conjunctiva
    palpebral conjunctiva
lacrimal apparatus (Fig. 19-10)
    lacrimal gland--on the dorsolateral aspect of the globe
    lacrimal lake--the area in the medial canthus for tear collection
lacrimal punctae--the openings (superior and inferior) of the lacrimal canals
lacrimal canal--the channel which connects each punctum to the lacrimal sac
lacrimal sac--the dilated area which receives the lacrimal canals
nasolacrimal duct--courses from the lacrimal sac to the nasal cavity near the nares

B. Clinical considerations

1. Entropion (inversion of the palpebral margins of the lids) may require surgical correction to prevent trauma to the cornea and excessive tearing. A number of procedures have been reported [3]. A common one involves removal of an elliptical piece of skin from the affected lid (the long axis of the removed part should be parallel to the palpebral border) and then suturing the wound.

2. Ectropion (eversion of the palpebral margins of the lids) may be corrected by a number of techniques [3]. A common method involves removal of a triangular portion of the lid margin or from the lateral palpebral commissure, and then suturing the defect. The increased tension often corrects the problem.

3. Enucleation is the most common surgical procedure involving the eye in carnivores. Incisions around the palpebral margins are followed by dissections around the globe which leave the soft tissues and extrinsic muscles in situ. The optic nerve is clamped and ligated (to control hemorrhage from vessels which accompany it) and then severed. In cases involving neoplasia, all related soft tissues should be removed (extirpation).

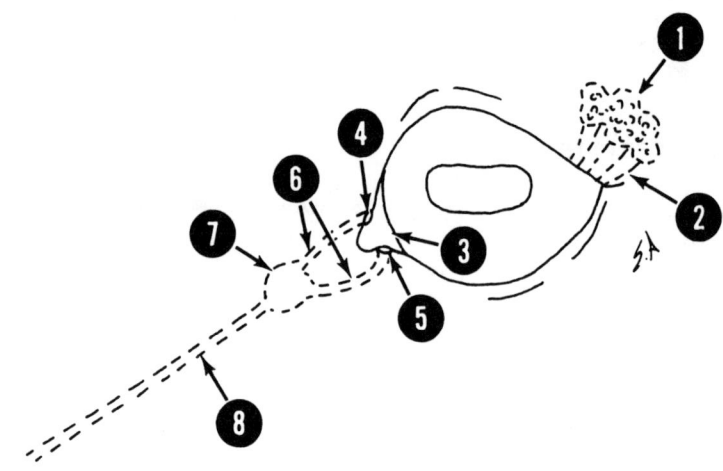

Figure 19-10

Parts of the Lacrimal Apparatus (schematic)

1. lacrimal gland
2. excretory ducts of lacrimal gland
3. lacrimal caruncle against which the lacrimal lake forms
4. superior lacrimal punctum
5. inferior lacrimal punctum
6. lacrimal canals (superior and inferior)
7. lacrimal sac
8. nasolacrimal duct

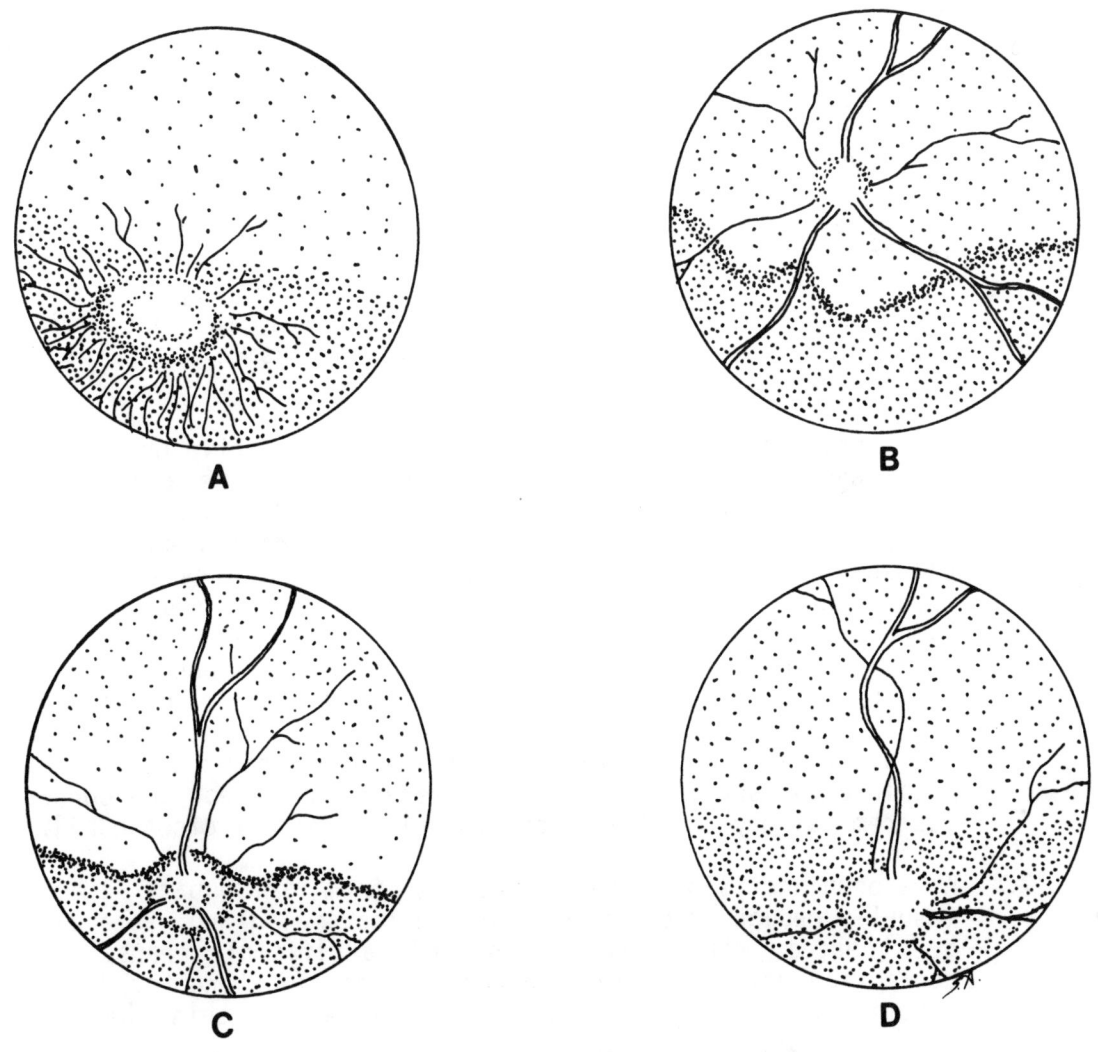

Figure 19-11

The Fundus of the Eye in the Horse (A), Cat (B), Dog (C), and Ox (D)
as Viewed Ophthalmoscopically

The optic disc is located in the pigmented portion of the fundus in the large domestic animals and in the nonpigmented portion (tapetum lucidum) in the cat. In the dog, its position varies; in larger dogs, it is in the tapetum lucidum, and in small dogs, it is located further ventrally in the pigmented portion. In the horse and cat, the vessels appear to radiate from the periphery of the disc while, in the dog and ox, they appear to radiate from its centrum.

After Habel, 1981 [11]

4. Cataracts are opacities of the lens and are classified in several ways. The condition is treated by removal of the lens - either by incising its capsule (extracapsular extraction) or by removing the capsule as well (intracapsular extraction). The latter technique may result in loss of the vitreous body. Juvenile cataracts are sometimes treated by cutting the anterior capsule and then allowing the aqueous humor to clear the opacity (discission) [3].

5. Glaucoma is a disease of the eye characterized by increased intraocular tension. It may be caused by increased production of the aqueous humor or by a blockage in the drainage system at the iridocorneal angle. Some drugs are useful in controlling the disease, and surgical correction includes lens removal, iridectomy, iridencleisis, and often, enucleation.

6. The third eyelid is formed by a fold of conjunctiva over a plate of cartilage. It is passively advanced across the cornea in most species by contraction of the retractor bulbi mm.; but in cats, striated muscle fibers from the lateral rectus m. and levator palpebrae superioris m. attach to it. The third eyelid has a deep gland and a superficial gland. Both of these have been called lymphatic tissue and Harder's gland(s) by some authors. Harder's gland is an eponym for the deep gland, which is absent in the dog. In addition to the glands, there are lymphatic nodules on the bulbar surface of the third eyelid. Any of these may become inflamed, but removal of the third eyelid should be avoided when possible in carnivores because it serves to protect the cornea, and its removal may predispose the animal to corneal disease [3].

7. Keratoconjunctivitis sicca results from inadequate lubrication (usually reduced secretion) from the lacrimal gland. Some cases may be treated with instillation of artificial tears. Surgical correction may be obtained in dogs by translocating the duct of the parotid salivary gland. (See Part III.A. of this chapter.) The parotid gland is the only salivary gland with a duct long enough and properly positioned to be used [3].

8. The lacrimal apparatus occasionally becomes clogged, resulting in tearing. It may be flushed by cannulating the lacrimal punctae or (in large animals) by cannulating its opening near the naris.

9. In examining the retina with an ophthalmoscope, the tapetum lucidum ("tapetal area") is the brightly colored, roughly triangular part which occupies most of the fundic area. The tapetum lucidum is absent in pigs. The tapetum nigrum ("nontapetal area") is the brown or black part along the ventral aspect of the tapetum lucidum. The optic disc ("papilla") is found near their junction and may be in either area. Vessels radiate from the center of the disc (dog, sheep, ox) or from the periphery (horse, cat; Fig. 19-11).

10. Subconjunctival injections may be made in the bulbar conjunctiva. A short, small gauge needle is used.

11. Severe corneal ulcers and abrasions are often treated by keratoplasty. The third eyelid or a flap of bulbar conjuntiva is used to cover a corneal defect while it heals.

12. Horner's syndrome involves enophthalmos, narrowed palpebral fissure, vasodilation, and miosis. It is indicative of injury to the sympathetic nerve supply to the head. Lack of smooth muscle innervation to the orbit and lids explains the enophthalmos and narrowed palpebral fissure in such cases. (There are smooth muscle fascicles as well as skeletal muscles in the eyelids.)

XIII. EAR (Fig. 19-12)

A. General features [1]

inner ear
   membranous labyrinth--semicircular ducts, ampullae, sacculus, maculae, cochlear duct, etc.
   osseous labyrinth--the bony channels housing the membranous labyrinth
      osseous semicircular canals--houses the semicircular ducts and ampullae
      cochlea--houses the cochlear duct
      internal acoustic meatus--the foramen which receives the vestibulocochlear nerve
middle ear
   vestibular ("oval") window--the aperture which receives the baseplate of the stapes
   cochlear ("round") window--the aperture, covered by a membrane, which absorbs the hydraulic shock waves caused by the stapedial vibrations
   tympanic membrane--the "eardrum" which spans the external acoustic meatus
   auditory ossicles
      malleus--attaches to the tympanic membrane
      incus--joins the malleus to the stapes
      stapes--the smallest bone in the body
   muscles of the auditory ossicles
      tensor tympani m.--attaches to the malleus (C.N. 5)
      stapedial m.--attaches to the stapes (C.N. 7)
   auditory tube--courses through the musculotubal canal
      pharyngeal ostium--the opening into the nasopharynx
      tympanic ostium--the opening into the middle ear
      diverticulum ("guttural pouch")--found in equidae only
external ear
   external acoustic meatus--the opening spanned by the tympanic membrane
      cartilage of the external acoustic meatus ("annular cartilage")
   auricle--the "pinna"
      auricular cartilage--the cartilage which imparts rigidity
      scutiform cartilage--the small plate of cartilage at the base of the auricular cartilage in the dog
         tragus--the angular projection at the ventral aspect of the external acoustic meatus

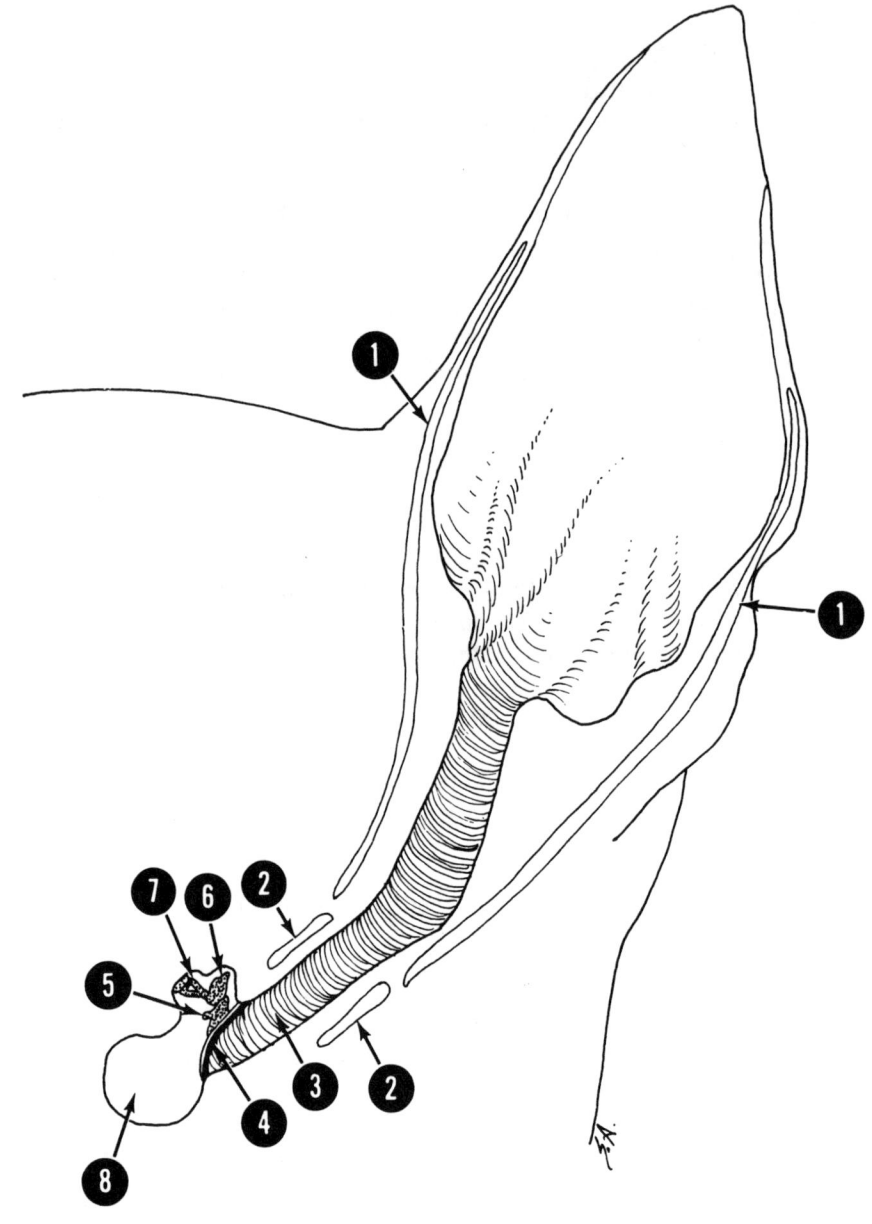

Figure 19-12

Some Features of the External Ear and Middle Ear
(sectional perspective)

1. Auricular cartilage
2. Cartilage of the external auditory meatus
3. Auditory canal
4. Tympanic membrane
5. Malleus
6. Incus
7. Stapes
8. Cavity of middle ear

B. Clinical considerations

1. The canal of the external ear has vertical and horizontal parts. Otoscopy in carnivores requires insertion into the vertical part, and then "turning the corner" several degrees to examine the tympanic membrane. This latter manipulation is facilitated by pulling gently on the pinna to straighten the auditory canal.

2. Otitis media and/or interna causes a characteristic head tilt toward the affected side. Chronic cases may require bullar osteotomies for drainage (see Part I.D.) [3].

3. Otitis externa can have several etiologies. In some breeds of dogs, a significant amount of hair grows in the canal. This may entrap wax and restrict air circulation enough that inflammation results. Periodic removal of the hair may control some cases. Other cases may require surgical resection of the lateral wall of the vertical portion of the ear canal (lateral resection) [3]. Major landmarks for this surgery include the tragus and the indentations at the cranial and caudal aspects of its base (tragohelicine incisure and intertragic incisure, repectively).

4. Ticks often congregate in the marginal cutaneous sac of the ears of carnivores, which is located along the caudal border of the auricle.

5. Ears are trimmed by some veterinarians for cosmetic purposes in the following breeds of dogs:

   Affenpinscher
   Miniature Pinscher
   Boston Terrier
   Bull Terrier
   Schnauzers
   Staffordshire Terrier (Pit bull)

   Briard
   Doberman Pinscher
   Great Dane
   Bouvier des Flanders
   Boxer

6. Blood may be collected from marginal ear veins in pigs (via needle aspiration) and cats (via a nick).

7. Hematomas of the auricles, resulting from trauma, may require surgical correction. These typically occur on the concave surface between the cartilage and skin. Correction may involve needle aspiration or surgical excision and elimination of dead space [3].

8. Myringotomy may be required to relieve intractable pain from pressure in the tympanic cavity [3].

References

1. International Committee on Veterinary Gross Anatomical Nomenclature. 1983. Nomina Anatomica Veterinaria, third ed. Published by the Committee, Ithaca, New York.

2. Getty, R. 1975. *Sisson and Grossman's The Anatomy of the Domestic Animals*, fifth ed. W. B. Saunders, Philadelphia.

3. Archibald, J., ed. 1974. *Canine Surgery*, second ed. American Veterinary Publications, Santa Barbara, California.

4. Amstutz, H. E. ed. 1980. *Bovine Medicine and Surgery*, second ed. American Veterinary Publications, Santa Barbara, California.

5. Case, A. A. 1957. Dehorning goats. *No. Am. Vet.* 38(12):356-359.

6. Vitums, A. 1954. Nerve and arterial blood supply to the horns of the goat with reference to the sites of anesthesia for dehorning. *JAVMA* 125:284-286.

7. Nickel, R., A. Schummer, E. Seiferle, and W. Sack. 1973. *The Viscera of the Domestic Mammals.* Paul Parey, Berlin.

8. McFarland, L. Z. 1970. *Veterinary Surgical Anatomy.* Department of Veterinary Anatomy, University of California, Davis.

9. Mansmann, R. A., E. S. McAllister, and P. W. Pratt, ed. 1982. *Equine Medicine and Surgery.* American Veterinary Publications, Santa Barbara, California.

10. Evans, H. E., and G. C. Christensen. 1979. *Miller's Anatomy of the Dog*, second ed. W. B. Saunders, Philadelphia.

11. Habel, R. E. 1981. *Applied Veterinary Anatomy*, second ed. Published by the author, Ithaca, New York.

AVIAN ANATOMY

Avian medicine and surgery is demanding and receiving a greater share of the veterinary professional effort. Although poultry practice has been well developed as a specialized discipline for many years, caged bird medicine and surgery is a relatively new field. In addition to exotic species kept as companions, increasing numbers of native wild birds are being examined and treated. Often these are birds of prey suffering traumatic injuries from gunshots or from other maladies, and it is a credit to our ecology-minded society that individuals care enough to bring them in for repair. In recent years, a number of clinically oriented references have emerged to assist practitioners in this expanding discipline [1-6].

There are numerous differences between mammalian and avian anatomy. The majority of these are in some way related to the relatively recent descent of birds from their reptilian ancestors or to the specializations required for flight, a physical skill which all birds either possess or have phylogenetically lost. Some of these specializations include [7]:

1. Feathers. Feathers act to conserve heat, streamline the body, and they have a high strength to weight ratio.

2. A light-weight skeleton. The skeletons of some birds are actually lighter than the total weight of their feathers. For example, the skeleton of a 4kg bald eagle may weigh less than 300g while its feathers may total over 600g [8].

3. A highly efficient digestive system. Weight is saved because of the short alimentary canal, lack of teeth, and small mandibular mass.

4. No urinary bladder. Birds excrete a semi-solid urine.

5. Seasonal reduction in the size of the reproductive organs in most species.

6. A respiratory system which passes air through the lungs twice during each respiratory cycle.

7. A large heart weight to body weight ratio.

Divergence from the mammalian anatomical pattern is very obvious in avian visceral body systems (digestive, respiratory, and urogenital), in the musculo-skeletal system, and in the integumentary system. However, the endocrine, circulatory, and nervous systems of birds and mammals are very similar.

Living birds vary in size from the 2.5g bee hummingbird to the 135kg male ostrich. The extinct elephant bird stood 3 m tall, weighed an estimated 450kg, and laid eggs with a volume of about 8 liters [8]. Even with a large variation in size, morphological similarity within the avian class is the rule. Consequently, even though much of the following discussion primarily concerns the domestic chicken and

Table 20-1

Major Living Orders of the Class Aves

The Class Aves contains about 8,600 living species of birds which are grouped into 27 orders, listed below:

Struthioniformes	ostriches
Rheiformes	rheas
Casuariiformes	cassowaries, emus
Apterygiformes	kiwis
Tinamiformes	tinamous
Sphenisciformes	penguins
Gaviiformes	loons
Colymbiformes	grebes
Procellariiformes	albatrosses, petrels, fulmars, shearwaters
Pelecaniformes	pelicans, cormorants, gannets, boobies
Ciconiiformes	herons, storks, ibises, spoonbills, flamingos
Anseriformes	swans, geese, ducks
Falconiformes	eagles, hawks, vultures, falcons, buzzards
Galliformes	quail, grouse, pheasants, domestic fowl
Gruiformes	cranes, rails, coots, gallinules
Charadriiformes	shore birds (gulls, plovers, terns, etc.)
Columbiformes	pigeons, doves
Psittaciformes	parrots, parakeets (budgerigars or "budgies")
Cuculiformes	cuckoos, roadrunners
Strigiformes	owls
Caprimulgiformes	goatsuckers, nighthawks, poorwills
Apodiformes	swifts, hummingbirds
Coliiformes	mousebirds
Trongoniformes	trogons
Coraciiformes	kingfishers, hornbills
Piciformes	woodpeckers
Passeriformes	perching birds

The orders which are most important to veterinary practitioners are the following:

- Anseriformes (food production)
- Galliformes (food production and experimental models)
- Columbiformes (food production and experimental models)
- Psittaciformes (pets)
- Passeriformes (pets and experimental models)

The individual species most important in research models are the chicken, duck, pigeon, turkey, and Japanese quail.

turkey, most of the morphological principles may also be applied to other orders and species of birds (Table 20-1). Sources of gross anatomical information include the works by Petrak [2], Nickel et al. [9], and King [10]. Radiographic studies have been made by Shively [7,11].

I. INTEGUMENTARY SYSTEM

Birds have several differences in their integumentary system compared to mammals.

A. Birds are covered with feathers instead of hair or fur.

1. Two major types of feathers occur (Fig. 20-1):

   a. Contour feathers comprise the majority of the visible feathers including most of the feathers covering the body as well as the flight quills of the wings (remiges; singular, remix) and of the tail (rectrices; singular, rectrix). The remiges can be divided into "primaries" (supported by the manus) and "secondaries" (supported by the antebrachium). The shaft of a typical contour feather may be divided into the rachis which supports the vane, and the calamus which is embedded in the skin. The vane consists of rami which bear proximal and distal barbules. The distal barbules have hooklets which fix onto the hookless proximal barbules of adjacent rami.

   b. Down feathers are tiny wisps which serve primarily as insulators. There is a complete gradation from contour feathers to down; "semiplume" is used to describe intermediate forms.

   c. In addition to contour and down feathers, a number of specialized types occur including filoplumes, bristle feathers, auricular feathers, oil gland feathers, and in some birds, powder feathers [10]. The differentiation of these has little value in veterinary medicine.

2. In most birds, contour feathers are arranged on the skin in numerous named tracts called pterylae. Neighboring areas which have only down feathers are termed apteria. The arrangement of the feather tracts in a number of species has been described [12].

3. Feather replacement is termed moulting and is seasonal in most species. Some species of birds lose many at one time and others replace them more systematically. New feathers require several weeks to grow. Growing feathers have a blood and nerve supply, but mature ones are avascular and aneural. Hemorrhage from injured, growing feathers can usually be controlled by plucking the feather [4].

4. Chickens may be rendered relatively immobile by a "wing lock" in which the wings are crossed over the back (twisted around each other), and some of the primary remiges of the caudal wing are

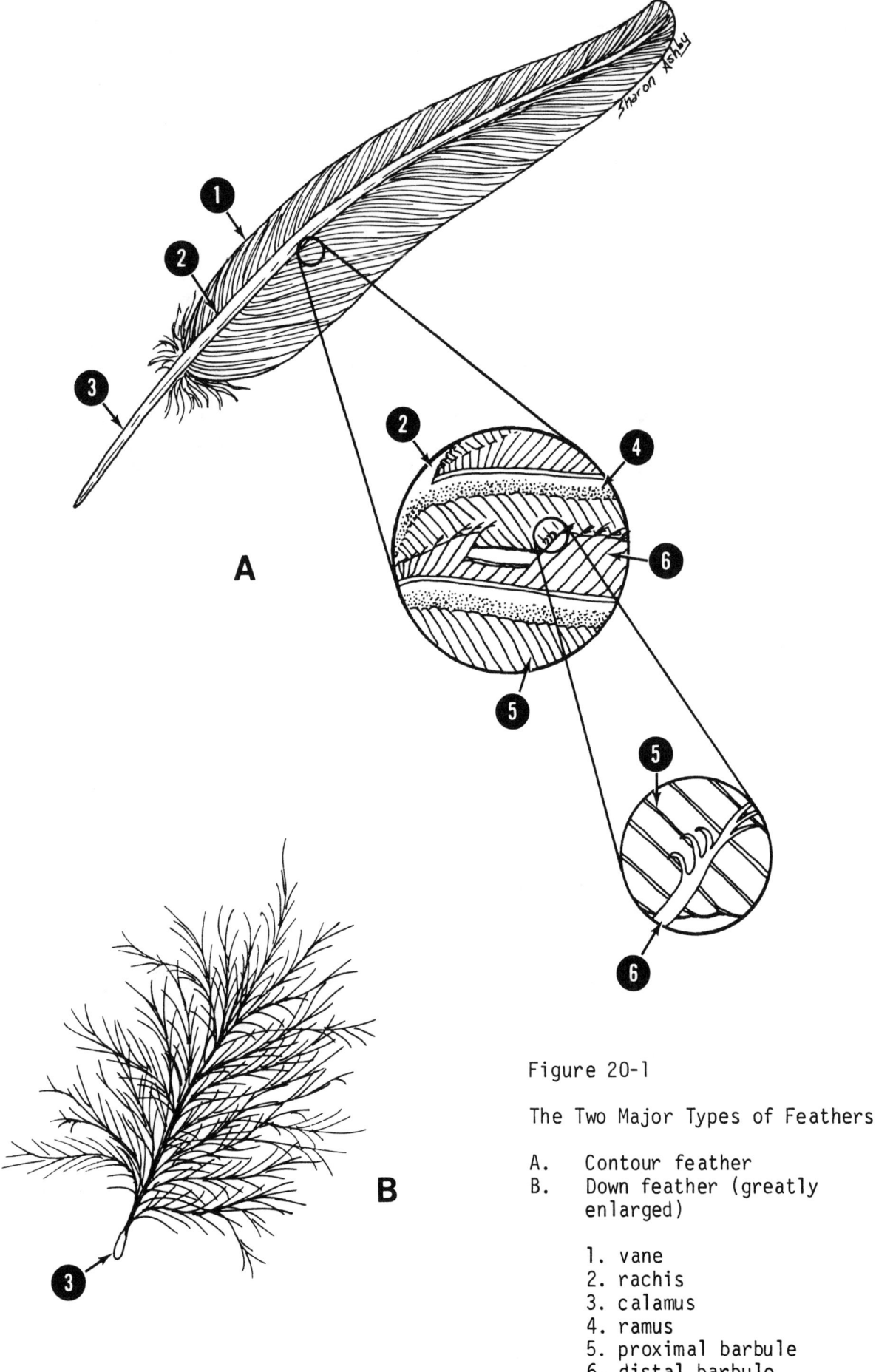

Figure 20-1

The Two Major Types of Feathers

A. Contour feather
B. Down feather (greatly enlarged)

1. vane
2. rachis
3. calamus
4. ramus
5. proximal barbule
6. distal barbule

passed cranially around the other (cranial) wing. This won't work in occasional individuals, and it won't work in turkeys.

5. Temporary pinioning (flight control) can be gained by clipping some of the flight quills of the wings. In small caged birds, most of the flight quills may have to be cut to prevent flight. This procedure is effective only until the next moult. Permanent limitation of flight may be surgically achieved in many ways (see Muscular System).

6. Feather disorders in caged birds include the following [4]:

    a. Feather picking--This vice is usually associated with stress and can sometimes be relieved by providing companionship (human or avian), providing a place for concealment in the cage, and following good principles of husbandry. Intractable cases may require a protective collar.

    b. Broken feathers--These may result from cages which are too small. These may bleed and mar the bird's appearance but are not health-threatening. They will not be replaced until a moult occurs unless they are physically removed.

    c. Bleeding feathers--Hemorrhage is usually the result of trauma to a young growing feather. Removal will usually stop the hemorrhage and pain.

    d. Ruffled feathers--This usually indicates that a bird is chilled and/or in negative caloric balance.

    e. Poor plumage--usually indicates a nutritional deficiency, improper housing, or in some cases, lice.

    f. Feather cysts--These contain curled feathers and cellular debris and are treated surgically.

B. Birds have very few glands associated with their skin. The uropygial gland near the base of the tail is the only major one. It is sebaceous and is important in feather maintenance (i.e., "preening gland") [2].

C. The legs and feet of most birds are covered with scales indicating their relatively recent evolution from reptiles (Fig. 20-2). In laying flocks, pale yellow legs indicate that a hen is laying, whereas brighter yellow scales indicate a nonlayer. Interdigital webbing in ducks and geese provides the surface area necessary for an efficient swimming stroke (Fig. 20-3).

D. A horny beak substitutes for the lips, cheeks, and teeth of mammals. It may be shortened by a process termed "debeaking" to reduce cannibalism in domestic flocks. Electro-cautery in specially designed "debeakers" is used. Caged birds may require occasional trimming and remodelling of the beak--especially those which have been infested with <u>Knemidocoptes</u> mites.

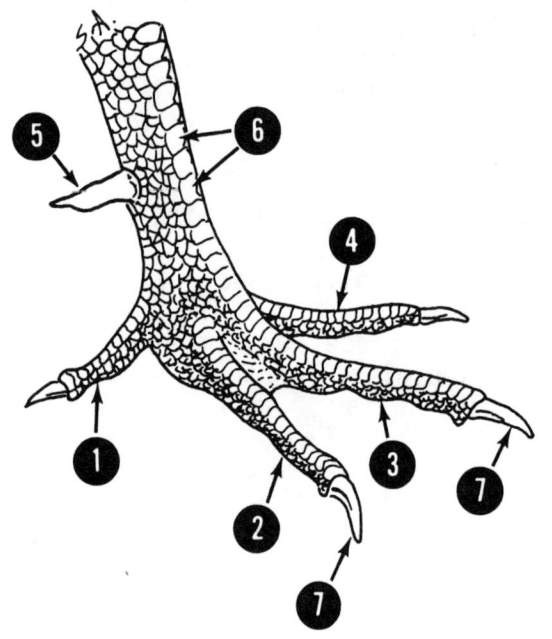

Figure 20-2

Left Foot of a Chicken

1. first digit
2. second digit
3. third digit
4. fourth digit
5. spur
6. scales
7. nails (claws)

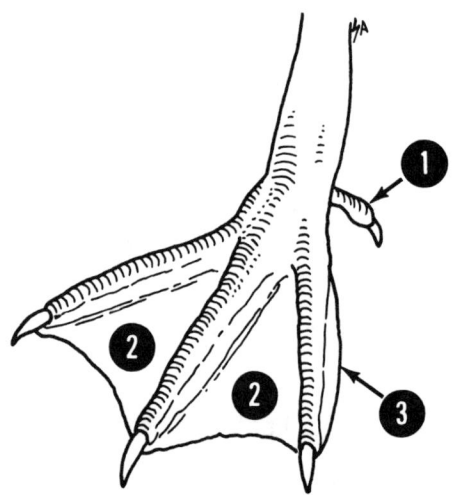

Figure 20-3

Foot of Duck

The reduced first digit (1) does not support any of the interdigital webbing (2). In some species of waterfowl, the webbing does not attach the weight-bearing digits together. Instead, it is reduced to a small flange of tissue on each side of each weight-bearing digit, similar to the one shown here on the abaxial side of the second digit (3).

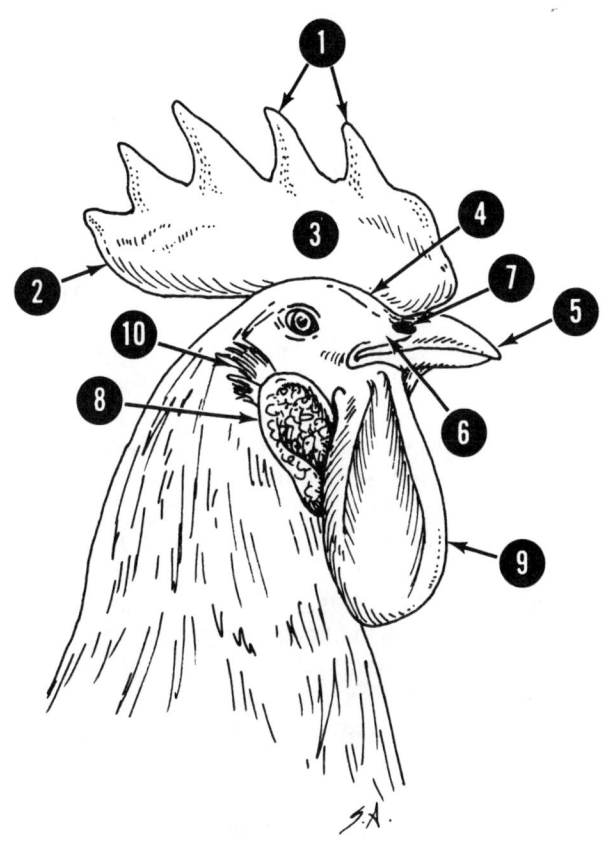

Figure 20-4

Head of a Male Chicken

1. points of comb
2. blade of comb
3. body of comb
4. base of comb
5. beak (superior and inferior)
6. cere
7. nostril
8. ear lobe
9. wattle
10. feathers over external opening of ear

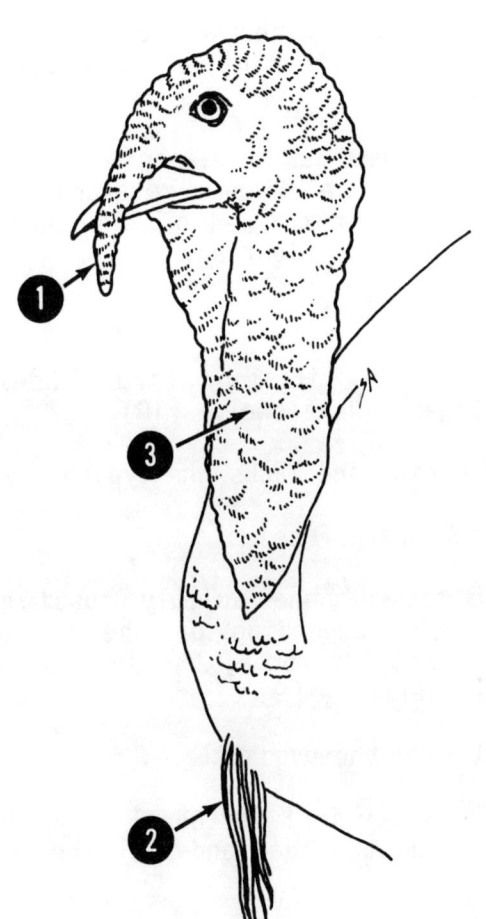

Figure 20-5

Head of a Turkey

1. frontal process (snood)
2. beard
3. non-feathered skin

E. A comb projects from the top of the head of chickens and is usually better developed in males. Several variations in shape occur including the rose, pea, strawberry, buttercup, and others. The typical single comb type has a base, body, blade, and points (Fig. 20-4). Removal of the comb to eliminate it as a target for pecking is termed "dubbing."

F. A pair of wattles is attached to the ventral aspect of the head and cranial cervical region in chickens (Fig. 20-4). Surgical removal of the wattles is termed "cropping." "Cropping" and/or "dubbing" may be indicated in some breeds or individuals kept in wire cages if the wattles or comb develop sufficiently to prevent proper feeding.

G. The ear lobe is an apterium below the external auditory meatus.

H. The cere is a fold of soft tissue at the base of the beak where the nares open. In pigeons, doves, and many psittacine birds, it is well developed. A hypertrophic cere is a common lesion associated with Knemidocoptes mite infestation in budgerigars. In adult budgerigars, a blue cere indicates a male and a pink or brown one is characteristic of a female [6]. Immature birds do not show this difference in color.

I. Much of the head and part of the neck of turkeys are covered with nonfeathered skin. The frontal process (snood) is an extension of this skin (Fig. 20-5) [10].

J. The beard is a complex structure attached to the neck of turkeys. Black filaments emerging from the beard are neither hairs nor feathers, and remain unclassified (Fig. 20-5) [10].

K. The spur is an epidermal structure used as a weapon by cocks which protrudes from the medial aspect of the distal metatarsus. It is supported by a bony process. Spurs may be trimmed or, in young birds, surgically excised to control injuries from fighting.

II. SKELETAL SYSTEM (Fig. 20-6)

A. The vertebral formula is $C_{14}T_7L-S_{14}Cd_6$ in many birds. Geese have seventeen cervical vertebrae and pigeons have twelve [10].

1. The atlas is in the shape of a ring and lacks the typical wings.

2. Several of the thoracic vertebrae are fused.

3. The lumbosacral region consists of one solidly fused mass of vertebrae called the synsacrum. Depending on the species, it includes the 14 lumbar and sacral vertebrae, the seventh thoracic vertebra, and the first caudal vertebra [9].

4. The last caudal vertebra is termed the pygostyle.

5. Chickens may be euthanized by a cervical vertebral separation. To effect this, place a thumb behind the head and cock the head back

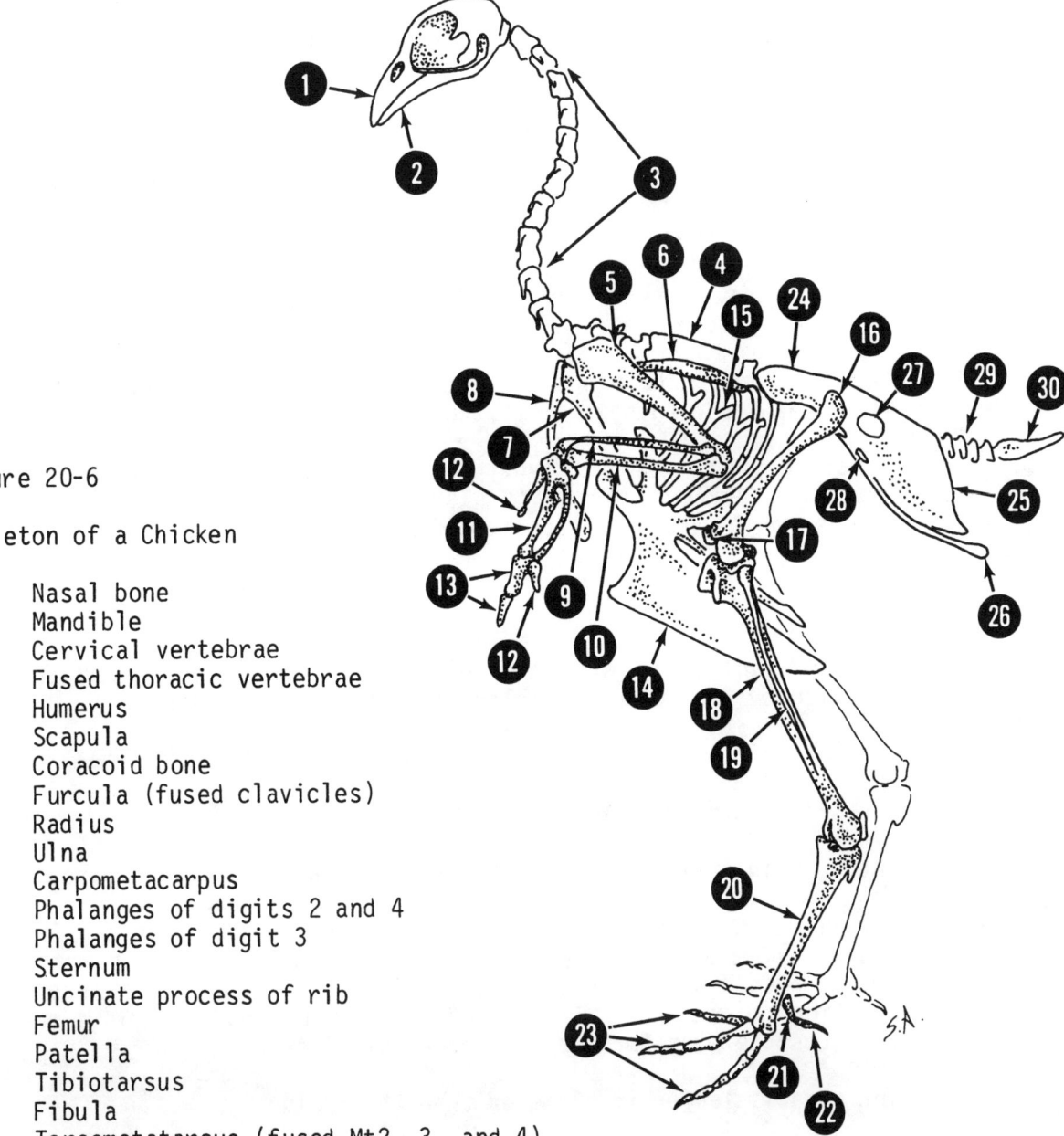

Figure 20-6

Skeleton of a Chicken

1. Nasal bone
2. Mandible
3. Cervical vertebrae
4. Fused thoracic vertebrae
5. Humerus
6. Scapula
7. Coracoid bone
8. Furcula (fused clavicles)
9. Radius
10. Ulna
11. Carpometacarpus
12. Phalanges of digits 2 and 4
13. Phalanges of digit 3
14. Sternum
15. Uncinate process of rib
16. Femur
17. Patella
18. Tibiotarsus
19. Fibula
20. Tarsometatarsus (fused Mt2, 3, and 4)
21. First metatarsal bone
22. Phalanges of digit 1
23. Phalanges of digits 2, 3, and 4
24. Ilium
25. Ischium
26. Pubis
27. Sciatic foramen
28. Obturator foramen
29. Caudal vertebrae
30. Pygostyle

by putting the fingers of the same hand under the beak. Then, with the feet (and wings) in the other hand, pull until a vertebral luxation occurs. Some terminal struggling is normal. Do not attempt this with turkeys (it makes them mad).

B. Ribs

1. Several of the ribs have two parts (vertebral and sternal). The sternal portions are termed sternocostal bones by some authors [9], and are homologous to ossified costal cartilages in mammals.

2. Some of the vertebral ribs bear an uncinate process which is a caudal projection not found in the ribs of any domestic mammal.

C. The sternum ("keel") is one solid mass of bone. It articulates with the coracoid bones and with several of the ribs.

D. The os coxae fuses to the synsacrum. It has obturator and sciatic foramina. The amount of space (spread) between its caudoventral extremities can be used by experienced poultrymen to assess if a hen is "in lay".

E. Wing

1. The left and right shoulder joints are held in a "sprung apart" position by the fused clavicles (= furcula = "wishbone").

2. The coracoid bone extends from the shoulder to the sternum.

3. The scapula is long and flat.

4. The glenoid cavity is formed by the scapula and coracoid bone.

5. The scapula, coracoid bone, and furcula come together to form a canal (foramen triosseum) through which the tendon of the supracoracoideus m. ("deep pectoral") passes to attain an insertion position on the dorsal aspect of the proximal humerus. This muscle elevates the wing for the "upstroke" of flight.

6. The ulna is larger in diameter than the radius.

7. There are only two separate carpal bones, a radial carpal bone and an ulnar carpal bone.

8. In the metacarpus, the distal row of carpal bones is fused to the second, third, and fourth metacarpal bones, and the whole mass is termed the carpometacarpus.

9. The third digit is the largest and usually contains two phalanges. The second and fourth digits typically contain a single phalanx. First and fifth digits are not present.

F. Leg

1. The tibia is fused to proximal tarsal bones to form the tibiotarsus. The tibiotarsus and the slender fibula form the skeleton of the "drumstick".

2. Metatarsals II, III, and IV are fused together and to the distal row of tarsal bones to form the tarsometatarsus. A bony process extends from the distal medial aspect of the tarsometatarsus to support the spur. Metatarsal I is very small and articulates with the distal end of the tarsometatarsus. It may be mistaken for the proximal phalanx of digit I.

3. The digits present are the first, second, third, and fourth. These typically contain 2, 3, 4, and 5 phalanges respectively. In domestic fowl, the first digit is oriented caudally and the other three are directed cranially. In some birds however, <u>two</u> digits are oriented caudally and two cranially.*

III. MUSCULAR SYSTEM

The muscular system of birds has many similarities to the general mammalian pattern and a few differences of significance. Only 5 points will be made.

A. The muscles of flight are the supracoracoideus m. ("deep pectoral") and the pectoralis thoracicus m. ("superficial pectoral"). These both attach to the sternum and to the humerus. The pectoralis thoracicus provides the "downstroke" of the wings for flight and supracoracoideus provides the "upstroke". Even though the supracoracoideus muscle originates from the sternum (and is located ventrally), it can affect the "upstroke" because its tendon passes through the foramen triosseum to attain a position of attachment on the dorsal aspect of the humerus [10].

B. Many perching birds and birds of prey have a type of "reciprocal" apparatus which dictates that flexion of the digital joints will occur whenever the tarsal joint is flexed. This happens because some of the flexor tendons pass over the rounded enlargement at the distal end of the tibiotarsus. Flexion of the tarsal joint applies tension to these tendons because they are stretched over a greater distance to their points of termination. This causes reciprocal flexion of the digital joints [7].

C. Mineralized tendons occur in the leg muscles of many species of birds and in the wing muscles of some. These should be recognized radiographically as normal [7].

D. Surgical pinioning (limiting the flight of a bird) may be done in several ways. Although tenotomies, tenectomies, neurectomies, and carpal arthrodesis have all been used, amputation through the carpal joint, or through the metacarpal region just distal to the carpus is the most

---

*In the parrot family, I and IV are directed caudally and II and III are directed cranially [2]. In the trogons, I and II are caudal and III and IV are cranial. Rarely (swifts) all 4 digits may be directed cranially.

widely accepted procedure. Removal of the distal limb removes the primary remiges. This procedure is done unilaterally to "unbalance" the bird during attempted flight [2,13,14].

E. Intramuscular injections may be made wherever convenient. In small pet birds, the pectoral mm. are commonly used and, in larger birds, the thigh muscles are large enough to be utilized.

IV. DIGESTIVE SYSTEM

A. Major parts of the digestive tube (Fig. 20-7)

1. The horny beak supported by bone replaces the lips, cheeks, and teeth.

2. The tongue is supported by an entoglossal bone which is part of the hyobranchial (hyoid) apparatus [2].

3. In parrots, gallinaceous birds, and a few other species, the esophagus has a diverticulum at the thoracic inlet, termed the crop, which is used for short term storage of ingesta [2].

4. The glandular stomach is the proventriculus.

5. The muscular stomach (ventriculus or "gizzard") functions to grind up ingested food. Grit or small pebbles are often swallowed by some species, and these appear to remain in the gizzard for a time [2].

6. The duodenum has closely related descending (proximal) and ascending (distal) parts with the pancreas wedged between them.

7. The rest of the small intestine is termed jejunoileum. A small bleb, Meckel's diverticulum, which developmentally opened into the yolk sac of the egg, may be found along this segment of the intestine.

8. The large intestine consists of a pair of blind-ended ceca and a short segment of intestine, termed colon by some and rectum by others.

9. The rectum opens into the cloaca which has three compartments. The initial expanded portion which continues the rectum caudally is the coprodeum. The area where the ureters and oviducts or deferential ducts open is the urodeum. The proctodeum is the last portion, and the cloacal bursa (bursa of "Fabricius") opens into its dorsal aspect. The external opening of the cloaca is termed the vent. An enlarged, moist, oval vent is characteristic of a hen in lay.

B. Accessory digestive organs

1. The liver has left and right lobes, and the gallbladder lies on the visceral surface of the right lobe. Two bile ducts typically enter

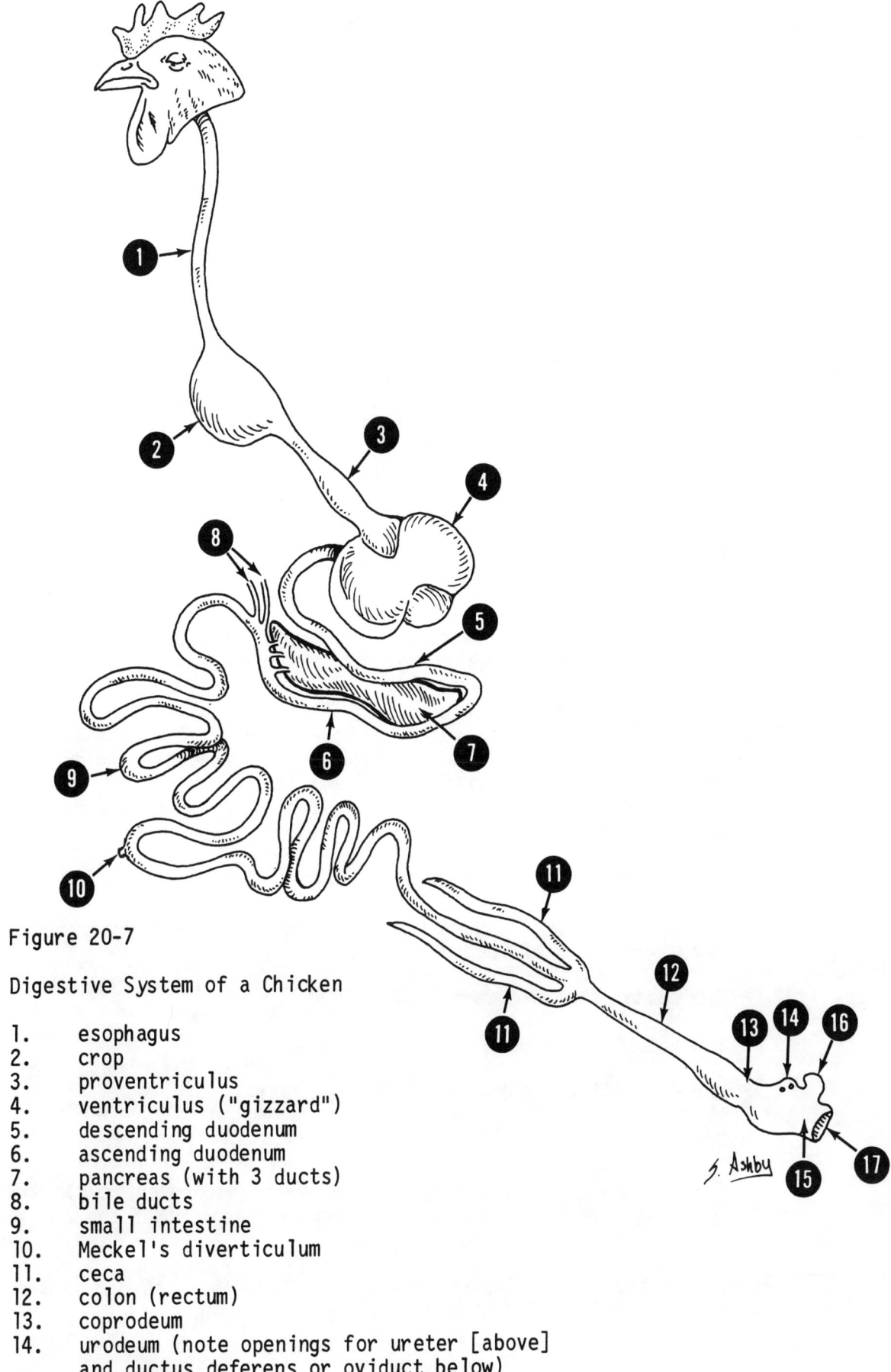

Figure 20-7

Digestive System of a Chicken

1. esophagus
2. crop
3. proventriculus
4. ventriculus ("gizzard")
5. descending duodenum
6. ascending duodenum
7. pancreas (with 3 ducts)
8. bile ducts
9. small intestine
10. Meckel's diverticulum
11. ceca
12. colon (rectum)
13. coprodeum
14. urodeum (note openings for ureter [above] and ductus deferens or oviduct below)
15. proctodeum
16. cloacal bursa
17. vent

the intestine near the distal part of the ascending duodenum--one directly from the liver (hepatoenteric duct), and one from the gallbladder (cysticoenteric duct). Some birds (like the pigeon) do not have gallbladders, and both ducts (hepatoenteric ducts) course directly from the liver to the duodenum [9].

2. The pancreas, which lies between the loops of the duodenum, may be divided into 3 or 4 regional parts. Three pancreatic ducts are typically present in chickens and pigeons, but only two in most ducks and geese. The pancreatic ducts enter the duodenum near the bile ducts [9].

V. RESPIRATORY SYSTEM

A. The nares are elongated slits in the upper beak.

B. The nasal cavity communicates with the oral cavity through the choanal opening. There is no soft palate. In fact, the hard palate has a slit (cleft) for communication with the nasal cavity.

C. The laryngeal mound is a conspicuous elevation on which the glottis (opening into the larynx) is positioned.

D. The tracheal rings are complete, signet-ring shaped, and overlap.

E. The small syrinx is the vocal organ and is located at the tracheal bifurcation. It includes cartilaginous components and two pairs of thin membranes [10].

F. The two unlobed lungs receive the primary bronchi from the syrinx. The bronchial architecture within the lung is quite complex and is believed by some to pass air through the lungs during both inspiration and expiration. The lungs do not expand and shrink during the respiratory cycle (see G, below).

G. Air sacs are connected to the lungs and include (Fig. 20-8) [10]:

1. Two cranial thoracic sacs (the axillary sacs listed by some authors are diverticula of these)

2. Two caudal thoracic sacs

3. Two abdominal sacs

4. One cervical sac (paired in many species)

5. One clavicular sac

The air sacs fill and empty during each respiratory cycle and air passes through the lungs as it is forced into and out of the air sacs.*

---

*Physiologically, most inspired air goes through the lungs into the air sacs during inspiration and then back through the lungs during expiration.

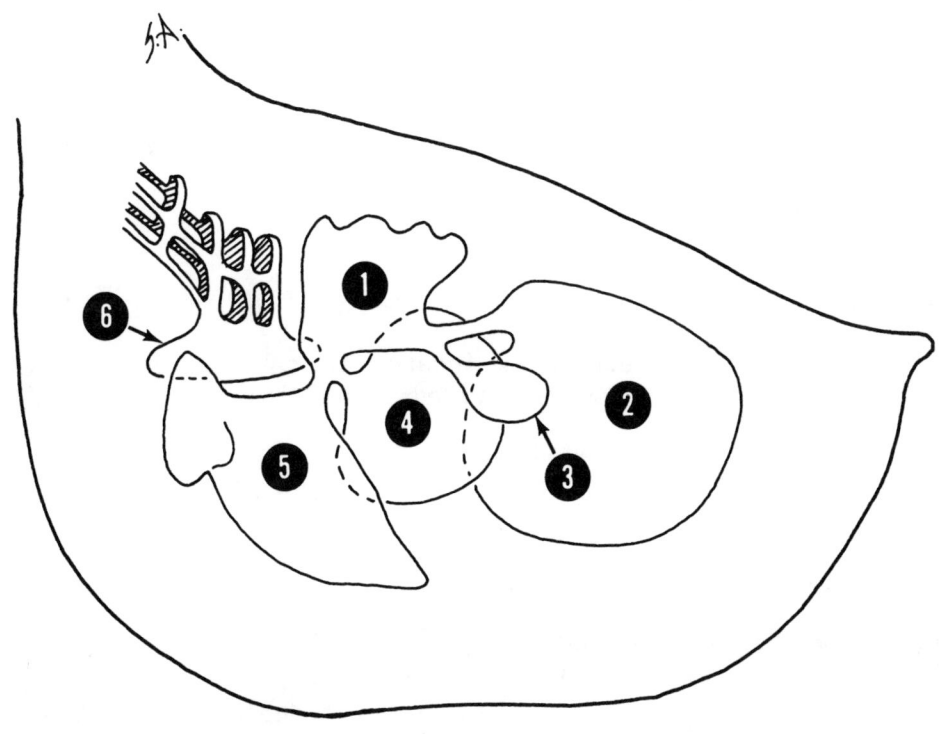

Figure 20-8

Air Sacs of a Chicken

1. lung
2. left abdominal sac
3. left caudal thoracic sac
4. left cranial thoracic sac
5. clavicular sac
6. cervical sac

After King, 1975 [10]

Oxygen-carbon dioxide exchange occurs in the lungs only. Several of the air sacs communicate with pneumatic medullary cavities in some of the bones (humerus, cervical vertebrae, etc., depending on the species). Air sacs are difficult to demonstrate grossly in a normal individual, and are often involved in respiratory pathology (air sacculitis). Radiographically, the air sacs provide negative contrast for evaluation of the viscera, but they may opacify if inflamed.

H. No diaphragm is present. Movement of the rib cage and sternum alter the intraabdominal-thoracic pressure and thus cause inspiration and expiration. This should be kept in mind to prevent suffocation when restraining small birds.

VI. UROGENITAL SYSTEM

　A. Urinary system

　　1. The kidneys are symmetrically located in cavities on the ventral aspect of the ilium. Each is divided into 3 lobes.

　　2. The ureters can be divided into a renal part passing along the kidney, and a pelvic part which runs from the kidney to the urodeum of the cloaca.

　B. Male reproductive system

　　1. The testes are symmetrically arranged and located within the body cavity. Surgical removal is termed caponization, and the resulting individual is a capon.* The pleuroperitoneal cavity is entered through a short incision between the last two ribs on the right side. In young cocks, the testes are very small and are located at the cranial aspects of the kidneys.

　　2. The epididymis is closely attached to the dorsomedial border of the testis.

　　3. The ductus deferens extends to the urodeum of the cloaca.

　　4. The copulatory apparatus of male chickens consists only of folds of cloacal mucosa. Some other birds have more sophisticated organs.

　　5. No secondary sex glands are grossly identifiable.

　C. Female reproductive system

　　1. Although both left and right ovaries and oviducts develop, for unknown reasons the left ones persist in most birds and the right

---

*Caponization is rarely done. In females, removal of the ovaries may be accomplished by a similar procedure termed poulardization.

ones regress. Occasionally, nonfunctional vestiges of the right oviducts are present. In some raptors, the right ovaries and oviducts are the functional ones.

2. The left ovary in an adult resembles a yellow bunch of grapes because of the numerous rounded follicles of different sizes. Evidently, sperm can be stored in many species since females can lay fertile eggs for some time after contact with males.

3. The left oviduct is about 65 cm long in a laying hen, opens into the urodeum, and can be divided into five regions which are not easily distinguished by the novice. Of academic interest is the time which an egg spends in each section [10]:

   a. Infundibulum (1/4 hr.)

   b. Magnum--secretes albumin (3 hr.)

   c. Isthmus--secretes shell membrane (1 1/4 hr.)

   d. Uterus--secretes the shell which is made primarily of calcium carbonate deposited on a protein-polysaccharide, organic matrix (20 3/4 hr.)

   e. Vagina--delivers the egg to the cloaca (a very short time)

4. The nonfunctional right oviduct may become cystic.

5. Occasionally, eggs are retained and may accumulate in the abdomen ("egg bound"). Surgical removal may be required.

6. Sexual differentiation in newly hatched chickens and turkeys can be made by highly skilled sexers who examine the vent. Some strains have been developed which show a sexual dimorphism in the degree of feather development at hatching. In older birds, secondary sex characteristics may often be used. For example, in chickens, cocks usually have a larger comb, are more likely to have a well-developed spur, and typically have contour feathers on their necks which are pointed (vs. being rounded) at the tips. Some caged birds are very difficult to sex. Techniques include surgical laparotomy to view the gonads directly, cytology, and steroid analyses of feces or plasma [2].

7. Chicken hens are heterogametic and are designated ZW. Roosters are homogametic and are designated ZZ [15].

VII. CIRCULATORY SYSTEM

A. A renal portal system exists whereby some venous blood returning from the legs and digestive tube filters through the kidneys en route back to the heart. The venous blood which enters the kidneys through the afferent renal vein is distributed to the tubules. The glomeruli receive only arterial blood [10].

B. The portal vein divides before entering the liver into left and right portal trunks. These enter the liver at two distinct loci.

C. The spleen is spherical or egg-shaped in chickens, but in aquatic birds, it is more triangular. It is located on the right side of the junction of the proventriculus and ventriculus.

D. Lymph nodes are absent in the chicken and turkey, but are present in most other species. The thymus and cloacal bursa (bursa of "Fabricius") are well developed.

E. Cardiocentesis in chickens may be performed by inserting a needle halfway between the cranial point of the keel and the dorsal aspect of the thorax. It may also be performed by a cranial approach. The bird is laid on its back, and the needle is directed caudally through the thoracic inlet.

F. Venipunctures in chickens may be done using the brachial ("wing") vein located on the medial side of the limb near the cubital joint. The brachial vein is very thin walled and hematomas often form. The external jugular veins and medial tarsometatarsal veins can also be used. The latter vessel is difficult to see through the scales of some species. It is best punctured as it crosses the medial aspect of the tarsal joint. Blood in most species can be collected by clipping a toenail.

G. Heart sounds are impossible to evaluate by standard means since the heart rate varies from 300/min (chicken) to 1000/min (canary).

VIII. NERVOUS SYSTEM

No differences of significance occur in the nervous system of birds compared to that of mammals. In the organs of special sense, the ear lacks a pinna and the eye includes 11-15 small bony plates in its sclera (scleral ossicles). Birds have well-developed eyes and exceptionally good vision. Many species possess color discrimination. The sciatic nerves on the caudomedial side of the leg are examined for enlargement and discoloration in Marek's disease (neural lymphomatosis).

IX. ENDOCRINE SYSTEM

A. The paired thyroid glands are located at the thoracic inlet adjacent to the common carotid arteries.

B. The ultimobranchial bodies are found a few millimeters caudal to the thyroid glands (in mammals they are incorporated into the thyroid gland as the "C" cells). They are pink in color, measure about 1.5 mm in diameter, and secrete (thyro-) calcitonin which lowers blood calcium levels. Their histological appearance is complex because they also contain lymphatic nodules, parathyroid tissue, and thyroid-like vesicles.

C. The parathyroid glands are immediately caudal to the thyroids and are represented by 2 small masses on each side (parathyroids III and IV). Parathyroid V is usually embedded in the ultimobranchial body.

D. The suprarenal glands lie against the cranial extremities of the kidneys.

References

1. Thomas, Barbara. 1982. Caged bird medicine: A bibliography. Swest. Vet. 35(2):141-142.

2. Petrak, M., ed. 1982. Diseases of Cage and Aviary Birds. Lea and Febiger, Philadelphia.

3. Steiner, C. V., and R. B. Davis. 1981. Caged Bird Medicine. Iowa State University Press, Ames, Iowa.

4. Fowler, M. E. ed. 1980. Diseases of caged birds and exotic pets. Section VIII in R. W. Kirk, Current Veterinary Therapy VII. W. B. Saunders, Philadelphia.

5. Feyerabend, C. 1970. Diseases of Budgerigars. T.F.H. Publications, Inc. Neptune City, New Jersey.

6. Stunkard, J. A., R. J. Russell, and D. K. Johnson. A Guide to Diagnosis, Treatment, and Husbandry of Caged Birds. Veterinary Medicine Publishing Co. Manhattan, Kansas.

7. Shively, M. J. 1978. Radiographic anatomy of the barred owl--Strix varia. Swest Vet. 31(2):143-150 (also in VM/SAC 74(4):552-558).

8. Perrins, C. 1976. Birds. Harry N. Abrams, New York.

9. Nickel, R., A. Schummer, E. Seiferle, W. Siller, and P. Wright. 1977. Anatomy of the Domestic Birds. Paul Parey, Berlin.

10. King, A. 1975. Aves. In Sisson and Grossman's The Anatomy of the Domestic Animals, ed. R. Getty. W. B. Saunders, Philadelphia.

11. Shively, M. J. 1982. Xerographic anatomy of the pigeon: Columbia livia domestica. Swest Vet. 35(2):101-111.

12. Lucas, A. M., and P. R. Stettenhein. 1972. Avian Anatomy Integument. Part I. Agriculture Handbook 362. U.S. Government Printing Office, Washington, D.C.

13. Sedgwick, C. J. 1967. Deflighting pet birds. Mod. Vet. Prac. 48(3):38-40.

14. Young, W. A. 1948. Amputation of birds in lieu of pinioning. JAVMA 112:224.

15. Pineda, M. H. and L. C. Faulkner. 1980. The biology of sex. In Veterinary Endocrinology. Lea and Febiger, Philadelphia.

ANATOMY OF THE PIG

Morphology of the pig is perhaps the most slighted specific subject in veterinary anatomy curricula. There are two major reasons for this:

1. The pig has a fatter carcass which does not lend itself to teaching fundamentals of anatomy as well as those of other species.

2. Less surgery is performed on pigs than on most of the other domestic species.

Although the pig has a number of species-specific anatomic peculiarities, most of them have little or no clinical significance. No comment is made in the following outline on the circulatory, nervous, or integumentary systems. However, in the skeletal system, endocrine system, and in the visceral system (digestive, respiratory, and urogenital) some of the more obvious distinctive features are noted.

I. SKELETAL SYSTEM

    A. Axial skeleton

        1. The vertebral formula is $C_7 T_{14-15} L_{6-7} S_4 Cd_{20-23}$.

        2. There are 6 sternebrae.

        3. The first seven ribs are true ("sternal") ribs, the last 7 or 8 are false ("asternal").

        4. An extra bone, the os rostrale (rostral bone), occurs in the nose. It is embedded in the rostral part of the nasal septum and gives rigidity which is helpful in rooting (Fig. 21-1/9) [1].

        5. The zygomatic processes of the frontal bone do not contact the zygomatic arches as they do in ruminants, and the paracondylar processes are especially well developed [2].

    B. Limbs

        1. The ulna and fibula are completely developed and do not fuse to the radius and tibia, respectively (in contrast to the situation in the other domestic ungulates).

        2. The generalized mammalian carpal pattern of 8 separate bones is present.

        3. The generalized mammalian tarsal pattern of 7 separate bones is present. The talus has both a proximal and a distal trochlea as in the ruminants.

4. First digits are absent, and digits 2 and 5 are reduced on all four limbs.

5. No distal sesamoid bones are present in the reduced (2 and 5) digits [3].

6. A metatarsal sesamoid bone, like that in ruminants, is present.

7. Epiphyseal lines remain radiographically detectable in the long bones and vertebral bodies for several years [2].

C. Abnormalities of the musculoskeletal system

1. A number of congenital and neonatal skeletal abnormalities have been reported in pigs.

    a. "Kinky-tails," resulting from fusion of adjacent coccygeal vertebrae, may or may not be associated with urogenital abnormalities [4,5].

    b. A single recessive trait may result in congenitally limbless pigs [6]. A lethal malformation of the pelvic limbs and sacrum, also associated with a recessive gene, has been reported in Denmark [7].

    c. Polydactyly has been reported [8], as has syndactyly [9]. Other congenital malformations, including clubfoot, absence of the fibula, and abnormal appendages resembling hooves have also been reported [10].

    d. Congenital splayleg (spraddleleg, myofibrillar hypoplasia) is a weakness primarily of the pelvic limbs, seen during the first week of life. Affected animals typically sit on their hindquarters with their front legs spread out. Some are able to move with difficulty, while others are unable to stand. Although the disease appears to be heritable, smooth, sloping floors may precipitate the problem in susceptible animals [2,11,12]. Spontaneous recovery may occur in a few days (providing the piglets receive adequate nutrition and are not trampled by the sow.)

2. Infectious polyarthritis is a significant and serious disease which may involve a number of bacterial agents. Several routes of entry for the organisms have been implicated including abrasions associated with roughened floors, tail docking, clipping of needle teeth, as well as the oral route [2].

3. Separation of the proximal femoral physis ("epiphysiolysis") may occur between 5 months and 3 years of age. This physis doesn't normally fuse until 3 or $3\frac{1}{2}$ years [2]. A similar separation has been reported in young sows involving the ischiatic tuberosities.

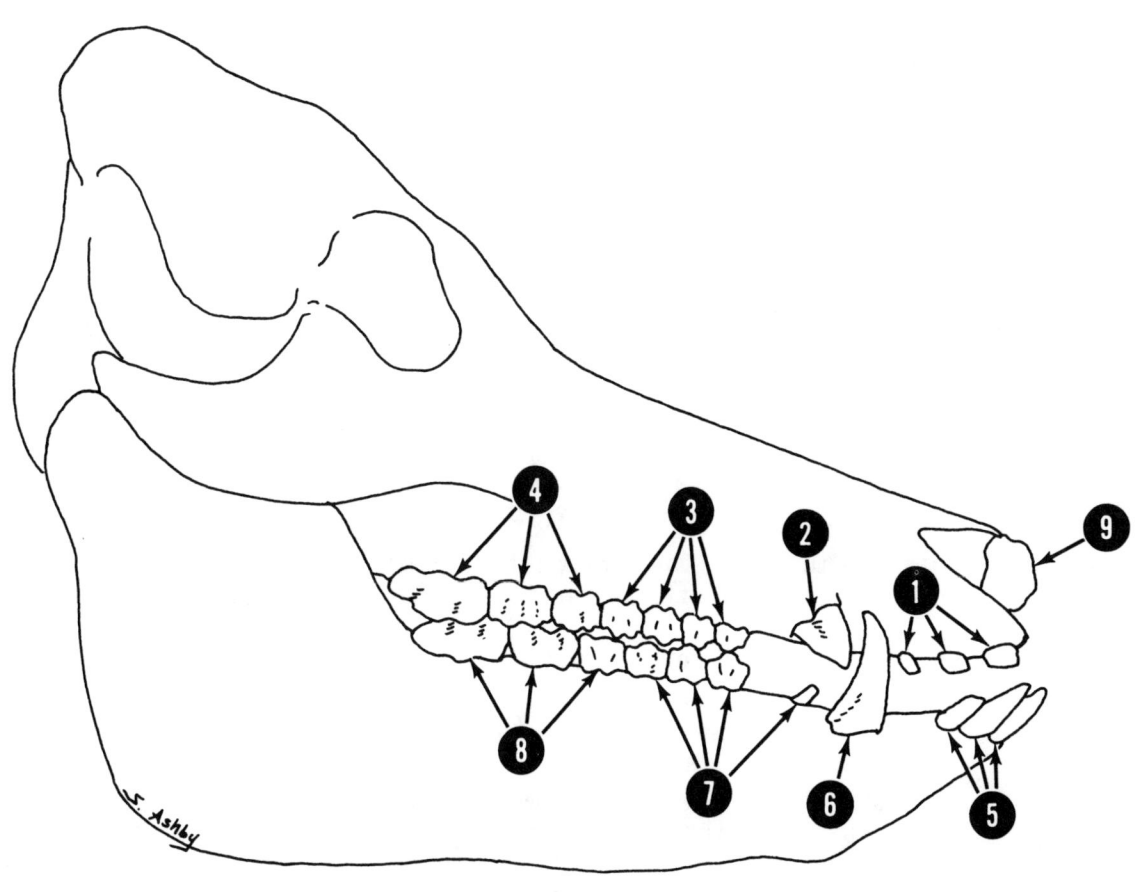

Figure 21-1

Dentition and Rostral Bone of the Pig

1. Right superior incisors (I1, I2, I3)
2. Right superior canine
3. Right superior premolars (P1, P2, P3, P4)
4. Right superior molars (M1, M2, M3)
5. Right inferior incisors (I1, I2, I3)
6. Right inferior canine
7. Right inferior premolars (P1, P2, P3, P4)
8. Right inferior molars (M1, M2, M3)
9. Rostral bone

4. Degenerative joint disease causing clinical lameness has been described in which no infectious organisms are involved [2]. This has also been described as arthropathy, arthrosis, polyarthrosis, osteoarthrosis, osteoarthritis, and osteochondrosis [2].

II. DIGESTIVE SYSTEM

A. The cheeks and lips are relatively stiff and nonprehensile.

B. A double lingual frenulum is present in contrast to the single one of other domestic mammals [1]. These are located just to each side of the median plane.

C. Dentition (Fig. 21-1):

1. Permanent dental formula: $2(I\frac{3}{3} C\frac{1}{1} P\frac{4}{4} M\frac{3}{3}) = 44$.

 This formula is the "complete" mammalian formula. In all other domestic species, the dentition is reduced in one or more areas.

2. Deciduous dental formula: $2(I\frac{3}{3} C\frac{1}{1} P\frac{3}{3}) = 28$.

 a. The deciduous canines and third incisors (Dc and Di3) are present at birth and often cause udder lacerations during suckling. They are commonly called "needle" teeth and are usually clipped by herdsmen soon after birth for the sow's comfort. Care should be taken to clip only the sharp tips of the teeth to prevent shattering them and causing gingivitis [2].

 b. The permanent dentition should be present by 18 months of age.

3. The inferior incisors are rodlike and project rostrally. They are used in rooting.

4. The canine teeth are commonly called "tusks" and never cease growing. They may be trimmed in breeding boars to reduce the risk of injury to handlers and other livestock.

5. The first inferior premolars are normally separated from the others by wide diastemata.

6. The molars increase in size from the rostral ones to the caudal ones (in contrast to those of a dog).

D. Tonsils of the pig include:

1. Lingual tonsils in the connective tissue cores of the filiform papillae at the base of the tongue.

2. Paraepiglottic tonsils at the bottom of the depressions on either side of the base of the epiglottis.

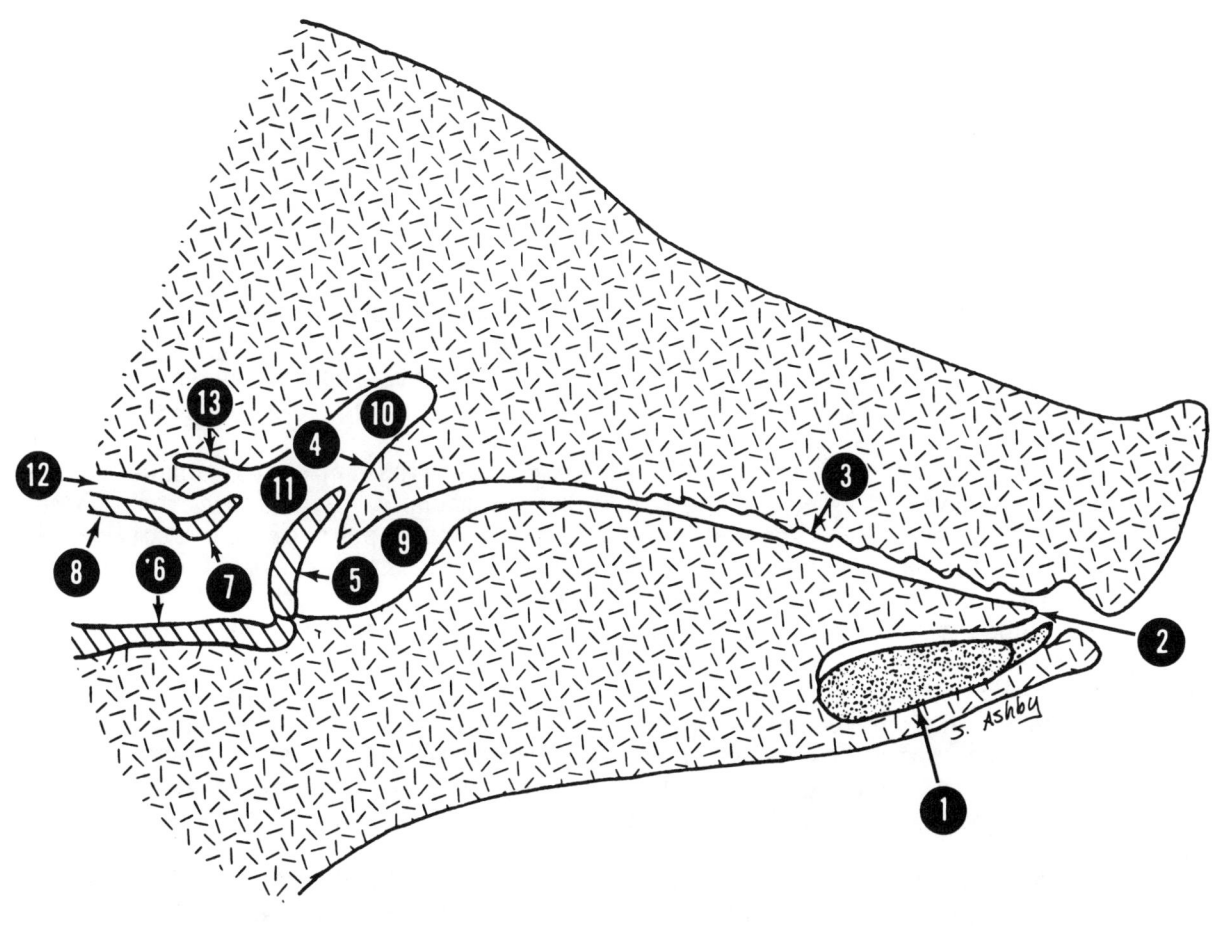

Figure 21-2

Sagittal Section of the Head of a Pig

1. Mandibular symphysis
2. Tongue
3. Hard palate
4. Soft palate
5. Epiglottis
6. Thyroid cartilage
7. Arytenoid cartilage
8. Cricoid cartilage
9. Oropharynx
10. Nasopharynx
11. Laryngopharynx
12. Esophagus
13. Pharyngeal diverticulum

3. A pharyngeal tonsil in the roof of the nasopharynx.

4. Tubal tonsils in the mucosa of the pharyngeal opening of the auditory tube.

5. Tonsil of the soft palate (on its ventral surface).

These are difficult to distinguish grossly. No palatine tonsil is present in the pig.

E. The major salivary glands are the paired parotid, mandibular, and sublingual glands.

F. A blind pharyngeal diverticulum is present in the laryngopharynx. This may "trap" an otherwise well placed balling gun (Fig. 21-2/13). Inadvertent drug deposition into this area or its injury due to improper handling of instruments may result in fatal necrotic pharyngitis [2].

G. The stomach has a gastric diverticulum extending from its fundus which distinguishes it from other simple stomachs. A constriction, more evident internally, separates it from the main part of the stomach. A nonglandular area extends from the cardia into the gastric diverticulum. The latter contains both glandular and nonglandular areas (Fig. 21-3). The mucosa of the stomach normally has a very hemorrhagic appearance.

H. At the pylorus, a torus pyloricus protrudes into the pyloric canal. Ruminants also have this structure. It consists of a fatty and fibrous prominence which extends into the lumen and diminishes the luminal diameter. In young animals, the torus pyloricus is poorly developed. It can be mistaken for a lesion by someone unfamiliar with it.

I. The intestinal arrangement matches the generalized mammalian pattern* except for modifications in the ascending colon and the fact that the porcine cecum is on the left side (Fig. 21-4).

1. The ileum joins the large intestine as if it were the stem of a T. The blind-ended cecum forms one branch of the T and the ascending colon forms the other one.

2. The ascending colon is tightly coiled to form a cone-shaped, ventrally directed spiral loop (ansa spiralis coli) and a distal loop. (The proximal loop, which precedes the spiral loop in ruminants, is absent.) The spiral loop consists of centripetal turns, a central flexure, and centrifugal turns [1].

(a) The initial part of the ascending colon (centripetal turns) passes around the central axis of this cone for about $3\frac{1}{2}$ turns in a clockwise direction (as viewed from above) to reach the ventrally located apex of the cone. The centripetal turns form the outside of the cone and are visible without dissection.

---

*In the generalized mammalian intestinal pattern, the descending duodenum and ascending colon are on the right side of the root of the mesentery; and the ascending duodenum and descending colon are on the left side. The transverse colon passes from right to left, cranial to the root of the mesentery.

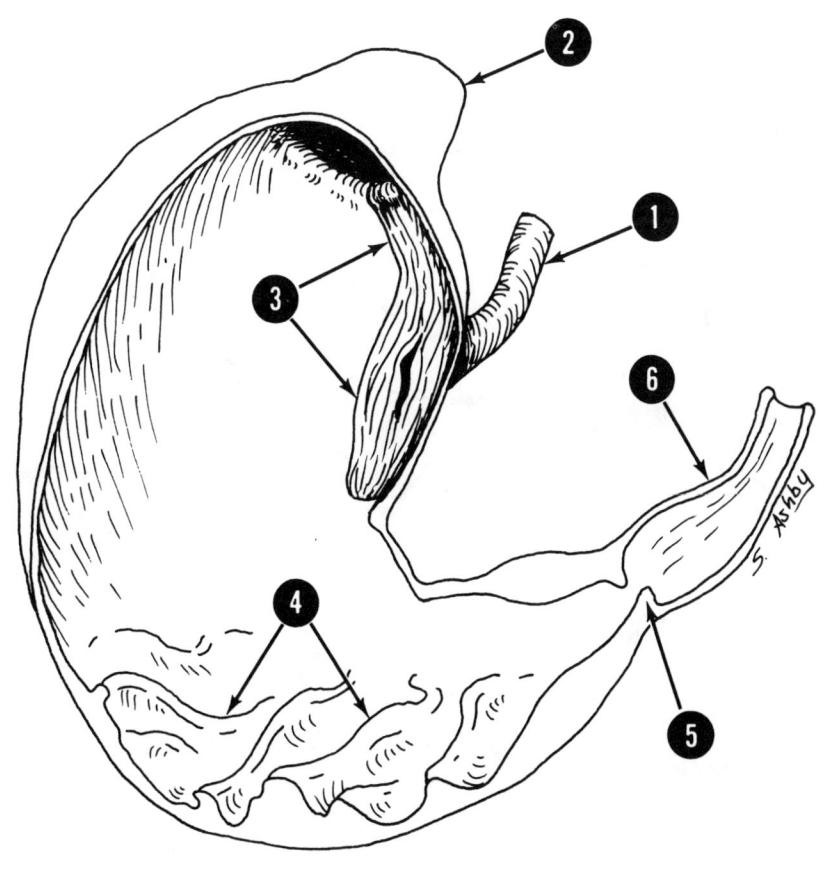

Figure 21-3

Sectional View of the Porcine Stomach

1. Esophagus
2. Gastric diverticulum
3. Non-glandular region
4. Rugae
5. Torus pyloricus
6. Duodenum

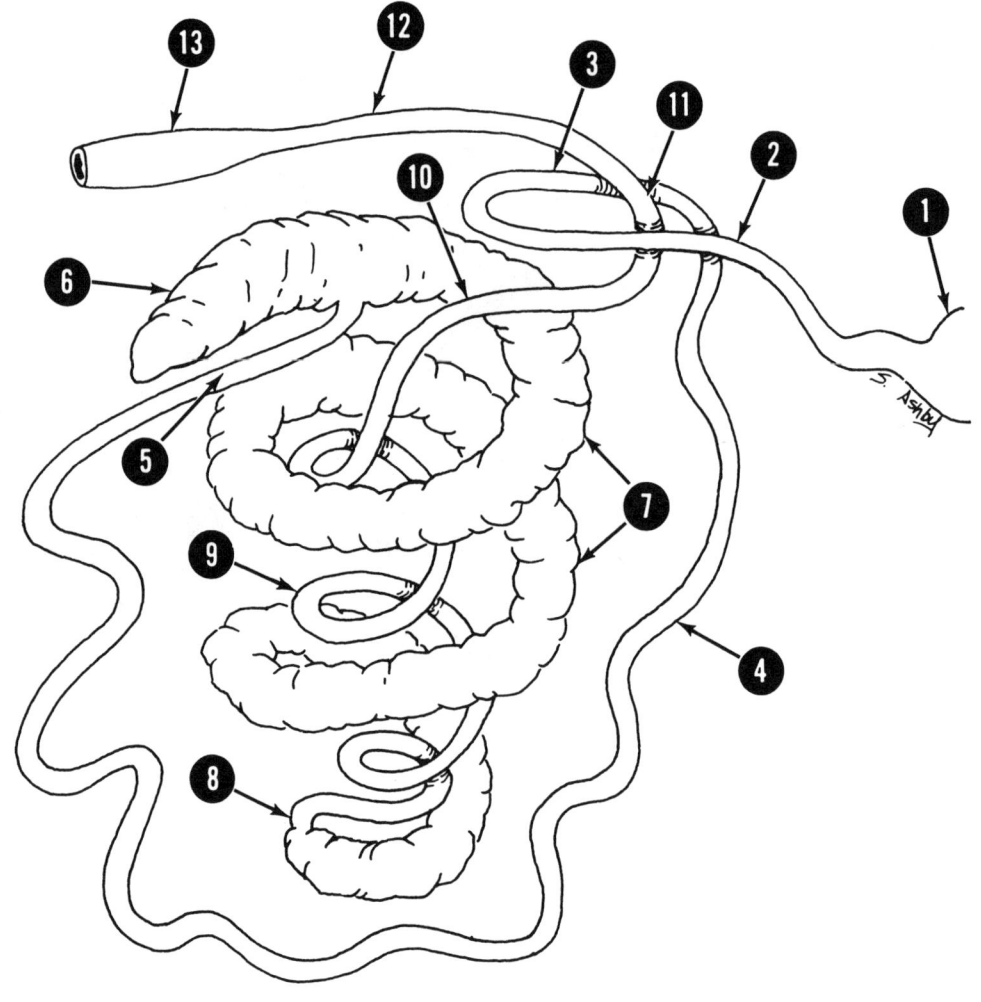

Figure 21-4

Arrangement of the Stomach and Intestines of the Pig
(right lateral aspect)

1. Stomach
2. Descending duodenum
3. Ascending duodenum
4. Jejunum
5. Ileum
6. Cecum
7. Centripetal turns of spiral loop of colon
8. Central flexure
9. Centrifugal turns of spiral loop of colon
10. Distal loop of colon
11. Transverse colon
12. Descending colon
13. Rectum

After Nickel, Schummer, Seiferle, and Sack, 1973 [1]

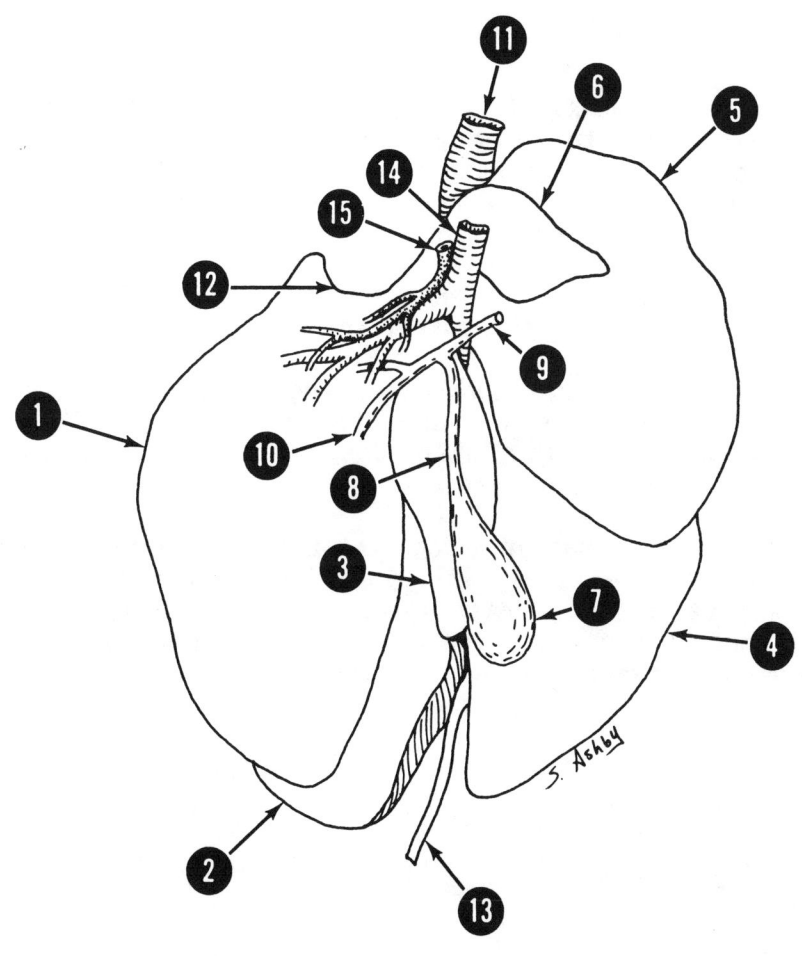

Figure 21-5

Porcine Liver (visceral surface)

1. Left lateral lobe
2. Left medial lobe
3. Quadrate lobe
4. Right medial lobe
5. Right lateral lobe
6. Caudate lobe
7. Gall bladder
8. Cystic duct
9. Bile duct
10. Hepatic duct
11. Caudal vena cava
12. Esophageal notch
13. Round ligament of the liver
14. Portal vein
15. Hepatic artery

- (b) At the apex of the coil, the ascending colon reverses direction to form the central flexure and then spirals dorsally in a counterclockwise direction to form the centrifugal turns. These are inside the centripetal turns and must be dissected to be seen.

- (c) The distal loop is not obviously separable from the centrifugal turns of the spiral loop. It joins the transverse colon.

- (d) The centripetal turns (and the cecum) are sacculated because of tenia. They are also larger in diameter than the centrifugal turns. The latter lack tenia except for some faint ones near the central flexure.

J. The liver resembles that of a dog except no papillary process is present on the caudate lobe: i.e., left lobe (medial and lateral), right lobe (medial and lateral), caudate lobe, and quadrate lobe (Fig. 21-5). It does not contact the right kidney (in adult animals) as it does in the other domestic mammals. The unusually long bile duct opens on the indistinct major duodenal papilla.

K. The pancreas completely surrounds the portal vein like that of the horse. The passageway for the portal vein through the pancreas is termed the anulus pancreatis. Only the duct of the dorsal pancreatic primordium remains (accessory pancreatic duct). It opens on the minor duodenal papilla.

L. Harelip, cleft palate, and atresia ani are the most common developmental defects of the digestive system [2].

III. RESPIRATORY SYSTEM

A. The nose is fused to and continuous with the upper lip. It is flattened and nearly hairless.

B. Several nasal cartilages assist the rostral bone in supporting the nose.

C. Post-mortem examination of the dorsal and ventral nasal conchae aids in the diagnosis of atrophic rhinitis (Fig. 21-6).

D. Paranasal sinuses include:

1. Maxillary sinus
2. Frontal sinus (by far the largest)
3. Lacrimal sinus
4. Sphenoid sinus
5. Dorsal and ventral conchal sinuses

E. The lungs have the same lobation and terminology as those of the dog. The left lung is divided into cranial and caudal lobes with the cranial lobe subdivided into cranial and caudal parts. The right lung has cranial, middle, caudal, and accessory lobes. The right cranial lobe is connected to the trachea by a tracheal bronchus like that found in ruminants (Fig. 21-7).

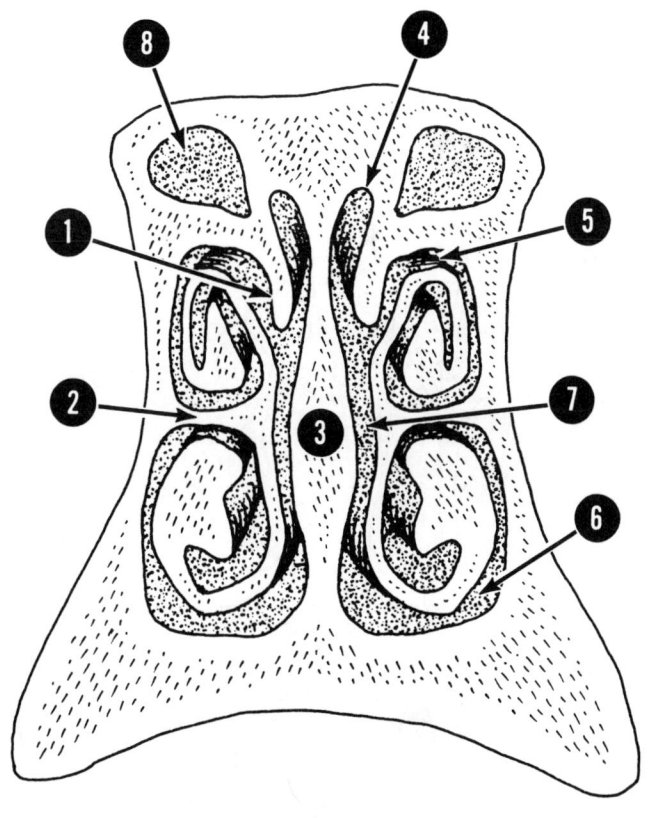

Figure 21-6

Transverse Section through the Head of a Pig at the Level of the Canine Teeth

1. Dorsal nasal concha
2. Ventral nasal concha
3. Nasal septum
4. Dorsal nasal meatus
5. Middle nasal meatus
6. Ventral nasal meatus
7. Common nasal meatus
8. Frontal sinus

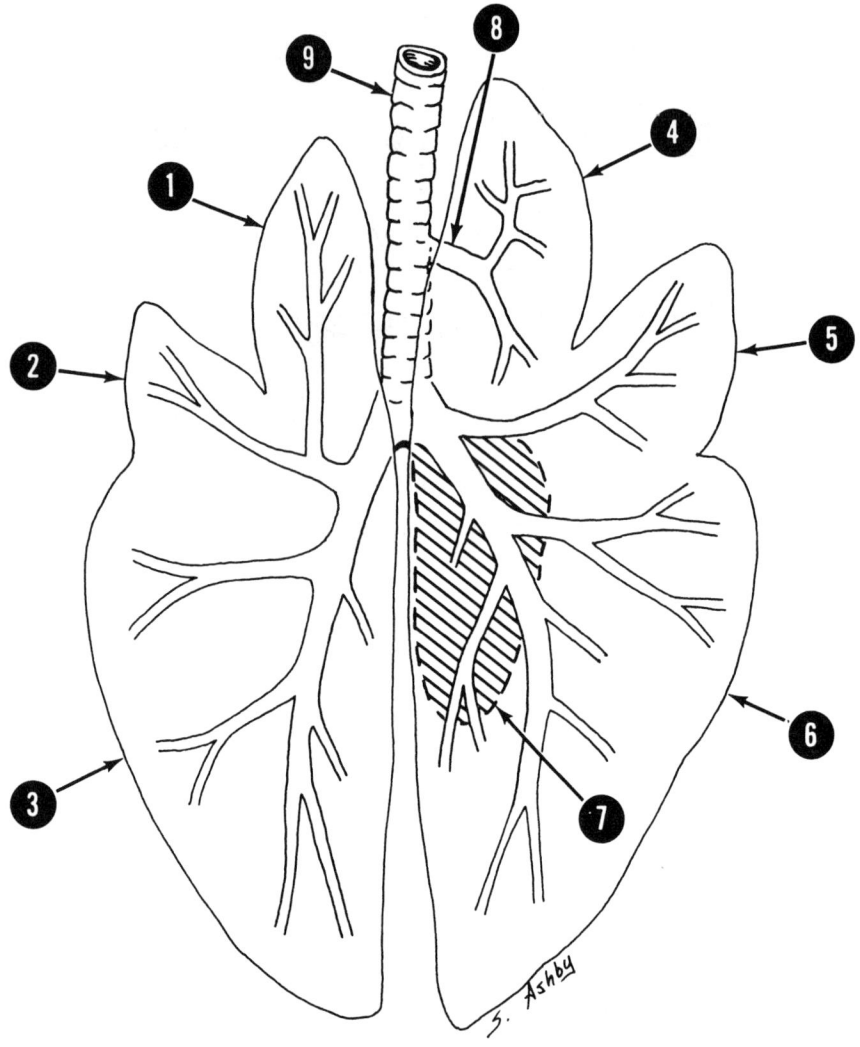

Figure 21-7

Lungs of a Pig (dorsal aspect)

1. Cranial part of cranial lobe of left lung
2. Caudal part of cranial lobe of left lung
3. Caudal lobe of left lung
4. Cranial lobe of right lung
5. Middle lobe of right lung
6. Caudal lobe of right lung
7. Accessory lobe of right lung (shaded)
8. Tracheal bronchus
9. Trachea

F. The mediastinum is not perforated, and so the two pleural cavities are separate and distinct.

IV. UROGENITAL SYSTEM

A. The kidneys are elongated and flattened in comparison to those of carnivores. Within each kidney, two major calyces drain into the pelvis. Each major calix drains several minor calices which invest the apical portions of the renal pyramids. Like the ox, the pig has no renal crest.

B. The scrotum, like that of a cat, is located just ventral to the anus. Pigs are usually castrated through two scrotal incisions. Some veterinarians prefer to incise just ventral (cranial) to the scrotum.

C. The accessory sex glands include vesicular, prostate, and very large, "cigar-shaped" bulbourethral glands (Fig. 21-8). The prostate gland has both a body and a disseminate part.

D. The penis is the fibroelastic type and has a sigmoid flexure. The paired retractor penis muscle attaches distal to the flexure. The glans penis appears to be twisted into a "corkscrew" configuration (Figs. 21-8, 21-9).

E. A preputial diverticulum is located in the dorsal wall of the prepuce. It is partially divided into two compartments by a median septum. Collections of debris and desquamated cells in this pouch give the boar its characteristic odor. Surgical resection of this pouch is sometimes indicated (see Chapter 15).

F. The sow, like the cow, has a suburethral diverticulum near the external urethral orifice (Fig. 21-10).

G. The uterine horns are very long (especially in parous individuals). The body of the uterus is short, and the cervix is very long.

H. Anomalies of the male urogenital system include cryptorchidism, aplasias and hypoplasias of the reproductive viscera, persistent frenulum and seminal defects [13]. Inguinal (and umbilical) hernias are among the most common defects of swine [2]. Aplasias, hypoplasias, and duplications are also found in sows. Intersexuality (hermaphroditism) is an important defect [2].

V. ENDOCRINE SYSTEM

A. The two suprarenal glands are elongated. Each one is positioned along the medial border of the ipsilateral kidney cranial to the hilus.

B. The thyroid gland is located ventral to the trachea near the thoracic inlet. The right and left lobes of the thyroid gland are fused ventrally.

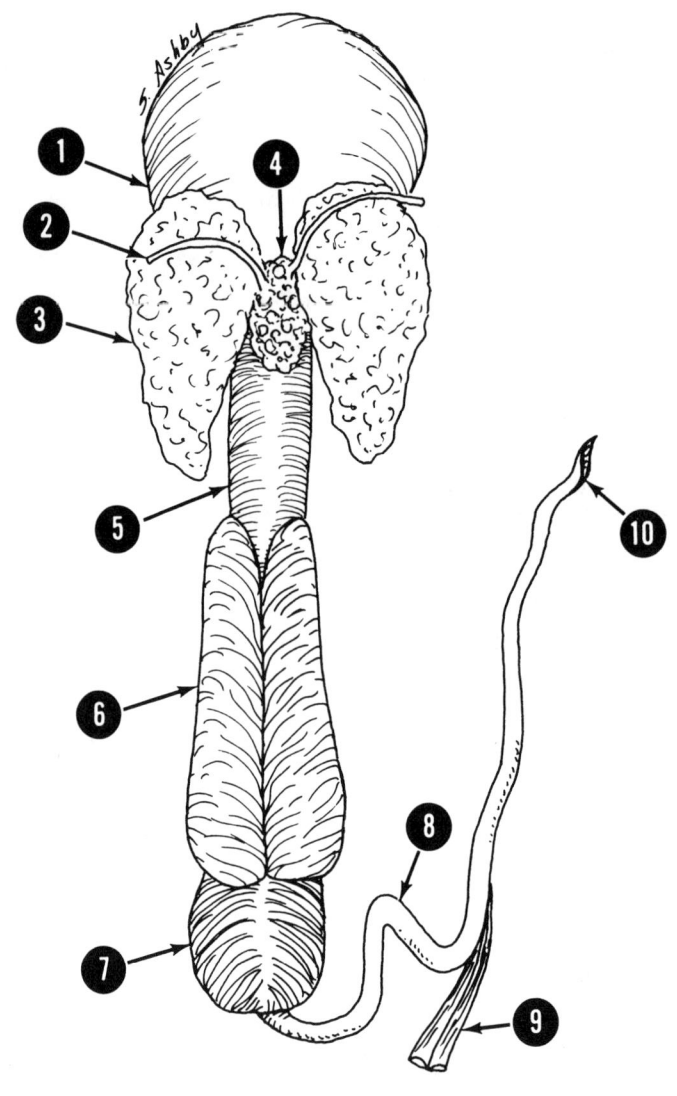

Figure 21-8

Accessory Sex Glands and Penis of Boar
(dorsal aspect with penis reflected to right)

1. Urinary bladder
2. Ductus deferens (transected)
3. Vesicular gland
4. Prostate gland (body)
5. Urethra (surrounded by urethalis m.)
6. Bulbourethral gland (surrounded by bulbourethralis m.)
7. Bulbospongiosus muscle
8. Sigmoid flexure of penis
9. Retractor penis muscle (transected)
10. Glans penis

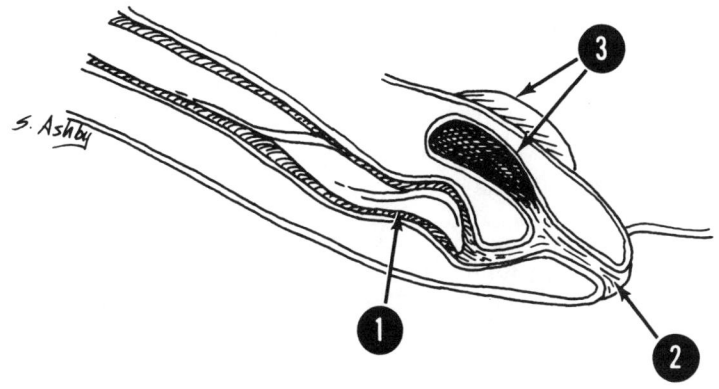

Figure 21-9

Glans Penis and Prepuce of Boar (sagittal section, right aspect)

1. Glans penis
2. Preputial orifice
3. Preputial diverticulum

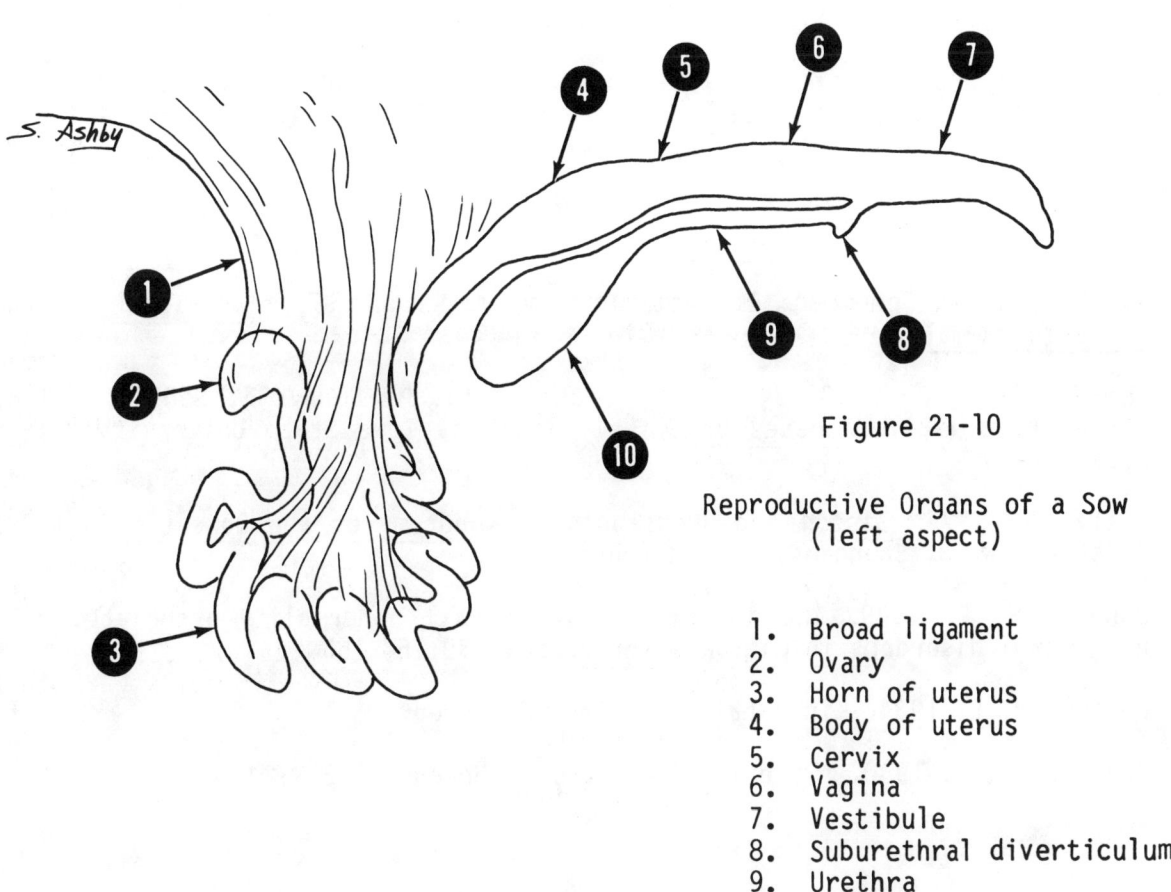

Figure 21-10

Reproductive Organs of a Sow
(left aspect)

1. Broad ligament
2. Ovary
3. Horn of uterus
4. Body of uterus
5. Cervix
6. Vagina
7. Vestibule
8. Suburethral diverticulum
9. Urethra
10. Urinary bladder

- C. The thymus is located along each common carotid artery. It is typically light in color but the cranial portions may be pigmented in black animals.

- D. There is only one parathyroid gland (external or III) on each side. It is not embedded in the thyroid gland, but is usually found within the cranial aspect of the thymus.

- E. The pineal and pituitary glands present no unusual features. The pituitary glands are removed at slaughterhouses to be further processed and used in pharmaceuticals.

VI. MISCELLANEOUS POINTS

- A. Blood is usually withdrawn from the right brachiocephalic vein. A 4-6" needle is inserted into the slight depression (on either side) at the base of the ventral aspect of the neck, just off the midline. It is directed at the opposite shoulder [14]. Clinicians often claim that they insert the needle into the cranial vena cava and occasionally they may well do so. A marginal vein in the ear may also be used for blood collection, as can the orbital sinus at the medial commisure if the pig is restrained in dorsal recumbancy. Additionally, pigs can be bled from the tail using a technique similar to the one used in cattle.

- B. A sow may have 10-18 teats. Twelve are typically required for breed registrations. In addition to normal teats, supernumerary and rectal (anal) teats have been described [15].

- C. The spleen is elongated, like that of a dog, and has a linear hilus.

- D. Tails are often docked in newborn pigs with sidecutter pliers (12-18 mm of tail should be left) [2]. This lowers the incidence of tail biting.

References

1. Nickel, R., A. Schummer, E. Seiferle, and W. Sack. 1973. _The Viscera of the Domestic Mammals._ Paul Parey, Berlin.

2. Leman, A. D., R. D. Glock, W. L. Mengeling, R. H. Penny, E. Scholl, and B. Straw, eds. 1981. _Diseases of Swine,_ fifth ed. Iowa State University Press, Ames, Iowa.

3. Getty, R. 1975. _Sisson and Grossman's The Anatomy of the Domestic Animals,_ fifth ed. W. B. Saunders, Philadelphia.

4. Donald, H. P. 1949. The inheritance of a tail abnormality associated with urogenital disorders in pigs. _J. Agric. Sci._ 39:164-165.

5. Nordby, J. E. 1934. Kinky-tail in swine. _J. Hered._ 25:171-174.

6. Johnson, L. E. 1940. "Streamlined" pigs. _J. Hered._ 31:239-242.

7. Ludvigsen, J. B. 1963. Afdelongen for forsog med svin Landoekon Forsoegslab. Kbh. 414.

8. Hughes, E. H. 1935. Polydactyly in swine. J. Hered. 25:415-418.

9. Ross, O. B., P. H. Phillips, G. Bohstedt, and T. J. Cunha. 1944. Congenital malformations, syndactylism, talipes, and paralysis agitans of nutritional origin in swine. J. Anim. Sci. 3:406-414.

10. Palludan, B. 1966. Swine in teratological studies. In Swine in Biomedical Research, edited by Bustad, McClellan, and Burns. Pacific Northwest Laboratory, Richlands, Washington.

11. Ward, P.S. 1978. The splayleg syndrome in new-born pigs: A review, I. Vet. Bull. 48:279-295.

12. Ward, P. S. 1978. The splayleg syndrome in new-born pigs: A review, II. Vet. Bull. 48:381-399.

13. Huston, R., G. Saperstein, D. Schoneweweis, and H. W. Leipold. 1978. Congenital defects in pigs. Vet. Bull. 48:645-675.

14. Schwartz, W. L., and J. E. Smallwood. 1977. Collection of blood from swine. Texas Veterinary Medical Journal 39(3):6-7.

15. Turner, C. W. 1952. The Mammary Gland. Lucas Brothers, Columbia, Missouri.

BIOLOGY OF LABORATORY ANIMALS

Laboratory animals include all of those creatures used in biomedical research. In the broad sense, these include a number of invertebrates, some lower vertebrates, and even some of our domesticated mammals. Obviously, the anatomy and other biological characteristics of such a diverse group is quite varied, and the subject is too complex to cover adequately here. This discussion will be limited to some of the salient features of several of the more common laboratory animals. For general references on these and other laboratory animals, veterinarians will find the works by Williams [1], Harkness and Wagner [2], Schuchman [3], and UFAW [4] very useful. They are concise, written from a medical viewpoint, and should form a useful addition to any practitioner's library. For more information concerning breeding and the reproductive system, the text by Hafez [5] may be consulted. A summary of anatomic, biological, and clinical data is presented in Tables 22-1 to 22-7.

MOUSE

The laboratory mouse is a member of the mammalian Order Rodentia which contains more species and subspecies than all of the other approximately 17 recognized orders of mammals combined. Mice are members of the Family Muridae which also includes rats, muskrats, and others. The laboratory mouse is a descendent of the common house mouse (Mus musculus) and bears the same scientific name [6]. In addition to Mus musculus, several types of wild mice may be encountered in research colonies including the field mouse (Microtus), grasshopper mouse (Onychomys), and the white-footed mouse (Peromyscus) [2]. More mice are used in biomedical research than any other animal. In fact, about 3 times as many mice are used as rats (the second most frequently used laboratory species) [1].

Mice have sleek, smooth-coated bodies, hairless tails, and erect, rounded ears. They have five digits on the hind feet and four on the front, with hairless foot pads. The dental formula is 2(I1/1 C0/0 P0/0 M3/3) = 16, and the dentition is monophyodontic. The incisors continually erupt and are worn down by abrasion.

Multilocular adipose tissue ("brown fat") occurs in many loci and especially prominent masses are found between the scapulae. Under laboratory conditions, these masses may be replaced with regular adipose tissue [4].

Deep within the orbit of the eye is a gland called the Harderian gland. This gland produces porphyrin and excretes it through a duct which opens at the base of the nictitating membrane [6].

The left lung is undivided, but the right one is divided into four lobes: cranial, middle, caudal, and accessory lobes. The thymus is also located in the thorax. It reaches maximal size near sexual maturity and involutes thereafter. Neonatal thymectomy was a common procedure in immunological investigations before discovery of the nude (athymic) mutant.

In the abdomen, the spleen is sexually dimorphic, with those of males often 50% larger than those of females.* Accessory splenic tissue is often embedded in the pancreas and the tip of the spleen is often bifurcated. The stomach has nonglandular and glandular portions. The cecum is an elongated blind sac similar to that of domestic ruminants [6].

The testes of males are located in individual scrotal sacs on either side of the urethra. The inguinal canals remain patent throughout life and the testes are often in a retracted position. A number of accessory sex glands are present including vesicular glands (largest), coagulating glands, ampullae, prostate, bulbourethral, and preputial glands [1]. The preputial glands are flattened, leaf-like glands on either side of the prepuce between the skin and abdominal wall. Males housed together may fight and inflict wounds on each other's genitals.

The uterus is Y-shaped with a body and two horns. A single cervix is present. The urethral orifice is separate from the vagina and is located ventral to it. The 5 pairs of mammary glands (3 thoracic and 2 abdominal) extend well up along the sides and back.

In the presence of males, females usually cycle every 4 days, but single females housed away from males cycle every 5-6 days. Large groups of females housed together become anestrous (the "Whitten" effect) [2]. An introduced male will cause most to go into heat on the third day. (The introductee should be in good shape!) Sometimes groups of females housed together will become pseudopregnant and not cycle for 15 days (Lee-Boot effect). Another reproductive phenomenon is the Bruce effect: a pregnant female exposed to a strange male during the period from the first to the fourth day of gestation will abort. If she remains with the second male long enough, she will reovulate and conceive again. These reproductive phenomena are best observed in outbred mice (isogenic strains do not always exhibit these characteristics) [1].

Gestation is 19-21 days. Females bred but not fertilized have a 13 day pseudopregnancy during which estrus does not occur. A litter typically consists of 4-12 young (up to 20 in some prolific breeds). The young are born hairless with their eyes closed. They nibble at solid food when their eyes open at about 11 days and weaning occurs at 3-4 weeks. Mice are sexually mature at 28-48 days of age.

Mice may be restrained by grasping the tail and then the loose skin at the base of the neck. As much of the skin should be gathered in as possible to prevent them from turning and biting. Picking them up by the tail without use of long, rubber-tipped forceps should be avoided since they can turn, climb up, and bite. Mice will usually urinate and defecate when they are handled [1].

---

*Histological sexual dimorphism is also seen in the kidneys and salivary glands. In males the epithelium of the glomerular capsule is cuboidal, but in females it is squamous. The ductal epithelium of the salivary glands of males is columnar; in females it is cuboidal.

Blood may be collected by clipping the tail or by cardiac puncture in anesthetized animals. A microhematocrit tube inserted into the medial canthus of the eye is another method (mouse should be anesthetized). Blood from the orbital sinus will enter the tube by capillary action. Intravenous injections may be made in the lateral tail veins using a 24-gauge or smaller needle.

Sexual differentiation is made by the relative distance between the genital papilla and the anus (this distance is larger in males than in females; Table 22-3).

A number of breeds and strains of mice have been developed. Isogenic mice have been produced by several (20 or more) generations of brother-sister matings. These will accept organ and skin grafts from any animal of the same strain. A complex system of coding (nomenclature) is used to designate each of these strains [7].

The following points may also be of value clinically [1]:

a. Mice are very susceptible to streptomycin toxicity. As little as 1.25 mg may be lethal.
b. Certain strains of inbred mice are very sensitive to chloroform and may die from its use as an anesthetic or from low-level, accidental exposure.
c. Chronic ulcerative skin lesions appear spontaneously in some inbred strains. They are usually fatal because of serum protein leakage.
d. Some females chew the hair off the backs and heads of their suckling babies. Some mice chew hair off the face of their cagemates.
e. Rectal prolapses occasionally occur in groups of young mice and are thought to be associated with heavy pin-worm infestations. Prolapses may be replaced with moistened cotton-tipped swabs. Pinworms may be treated with a variety of drugs (piperazine adipate 4-7 mg/ml in drinking water).
f. Many tumors occur, and they are often benign, making surgical removal highly effective. Mammary tumors can occur in unusual places because of the extensive distribution of the mammary tissue.

A standard reference on the biology of the mouse is the work edited by Green [8]. For anatomy only, the work of Cook [9] may be consulted.

RAT

Like mice, rats are members of the Order Rodentia and the Family Muridae. Laboratory rats are descendents of the Norway rat (Rattus norvegicus) and bear the same scientific name. Many strains have been developed, but most belong to one of three main groupings: Wistar albinos, Sprague-Dawley albinos, and Long-Evans hooded rats [4]. Rats rank second only to mice in the numbers used in biomedical research. In fact, these two murine species are used 14 times as often as all other laboratory animal species combined [10].

Some of the more distinctive features of rat anatomy include the absence of tonsils, the lack of a gallbladder, and the presence of multilocular

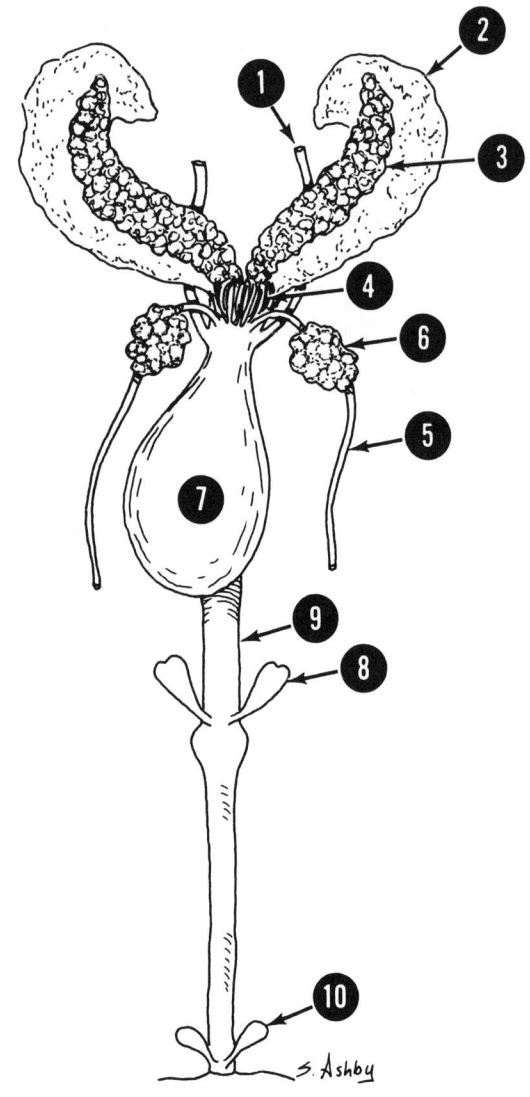

Figure 22-1

Reproductive System of a Male Rat (ventral aspect)

1. Ureter (severed)
2. Vesicular gland
3. Coagulating gland*
4. Ampulla
5. Ductus deferens
6. Prostate gland
7. Urinary bladder
8. Bulbourethral gland
9. Urethra
10. Preputial gland

*In some laboratory animals, especially members of the families Cricetidae and Muridae, the cranial lobe of the prostate is elongated, closely applied to the vesicular glands, and is known as the coagulating gland.

Modified from Baker et al., 1979 [11]

adipose tissue ("brown fat") around the head and neck which resembles glandular tissue. They have four toes on their front feet and five on their hind feet with hairless pads like those of mice. Rats have extraorbital lacrimal glands on the cheek below each eye [1]. The dental formula is 2(I1/1 C0/0 P0/0 M3/3) = 16 and is monophyodontic. The four incisors continuously erupt as they are worn by appositional abrasion at their occlusal surfaces. Malocclusion results in overgrowth similar to that seen occasionally in horses.

Rats are omnivorous and have a simple stomach which is divided into two regional areas like that of horses. The cecum is well developed and has a rumen-like function in the digestion of cellulose. Cecal enlargement in germ-free rats may result in fatal cecal torsion. The lungs resemble those of a mouse. They lack lobation on the left lung and the right one has cranial, middle, caudal, and accessory lobes.

Male rats (boars) have an os penis, numerous accessory sex glands, (Fig. 22-1) and a persistently patent inguinal canal. Females (sows) have a double cervix with two distinct cervical canals, but they both open into the same (unpaired) uterus (see rabbit). Estrus of 9-12 hours' duration occurs every 4-5 days until conception. Gestation is 21-23 days and 8-12 hairless pups comprise a litter. There are usually 12 mammary glands, three pairs in front and three behind with a space between them [1].

Newborn pups weigh about 5 g, have closed eyes and ears, and have no erupted teeth. As in mice, sex differentiation in neonates can be accomplished by comparing the relative distance between the genital and anal orifices. Pups are well haired by the tenth day, nibble at food by day 16, and can be weaned by 21 days. Puberty occurs by 2 months of age.

Rats are nocturnal and must be provided with regular light-dark cycles for normal behavior and physiology. Most laboratory rats are docile and easily handled. To handle a rat, grasp its tail at the base and when the rat stretches away, encircle its chest with the other hand. By placing a thumb and index finger around the neck, the head can be controlled. Plastic cylinders and other types of "squeeze" restraint may be of value in some special procedures. Rats can be picked up by their tails, but one should hold them near the base (of the tail) because the skin may slip off the tip.

Blood may be collected from rats by cardiac puncture of anesthetized individuals, by jugular venipuncture, or from the orbital sinus (as in mice) using a microhematocrit tube. Small volumes (1 ml) may be obtained by amputating the tip of the tail. Prior immersion of the tail in warm water will facilitate this procedure. Blood may also be collected from the femoral vein. Intravenous injections may be made into the caudal veins which are located dorsally, laterally, and ventrally in the tail. Alternate routes are the saphenous vein on the medial aspect of the thigh, the dorsal vein of the penis, the lingual vein, and the blood collection routes mentioned above.

The most significant infectious disease of laboratory rats is murine respiratory mycoplasmosis (Mycoplasma pulmonis). The principal signs are sneezing, hunched posture, rales, and a roughened hair coat. Tetracyclines in the drinking water may reduce the severity of the disease in a colony (400 mg/liter). The following points may also be of value clinically [1]:

a. Bulging eyes (sialodacryoadenitis) is caused by a virus which causes swelling of the lacrimal and sometimes of the salivary glands. Recovery is usually spontaneous in 10-14 days, although some may need artificial tear instillation during the acute stage to prevent drying of the cornea.

b. Red tears (chromodacryorrhea) is a "normal" phenomenon caused by porphyrin production by the Harderian gland. The dried secretion may resemble crusts of blood around the eyes and nose and the discoloration may be spread by grooming to produce a reddish brown "cape."

For additional information on the medical aspects of R. norvegicus, the reader is referred to references 1-4, as well as to the works by Baker et al[10,11]. For anatomical information, the books by Greene [12] and Hebel and Stromberg [13] may be consulted.

HAMSTER

Hamsters belong to the mammalian Order Rodentia and the Family Cricetidae. There are several species of hamsters, but only two have been widely used in the United States as pets or laboratory animals: the golden (Syrian) hamster (Mesocricetus auratus) and the Chinese or striped-back hamster (Cricetulus griseus). Hamsters are native to Europe and Asia. They were first domesticated about 1930 and are the third most widely used laboratory animal (behind mice and rats) [14].

Hamsters are between mice and rats in size and they have short stubby tails. They have four toes on the front feet and five on the back feet with hairless foot pads. Golden hamsters are about 15 cm in length while the smaller Chinese hamsters are about 10 cm long. The sexes can be distinguished in several ways. The caudal aspects of males are elongated and slightly rounded because of the testes. This can be determined from above without handling the animals, or the animals can be picked up and examined directly. The genitoanal distance is another method of sexual differentiation especially useful in young animals. Finally, males possess two well developed hip glands which are marked by darkly pigmented spots on the hip region with roughened skin and coarse hairs. In the female, these are poorly developed. The total significance of these glands is not understood, but they apparently are used for territorial marking and actively secrete during periods of sexual excitement.

Like rats, hamsters have extraorbital lacrimal glands on their cheeks. They also have a well developed cheek pouch on each side for storing and transporting food. These are evaginations of the lateral buccal wall and are quite distensible. The pouches offer unique features that make the hamster extremely useful in studies of vascular physiology and oncology. The dental formula is 2(I1/1 C0/0 P0/0 M3/3) = 16, which is identical to that of the rat and mouse and is also monophyodontic. The left lung is undivided and the right lung has three lobes. The stomach has glandular and nonglandular regions which are separated by a narrow passageway (Fig. 22-2). The cecum is large and the colon is long with a simple coil in its ascending part, like that of a guinea pig. Each kidney has a remarkably long papilla which extends out into the ureter. Males have extremely large testes in relation to their body size. Large fat deposits are present just cranial to the testes. The vesicular glands are very well developed.

In golden hamsters, the estrous cycle is about 94 hours. The end of estrus is marked by an opaque, white, postovulatory discharge which fills the vagina and even protrudes from it. (This has been mistaken for vaginitis [1].) Females are commonly bred on the evening of the third day after the appearance of this discharge. Receptive females in the presence of a male assume a distinctive posture termed "lordosis." Gestation is 15-18 days and the usual litter size is 6-8. Females usually have 12-14 nipples, but some have more. The newborn are hairless with closed ears and eyes. Cannibalism is common in young females. Females do have the ability to conceal a newborn litter in their cheek pouches. They may do so when excited and later return them to the nest [2]. Pseudopregnancies of 8-10 days duration result from infertile matings. Young are weaned at 21-28 days of age, and become sexually mature at 6-8 weeks.

Hamsters are nocturnal animals and are often pugnacious. They may be restrained by picking them up with a thumb and index finger encircling the neck as described for rats. They may also be pressed down on a flat surface and the loose skin gathered up into the hand. Make sure the animal is awake because startled hamsters frequently bite.

The following points may also be of value clinically:

a. Hamsters are very susceptible to both penicillin and streptomycin. In fact, a single dose of 1000 i.u. of potassium penicillin will kill some 50 g hamsters in a few days. This is not a direct toxicity (as in the mouse) but results from a secondary gram-negative overgrowth [1].
b. Hamsters that appear to be dead should be suspected of hibernating and warmed up gradually [1]. Hibernation may be induced by a set of conditions including ample food supply, short photoperiods, and lowered temperatures [4].
c. The most significant hamster disease is "wet-tail" (also called "proliferative ileitis"). The cause is thought to be Camphylobacter sp. The disease is characterized by lethargy, anorexia, and wet rear ends. Sometimes there is diarrhea; sometimes the feces are formed but accompanied by a watery discharge. The recommended treatment is 400 mg/l tetracycline in the drinking water for 10 days [1].

The standard source of reference for the hamster is the book edited by Hoffman et al [15].

GUINEA PIG

Guinea pigs belong to the Order Rodentia and the Family Cavidae. They bear the scientific name Cavia porcellus and are native to South America.

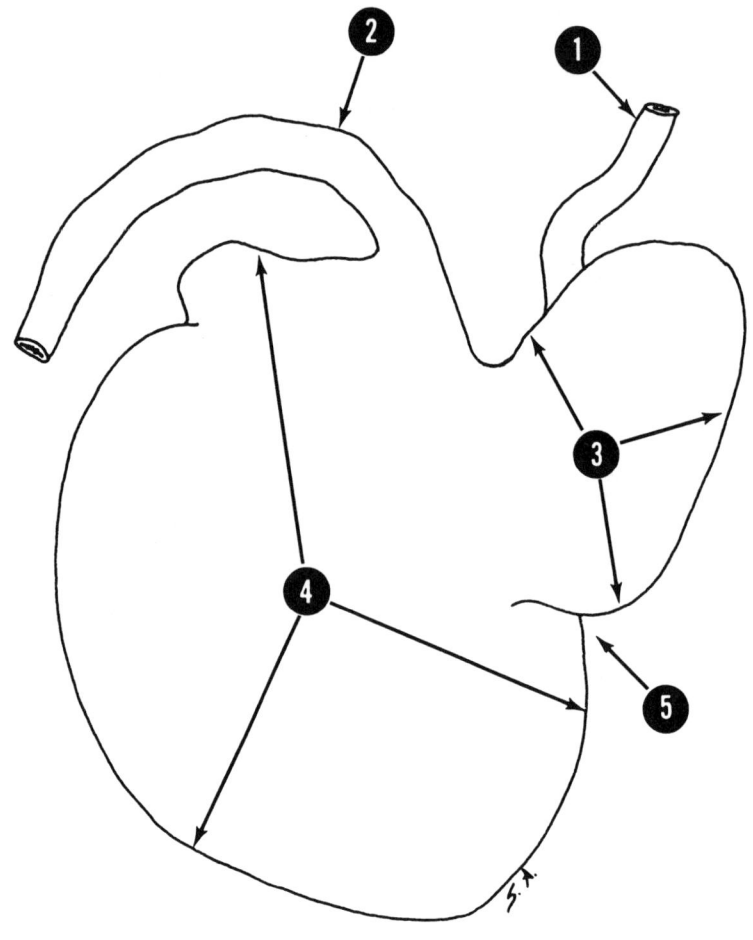

Figure 22-2

Stomach of a Hamster (visceral surface)

1. Esophagus
2. Duodenum
3. Nonglandular portion of stomach (also called "forestomach" or "esophageal diverticulum")
4. Glandular portion of stomach
5. Constriction separating glandular and nonglandular portions of stomach

Three types are recognized: English (short, coarse hair); Abyssinian (short, coarse hair arranged in numerous whorls); and Peruvian (long, fine, silky hair which may or may not be arranged in whorls). Most guinea pigs used in the laboratory are of the English type, and the Abyssinian and Peruvian varieties are primarily kept as pets for show and fancy. In terms of numbers, guinea pigs are the fourth most commonly used laboratory animal (behind mice, rats, and hamsters) [16].

The guinea pig has no externally obvious tail. Sexual differentiation can be made by applying pressure just cranial to the genital orifice. In males this will cause the penis to protrude. In contrast to other laboratory rodents, guinea pigs have only four digits on each thoracic limb and only three on each pelvic limb, but like the mouse, rat, and hamster, they have hairless foot pads. Also distinctive is the single pair of mammary glands. The dental formula is 2(I1/1 C0/0 P1/1 M3/3) = 20, and they are the only common laboratory rodent with premolars. The cecum is very large and distinctly sacculated and the colon is long with a simple spiral loop in its ascending portion (Fig. 22-3)

In males, the vesicular glands are very well developed (Fig. 22-4) and like the hamster, guinea pigs have large fat deposits cranial to the testes. Females are polyestrous with approximately 16 day cycles. If receptive, they exhibit a lordotic response in the presence of a male. Gestation is about 68 days and the litter size is 1-4. In marked contrast to other laboratory animals, newborn guinea pigs are fully haired with open eyes and can be weaned immediately. Sexual maturity occurs at 2-3 months.

Guinea pigs rarely bite, but they squeal noisily when alarmed or hungry. They may be handled by placing a hand over the thorax similar to the technique used for rats. However, in large or pregnant animals, the thorax should be supported from below because the pressure required for restraint from above may injure the lungs [2]. The hindquarters should be controlled with the opposite hand to prevent being scratched by the hind feet. For intravenous drug administration, the cephalic vein may be used.

The following may also be of value clinically [1]:

a. Guinea pigs often produce hypersensitive reactions in humans including upper respiratory signs and lacrimation.
b. Antibiotics specific for gram-positive organisms may produce a secondary toxicity due to a gram-negative overgrowth. Included are penicillin, erythromycin, and lincomycin. Oral neomycin and polymixin B (5 mg and 3 mg, respectively) twice a day for a few days will often protect the animal after a penicillin injection.
c. A fractured tibia is common (resulting from being dropped by a child or getting the leg caught in the caging). Simple splints often work well. These fractures should be clinically distinguished from pathologic fractures associated with scorbutic rickets (vitamin C deficiency).

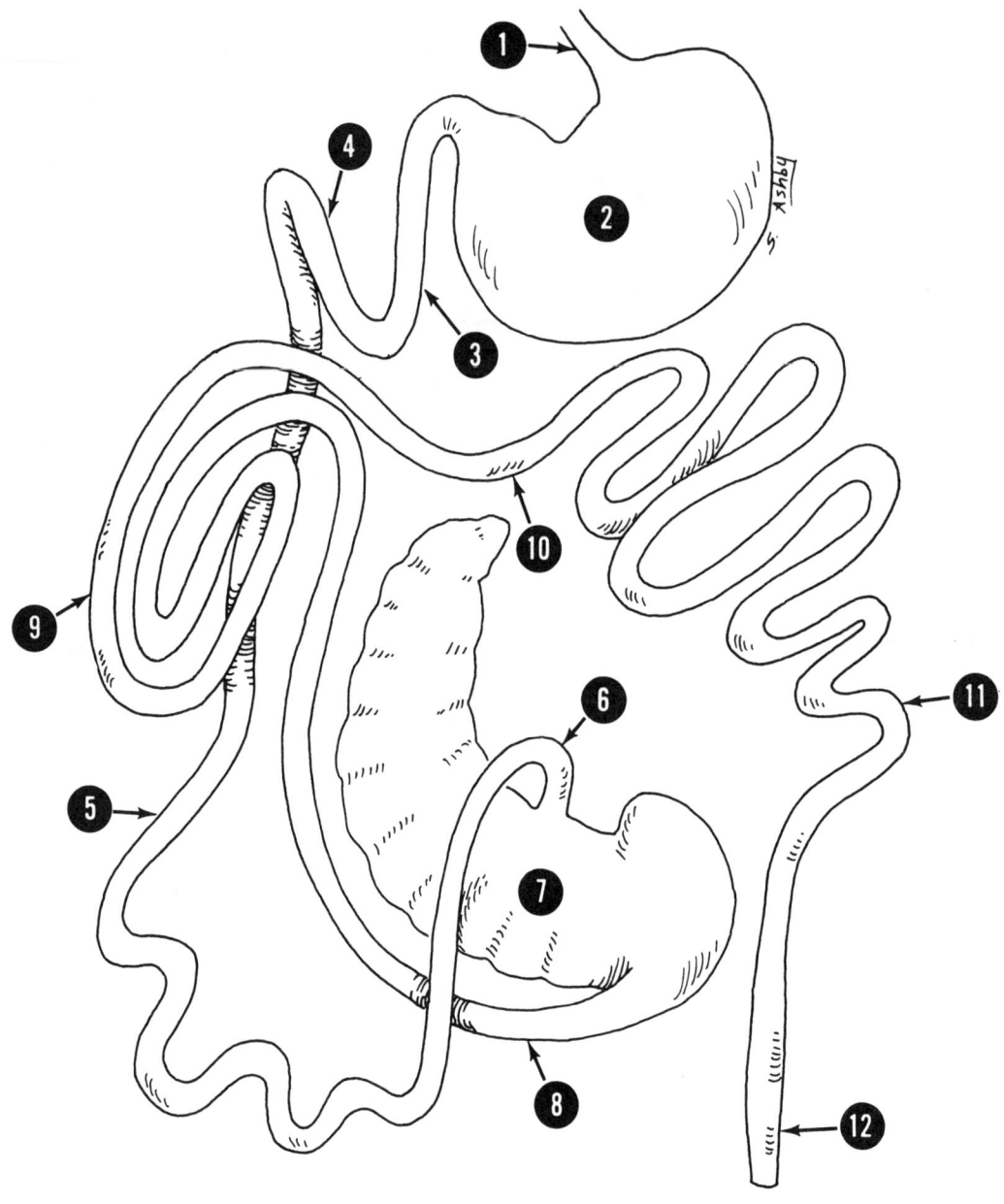

Figure 22-3

Stomach and Intestines of a Guinea Pig (ventral aspect)

1. Esophagus
2. Stomach
3. Descending duodenum
4. Ascending duodenum
5. Jejunum (shortened for illustrations)
6. Ileum
7. Cecum
8. Ascending colon
9. Spiral loop of ascending colon
10. Transverse colon
11. Descending colon
12. Rectum

Modified from Shively and Stump, 1975 [17]

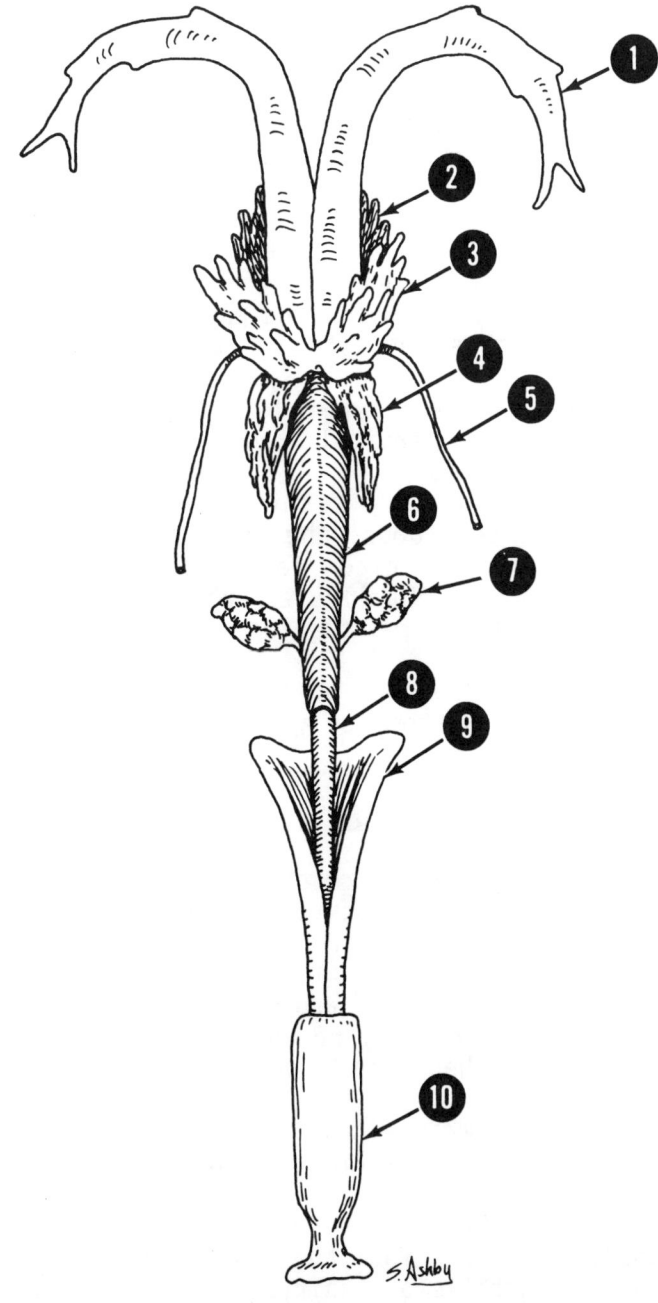

Figure 22-4

The Reproductive System of a Male Guinea Pig (dorsal aspect)

1. Seminal vesicle
2. Coagulating gland
3. Dorsal lobe of prostate gland
4. Ventral lobe of prostate gland
5. Ductus deferens
6. Urethra (surrounded by urethralis muscle)
7. Bulbourethral gland
8. Urethra (surrounded by corpus spongiosum)
9. Corpus cavernosum
10. Prepuce (surrounding glans penis)

Modified From Cooper and Schiller, 1975 [19]

- d. Mature boars may develop a scrotal plug of sebaceous material between the halves of the scrotum. It can be manually removed.
- e. Sows suffer a number of pregnancy related problems because of the large size of the fetuses. They may develop pregnancy ketosis (acetonemia) and those not bred until after six months of age may need cesarean sections because the pelvic symphysis may be permanently fused. Pregnant females are very susceptible to heatstroke. Some suffer clotting problems because the large size of the fetuses pushes the stomach against the liver, blocks bile drainage, and impedes vitamin K absorption.
- f. Lymphadenitis, often caused by Streptococcus spp., is common, especially in the cervical region. Some respond to antibiotic therapy; others do not.
- g. Guinea pigs need dietary vitamin C. Although it is available in commercial pelleted foods, the relatively short shelf life of this vitamin (90-120 days) often leads to insufficient dietary intake. Pet animals are occasionally fed rabbit chow inadvertently, and may develop scurvy if not fed supplemental fresh greens.

A standard source of reference on the guinea pig is the book by Wagner and Manning [18]. For anatomy only, the work of Cooper and Schiller may be consulted [19].

MONGOLIAN GERBIL (by Dr. F. J. Stein)

The mongolian gerbil, commonly called gerbil or jird, is a relatively new addition to the laboratory animal group that has rapidly increased in popularity because of unique anatomical and physiological characteristics. The gerbil is also a popular pet. It belongs to the Order Rodentia and the family Cricetidae and bears the scientific name Meriones unguiculatus. These small, friendly rodents originated in the desert regions of eastern Mongolia and northeastern China [2].

The gerbil is easy to maintain and manage in captivity and can tolerate a wide range of temperatures and environmental conditions. The maximum weight of a mature male is just over 100 g and the female is slightly smaller. Gerbils are most often native agouti brown in color, but some black strains have been developed. They have four toes on their front feet and five on the back. Their foot pads and tails are hairy.

Restraint is relatively simple and techniques described for the rat are entirely adequate. One should be aware, however, that they are more adept at quick, jerky movements, and once free, they may be hard to catch. One should be careful in handling the tail as the skin is loosely attached and may slip off, leaving the caudal muscles and vertebrae exposed.

Because its desert origins, have induced a well-developed ability to concentrate urine, the gerbil has a very low requirement for water. Gerbils consume only one quarter to one half as much water as other laboratory rodents. They are easily maintained without supplements on laboratory rodent pellets. Sunflower seeds can be added as a treat. Gerbils have the same monophyodontic dentition as rats, mice, and hamsters.

Sex differentiation can be made by comparing anogenital distances. As with other rodents, the scrotum of the young male is not prominent. The female, like the female rat, has two separate cervical canals, but both open into a common uterine body. There is a sebaceous gland on the abdominal midline of both sexes that is used for territorial markings. This gland is more prominent on the male and can be used for sex determination in older animals.

Both sexes reach maturity at 10 to 12 weeks. The female has a reproductive life of 12 to 15 months, and both sexes have a life expectancy of 2 to 4 years. Gerbils usually mate for life and should be paired before reaching sexual maturity. Females have an estrus of less than 24 hours' duration every 4 to 6 days. Gestation is 24 to 26 days with parturition usually occurring at night. Four or 5 hairless young comprise a litter. Weaning at 21 days of age is normal. Like other rodents, gerbils have a 24-hour postpartum estrus; however, a nursing female will delay implantation for 4 to 17 days after this mating.

The easily accessible abdominal sebaceous gland on the ventral midline is used frequently in research to study the effect of various gonadal hormones on sebaceous gland activity. The adrenal glands of the gerbil are three times as large as those of the rat on an organ to body weight ratio and are used to study endocrine gland metabolism. The gerbil is an excellent model to study epilepsy since 20% of any population will undergo predictable and reproducible seizures when placed in a novel environment. Strains have been developed where 100% of the population have seizures. Another feature that makes the gerbil a desirable research animal is its ability to ready acceptance of both homologous and heterologous tumor grafts. It also has high serum lipid and cholesterol levels without developing atherosclerosis, and it can tolerate much higher radiation exposures than most other animals [2].

The following points may be clinically useful [1]:

a. Like mice, gerbils are very susceptible to a direct streptomycin toxicity (a single dose of 25 to 50 mg is often fatal).
b. A roughened hair coat is often the result of environmental humidity over 50%.
c. Bald noses may result from excessive digging or pushing the nose through the cage bars. Sometimes these develop Staphylococcus. infections which may appear smooth and shiny or scabby. Daily topical nitrofurazone dressing and 250 mg tetracycline in 100 ml of drinking water may be helpful.
d. Basophilic stippling of red blood corpuscles is a normal phenomenon and should not be confused with Eperythrozoon infection.
e. The epileptiform seizures are sometimes initiated by sudden handling or fright. They only last a few seconds and no treatment is necessary.

Additional information concerning gerbils is available in the first four references [1-4].

RABBIT

Domesticated rabbits are descendents of the European wild rabbit and bear the scientific name Oryctolagus cuniculus. They are members of the mammalian Order Lagomorpha and the Family Leporidae.

The dental formula is 2(I2/1 C0/0 P3/2 M3/3) = 28. The second pair of superior incisors is very small and is positioned directly caudal to the principal pair. These reduced incisors cannot be seen without opening the mouth and they constitute the scientific basis for placing rabbits (along with the hares and pikas) in a separate order instead of including them in the Order Rodentia [21].

The names "hare" and "rabbit" have been used as though they are synonymous, but technically they are not. Young hares are born in the open, fully haired, with open eyes and are able to run within a few minutes of birth. Rabbits, on the other hand, are born in a nest, blind, naked, and helpless. Hares are usually larger than rabbits and typically (but not always) have black ear tips. The actual anatomical differences are found in the skull and include subtle differences in the zygomatic arch, the hard palate, and the interparietal bone. The names "jackrabbit" and "snowshoe rabbit" have been incorrectly applied to hares and the name "Belgian hare" has been incorrectly applied to a rabbit.

In addition to their peculiar dentition, rabbits have a Y-shaped glabrous groove which extends from the oral margin of the superior lip to and around the nose, and the superior lip is cleft. (The term "hare-lip" was derived from this feature.) When the mouth is closed, the incisors are separated from the rest of the oral cavity by labial folds. Other obvious external features include elongated ears which are several times as long as they are wide. The pelvic limbs are longer than the thoracic limbs and are specialized for running. There are five digits on the front feet and four on the back. In addition, the feet are covered with hair (no foot pads).

In the thorax, the mediastinum is strong enough to withstand unilateral thoracotomies without collapsing. The lung lobation resembles that of dogs. The tracheal bifurcation is quite delicate and can easily be ruptured by an endotracheal tube or a misplaced stomach tube [1].

In the abdomen, the ileum is enlarged at its termination into the sacculus rotundus. This area contains lymphatic tissue and has a pale appearance. The cecum is very large and terminates in an appendix. The initial part of the cecum has a large diameter and is sacculated. The distal portion becomes smaller and is not sacculated (Fig. 22-5) [21].

Male rabbits are commonly called bucks, and they are usually smaller than females (does). In contrast to most other laboratory animals, they lack an os penis and have the penis positioned caudal to the scrotum.

Reproductively, does are polyestrous and are induced ovulators. After a gestation period of 4-5 weeks they bear 3-9 young (kits) which reach puberty in 3-8 months. Abortion and resorption of embryos is common. Does have two cervices, two distinct uteri, and 4-5 pairs of nipples. Bucks do not develop nipples.

There is an inguinal gland on each side of the vulva that produces a brown odiferous secretion. Males also have these glands. Both sexes have a chin gland, but it is better developed in the males [1].

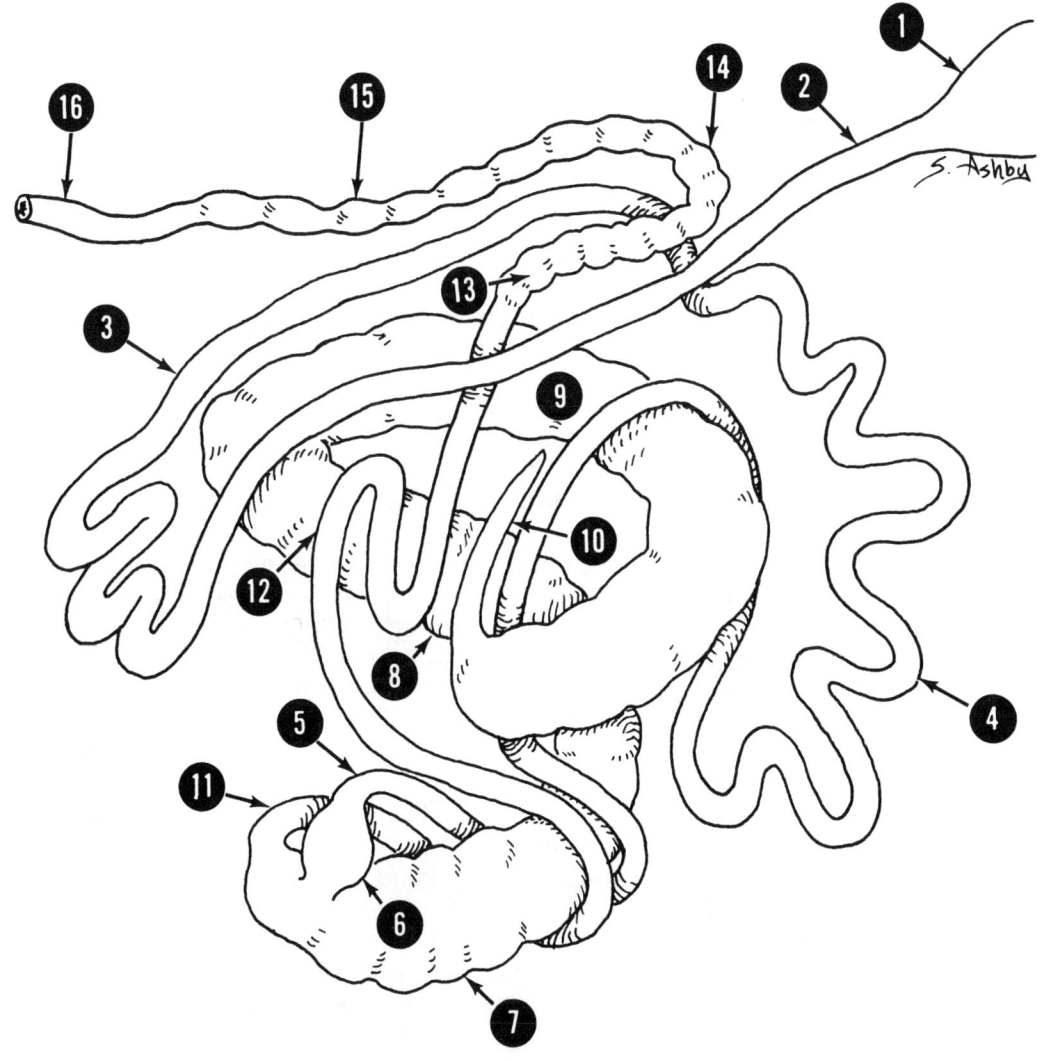

Figure 22-5

The Intestines of a Rabbit (right aspect)

1. Pyloric region of stomach
2. Descending duodenum
3. Ascending duodenum
4. Jejunum
5. Ileum
6. Sacculus rotundus
7. First gyrus of cecum
8. Second gyrus of cecum
9. Third gyrus of cecum
10. Appendix of cecum
11. Initial part of ascending colon
12. Central loop of ascending colon
13. Distal loop of ascending colon
14. Transverse colon
15. Descending colon
16. Rectum

Modified from Popesko, 1978 [22]

To pick up a rabbit, the loose skin over the neck and shoulders is grasped in one hand and the other hand is used to support the hindquarters. Failure to support the pelvic limbs may result in serious scratches to the handler and/or a broken back to the rabbit because of the struggling which often occurs. Rabbits kept as pets for children may be declawed by procedures similar to those used in cats [1].

Blood may be collected from rabbits via the conventional cardiac or venous routes and the marginal ear veins may also be nicked. Sexual differentiation may be made as indicated in Fig. 22-6.

The following points may be of value clinically [1]:

a. Orphaned baby rabbits need be fed only once each day. Cow's milk with 9-15% casein added or bitch's milk is satisfactory.
b. The redundant skin on the ventral aspect of the neck is susceptible to a moist dermatitis termed "slobbers." Damp bedding, water crocks, and drooling from malocclusion are initiating factors.
c. Malocclusion of the incisors may require frequent trimming.
d. A serous or mucopurulent discharge from the nose may be indicative of "snuffles" (Pasteurella multocida infection).
e. Rabbits are avid ingestors of their own feces (coprophagy, reingestion, pseudorumination). (This also occurs to some extent in rats, guinea pigs, and some other rodents.) Fecal pellets which are reingested are softer than noningested pellets and are covered with mucus. They are taken directly from the anus and swallowed whole. The habit is believed to improve nitrogen utilization and to recover certain B-vitamins, but is not necessary for the animal's well-being.
f. Neutrophils have intracytoplasmic eosinophilic granules which are easily confused with those of eosinophils [2].
g. Ear mites (Psoroptes cuniculi) are common and may result in severe otitis.

For additional information on rabbits, the first four references may be consulted as well as the work of Weisbroth et al [22]. For radiographic anatomy, the work of Shively is available [24,25].

NONHUMAN PRIMATES (by Dr. F. J. Stein)

Nonhuman primates (NHP) are members of the Order Primates. Primates have long digits with divergent and mobile thumbs on both fore and hind limbs. They have simplex uteri with no uterine horns.

Most nonhuman primates used in research belong to the Suborder Anthropoidea (true primates). This group is further divided into two groups: old-world monkeys and new-world monkeys. These groups are differentiated by anatomical characteristics.

Old-world monkeys are catarrhine (narrow nasal septum), and have cheek pouches, a distinctive sex skin, and ischial callosities. They are also sexually dimorphic (body size and size of upper canines). The sex skin

Figure 22-6

Sexual Differentiation in Rabbits

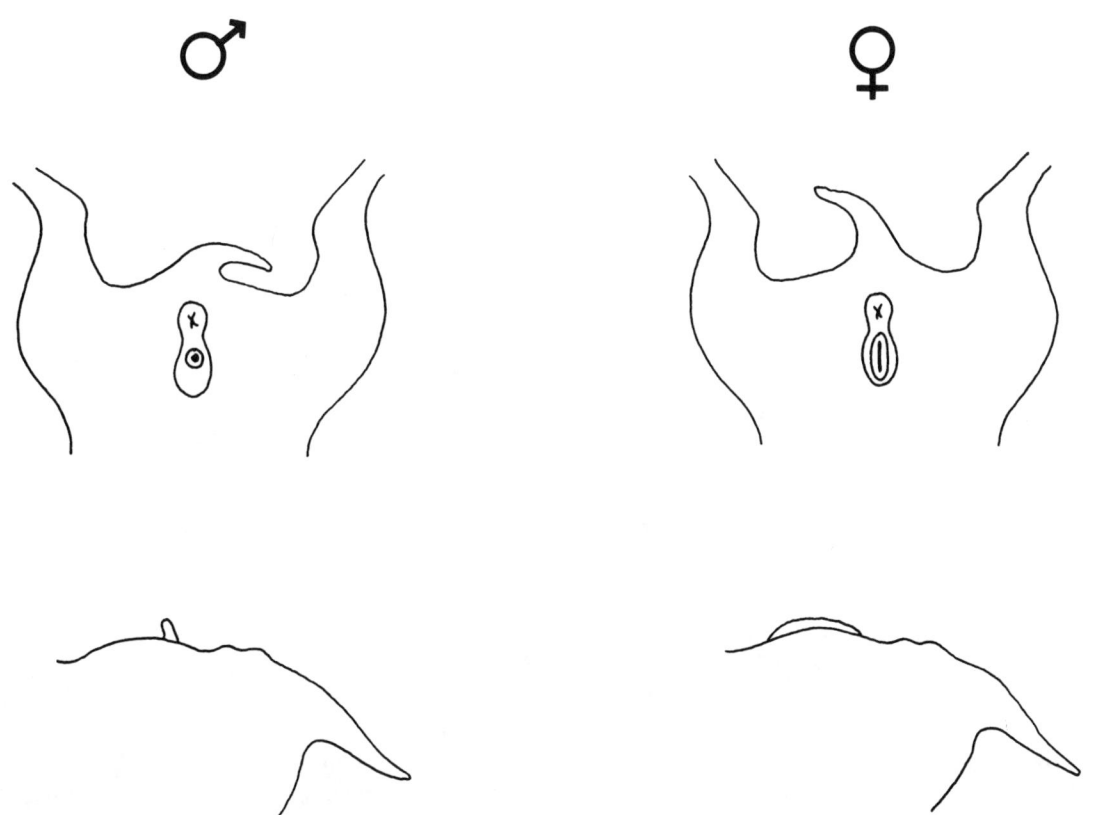

Young Rabbits (see above)

In males, the penis is a rounded protrusion more than 1.2 mm cranial to the anus and a pair of reddish brown spots are present near the anus. In females, the vulva is a slit-like opening less than 1.2 mm from the anus and no specks are present.

Mature Rabbits

MALE	FEMALE
1. Protrude penis by manipulating skin of prepuce.	1. There is a common orifice for both the vagina and urethra (like dog and cat).
2. Palpate for testicles.	2. No structure like a "penis" can be protruded from the urogenital orifice.
3. Anogenital distance is longer.	3. Anogenital distance is shorter.

From Schuchman, 1980 [3]

surrounds the genitals, tail, and thighs. It becomes bright red and tumescent during estrus, with maximum swelling at ovulation. Additionally, all old-world primates exhibit menstrual bleeding, which is an excellent criterion, along with sex skin changes, for monitoring the estrous cycle of the female. Another characteristic of most old world primates (especially the macaques) is a post-implantation bleeding which occurs about 20 days after implantation. This is usually less severe than that which occurs during menses and should not be confused with it.

New-world monkeys are platyrrhine (wide nasal septum); lack ischial callosities, sex skin, and menses; and some have prehensile tails.

Old-world monkeys commonly used in research include the macaques (Macaca sp.), the baboons (Papio sp.), and the chimpanzees (Pan sp.). Of all primates, the rhesus monkey (Macaca mulatta) is the most widely used in research. Adult male rhesus monkeys weigh up to 14 kg and females weigh 3-8 kg. The gestation period is 156-180 days. Females have a post-implantation blood loss that has sometimes been confused with menses. Other macaques used in research include the cynomolgus monkey (crab-eating macaque, M. fascicularis), stump-tailed macaque (M. aretoides, redder sex skin during sexual activity than other macaques), pig-tailed macaque (M. nemestrina, larger than rhesus); and barbary ape (M. sylvana, no tail).

Of the baboons, Papio cynocephalus is the one most often used in research. They have gestation periods of 175 days. The males weigh up to 26 kg and the females 13 kg. The upper canines are well developed in the male.

Of the great apes (gorillas, orangutans, chimpanzees, and gibbons) only the chimpanzee is commonly used in biomedical research. The chimpanzees include the pygmy chimp (Pan panisius) and the common chimp (Pan troglodytes). The common chimp is used in research requiring a model very similar to man. Males weigh 50 kg and females 40 kg. The gestation period of the chimp is 7 months.

New-world monkeys used in research include the squirrel monkey (Saimiri sciureus), which is the second most widely used research primate. It weighs up to 1,000 g and has a 165- to 170-day gestation period. The owl monkey (Aotus trivirgatus) is nocturnal, does not breed well in captivity, and is used for studies of viral diseases and human malaria. Its gestation period is 120 to 140 days; and it has a throat sac that can be inflated to produce resonant sounds.

Marmosets and tamarins belong to the Family Callitrichidae. Those used in research belong primarily to the genera Callithrix and Saguinus. Weight varies from 70 to 1,000 g The gestation period is 146 days, and twins or triplets are normal. There is joint placentation and multiple offspring are chimeric. This feature makes marmosets and tamarins excellent models for immunologic research.

Common sites for venipuncture of all primates include the jugular, saphenous, and femoral veins. The femoral vein is the most frequently used site.

There are numerous zoonotic diseases of primates that are important in laboratory animal medicine. Three should be mentioned because of their serious public health significance. Probably the most important of these, because of the large numbers of nonhuman primates that may be infected, is tuberculosis (TB), caused by Mycobacterium spp. Those species that most frequently infect nonhuman primates in their order of importance are M. tuberculosis, M. bovis, and M. avium. TB is more common in old-world NHP than new-world NHP, and once contracted is very contagious and will spread rapidly throughout a colony. There is no treatment for TB that is 100% effective and treatment quite often masks the disease resulting in carrier animals. Control of TB in NHP is therefore best obtained by destruction of infected animals.

Several different methods have been utilized for detection of TB, and these include radiography, skin testing, serology, and culture. A combination of these methods may be used. The current method of choice is skin testing with 0.10 ml of mammalian tuberculin, diluted 1:10 and injected intradermally in the upper eyelid. The injection site is checked at 24, 48, and 72 hours for any swelling or redness. Although an early false reaction may be encountered due to trauma inflicted during the injection procedure, any reaction should be considered positive. In extremely valuable animals, when the reaction appears to be minimal and possibly due to trauma, a confirmatory test may be performed in the opposite eyelid or on a shaved area of cranial abdominal skin. Any reaction on the confirmatory test should be considered positive, and the animal should be destroyed. Additionally, a recently infected animal may have a false negative reaction. Newly acquired animals should be tested once every two weeks until all animals have at least three consecutive negative reactions. Testing should then be done quarterly and repeated biweekly if a positive reaction is encountered until the animal shows three consecutive negative response.

The other two highly significant zoonotic diseases are Marburg virus and Herpes B virus. Both are fatal to man. Little is known about the Marburg virus, especially its reservoir in nature. Although African green monkeys were involved in the original outbreak of this disease in 1967, these monkeys have not been involved in subsequent human cases. While Herpes B affects newly infected monkeys (especially macaques) in much the same way that Herpes simplex affects humans, there are no diagnostic lesions for the identification of monkeys infected with Marburg virus. All newly acquired primates should be maintained under strict quarantine for a minimum of 90 days. Any animal that becomes sick or dies should undergo a complete diagnostic examination with particular emphasis given to the above diseases.

Much of the information on diseases of nonhuman primates is in the current literature, but the somewhat dated work by Ruch [26] is well respected. Other useful references on anatomy, physiology, behavior, and diseases may be found in the texts by Hill [27], Hafez [20], and Bourne [29].

References

1. Williams, C. 1976. Practical Guide to Laboratory Animals. C. V. Mosby, Saint Louis.

2. Harkness, J. E., and J. E. Wagner. 1977. *The Biology and Medicine of Rabbits and Rodents.* Lea and Febiger, Philadelphia.

3. Schuchman, S. M. 1980. Individual care and treatment of rabbits, mice, rats, guinea pigs, hamsters, and gerbils. In *Current Veterinary Therapy VII*, edited by Kirk. W. B. Saunders, Philadelphia.

4. *The UFAW Handbook on the Care and Management of Laboratory Animals*, fourth ed. 1972. Williams and Wilkins, Baltimore.

5. Hafez, E. S. 1970. *Reproduction and Breeding Techniques for Laboratory Animals.* Lea and Febiger, Philadelphia.

6. McPherson, C. W., and G. L. Van Hoosier. 1973. *The Mouse: Biology and Use in Research.* American College of Laboratory Animal Medicine and Washington State University College of Veterinary Medicine, Seattle, Washington.

7. Foster, H. L., J. D. Small, and J. G. Fox. 1981. *The Mouse in Biomedical Research, Vol. 1, History, Genetics, and Wild Mice.* Academic Press, New York.

8. Green, E. L., ed. 1966. *Biology of the Laboratory Mouse*, second ed. McGraw-Hill, New York.

9. Cook, M. J. 1965. *The Anatomy of the Laboratory Mouse.* Academic Press, New York.

10. Baker, H. J., and W. S. Bivin. 1977. *The Laboratory Rat.* American College of Laboratory Animal Medicine and Washington State University College of Veterinary Medicine, Seattle, Washington.

11. Baker, H. J., J. R. Lindsey, and S. H. Weisbroth. 1979. *The Laboratory Rat, Vol. 1, Biology and Diseases.* Academic Press, New York.

12. Greene, E. C. 1955. *Anatomy of the Rat.* Hafner Publishing Co., New York.

13. Hebel R., and M. W. Stromberg. 1976. *Anatomy of the Laboratory Rat.* Williams and Wilkins, Baltimore.

14. Clark, J. D. 1975. *The Hamster.* American College of Laboratory Animal Medicine and Washington State University College of Veterinary Medicine, Seattle, Washington.

15. Hoffman, R. A., P. F. Robinson, and H. Magalhaes. 1968. *The Golden Hamster.* Iowa State University Press, Ames, Iowa.

16. Clark, J. D., and H. J. Baker. 1975. *Guinea Pig.* American College of Laboratory Animal Medicine and Washington State University College of Veterinary Medicine, Seattle, Washington.

17. Shively, M. J., and J. E. Stump. 1975. The systemic arterial pattern of the guinea pig. *Anat. Rec.* 182:355-366.

Table 22-1
Anatomic Data on Common Laboratory Animals

	Mouse	Rat	Hamster	Guinea Pig	Gerbil	Rabbit
Dental Formula	$2(I\frac{1}{1}C\frac{0}{0}P\frac{0}{0}M\frac{3}{3})=16$	(like mouse)	(like mouse)	$2(I\frac{1}{1}C\frac{0}{0}P\frac{1}{1}M\frac{3}{3})=20$	(like mouse)	$2(I\frac{2}{1}C\frac{0}{0}P\frac{3}{2}M\frac{3}{3})=28$
Vertebral formula	$C_7 T_{13} L_6 S_4 Cd_{18}$	$C_7 T_{13} L_6 S_4 Cd_{27-31}$	$C_7 T_{13} L_6 S_4 Cd_{13-14}$	$C_7 T_{13-14} L_6 S_{3-4} Cd_7$	$C_7 T_{13} L_6 S_4 Cd_{17}$	$C_7 T_{12-13} L_7 S_4 Cd_{16}$
Digits $\frac{manus}{pes}$	$\frac{4}{5}$	$\frac{4}{5}$	$\frac{4}{5}$	$\frac{4}{3}$	$\frac{4}{5}$	$\frac{5}{4}$
Character of foot pads	glabrous	glabrous	glabrous	glabrous	hairy	hairy (no pads)
Presence of tail	+	+	(very short)	–	+	+
Hair on tail	–	–	–	–	+	+
Left lung lobation	undivided	undivided	undivided	divided cranial lobe, caudal lobe	(like guinea pig)	(like guinea pig)
Right lung lobation	cranial, middle caudal, and accessory lobes	(like mouse)	cranial, middle and caudal lobes	(like mouse)	(like mouse)	(like mouse)
Unusual features of alimentary canal	–	–	stomach grossly divided into two compartments	cecum resembles that of horse	–	ileum joins sacculus rotundus, cecum has appendix
Conformation of uterus and vagina	Y-shaped uterus with single cervix	2 cervices which open into same uterus	each horn of the uterus has a separate cervical opening into the vagina	(like mouse)	(like rat)	2 cervices and 2 distinct uteri
Unique superficial glands	–	extraorbital lacrimal glands	hip gland (well developed) in males	–	abdominal sebaceous gland	inguinal gland chin gland
Other peculiar anatomic characteristics	sexually dimorphic spleen	absence of gallbladder & tonsils	cheek pouches, single long renal papilla, up to 22 teats	single pair of mammary glands, only 3 digits on each pes	relatively large suprarenal glands, incomplete cerebral arterial circle, basophilic stippling of RBC's	elongated ears, second superior incisors located directly behind first ones, eyes largest (relatively) of all mammals

Table 22-2

Biological Data on Common Laboratory Animals

	Mouse	Rat	Hamster	Guinea Pig	Gerbil	Rabbit
Weight at birth	1.5 g	5.5 g	2 g	100 g	3 g	100 g
Puberty	35 days	(F)50-60 days (M)3 months	(F)28-31 days (M)45 days	(F)20-30 days (M)70 days	(F)2½-4 months (M)70 days	4-9 months
Estrous cycle (days)	4	4	4	16-19	4	15-16
Gestation	19-21 days	21-23 days	16 days	62-72 days	24 days	28-36 days
Separation of adults during parturition and weaning	No	No	Yes	No	No (mates for life)	Yes
Number per litter	4-12	8-12	4-10	1-4	4-5	7
Eyes open (days)	11-14	14-17	15	Prior to birth	16-20	10
Wean at (days)	21	21	25	14-21 or 160 g	21	42-56
Postpartum estrus	Within 24-48 hours	Within 24-48 hours	Within 24 hours	Within 24 hour	Within 24 48 hours	Immediate
Breeding life	12-18 months	14 months	11-18 months	3-4 years	15-20 months	1-3 years maximum 6 years

Table 22-2 (Continued)

	Mouse	Rat	Hamster	Guinea Pig	Gerbil	Rabbit
Adult weight	(F) 30 g (M) 30 g	(F) 300 g (M) 500 g	(F) 120 g (M) 108 g	(F) 850 g (M) 1000 g	(F) 75 g (M) 85 g	(F) 4.0 kg (M) 4.3 kg
Life span (years)	1-3	2-3	2-3	4-5	4	5-7
Body temperature (°F)	96.4-100	99.5-100.6	97-101	100.4-102.5	100.8	101-103.2
Diet	Commercial rodent chow	Commercial rodent chow	Commercial rodent chow	Commercial guinea pig chow, good quality hay, kale, cabbage, fruits (cannot rely on vitamin C levels of commercial ration)	Commercial rodent chow (lowest fat possible), sunflower seeds	Commercial rabbit pellets, greens in moderation
Room temperature (°F)	70-80	76-78	65-75	65-75	65-80	62-68
Humidity (percent)	50	50	50	50	under 50	50

*All species listed are seasonally polyestrous.

Modified from Schuchman, 1980 [3]

Table 22-3

Sexual Determination in Laboratory Rodents

Mature Mice, Rats, Hamsters, Guinea Pigs, and Gerbils

Male	Female
1. Anogenital distance longer in the male.*	1. Anogenital distance shorter in the female.
2. Manipulate "genital papilla" (prepuce) to protrude penis.	2. Have three external openings in the inguinal area: (a) anus (most caudal opening); (b) vaginal orifice (middle opening); (c) urethral orifice at tip of urethral papilla (most cranial opening).
3. Palpate for testicles either in a scrotal sac (if present) or subcutaneous inguinal region.	In these animals the urethral papilla is located outside the vagina (unlike the dog or cat).
4. Males have only two external openings in the inguinal area: (a) anus; (b) urethral orifice at tip of penis.	In very fat females or young females, the vaginal orifice may be hidden by folds of skin (the former) or sealed (latter). Gentle manipulation of the skin in this area will divulge the orifice.
In very fat males there may be a depression between the penis and anus. This depression can be obliterated by manipulating the skin in that area.	

*Not useful in the guinea pig

Modified from Schuchman, 1980 [3]

Table 22-4

Blood Collection Routes

	Mouse	Rat	Hamster	Guinea Pig	Gerbil	Rabbit	Non-Human Primates
1. Tail Clip	+	+	+ (1 or 2 drops)	-	+	-	-
2. Cardiocentesis	+	+	+	+	+	+	+
3. Orbital sinus puncture with capillary tube	+	+	+	+	+	-	-
4. Jugular venipuncture	-	+	+	-	-	+	+
5. Femoral or saphenous venipuncture	-	+ -	-	+	-	+	+
6. Cephalic venipuncture	-	-	-	-	-	-	+
7. Other methods	---	Clip toenail	Split foot pad	Clip toenail	---	nick lateral ear vein	---

Note: Terminal blood collection in small laboratory animals may be done by decapitation. It should also be noted that some vessels which are adequate for intravenous administration of drugs are too small to serve as satisfactory blood collection routes.

Table 22-5

Comparative Anatomy of the Male Reproductive System

	Mouse	Rat	Hamster	Guinea Pig	Gerbil	Rabbit	Nonhuman Primate
Ampulla	+	+	+	-	+	+	-
Seminal Vesicles	+	+	+	+	+	+	+
Prostate gl.	+	+	+	+	+	+	+
Paraprostate gl.	-	-	-	-	-	+	-
Bulbourethral gl.	+	+	+	+	+	+	-
Os penis	+	+	+	+	+	-	+
Urethral gl.	+	+	+	-	+	-	-
Preputial gl.	+	+	+	P	-	-	D
Inguinal gl.	-	-	-	-	-	+	-

Note: P = poorly developed
D = diffuse

Modified from Hafez, 1970 [5]

Table 22-6

Hematological Values in Common Laboratory Animals

Test	Mouse	Rat	Golden Hamster	Guinea Pig	Gerbil	Rabbits New Zealand White	Rabbits Dutch Belted
Erythrocytes (RBC) ($\times 10^6/mm^3$)	8-13	7-9	4.0-10.0	3.3-6.8	7.87-9.97	4.3-6.8	4.8-6.3
Hemoglobin (g/dl)	11-15	12-14	13.1-19.2	11.4-17.2	15.2-16.8	9.4-13.9	12.2-16.3
Hematocrit (%)	39-43	40-50	39.2-58.8	37-50	46.0-52.0	31.6-50.0	34.8-48.9
Luekocyte (WBC) ($\times 10^3/mm^3$)	6-12	8-15	5.2-10.6	5.5-17.5	6.51-21.6	6.0-13.0	4.0-13.0
Neutrophils (%)	13.2-21.6	4.4-49.2	17.1-35.2	20.3-56	2.0-23.0	36.0-52.0	30.0-50.0
Eosinophils (%)	0.29-0.41	0.0-1.96	0.22-1.54	0.18-0.70	0.0-4.0	0.5-3.5	0.5-5.0
Basophils (%)	0.13-0.85	0.0-0.6	0.0-5.0	0.01-0.12	0.0-1.0	2.0-7.0	2.0-8.0
Lymphocytes (%)	62.4-82.8	50.2-84.5	50.9-92.3	40.0-80.4	73.0-97.0	30.0-53.0	28.5-52.5
Monocytes (%)	0.98-2.47	0.01-0.04	0.4-4.4	1.0-5.3	0.0-3.0	4.0-12.0	2.0-16
Sedimentation Rate (mm/hr)	0.0-0.9	0.68-1.76	0.3-0.96	1.1-2.2	--	--	--

Modified from B. M. Mitruka, H. M. Rawnsky, and B. V. Vaderha. Clinical, Biochemical and Hematological Reference Values in Normal Experimental Animals (Masson Publishing USA, Inc., New York) and Syllabus for the Laboratory Technologist, Publication 72-2 (American Association for Laboratory Science, 210 Hammes Ave., Suite 205, Joliet, Illinois 60435).

Table 22-7

Biochemical Values in Common Laboratory Animals

Test	Mouse	Rat	Golden Hamster	Guinea Pig	Gerbil	Rabbits New Zealand White	Rabbits Dutch Belted
Platelets (x 10^3/mm^3)	150-500	450-850	300-573	260-740	---	180-630	126-490
Blood Glucose (mg/dl)	63-176	50-135	32.6-118	82-107	40-141	50-93	69-159
BUN (mg/dl)	14-28	5-29	12-26	9-31.5	17-31	9-32	13-40
Calcium (mg/dl)	3.2-8.5	7.2-13.9	7.4-12	8.3-12	3.7-6.2	5.6-12.1	5.6-12
Sodium (mEq/l)	128-145	143-156	106-146	120-146	141-171	100-145	138-156
Potassium (mEq/l)	4.85-5.85	5.4-7	4-6	3.8-7.95	3.3-6.3	3.6-6.9	4.4-7.4
Chloride (mEq/l)	105-110	100-110	86-112	90-115	93-118	98-116	102-120
Bicarbonate (mEq/l)	20-31.5	12.6-32	33-44	13-30	---	16.2-31.8	16.2-31.8
Phosphorus (mg/dl)	2.30-9.2	3.11-11	3.5-8	3-7.6	3.7-7.2	4.4-7.8	3.1-8.1
Magnesium (mg/dl)	0.8-3.9	1.6-4.4	2-3.5	1.8-3	17-31	2.1-4.3	2-4.1
Total Protein (g/dl)	4.0-4.7	4.7-8.15	4.3-7.7	5-6.8	4.8-16.8	5.3-7.9	5.7-9.8
Albumin (g/dl)	2.5-4.8	2.7-5.1	2.6-4.1	2-4	1.8-10.7	2.5-5.3	3-6

Modified from B. M. Mitruka, H. M. Rawnsky, and B. V. Vaderha. Clinical, Biochemical and Hematological Reference Values in Normal Experimental Animals (Masson Publishing USA, Inc., New York), and Syllabus for the Laboratory Technologist, Publication 72-2 (American Association for Laboratory Science, 210 Hammes Ave., Suite 205, Joliet, Illinois 60435).

18. Wagner, J. E. and P. J. Manning. 1976. The Biology of the Guinea Pig. Academic Press, New York.

19. Cooper, G., and A. Schiller. 1975. Anatomy of the Guinea Pig. Harvard University Press, Cambridge, Massachusetts.

20. Williams, W. 1974. Anatomy of the Mongolian Gerbil (Meriones unguiculatus). Tumblebrook Farm, Inc., West Brookfield, Massachusetts.

21. Flatt, R. E. 1975. The Rabbit. Amercian College of Laboratory Animal Medicine and Washington State University College of Veterinary Medicine.

22. Popesko, P. 1978. Atlas of topographic anatomy of the domestic animals. W. B. Saunders, Philadelphia.

23. Weisbroth, S. H., R. E. Flatt, and A. L. Kraus. 1974. The Biology of the Laboratory Rabbit. Academic Press, New York.

24. Shively, M. J. 1981. Xeroradiographic anatomy of the domesticated rabbit (Oryctolagus cuniculus), Part I, Head, Thorax, and Thoracic Limb. Lab Anim. 10(4):36-46, (reprinted from Swest Vet. 32(3):219-233).

25. Shively, M. J. 1982. Xeroradiographic Anatomy of the Rabbit, Part II, Abdomen, Pelvis, and Pelvic Limb. Lab Animal 11(1):24-32 (reprinted from Swest Vet. 33(1):57-67).

26. Ruch, T. C. 1959. Disease of Laboratory Primates. W. B. Saunders, Philadelphia.

27. Hill, W. C. O. 1974. Primates: Comparative Anatomy and Taxonomy. 7 vols. John Wiley, New York

28. Hafez, E. S. 1971. Comparative Reproduction of Nonhuman Primates. Charles C. Thomas, Springfield, Illinois.

29. Bourne, G. H., ed. 1969-1973. Anatomy, Behavior and Diseases of Chimpanzees. 6 vols. from 1969-1973). University Park Press, Baltimore.

INTEGUMENTARY SYSTEM

The skin surrounds the body and serves as a physical barrier against the environment. Some of its specific functions include the following:

a. temperature regulation
b. sensation (temperature, pressure, pain, touch)
c. protection from dessication and microbes

In addition to these general functions, the skin serves the body in a number of more specialized ways. Odiferous glands in the skin serve as species and individual markers. Epidermal modifications in various loci serve as weapons (horns, hooves, claws) or as shock absorbing coverings for the digits.

I. Common Integument

The common integument of domestic animals consists of two major layers:

epidermis--the outer, ectodermally derived layer of the skin which consists of 4 or 5 histologic layers.

dermis (corium)--the deeper, connective tissue component of the skin. Underneath the dermis is the subcutaneous layer of connective tissue ("hypodermis"). It is continuous (synonymous) with superficial fascia and serves as a major locus for the accumulation of adipose tissue. These accumulations characteristically occur in the ventral thoracic region of oxen, in the dorsal cervical region of horses, in the inguinal and lumbar regions of carnivores, and over most of the body in pigs [1].

The skin is usually thicker on the dorsum than on the ventrum and on older animals than on the young, and it is thicker in some species than others. Two major types of glands are present. Sebaceous glands produce an oily (fatty) secretion which protects the skin and hair coat. The sweat glands function in thermal regulation, water and electrolyte balance, maintenance of surface pH, and production of individual and species specific odors. Consideration of the specialized cutaneous glands is given in Part III.

A number of general modifications of the skin occur [1]:

1. nasal plane (carnivores and small ruminants), nasolabial plane (ox), rostral plane (pig) (Fig. 23-1/1-3)
2. dewlap (palear) of the ox
3. collar (plica transversae colli) of the sheep
4. tassels (appendices colli--also called "wattles") in some goats and more rarely in some sheep and pigs (Fig. 23-1/6).

More specialized modifications of the skin are considered in Part IV.

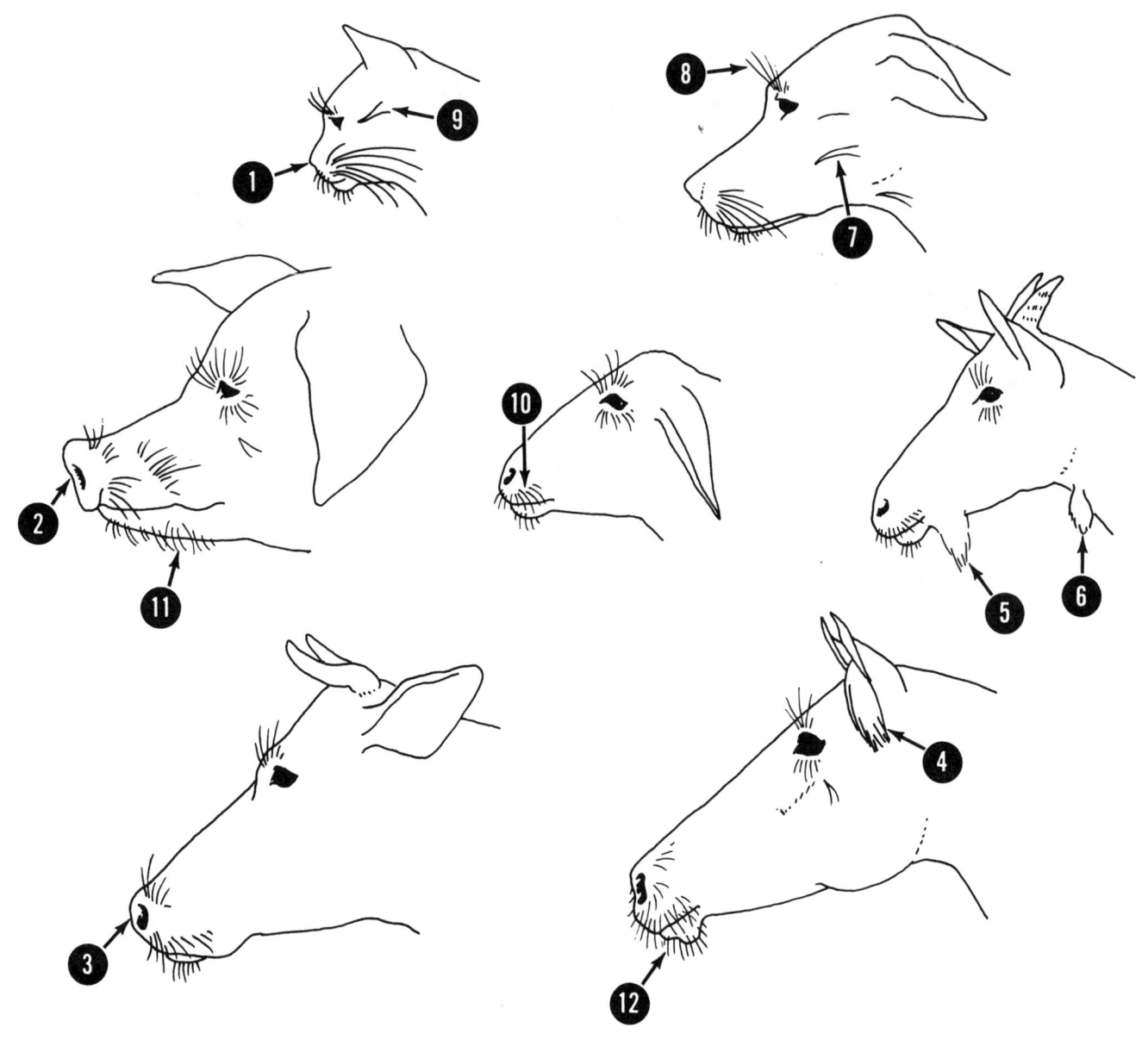

Figure 23-1

Integumentary Modifications Associated with the Head

1. nasal plane of cat (also present in dog, sheep, and goat)
2. rostral plane of pig
3. nasolabial plane of ox
4. forelock of horse
5. beard of goat
6. tassel of goat
7. tactile hairs of cheek
8. tactile hairs of supraorbital region
9. tactile hairs of zygomatic region
10. tactile hairs of superior lip
11. tactile hairs of inferior lip
12. tactile hairs of chin

II. Hair

   A. Types of hair

      1. guard hair (capilli)--the characteristic outer coat hair of most domestic animals except the sheep and pig.
      2. wool hair (pili lanei)--the fine, dense undercoat hair of most domestic animals (forms most of the hair coat of sheep)
      3. bristles (setae)--thick stiff hairs which form the hair coat of pigs as well as the following:

         cilia--eyelashes
         vibrissae--hairs of the nostrils
         tragi--hairs at the entrance to the auditory canal and on the inside of the pinnae
         beard (barba)--the long hairs in the submandibular region of goats
         mustache--the long hair on the superior lip which occasionally develops in horses

      4. long (horse) hairs - very long hairs found primarily in certain regions of the equine body.

         cirrus capitis (forelock)
         juba (mane)
         cirrus caudae (tail hair)
         cirrus metacarpeus ⎫ "feathers"
         cirrus metatarseus ⎭

      5. tactile hairs--well-developed, stiff hairs which function in a sensory capacity. They are divided by location into the following (not all species have all of these; Fig. 23-1/7-12):

         tactile hairs of the superior lip
         tactile hairs of the inferior lip
         tactile hairs of the chin
         tactile hairs of the cheek
         tactile hairs of the zygomatic region
         tactile hairs of the infraorbital region
         tactile hairs of the supraorbital region
         tactile hairs of the carpal region

   B. Arrangement of hair

   In the horse and ox, the hairs are evenly distributed over the body, but in the pig and carnivores the hairs are arranged in groups. Most hairs in a given region of the body are oriented parallel to each other and form characteristic tracts (flumina pilorum) for each species. These tracts meet at points (vortices pilorum) or lines (linea pilorum).

   C. Color of hair

Hair color is dependent on its pigment content, air content, and surface structure. Hairs which lack pigment are white. Those which are heavily pigmented are black. Red, brown, (etc.) hairs result from intermediate levels of pigment. Total lack of pigment in both hair and skin (albinism) is rare in domestic animals, but locally depigmented areas are common (especially on the limbs). The appearance of gray hair with increasing age is termed canities.

III. Specialized glands of the skin

A number of species have sex specific glands which produce the characteristic scents that occur in the skin of domestic mammals. They are usually coiled, tubular, apocrine glands or modified sebaceous glands. The secretions of most of these glands contain pheromones, believed to be used in territorial marking and individual recognition. Domestication has probably reduced the significance of some of these communications. A summary of the species occurrence of these glands is presented in Table 23-1. Several of these are found in only one domestic species, some are found in two or more, and some are present in all species [1].

- glands of the infraorbital sinus--occur in sheep. They are better developed in rams than in ewes, and their sticky secretion exudes from the infraorbital sinus, a depression just rostral to the eye.

- circumoral glands--occur in cats only. The function of these hypertrophic sebaceous glands remains unknown.

- mental (chin) gland--found in pigs. Located in a small area of the skin which projects about 0.5 cm above the surrounding skin. This eminence, known as the mental organ, has both a marking and a tactile function.

- carpal glands--found in pigs. These are found in a caudomedial position just proximal to the carpus. They open at the surface through several small orifices on a slightly elevated 2 x 5 cm area of skin. Their function appears to be the production of a sexual pheromone useful in libido and in marking sows as property of a given boar.

- glands of the interdigital sinus--found in sheep. These glands are present in all four limbs and secrete into an interdigital sinus located in the soft tissue near the level of the proximal interphalangeal joint. A single orifice drains the sinus in each limb, and it opens just proximal to the hoof on the dorsal aspect between the digits.

- glands of the inguinal sinus--occur in sheep. They are found on either side of the base of the udder or scrotum and their secretion exudes through skin invaginations.

- horn gland--occurs in goats and some sheep. It is located just caudal to the base of the horns (and in a similar location in hornless sheep).

- caudal (coccygeal) glands--found in carnivores. In cats, the glands are located on the dorsal aspect of the root of the tail, and in dogs

Table 23-1

Summary of the Specialized Cutaneous Glands in Domestic Mammals

	Cat	Dog	Pig	Sheep	Goat	Ox	Horse
glands of the infraorbital sinus	−	−	−	+	−	−	−
circumoral glands	+	−	−	−	−	−	−
mental (chin) gland	−	−	+	−	−	−	−
carpal glands	−	−	+	−	−	−	−
glands of the interdigital sinus	−	−	−	+	−	−	−
glands of the inguinal sinus	−	−	−	+	−	−	−
horn gland	−	−	−	+	+	−	−
caudal (coccygeal) gland	+	+	−	−	−	−	−
subcaudal gland	−	−	−	±	+	−	−
glands of the anal sac	+	+	−	−	−	−	−
glands associated with the nose	−	−	+	+	+	+	−
preputial glands	+	+	+	+	+	+	+
circumanal glands	+	+	+	+	+	+	+
ceruminous glands	+	+	+	+	+	+	+

<u>Note</u>: Those glands listed at the top of this table are found in only one of the domestic mammals. Those grouped in the middle are found in two or more species, and those at the bottom are present in all domestic mammals.

they are located over the ninth caudal vertebra. Different colored coat hairs may grow from this region. The glands are better developed in long-haired dogs than in those with short coats, and they are more prominent in males than in females.

subcaudal gland--found in goats. This gland consists of two glandular pockets under the base of the tail which are believed to be the source of the characteristic odor of the buck [1] (some authors blame the horn gland). Sheep have a gland in the same general area called the subcaudal infracaudal organ.

glands of the anal sac--occur in both dogs and cats. They are located in the walls of the anal sacs, and their secretion is temporarily stored in the anal sacs. Each of the two anal sacs is drained by a single duct (see Chapter 11).

glands of the nasal skin--occur in artiodactyles. These are named to correspond to the species specific name of the cutaneous modification involving the nose. Accordingly, those in pigs are termed glands of the rostral plane. In cattle, they are termed the glands of the nasolabial plane and in small ruminants they are termed glands of the nasal plane. The nasal plane of the carnivores is aglandular. The horse has no particular modification of the skin around the mouth and nose.

preputial glands--occur in all male domestic mammals.

circumanal glands--occur in dogs. Neoplasia of these glands results in perianal adenoma.

ceruminous glands--occur in all domestic mammals. These glands are located in the wall of the external auditory canal, and their secretion is believed to assist the tragi in preventing foreign bodies from entering the ear. The ceruminous glands are especially well developed in pigs and carnivores.

IV. Mamma

The mammary gland is a modified sweat gland which is fully developed and functional only in females. The term mamma refers to the glandular complex associated with one papilla (teat). The term udder designates collectively all of the mammae in ruminants and horses. The term is frequently used in reference to the sow, as well.

A. General features of the mamma (Fig. 23-2) [2]

papilla of the mamma--teat
sphincter muscle--the muscle which guards the opening(s) of the teat
body of the mamma
parts of the glandular complex
    intermammary groove--the midline separation between mammae
    glandular lobes
        glandular lobules

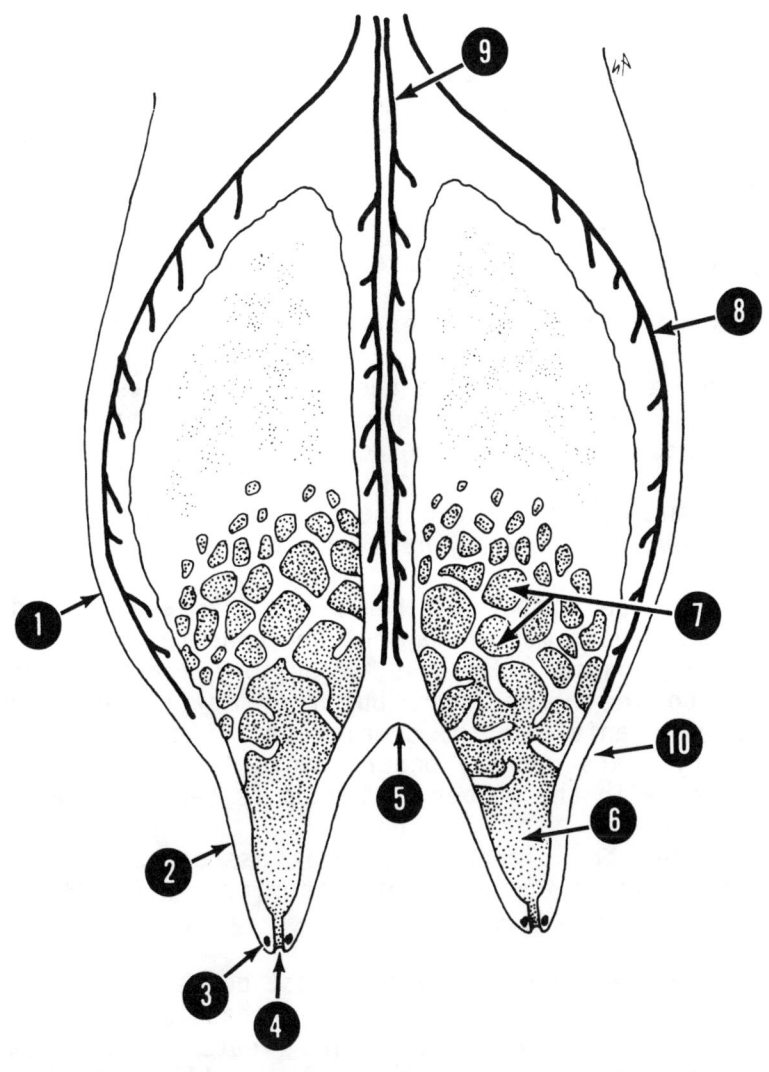

Figure 23-2

Transverse Section through Caudal Mammae of Cow

1. body of mamma
2. teat
3. sphincter muscle
4. papillary duct ("teat canal") and ostium
5. intermammary groove
6. papillary part of lactiferous sinus ("teat sinus")
7. glandular part of lactiferous sinus ("gland sinus")
8. lateral lamina of mammary suspensory apparatus
9. medial lamina of mammary suspensory apparatus
10. level of "Furstenberg's venous ring"

   lactiferous ducts--channels which enter the lactiferous sinus
   lactiferous sinus--the milk collecting cavity
     glandular part--"gland cistern" or "gland sinus"
     papillary part--"teat cistern" or "teat sinus"
   papillary duct--"teat canal" or "streak canal"
   papillary ostium--the opening of the papillary duct
  suspensory apparatus--the connective tissue which supports the mammary gland
   lateral lamina
   medial lamina--suspensory lig of the udder
  accessory mammae--those which have no connected glandular tissue

B. Comparative and clinical considerations

1. Comparative data regarding the number of teats, number of glandular complexes per teat, and position of the mammae in the various domestic species are presented in Table 23-2.

2. Male animals usually have the same number and position of teats as do females, but they may have more or fewer.

3. Sometimes the number of teats is increased (polythelia). These additional teats may or may not be connected to a glandular complex (accessory mamma). In cows, accessory teats are usually located caudal to the other four, but they may occur between the normal teats or cranial to the cranial pair. In bulls, rams, and bucks, accessory teats usually occur cranial to the base of the scrotum. An increase in the number of mammae is termed polymastia.

4. As a rule, the glandular complex associated with each papillary duct is distinct and does not communicate with other cavity systems (even others of the same mamma).

5. The skin covering the mammae of most domestic species is similar to that on other parts of the body. In cattle, it is thinner and more sparsely covered with hair. The teats of the sow and cow are glabrous, but those of the mare, small ruminants, and cats are sparsely covered with hair.

6. The mammary suspensory apparatus varies considerably among the domestic species. It is best developed in the cow, and includes medial and lateral laminae which detach lamellae into the parenchyma of the glandular tissue (Fig. 23-2). Both laminae are paired, and they attach proximally to the symphysial tendon (the medial tendon of insertion of the gracilis and adductor mm), and to the fascia of the external abdominal oblique m. The medial lamina is primarily elastic connective tissue, and it forms a double septum between the right and left glands. The lateral lamina is primarily fibrous connective tissue. Because of the difference in the connective tissue types of the lamina, a full udder tends to drop more centrally than laterally. Consequently, the teats of a full udder tend to angle laterally rather than hang vertically.

7. The complete internal separation which occurs in the four quadrants of the cow's udder is of practical significance in "milking out" and in udder pathology [1].

8. At the transition between the papillary and glandular parts of the lactiferous sinus, there is a distinct constriction formed by connective tissue. Circularly arranged venous channels in this connective tissue are sometimes called "Furstenberg's venous ring."* This venous ring and muscular fibers around the papillary ostium prevent milk outflow except during milking or sucking.

9. The blood supply to the cow's udder is primarily from the external pudendal a. (Fig. 23-3). This vessel gives off a basal branch to the caudal mammary tissue, and then typically divides into cranial and caudal mammary arteries. Left and right vessels anastomose to form a vascular ring around the base of the udder. A small branch of the internal pudendal a. courses ventrally to join the arterial input caudally. Cranially, the cranial mammary arteries (also known as superficial caudal epigastric aa.) anastomose with the tiny superficial cranial epigastric aa. The venous return follows the arterial input (external pudendal v., internal pudendal v., and superficial cranial epigastric v). The very large abdominal veins, commonly called "milk veins" by herdsmen, are the superficial caudal epigastric veins and their cranial continuations, the superficial cranial epigastric veins. These vessels can be used for intravenous injections (although herdsmen may object). The innervation of the cow's udder is through the iliohypogastric and ilioinguinal nerves (skin of cranial part), and the genitofemoral and pudendal nerves (skin of caudal part).

10. In the small ruminants, the blood supply to the udder is entirely through the external pudendal artery. The innervation is similar to that in the ox.

11. In the bitch, the number of glandular complexes varies according to breed and individual, and may also vary on the two sides. The teats may also alternate positions so that they are more accessible to a nursing litter. Male dogs usually have the same number of teats as bitches. The blood supply includes branches of the internal thoracic aa., intercostal aa., superficial cranial epigastric aa., cranial abdominal aa., and external pudendal aa. The major venous drainage for the cranial 2-3 pairs of mammae is via the superficial cranial epigastric vein, and for the caudal 2-3 pairs is via the external pudendal vein. Lymphatic drainage from the cranial 2-3 pairs is through the axillary lymph nodes and from the caudal 2-3 pairs is through the superficial inguinal lymph nodes.

---

*"Furstenberg's venous ring" should not be confused with "Furstenberg's rosette," a fold of mucosa at the proximal end of the teat canal.

Table 23-2

Comparison of the Mammae of Domestic Mammals

	Number of teats	Glandular complexes per teat*	Position of mammae
Cat	8	5-7	thoracoabdominal
Dog	8-10	6-20	thoracoinguinal
Pig	10-18	2-3	thoracoinguinal
Sheep	2	1	inguinal
Goat	2	1	inguinal
Ox	4	1	inguinal
Horse	2	2	inguinal

*(Also represents the number of papillary ducts and papillary ostia per teat.)

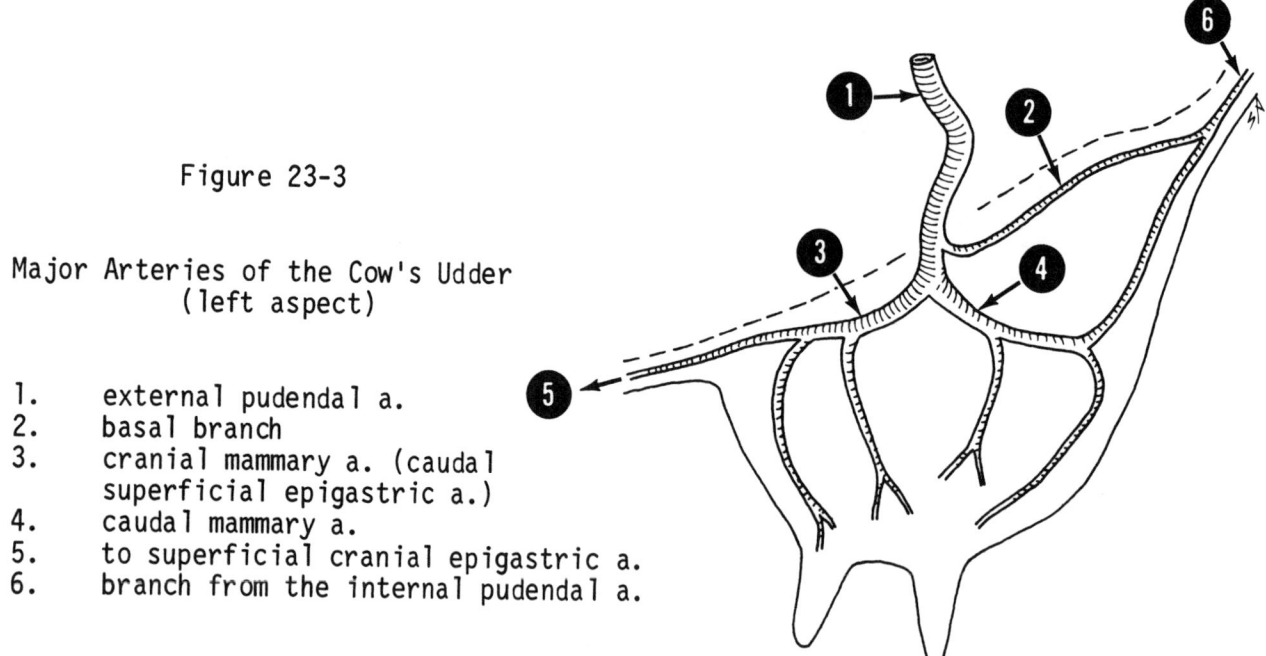

Figure 23-3

Major Arteries of the Cow's Udder (left aspect)

1. external pudendal a.
2. basal branch
3. cranial mammary a. (caudal superficial epigastric a.)
4. caudal mammary a.
5. to superficial cranial epigastric a.
6. branch from the internal pudendal a.

12. The mammary glandular complex of the cat resembles that of the dog except that queens typically have a constant number (4 pair) and male cats usually have only 2 rudimentary teats.

V. Highly Modified Hairless Cutaneous Organs

A number of highly specialized cutaneous organs occur in domestic mammals including pads (tori), digital organs (claws and hooves), and horns. These structures are hairless, highly keratinized, and are often devoid of glands. They serve as shock absorbers for the feet, as weapons of defense, and in some cases, as digging instruments.

A. Pads

Pads may be divided into three general groups:

> digital pads (tori digitalis)--those that are associated with the distal ends of the digits. In the ungulates, these may be termed tori ungulae (hoof pads or bulbs).
> metacarpal and metatarsal pads (tori metacarpeus, metatarseus) - those that are located near the distal end of the metacarpus and metatarsus.
> carpal and tarsal pads (tori carpeus, tarseus).

These are present in varying functional or rudimentary degrees in the domestic mammals.

In carnivores, the digital pads are well developed and their number corresponds to the number of digits present. The metacarpal and metatarsal pads are also well developed and weight bearing. Evidence of their formation from the fusion of three separate primordia can be deduced from their general shape. The carpal pads of carnivores are present but are generally nonfunctional (those of cats may be useful in climbing). Carnivores lack tarsal pads.

The pads of ungulates are not as well developed as those of carnivores. All domestic ungulates have digital pads represented by the softer horn and underlying tissue on the sole surface of the digit. The other pads (metacarpal, metatarsal, carpal, and tarsal) are absent in all species except the horse where they are represented by functionless rudiments (ergots and chestnuts).

The ergots of horses (calcar metacarpeum and calcar metatarseum) are believed by some to be homologues of the metacarpal and metatarsal pads of carnivores [1]. Other authors regard them as vestiges of the second and fourth digits [3]. Ergots are small, horny protrusions on the palmar (plantar) aspects of the limb at the level of the "fetlock" joint. They are typically buried in the "feathers" (cirrus metacarpeus, metatarseus). Ergots are especially well developed in draft horses and mules. A small fibrous band (lig. of the ergot), 3-5 mm wide, extends distally and slightly dorsally from the base of the ergot, across the digital vessels, and blends below with the digital fascia.

In horses, the rudimentary carpal and tarsal pads are commonly called chestnuts [1]. Some authors consider them to be vestiges of first digits [3]. In the thoracic limb, they are located on the caudomedial aspect of the limb just proximal to the carpus. In the pelvic limb, they are located on the plantaromedial aspect just distal to the tarsus. There is considerable variation in the size and development of chestnuts. Photographs and measurements of their individual character are used as identification characteristics by some horse racing associations. The chestnuts of the thoracic limbs are usually larger than those of the pelvic limbs. The latter are occasionally absent in horses, typically absent in donkeys, and they are very small in mules [3].

B. Claws

The claws of carnivores cover and extend the unguicular process of the distal phalanges. They resemble hollow, curved, flattened cones. The base of the nail fits inside the unguicular crest and the germinal epithelium which produces the claw is located there. The claws of cats are compressed laterally more than those of dogs, and those on the thoracic limbs are better developed than those on the pelvic limb.

The claws of dogs cannot be withdrawn, and their tips normally become blunted through wear. Depending on the exercise an individual animal gets and the type of surface it runs on, the claws may or may not require periodic trimming. If they are trimmed too short, the underlying dermis may be invaded, which causes hemorrhage and pain. Such animals are said to have been "quicked", and they may object to future trims. Trimming a claw markedly too short can result in exposure of the distal phalanx. The only treatment that is usually required is control of the hemorrhage with styptic agents.

In feline onychectomies, the whole distal phalanx is usually removed by amputation through the distal interphalangeal joint. This insures that all of the germinal epithelium is removed and thus prevent subsequent regrowth of the claw. Removal of the whole distal phalanx does not hinder the gait because the distal phalanx is functional only when the claws are protruded.

C. Horns

Horns are retained throughout life (in contrast to antlers which are shed annually). Horns are present in all three species of domestic ruminants, and even "hornless" breeds have vestiges of them. Horns develop on processes of the frontal bone termed cornual processes. In cattle, these processes develop as direct proliferation of the bone, but in small ruminants, they begin as separate centers of ossification which later fuse to the frontal bone. Horns of goats and sheep are located directly behind the orbits, but those of oxen are located at the caudal aspect of the head.

Horns are highly keratinized epidermis, consisting of a base, body, and apex. They grow from germinal epithelium associated with the dermis (corium) at the base of the cornual process and also at the cornual apex. At both the base and apex of the horn, the dermis has papillae and the overlying germinal epithelium produces tubular horn. Intertubular horn is produced by germinal epithelium between papillae. The dermis of the body of the horn is smooth (has no papillae). The external surface of the horns of bulls are relatively smooth while those of cows and small ruminants are circumferentially grooved to correspond to growth spurts related to periodic differences in body metabolism. In cows these rings are sometimes called pregnancy grooves because a constriction is produced from slowed growth near the end of gestation and during lactation. Assuming an annual pregnancy, the number of rings plus the age at the first pregnancy will give the current age. In sheep and goats, the cornual rings are more distinct and 9-12 are produced each year.

Dehorning is discussed in Chapter 19, Head. Removal of the horn in adult ruminants exposes the frontal sinus because the cornual processes are pneumatic. Developmentally, the horns are solid. Pneumatization begins at about 6 months of age and continues throughout life until all but the very tip is hollow. Fracture of the cornual process sometimes occurs.

D. Equine hoof (Figs. 23-4, 23-5)

The hoof of the horse is more highly developed and complex than those of the other domestic ungulates. The hoof has three layers (epidermal, dermal, and subcutaneous), and is divided into six regional parts:

1. Periople (limbus ungulae)--the narrow region at the proximal border of the hoof. The germinal epithelium in this region produces the stratum externum of the hoof wall which corresponds to the cuticle of the human nail.

2. Coronet--the wider band just distal to the periople. The germinal epithelium here produces the stratum medium of the hoof wall.

3. Wall--the dorsal, medial, and lateral portions of the hoof distinguished by the presence of dermal and epidermal lamellae. The equine hoof has about 600 interdigitating, grossly visible, primary lamellae, and each of these bear microscopic secondary lamellae. This increases the total surface area of dermal-epidermal contact to an estimated average of 9 square meters per hoof. The wall has a number of named subparts [2]:

    lamina (hoof plate, wall horn)--the cornified epidermis produced by the periople, coronet, and wall.
    stratum externum--the epidermis produced by the periople. It is a thin, glossy layer which becomes opaque when wet. It is fully developed in foals, but is largely worn off the hoof wall in adults.

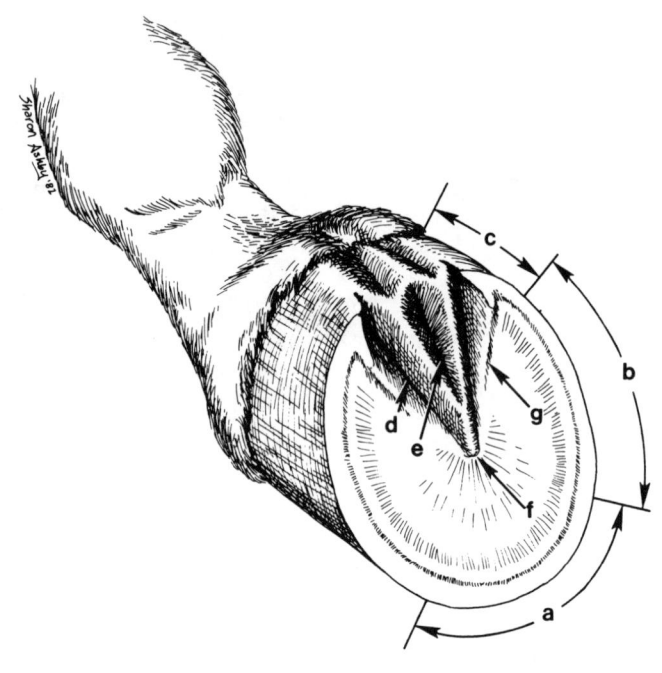

Figure 23-4

Equine Hoof (solar aspect)

- a. "toe"
- b. "quarter"
- c. "heel"
- d. medial (or lateral) paracuneal groove ("collateral sulcus")
- e. central cuneal groove ("central sulcus of frog")
- f. cuneal apex ("apex of frog")
- g. medial (or lateral) crus ("bar") of hoof wall

From Shively, 1982 [5])

Figure 23-5

Sectional Perspective of the Wall of the Equine Hoof

1. stratum externum (produced by the periople)
2. stratum medium (produced by the coronet)
3. stratum internum (interdigitating with 4)
4. laminar corium
5. bone of distal phalanx

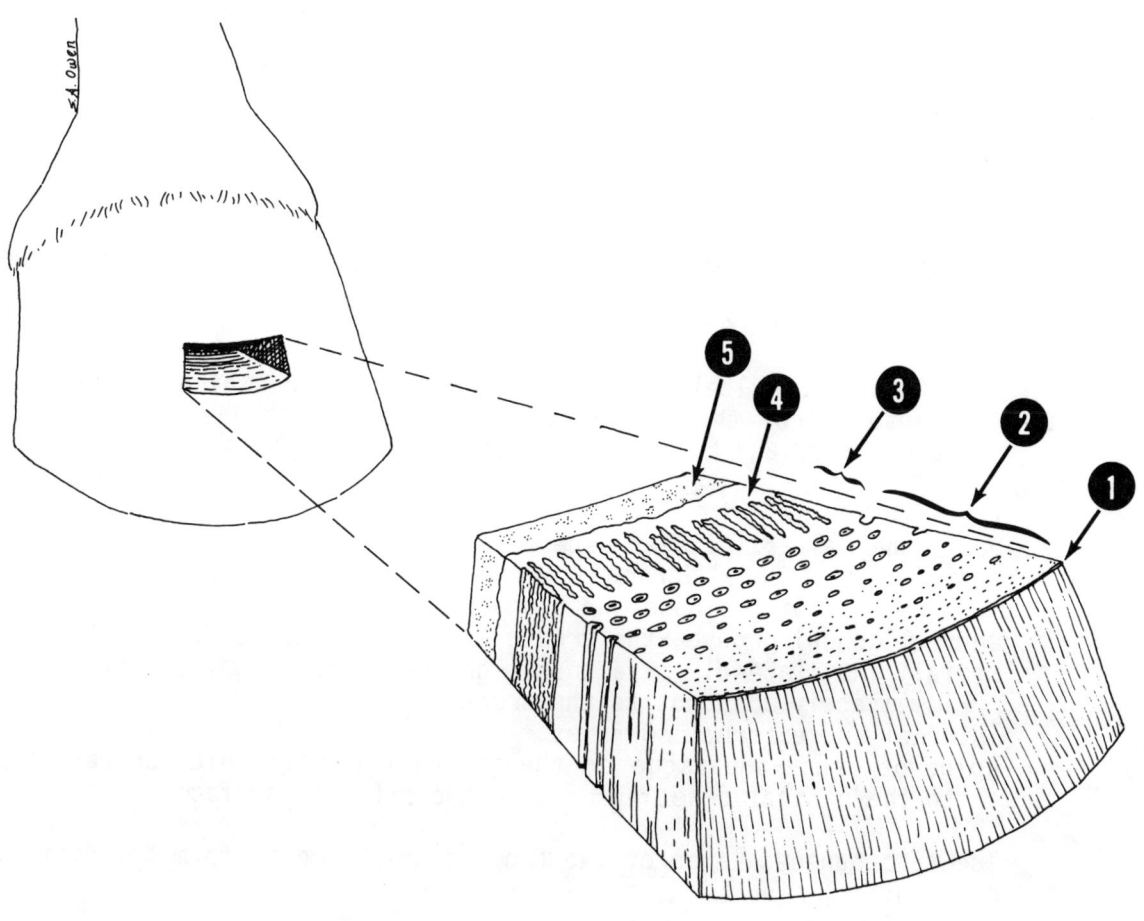

After Stump, 1967 [4]

       stratum medium--the epidermis forming the bulk of the hoof wall. It is produced by the coronet.
       stratum internum--the epidermal lamellae.
       white zone--the junction of the wall horn and the sole. The term zone was adopted to avoid confusion with the linea alba of the abdomen.
   coronary and solar borders--the proximal and distal borders of the hoof wall.
   medial and lateral palmar (plantar) borders--the portion of the horny wall which corresponds to the frequently used "heels."
   medial and lateral "bars"--the bar (pars inflexa) is the part of the horny wall that extends from the palmar (plantar) border in a dorsal and axial direction along the paracuneal groove.
   dorsal part of the horny wall--the portion which corresponds to the frequently used "toe."
   medial and lateral collateral parts--the portions of the horny wall which correspond to the frequently used "quarters."

4. Sole--the portion of the hoof between the wall and frog. It has the following parts [2]:

   body--divided by the apex of the frog into medial and lateral crura which project palmarly (plantarly) to form the medial and lateral angles of the sole
   parietal and central borders--the borders adjacent to the wall and frog respectively
   internal and external surfaces

5. Frog (cuneus ungulae)--the wedge-shaped structure which invaginates the sole from the palmar (plantar) aspect. It lies between the sole, bars, and bulbs. It has the following parts [2]:

   apex--the dorsal tip
   base--the palmar (plantar aspect)
   medial and lateral crura--the medial and lateral ridges which project from the base and blend dorsally to form the apex.
   central cuneal groove--the groove which lies between the crura
   medial and lateral paracuneal grooves--the grooves which lie immediately adjacent to the crura
   internal and external surfaces
   spine of frog--the ridge on the internal surface which corresponds to the central cuneal groove on the external surface

The subcutaneous layer of the frog is thickened to form the digital cushion.

6. Bulb (torus ungulae)--the region of the hoof which lies just proximal to the frog. It consists of a base, apex, medial and lateral parts, and has internal and external surfaces [2].

The hooves of thoracic and pelvic limbs can be distinguished by several criteria [1]:

	hoof of thoracic limb	hoof of pelvic limb
ratio of wall height at toe vs. heel	3:1	2:1
angle formed by dorsal wall and ground surface	45-50°	50-55°
shape of sole	rounded	pointed dorsally

The medial quarter of the hoof wall is normally steeper than the lateral one. The wall grows at a rate of about 8-10 mm/month. At the toe, about a year is required for complete replacement, but only 4-5 months are required at the heels. The frog and sole are replaced every two months [1].

A number of terms are clinically used to describe the conformation of the equine hoof and foot.* "Toe," "quarter," and "heel" have already been equated to their official (but rarely used) names. Other terms used to describe the equine foot include [4]:

Foot axis--the inclination of the foot (hoof) with reference to the ground surface (Fig. 23-6). This is observed and/or measured from the front and from the side. As viewed from the front (i.e., dorsopalmarly), the foot axis should be perpendicular to the ground surface. From a lateral perspective, the angle of the dorsal hoof wall to the ground surface should be 45-50° for front feet and 50-55° for back feet. Although foot angles can be altered by corrective trimming, major changes often produce pathologic conditions after a period of time.

Pastern axis--The inclination of the proximal phalanx ("pastern") with reference to the ground surface as observed from dorsal and lateral perspectives. These are observed in the same two planes as the foot axes and should form continuous lines with them (Fig. 23-6).

Level foot--a foot in which the medial and lateral aspects of the hoof wall (quarters and heels) are the same length. This is the ideal normal and is necessary to form a perpendicular foot axis as observed dorsopalmarly.

Broken foot--a foot in which the laterally observed foot axis and pastern axis are not identical (i.e., a foot in which the angle of the dorsal hoof wall as it meets the ground is not identical to the angle of the proximal phalanx ["pastern"] when viewed laterally) (Fig. 23-7A).

Coon foot--a form of broken foot in which the dorsal hoof wall is more vertically oriented than the proximal phalanx ("pastern") (Fig. 23-7B).

Club foot, steep foot, upright foot--a foot with a dorsal hoof wall angle of 60° or more which imparts a cylindrical shape to the foot (Fig. 23-7C). The foot may or may not be broken. If unbroken, the upright foot and pastern axis will tend to shorten the stride and give a rougher ride than normal.

---

*"Foot" as used here includes the hoof and its contents.

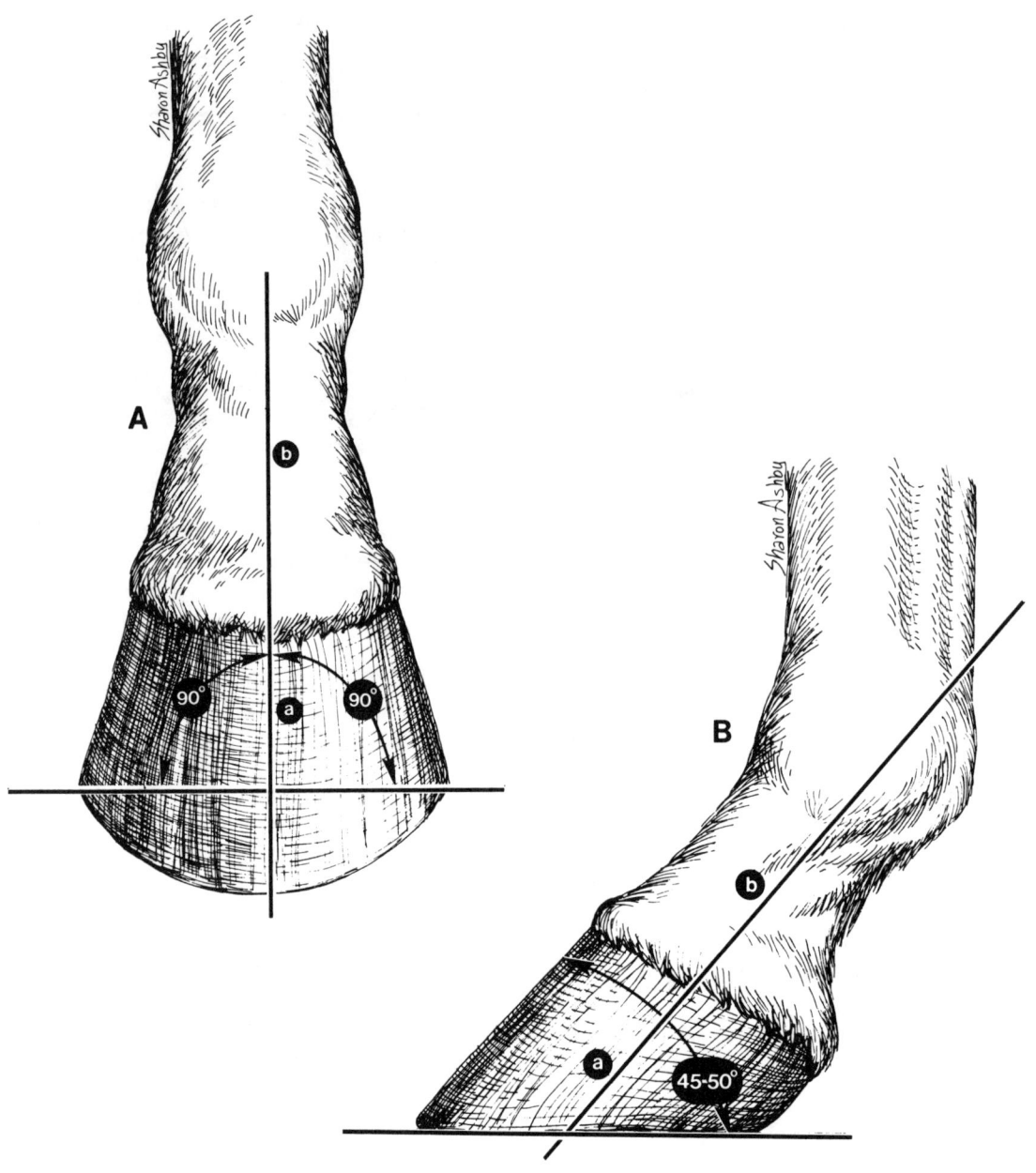

Figure 23-6

Foot and Pastern Axis of Horse
(dorsal aspect--A; lateral aspect--B)

a. foot axis

b. pastern axis

From Shively, 1982 [5]

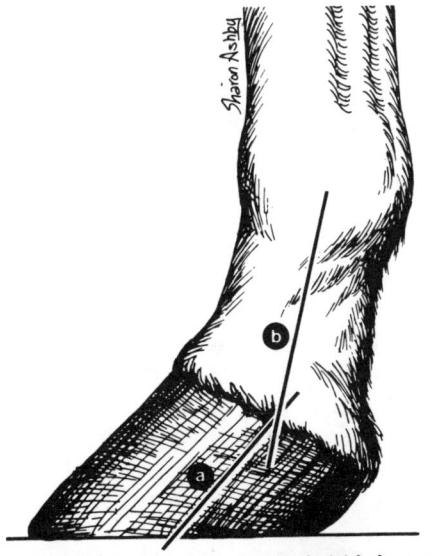
A. Broken foot in which the foot axis (a) is less upright than the pastern axis (b)

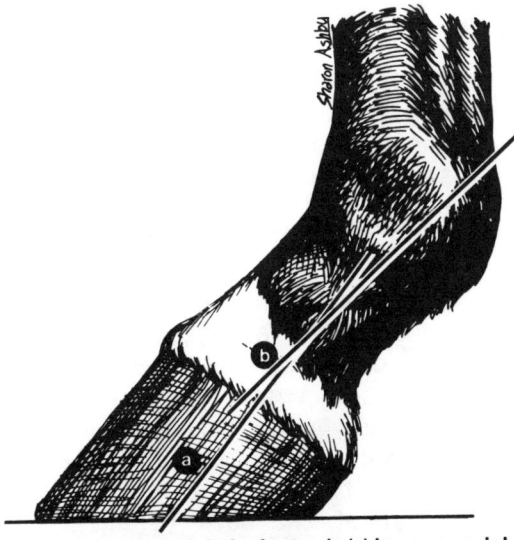
B. Broken foot in which the foot axis (a) is more upright than the pastern axis (b) ("coon foot")

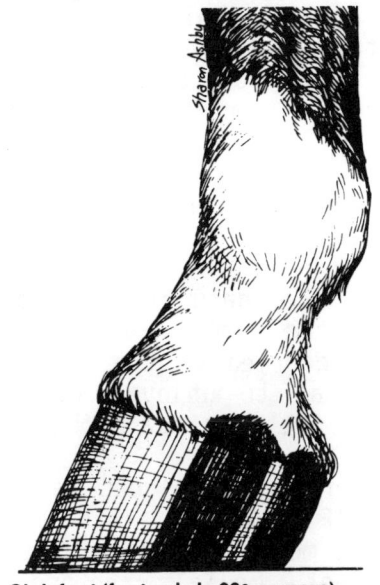
C. Club foot (foot axis is 60° or more)

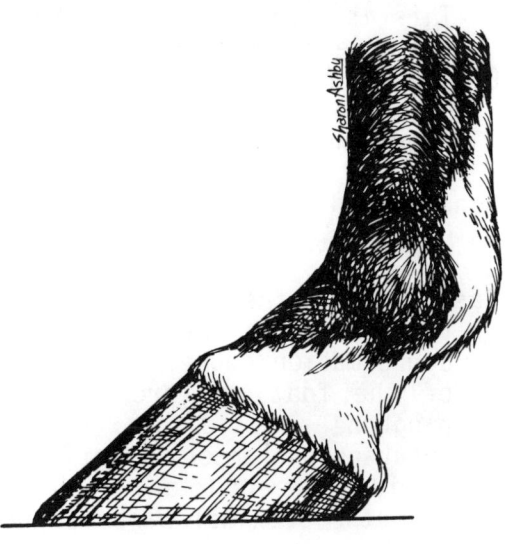
D. Sloping foot (foot axis is less than 45°)

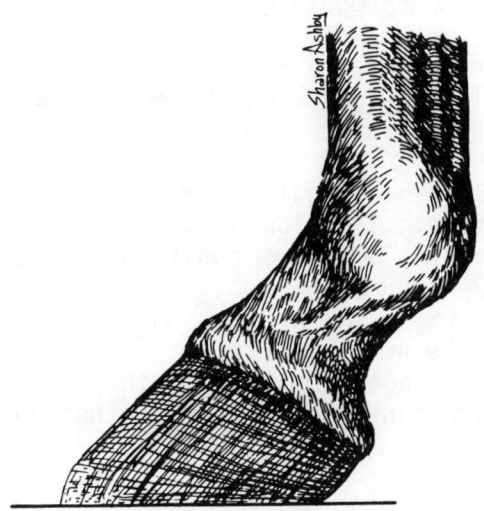
E. Bull-nosed foot

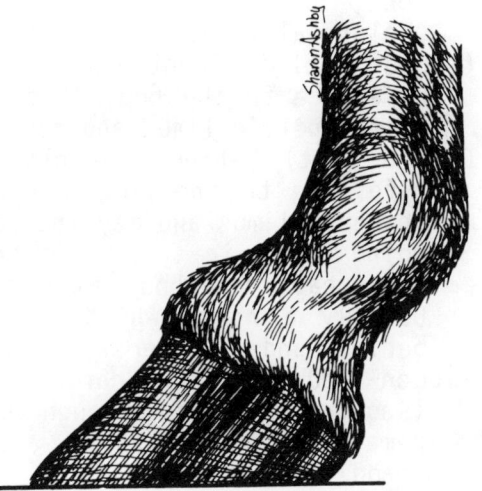
F. Buttress foot

Figure 23-7 Abnormal Conformation of the Equine Digit
From Shively, 1982 [5]

Low foot, sloping foot--a foot with a lower than normal dorsal hoof wall angle (Fig. 23-7D). The foot may or may not be broken. If unbroken, the low foot and pastern axis will usually lengthen the stride and smooth out the ride compared to that of a horse with normal conformation.

Bull-nosed foot--a foot which has been rasped down at the toe to fit a shoe (Fig. 23-7E). This practice predisposes the horse to lameness because it induces quicker breakover.

Buttress foot--a foot with a noticeable swelling on the dorsal aspect of the coronary region ("coronary band region") due to exostosis on the extensor process of the distal phalanx ("coffin bone") (Fig. 23-7F). This may result from a healed fracture or from low ringbone.

Flat foot--the natural concavity of the sole is absent. It should be noted that the soles of the front feet are naturally flatter than those of the back feet.

Dropped sole, pumiced foot--an excessively flat foot in which the sole has dropped to or beyond the weight-bearing surface of the hoof wall. This is typically associated with chronic laminitis and results from the sole being forced down by the rotation of the distal phalanx.

Off level foot--a foot with one quarter lower or higher than the opposite quarter. This may be caused by improper trimming or by uneven wear.

Abnormal placement of the feet result in the following conformational defects [5]:

Base narrow--the left and right feet are naturally placed closer together than the proximal parts of the limbs (Fig. 23-8B). This conformation causes more weight to be carried on the lateral aspect of the foot and predisposes the animal to unlevel feet, lateral ringbone and sidebone, and windpuffs of the metacarpophalangeal and metatarsophalangeal ("fetlock") joints.

Base wide--the left and right feet are naturally placed farther apart than the proximal parts of the limbs (Fig. 23-8C). This conformation causes more weight to be carried on the medial aspect of the foot and predisposes the animal to unlevel feet, medial ringbone and side bone, and windpuffs of the metacarpophalangeal and metatarsophalangeal ("fetlock") joints.

Camped (out) in front--the front feet are placed too far cranially with reference to the body (Fig. 23-9B). This position shifts more weight to the pelvic limbs and may indicate thoracic limb lameness.

Camped (out) behind--the hind feet are placed too far caudally with reference to the body (Fig. 23-9C). This shifts more weight to the thoracic limbs and may indicate a pelvic limb lameness.

Standing under in front (or behind)--the feet are positioned too far underneath the body (the opposite of camped out; Figs. 23-9B,C). Usually a horse which is camped in front will be standing under behind (and vice versa) because of the weight shift.

Pigeon-toed (toe-in conformation)--the toes tend to point medially (sagittal planes through the feet converge cranially instead of remaining parallel; Fig. 23-10A). This usually causes a horse to "paddle" when walking [6].

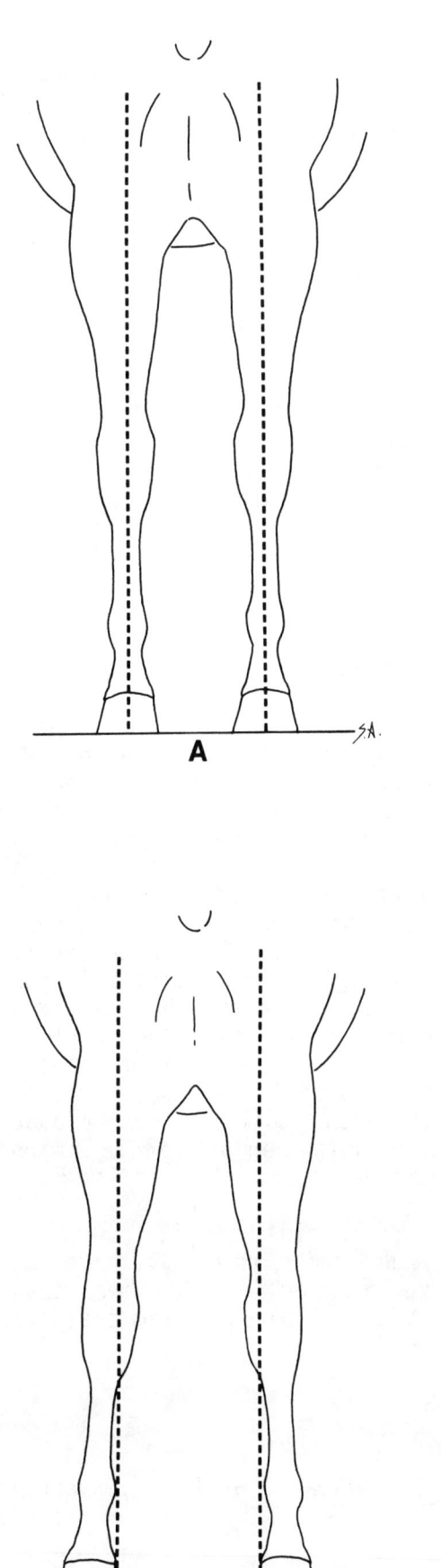
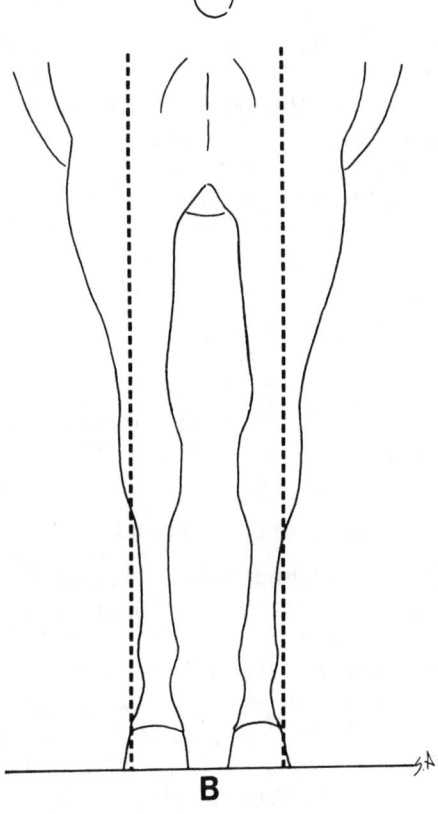

Figure 23-8

Width of the Base

A. normal
B. base narrow
C. base wide

From Shively, 1982 [5]

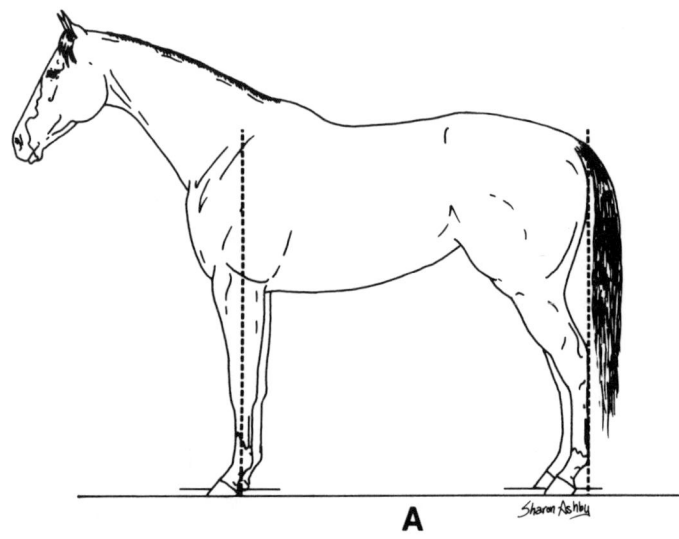

Figure 23-9
Cranial-Caudal
Placement of Feet

A. normal
B. camped in front, standing under behind
C. standing under in front, camped behind

From Shively, 1982 [5]

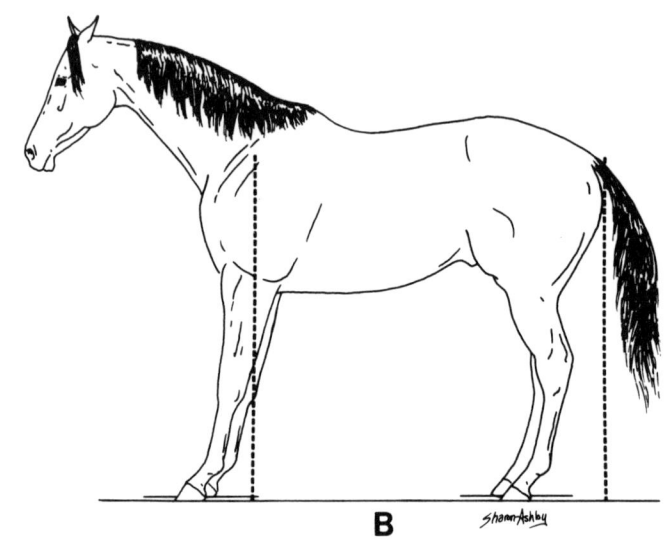

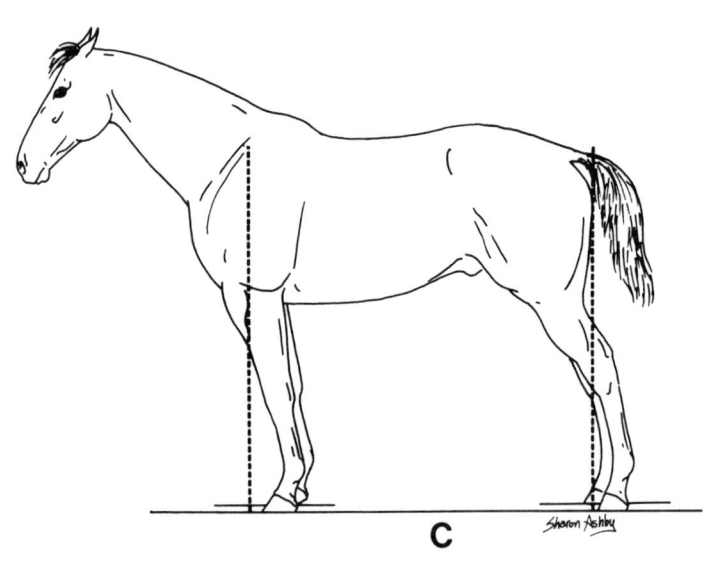

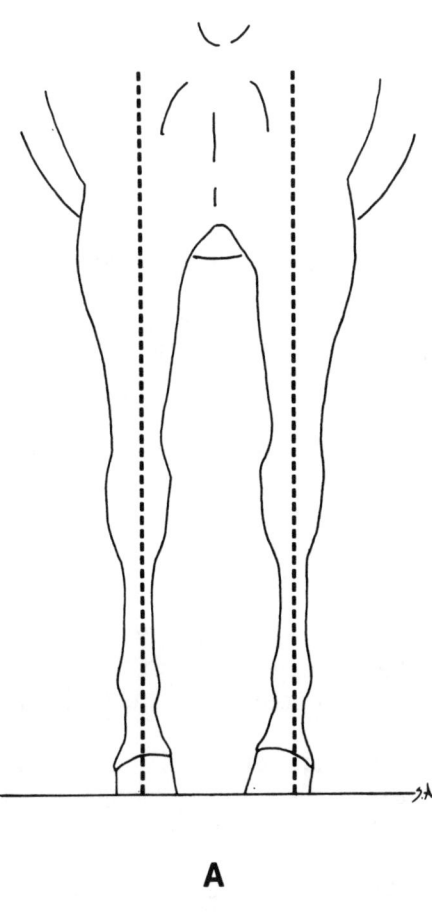
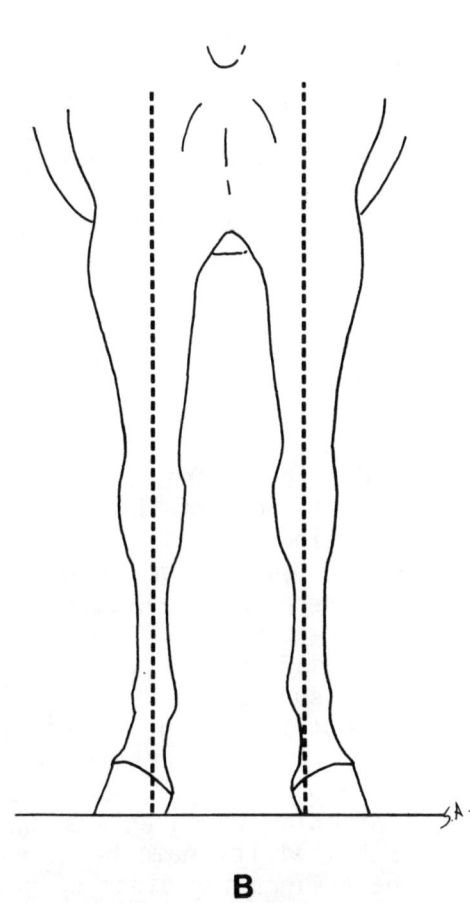

Figure 23-10

Rotation of Feet

A. pigeon-toed (toe-in)

B. splay-footed (toe-out)

From Shively, 1982 [5]

Splay-footed (toe-out conformation)--the toes tend to point laterally (sagittal planes through the feet diverge cranially instead of remaining parallel; Fig. 23-10B). This usually causes a horse to "wing" when walking [6].

A few of the specific disease conditions which affect the hoof include [7]:

Brittle feet--feet with cracks in the hoof wall due to dryness. Brittle feet may be improved by daily application of hoof dressings.

Canker--a relatively rare chronic hypertrophy of the horn-producing tissues of the foot. It is believed to be the result of an infection from unclean stables and affects the hind feet more frequently than the front.

Corn--a contusion of the sole near the junction of the sole with the hoof wall at the medial or lateral angle of the hoof. This is usually due to improper shoeing and may be classified as dry, moist, or suppurative.

Contracted foot, contracted heels--a foot which is narrower than normal, especially in the palmar or plantar aspect. This may be caused by a lack of frog pressure and often occurs in horses which are improperly shod. The front feet are more commonly affected than the back, and occasionally the contraction is so severe that lameness results (hoof-bound).

Founder or laminitis--inflammation of the laminae of the foot from any of a variety of causes. The pathoetiology is not completely understood, and there are several subtypes based on the inciting insult. Some of the more common ones include:
  Grain or grass founder--laminitis from ingestion of an excessive amount of grain or lush pasture grass.
  Water founder--laminitis from ingestion of a large amount of cold water.
  Road founder--laminitis due to concussion of the feet on a hard surface.
  Post-parturient laminitis--laminitis from the toxemia associated with postparturient endometritis.

Gravel--a drainage tract at the heel area (sometimes at the toe) from an infection which enters through a crack in the white zone (line). It received its name because it was originally (incorrectly) thought to be a migrating piece of gravel.

Hoof-bound--a lameness resulting from chronic contracted heels. In this condition, the hoof wall presses so tightly against the distal phalanx that pain results.

Quittor--a chronic purulent inflammation of a cartilage of the hoof ("lateral cartilage"), characterized by draining tracts at or just proximal to the coronary region. Quittor is usually related to traumatic injury.

Seedy toe--separation of the dermal ("sensitive") and epidermal ("insensitive") laminae commonly occurring as a sequel to chronic laminitis.

Thrush--a degenerative condition of the cuneus ungulae ("frog") and its paracuneal ("collateral") sulci associated with filth and characterized by black necrotic material in the affected areas.

Toe crack, quarter crack, heel crack--cracks in the hoof wall beginning at the solar border (resulting from improper or lack of trimming) or at the coronary border (resulting from a defect in hoof formation). These are sometimes called sand cracks and "toe," "quarter," or "heel" implies the location.

E. Hoof of the Ruminants and Pig

The hooves (claws) of the artiodactyles resemble those of the horse except they have no bars, frog, or secondary lamellae. In the ox, the hooves of the thoracic limb are broader, blunter, and shorter than those of the pelvic limb. There is also a wider interdigital cleft between the claws of the thoracic limb.

The bovine hoof and foot are subject to a number of maladies [8]:

Foot rot (infectious pododermatitis)--proliferative inflammation of the interdigital space, coronary region, and region of the proximal phalanx.
Interdigital dermatitis--a superficial, wet inflammation of the interdigital space.
Overgrown hooves--unusually long hoof wall, usually on the lateral claw. This is often associated with base narrow conformation and the elongated lateral wall curls under the sole.
Cracks in the hoof wall--loss of elasticity due to drying is a predisposing factor.
Ulceration of the sole--affects heavier animals more than lighter ones. Straight tarsi may predispose the animal to the condition in the pelvic limbs because the feet are overly stressed due to lack of shock absorption in other parts of the limb.
Interdigital fibroma--may result from proliferation associated with foot rot or interdigital dermatitis.

Reference

1. Schummer, A., H. Wilkens, B. Vollmerhaus, and K. Habermehl. 1981. The Circulatory System, the Skin, and the Cutaneous Organs of the Domestic Mammals. Translated by W. Siller and P. Wight. Paul Parey, Berlin.

2. International Committee on Veterinary Gross Anatomical Nomenclature. 1983. Nomina Anatomica Veterinaria, third ed. Published by the Committee, Ithaca, New York.

3. Getty, R. 1975. Sisson and Grossman's The Anatomy of the Domestic Animals, fifth ed. W. B. Saunders, Philadelphia.

4. Stump, J. E. 1967. Anatomy of the normal equine foot including microscopic features of the laminar region. JAVMA 151(12):1588-1598.

5. Shively, M. J. 1982. Equine-English dictionary: Part I, Standing conformation. J. Equine Prac. 4(5):10-27.

6. Shively, M. J. 1982. Equine-English dictionary: Part II, Locomotion (ways of going). J. Equine Prac. 4(8):11-20.

7. Shively, M. J. 1983. Equine-English dictionary: Part III, Lameness. J. Equine Prac. 4(10):31-40.

8. Amstutz, H. E., ed. 1980. Bovine Medicine and Surgery, second ed. American Veterinary Publications, Santa Barbara, California.

INDEX

Abdomen, 231
    regions, 231, 232
    quadrants, 231, 232, 233
Abdominal wall, 231, 234
Abnormal origin of right subclavian a., 314
Abomasopexy, 242
Abomasum, 240
    displaced, 242
Absence of caudal vena cava, 315
Accessory of sex glands, 349, 350
Acetabular lip, 176
Acetabuloplasty, 130
Acetabulum, 125, 126
    depth, 174
    wedging, 174
Adrenalectomy, 300
Air sac, 482, 483
Air sacculitis, 484
Ampulla, 344
Anal canal, 255
Anal paralysis, 219
Anal sac, 255
Anatomic nomenclature, 1
Aneurysm
    of cranial mesenteric a., 301
    poststenotic, 281
Angiology
    central, 293
    cephalic, 452
    plevic limb, 199
    thoracic limb, 87
Anisognathism, 380
Anodontia, 386
Anomalous pulmonary v., 315
Antler, 548
Aortic stenosis, 279
Aotus trivirgatus, 524
Appendix colli, 537
Arch
    vertebral, 404
    zygomatic, 429
Arthrocentesis (see synoviocentesis)
Artery
    abaxial palmar proper digital aa., 96
    aorta, 293, 299
    aortic arch, 293, 294
    ascending aorta, 293
    axial palmar proper digital aa., 96
    axillary a., 87
    bicarotid trunk, 293
    bicipital a., 89
    brachial a., 89
    brachiocephalic trunk, 293
    bronchoesophageal a., 298
    caudal abdominal a., 306
    caudal auricular a., 454
    caudal circumflex humeral a., 89
    caudal epigastric a., 305
    caudal femoral a., 201
    caudal gluteal a., 306
    caudal interosseous a., 90
    caudal mesenteric a., 301
    caudal pancreaticoduodenal a., 300
    caudal tibial a., 201
    cecal a., 304
    celiac a., 265, 300, 302
    circumflex branch, 293
    collateral unlar a., 89
    common carotid a., 293, 452, 453
    common digital aa., 91
    common interosseous a., 90
    costocervical trunk, 295
    cranial abdominal a., 300
    cranial a. of penis, 305
    cranial circumflex humeral a., 87
    cranial gluteal a., 306
    cranial interosseous a., 90
    cranial mammary a., 305
    cranial mesenteric a., 300, 304
    cranial pancreaticoduodenal a., 300
    cranial rectal a., 301
    cranial tibial a., 201
    cremasteric a., 305
    deep antebrachial a., 90
    deep brachial a., 89
    deep cervical a., 295
    deep circumflex iliac a., 301, 305
    descending aorta, 298
    descending genicular a., 201
    digital aa., 91, 202
    distal caudal femoral a., 201
    distal perforating branch, 202
    dorsal a. of penis, 305
    dorsal costoabdominal aa., 298
    dorsal intercostal aa., 298
    dorsal metacarpal aa., 91
    dorsal pedal a., 202
    dorsal scapular a., 295
    ductus arteriosus, 308
    external carotid a., 454
    external iliac a., 301
    external pudendal a., 305
    external thoracic a., 87
    facial a., 454
    femoral a., 199
    fourth palmar common digital a., 96
    gastroduodenal a., 300
    gonadal a., 301
    hepatic a., 300
    ileal a., 304
    iliacofemoral a., 305
    iliocolic a., 300

iliolumbar a., 306
internal carotid a., 452
internal iliac a., 306
internal pudendal a., 306
internal thoracic a., 295
jejunal a., 300
lateral circumflex femoral a., 199
lateral digital a., 91, 202
lateral palmar a., 91
lateral palmar metacarpal a., 96
lateral plantar a., 202
lateral plantar metatarsal a., 203
lateral thoracic a., 89
left colic a., 301
left coronary a., 293
left gastric a., 300
left gastroepiploic a., 295, 300
left subclavian a., 293, 296
lingual a., 454
linguofacial trunk, 454
lumbar a., 301
maxillary a., 454
medial circumflex femoral a., 305
medial digital a., 91, 202
medial palmar a., 96
medial palmar metacarpal a., 96
medial plantar a., 202
medial plantar metatarsal a., 203
median a., 90
median sacral a., 306
metacarpal aa., 91, 96
metatarsal aa., 202
middle a. of penis, 305
middle caudal a., 306
middle caudal femoral a., 201
middle colic a., 301
nutrient a., 90, 201
obturator a., 305
occipital a., 454
of bovine manus, 94
of bovine pes, 203, 206
of cow's udder, 545
of equine manus, 91
of equine pes, 202, 204
of head, 425
of pelvic limb, 199, 200
of penis, 357
of rumen, 300
of thoracic limb, 87, 88
of thorax and abdomen, 293
ovarian, 301
palmar branch, 91
palmar metacarpal a., 91
paraconal interventricular branch, 293
perforating branch
    distal, 203
       of dorsal pedal a., 202
    proximal, 203

perforating tarsal a., 202, 203
phrenic aa., 298
phrenicoabdominal a., 298
plantar metatarsal aa., 202
popliteal a., 201
prostatic a., 306
proximal caudal femoral a., 201
proximal radial a., 91
pudendoepigastric trunk, 303
pulmonary a., 307
pulmonary trunk, 307
radial a., 90
renal a., 301
right colic a., 301
right coronary a., 293
right gastric a., 300
right gastroepiploic a., 300
right subclavian a., 293
ruminal a., 300
saphenous a., 201
second palmar common digital a., 91, 96
second plantar common digital a., 203
short gastric a., 264, 265
splenic a., 300
subscapular a., 89
subsinuosal interventricular branch, 293
superficial branchial a., 90
superficial caudal eigastric a., 305
superficial cervical a., 295
superficial circumflex iliac a., 201
superficial temporal a., 454
suprascapular a., 89
supreme intercostal a., 295
terminal arch, 91
testicular a., 301
third dorsal metacarpal a., 96
third dorsal metatarsal a., 202
third palmar common digital a., 91
third plantar common digital a., 203
thoracic vertebral a., 295
thoracodorsal a., 89
transverse cubital a., 89
ulnar a., 90
umbilica a., 308, 334
urogenital a., 306
uterine a., 305
vaginal a., 306
ventral labial a., 305
ventral scrotal a., 305
vertebral a., 295
Arthrocentesis (see synoviocentesis)
Arthrodesis
    carpal, 73
    interphalangeal, 81, 82
Arthrology
    pelvic limb, 167
    thoracic limb, 67
Arytenoid cartilage, 451

Ascent of the spinal cord, 415
Aseptic necrosis of the femoral head, 176
Atlantoaxial subluxation, 413
Atlas, 406, 407
Atresia ani, 498
Atrium
    of heart, 277
    of rumen, 246
Atrophic rhinitis, 498
Auditis laryngeus, 450
Auditis pharyngeus, 450
Auditory ossicle, 465
Auditory tube, 449
Auricle, 277
Auscultation
    heart, 279
    lungs, 276
    omasum, 248
    reticulum, 247
    rumen, 246
Aves, 470
Avian anatomy, 469
Avulsion
    brachial plexus, 103
    origin of popliteus m., 164
    tibial tuberosity, 179
Axis, 406
Axis of limb, 30
Baboon, 524
Balling gun, 494
Balling up, 359
Bandy-legged, 74
Barbary ape, 524
Basal border of lung, 273
Base narrow, 556
Base wide, 556
Basophilic stippling of RBC, 519
Beak, 473
Beard, 476
Bench knees, 74
Biopsy
    kidney, 330
    liver, 258
Bishoping, 401
Blood collection
    birds, 486
    domestic mammals, 96, 203
    lab animals, 531
Bone
    acetabular b., 126
    atlas, 406, 407
    auditory ossicles, 465
    axis, 406
    basihyoid b., 436
    calcaneus, 137
    cannon b., 26
    carpal b., 23, 25, 27
    carpometacarpus, 478
    ceratohyoid b., 436
    chonchae, 433
    clavicle, 13
    coffin b., 31
    coracoid b., 478
    diaphysis, 16
    distal phalanx, 30, 32, 35
    distal sesamoid b., 33, 35
    dorsal sesamoid b., 33
    entoglossal b., 480
    eiphyoid b., 436
    epiphysis, 16
    ethmoid b., 433
    fabellae, 146
    femur, 130, 132, 133, 134
    fibula, 137, 138, 139, 140
    fibular tarsal b., 137
    frontal b., 433
    furcula, 478
    hemipelvis, 125
    humerus, 13. 14
    hyoid b., 433
    ilium, 125
    incisive b., 433
    incus, 465
    interparietal b., 432
    ischium, 125
    lacrimal b., 433
    large metatarsal b., 26
    long pastern b., 31
    malleus, 465
    mandible, 433
    maxilla, 433
    metacarpal b., 24, 27, 29
    metaphysis, 16
    metatarsal b., 143
    metatarsal sesamoid b., 146
    middle phalanx, 30, 35
    nasal b., 433
    navicular b., 36
    occipital b., 432
    of head, 432
    of pelvic limb, 125
    of thoracic limb, 11
    of vertebral column, 18
    os coxae, 125, 478
    palatine b., 433
    parietal b., 433
    patella, 135
    pelvis, 126, 127, 128
    proximal phalanx, 30, 35
    proximal sesamoid b., 33, 35, 36
    pterygoid b., 432
    pubis, 125
    radius, 17, 18
    rostral b., 433
    sacrum, 408, 409
    scapula, 11, 12

scleral ossicles, 486
second metatarsal b., 146
sesamoid b., 33, 146
sesamoid of abductor digit I, 24
sesamoid of popliteus m., 146
sesamoids of gastrocnemius m., 146
short pastern b., 31
small metacarpal b., 26
small metatarsal b., 146
sphenoid b., 432
splint b., 26
stapes, 465
sternocostal b., 478
stylohyoid b., 436
talus, 137
tarsal b., 137, 145
tarsometatarsus, 479
temporal b., 432
thoracic limb, 11
thyrohyoid b., 436
tibia, 136, 138, 139
tibial tarsal b., 137
tibiotarsus, 479
tympanohyoid b., 436
ulna, 21, 22
vertebrae, 404
vomer, 433
wishbone, 478
zygomatic b., 433
Bone spavin, 188
Bots, 243
Bow legs, 74
Bowed tendon, 61
Brachial plexus, 101, 103
Brachygnathia, 401
Brittle feet, 560
Broad ligament, 375
Broken foot, 553
Broken penis, 359
Bronchus, 271
Brown fat, 597, 511
Buck Knees, 74
Bucked shins, 30
Budgerigar, 476
Bulb of hoof, 552
Bull-nosed foot, 556
Bursa
    bicipital, 67
    cloacal, 480
    cunean, 158
    intertubercular, 67
    nuchal, 418
    navicular, 82
    of Fabricius, 480
    of calcaneus, 162
    of superficial digital flexor muscle, 162
    omental, 238
    ovarian, 238, 366
    podotrochlear, 33, 82, 83
    subcutaneous bursa of olecranon, 54
    supraspinous, 418
    subtendinous bursa of triceps brachii, 54
    testicular, 240
    trochanteric, 151
Bursitis
    bicipital, 67
    capped hock, 143, 162
    cunean, 158
    nuchal, 418
    of hock, 143
    of the point of the elbow, 23
    olecranon, 23, 54
    podotrochlear, 82
    shoe boil, 23, 54
    supraspinous, 418
    trochanteric, 151
Buttress foot, 556
Cakala block, 416
Calcar metacarpeum, 547
Calcar metatarseum, 547
Calculi
    urethral, 337
    urinary, 334, 337, 357
Calf knees, 74
Callithrix sp., 524
Camped (in front, behind), 556, 558
Camphylobacter, 513
Canal
    auditory, 466, 467
    carpal, 70
    optic, 432
    hypoglossal, 432
    infraorbital, 433
    inguinal, 345
    lacrimal, 461
    musculotubal, 432
    nasolacrimal, 432
    of gartner, 373
    of sole, 31
    semicircular, 465
    tarsal, 204
    teat, 544
    vertebral, 404
Canine hip dysplasia, 174
Canker, 560
Cap, 401
Capped hock, 143, 162
Cape, 512
Capon, 484
Caponization, 484
Capped elbow, 54
Cardiocentesis, 486
Carpal angulation, 74
Carpal canal, 73
Carpal canal syndrome, 73
Carpal deviation, 74

Carpitis, 73
Carpometacarpus, 478
Cartilage
    annular, 465
    auricular, 465
    costal, 267
    epiphyseal, 22
    of hoof, 31, 32, 82
    of larynx, 451
    of third eyelid, 461
    scapular, 11
    scutiform, 465
    ungual, 82
Castration, 343
    closed, 349
    open, 349
Cataract, 464
Catheterization
    female urethra, 337
    male urethra, 337
Cavia porcellus, 513
Cavity
    abdominal, 231
    cranial, 429
    glenoid, 11
    oral, 404
    pelvic, 126
    pericardial, 277
    peritoneal, 286
    pleural, 267
    nasal, 442
    thoracic, 267
    vaginal, 347
Cecal impaction, 252
Cecum, 249, 252
Center of ossification, 13
    acetabular bone, 126, 127
    carpal bones, 24
    femur, 131
    fibula, 137, 139, 140
    humerus, 14. 17
    ilium, 126, 127
    ischium, 126, 127
    metacarpal bones, 26
    metatarsal bones, 144
    os coxae, 126, 127
    patella, 136
    pelvis, 126, 127
    phalanges, 31
    primary, 13
    pubis, 126, 127
    radius, 17
    scapula, 12, 13
    secondary, 13
    tarsal bones, 143
    tibia, 136, 139
    ulna, 22
Cere, 476
Cervical vertebral instability, 413

Cervical vertebral separation, 476
Cervix, 367
Cesarean section, 369
Cheek pouch, 512
Cheeks, 441
Cheiloplasty, 441
Chestnut, 548
Chimpanzee, 524
Chloroform toxicity, 509
Choanae, 432
Choke, 288
Cholecystoduodenostomy, 259
Chondromalacia, 135
Chondroplasty of the femoral trochlea, 182
Chromodacryorrhea, 512
Chylothorax, 290, 322
Circulation
    fetal, 308
    pulmonary, 307
Claw, 61, 548, 561
Cleft palate, 498
Clitoris, 375
Cloaca, 480
Cloacal bursa, 480
Club foot, 553
Coarctation of the aorta, 314
Collar, 537
Collateral cartilage, 31, 560
Colon, 252
Comb, 476
Common atrium, 285
Common integument, 537
Conformation
    equine base, 556, 557
    equine carpus, 74, 75
    equine digit, 553, 554, 555
    equine pelvic limb, 189, 190, 191
Contagious equine metritis, 375
Contracted foot, 560
Contracted heels, 560
Contracted tendons, 60, 61
Coon foot, 553
Coprodeum, 480
Coprophagy, 522
Corium, 537
Corn, 560
Cornea, 458
Corneal ulcer, 465
Coronet, 549
Corpus Cavernosum, 352
Cow-hocked, 189
Crab-eating macaque, 524
Cranial drawer sign, 179
Cribriform plate, 433
Cricetulus griseus, 512
Cricoid cartilage, 451
Crop, 480

Cryptorchid, 344
Cuneus ungulae, 552
Curb, 187
Curby conformation, 189, 190
Cut out under the knees, 74
Cynomologus monkey, 524
Cysterna chyli, 323
Cystocentesis, 334
Cystography, 334
Debeaking, 473
Declawing, 82
Dehorning, 436
Dens in dente, 386
Dental aging
    dog, 382, 384
    goat, 391
    horse, 393, 394
    ox, 390
    sheep, 390
Dental formulae, 380, 381
Dental pad, 387
Dental star, 391
Dentistry, 401
Dentition
    carnivores, 382
    horse, 386
    in wear, 390, 393, 401
    level, 387, 401
    pig, 386, 492
    ruminants, 387
    terms applied to, 380
Dermatome
    pelvic limb, 223, 226
    thoracic limb, 119, 120
Dermis, 537
Descent of the testes, 347
DeVita pin, 172
Dewclaw, 30
Dewlap, 537
Dextrocardia, 286
Diaphragm, 286
Diaphragmatic hernia, 288
Dioctophyma renale, 331
Directional terms, 2, 3
Dirofilariasis, 281, 308
Displacement (in fractures), 131, 134
Diverticulum
    cornual, 444
    gastric, 242, 494
    Meckel's, 480
    nasal, 442
    nuchal, 444
    of auditory tube, 449
    pharyngeal, 494
    postorbital, 444
    preputial, 501, 503
    suburethral, 373, 501
Dog-style locomotion, 151

Dorsal buckling, 60
Double aortic arch, 314
Double caudal vena cava, 315
Double cranial vena cava, 315
Duodenum, 248
Downer cow, 210
Drawer sign, 179
Dropped sole, 556
Dubbing, 476
Duct
    accessory pancreatic d., 260
    bile d., 259
    common hepatic d., 259
    cystic d., 257, 259
    cystoenteric d., 482
    deferential d., 344
    efferential d., 341
    ejaculatory d., 344
    hepatic d., 259
    hepatocystic d., 259
    hepatoenteric d., 482
    lactiferous d., 544
    mandibular d., 440
    mesonephric d., 367
    nasolacrimal d., 461
    of epididymis, 341
    of the anal sac, 256
    pancreatic d., 260
    papillary d., 544
    paramesonephric d., 345
    parotid d., 439
    salivary d., 439, 440
    Santorini's, 260 d.
    sublingual d., 440
    thoracic d., 289, 322
    tracheal d., 322
    Wirsung's d., 260
    Wolffian d., 367
    zygomatic d., 439
Ductus deferens, 344
Ductus venosus, 309
Duodenum, 248
Dural ossification, 414
Ear, 465, 466
Ear trim, 467
Ectopia cordis, 286
Ectopic ureter, 331, 335
Ectropion, 461
Egg bound, 485
Ejaculation, 358
Enamel spot, 391
Enosotosis, 135
Enterotomy, 249
Entoglossal bone, 480
Entropion, 461
Enucleation, 461
Epidermis, 537
Epididymis, 341

Epididymitis, 343
Epidural anesthesia
    high (cranial), 414
    low (caudal), 414
    lumbar, 415
Epiglottis, 451
Epilepsy (gerbil), 519
Epiphyseal cartilage, 22
Epiphysiolysis, 490
Epoophoron, 367
Ergot, 547
Esophagus, 288
Epispadia, 336
Eustachian auditory tube, 449, 465
External ear, 465
Exungulation, 121
Eye, 458, 459
Eyelid, 461
facial paralysis, 458
Farquharson block, 416
Fascia
    fascia lata, 151
    orbital, 460
Feather, 471
    disorders, 473
    types, 471
Feline urological syndrome, 337
Femoral triangle, 157
Femoropatellar desmotomy, 182
Fenestration
    of intervertebral disc, 424
    of mediastinum, 270
Fibroma, 561
Fibrotic myopathy, 156
Fistulous withers, 481
Fabella, 146
Flat foot, 556
Flexion bandage, 172
Flexor deformity, 60, 61
Flexor retinaculum, 73
Flexure
    colic, 253
    diaphragmatic, 253
    duodenal, 248
    duodenojejunal, 248
    pelvic, 253
    sigmoid, 354
    sternal, 253
Foot axis, 553, 554
Foot rot, 561
Foramen
    alar for., 432
    cribriform for., 433
    epiploic for., 238, 240
    foramen lacernum, 429
    foramen magnum, 432
    foramen of sole, 31
    foramen orbitorotundum, 432
    foramen ovale, 308
    foramen triosseum, 478, 479
    greater sciatic for., 167
    infraorbital for., 433
    intervertebral for., 404
    jugular for., 429
    lacrimal for., 433
    lesser sciatic for., 167
    mandibular for., 436
    maxillary for., 433
    mental for., 433
    nutrient for., 134
    obturator for., 125
    oval for., 432
    palatine for., 429
    round for., 432
    sacral for., 408
    sciatic for., 167, 168
    stylomastoid for., 433
    supracondylar for., 16
    supratrochlear for., 16
    vertebral for., 404
Fossa
    acetabular, 125
    clitoridis, 375
    coronoid, 16
    extensor, 130, 134, 135
    infraspinous, 11
    Ovulation, 363
    of gallbladder, 256
    of glans penis, 354
    olecranon, 16
    paralumbar, 236
    pterygopalatine, 429
    radial, 16
    supracondylar, 130
    sypraspinous, 11
    temporal, 429
    trochanteric, 130, 131
Fossa ovalis, 277
Founder, 560
Fracture
    accessory carpal bone, 73
    chip, 73
    displacement in, 131
    femoral head, 176
    femoral shaft, 131
    overriding in, 131
    proximal phalanx, 36, 79
    proximal sesamoid bone, 36, 79
    pelvis, 126
    proximal phalanx, 79
    scapula, 13
    slab, 73
    splint, 26
    "T" (humeral condyle), 14, 16
    "Y" (humeral condyle), 14, 16
Fragmented coronoid process, 22, 69

Frog, 552
Frontal process (of turkey), 476
Full mouth, 401
Furcula, 478
Furstenberg's rosette, 545
Furstenberg's venous ring, 545
Gallbladder, 259
Galvayne's groove, 400
Ganglion
    cervicothoracic, 289
    middle cervical, 289
    stellate, 289
Gastric distension, 243
Gastric torsion, 243
Gastrotomy, 242
Gemination, 386
Gerbil, 518
Gizzard, 480
Gland
    abdominal sebaceous, 519
    adrenal, 236
    anal, 255
    Bartholin, 373
    bulbourethral, 351
    carpal, 540
    caudal, 540
    ceruminous, 542
    chin, 540
    ciliary, 461
    circumanal, 255, 542
    circumoral, 540
    coccygeal, 540
    coagulating, 508, 510
    dorsal buccal, 439
    extraorbital lacrimal, 511
    Harder's, 464, 507
    hip, 512
    horn, 540
    inguinal, 520
    lacrimal, 461
    mammary, 542
    mandibular, 440
    Meibomian, 461
    mental, 540
    of anal sac, 255, 542
    of infraorbital sinus, 540
    of inguinal sinus, 540
    of interdigital sinus, 540
    of Moll, 461
    of nasal skin, 542
    of skin, 540, 541
    of the paranal sinus, 255, 542
    of the third eyelid, 461
    of Zeis, 461
    parathyroid, 486, 504
    parotid, 439
    preputial, 542
    prostate, 349
    salivary, 439
    subcaudal, 542
    sublingual, 440
    suprarenal, 236
    tarsal, 461
    thyroid, 501
    uropygial, 473
    vesicular, 351
    vestibular, 373
    zygomatic, 439
Glaucoma, 464
Goat knees, 74
Goose-step, 110
Gorman approach, 131, 133, 173
Gravel, 560
Great ape, 524
Green osselet, 81
Groove (sulcus)
    abomasal, 247
    brachial, 13
    coronary, 277
    extensor, 136
    Galvayne's, 400
    gastric, 247
    intermammary, 542
    intertubercular, 13
    interventricular, 277
    jugular, 43
    longitudinal
        metacarpal bone, 26
        metatarsal bone, 144
    obturator, 126
    omasal, 247
    of rumen, 243
    on lateral malleolus, 137
    on radius, 18
    parietal (horse), 32
    reticular, 247
    ruminoreticular, 243
Gubernaculum, 347
Guinea pig, 513
Guttural pouch, 449
Hair, 539
    arrangement, 539
    color, 539
    types, 539
Hamster, 512
Hardware disease, 246
Hare, 520
Harelip, 498, 520
Haustra, 252, 253
Head
    of a long bone, 22
    skull, 429
Heart, 277
    auscultation, 279
    developmental anomalies, 285
    radiography, 281

Heel crack, 561
Heel, 552
Hemal arch, 410, 411
Hemal node, 321
Heamtoma
    aural, 467
    of penis, 359
    perivaginal, 372
Hemilaminectomy, 424
Hemivertebra, 410
Hepatectomy, 258
Hermaphroditism, 501
Hernia
    diaphragmatic, 288
    inguinal, 345
    scrotal, 345
    umbilical, 236
Herpes "B" virus, 525
Hibernation, 513
Hip dysplasia, 174
Hoof, 549, 561
Hoof-bound, 560
Hook, 125
Horn, 548
Horner's syndrome, 465
Hyobranchial apparatus, 480
Hydronephrosis, 331
Hymen, 372
Hypertrophic osteoarthropathy, 33
Hypertrophic osteodystrophy, 23
Hypodermis, 537
Hypospadia, 336
Ileum, 248
Ilium, 125
Imbrication, 182
Impaction, 252
In lay, 473
Incision
    flank, 236
    grid, 236
    intercostal, 270, 298
    midline, 234, 235
    midsternal, 271
    paracostal, 234, 236
    paralumbar, 236
    paramedian, 234, 235
        pararectus, 236
        perrectus, 236
    parapatellar, 182
    scrotal, 343
    transthoracic, 271
Incontinence (urinary), 335
Incus, 465
Infectious pododermatitis, 561
Infrapatellar fat (pad), 181
Infundibulum (of oviduct), 485
Infundibulum (of equine incisor), 391
Inguinal canal, 345

Inguinal hernia, 345
Inguinal ring. 345
Inner ear, 465
Insufficiency of heart valves, 279
Integumentary modifications, 538
Integumentary system, 537
Intercostal space, 267
Interrupted aortic arch, 315
Intersexuality, 501
Interventricular septal defect, 285
Intervertebral disc, 413, 416, 424
    fenestration of, 424
Intervertebral disc disease, 410
    corrective surgery, 424
    radiography, 410
Intestinal anastomosis, 249
Intramedullary pinning
    humerus, 14, 17
    manipulations of hip during, 173
    normalgrade, 16
    retrograde, 16, 131
Intramuscular injections, 155, 218
Intravenous regional anesthsia, 208
Intussusception, 252
Inverted "L" block, 416
Iris, 460
Ischial callosity, 522
Isthmus of oviduct, 485
Jejunoileum, 480
Jejunum, 248
Jird, 518
Joint
    antebrachiocarpal jt., 70
    atlantoaxial jt., 413
    calcaneoquartal jt., 186
    carpal jt., 69, 71
    carpometacarpal jt., 70
    centrodistal jt., 186
    coffin jt., 82
    coxal jt., 169
    "coxofemoral" jt., 169
    cubital jt., 68
    distal interphalangeal jt., 81
    elbow jt., 68
    femoropatellar jt., 177
    femorotibial jt., 176
    fetlock jt., 81
    genual jt., 176
    hip jt., 169
    humeral jt., 67
    humeroradioulnar jt., 68
    intercarpal jt., 70
    intermetacarpal jt., 74
    intermetatarsal jt., 189
    intertarsal jt., 183
        distal, 186
        proximal, 186
    luxation (see individual jt.)

metacarpophalangeal jt., 77
metatarsophalangeal jt., 189
middle carpal jt., 70
of pelvic limb, 167
of thoracic limb, 67
of vertebral column, 416, 425
pastern jt., 81
pouch, 187
proximal interphalangeal jt., 81
radiocarpal jt., 70
radiography
    carpal jt., 70
    coxal jt., 174
    cubital jt., 68
    genual jt., 181
    shoulder jt., 68
    tarsal jt., 188
radioulnar jt., 69
    distal, 69
    proximal, 69
sac, 181
sacroiliac jt., 167
scapulohumeral jt., 67
shoulder jt., 67
stifle jt., 176
talocalcaneal jt., 183
talocalcaneocentral jt., 183
talocrural jt., 183
tarsal jt., 183, 184, 165
tarsocrural jt., 183
tarsometatarsal jt., 186
tibiofibular jt., 183
tibiotarsal jt., 183
ulnocarpal jt., 70
Jugular groove, 43
Jugular trunks, 322
Keel, 478
Keratoconjunctivitis, 439, 464
Keratoplasty, 465
Kidney, 325
    biopsy, 330
    location, 325
    size, 300
Kinky tail, 490
Knee, 70
Knee narrow, 74
Knee sprung, 74
Knemidocoptes mites, 473
Knock knees, 74
Knowle's toggle pin, 172
Kyphosis, 410
Laboratory animals, 507
    anatomic data, 527
    biochemical values, 534
    biological data, 528
    blood collection, 531
    hematological values, 533
    male reproductive system, 532

    sexual determination, 523, 530
Lacertus fibrosus, 51
Lacrimal apparatus, 461, 462
Lacrimal sac, 461
Large intestine, 249
Lamina, 549
Laminectomy, 424
Laminitis, 33, 560
Large colon, 253
Larynx, 451
Laryngeal hemiplegia, 289, 452
Laryngeal mound, 482
Laryngopharynx, 450
Laryngospasm, 451
Lateral ventricle, 451
Lee-Boot effect, 508
Legg-Calve-Perthe's disease, 176
Lens, 460
Level foot, 553
Ligament
    accessory lig. of deep dig. flexor mm., 60, 62
    accessory lig. of femur, 169
    accessory lig. of sup. dig. flexor mm., 60, 62
    anterior cruciate lig., 176, 179
    broad lig. of uterus, 238. 375
    broad sacrotuberous lig., 167
    caudal cruciate lig., 177
    check lig.
        of thoracic limb, 60
        tarsal, 163
    collateral lig. (see involved joints)
    collateral sesamoidean lig., 82
    coronary lig., 238
    cranial cruciate lig., 176, 179
    cranial pubic lig., 169
    cricothyroid lig., 451
    distal digital annular lig., 85
    distal interdigital lig., 82, 84
    dorsal longitudinal lig., 416
    falciform lig., 237, 240
    femoropatellar lig., 177
    fibular collateral lig., 176, 186
    gastrohepatic lig., 237
    gastrophrenic lig., 237
    gastrosplenic lig., 237
    glenohumeral lig., 67
    hepatoduodenal lig., 237
    hepatorenal lig., 238
    inguinal lig., 231, 345
    intercapital lig., 418
    intercornual lig., 369
    interdigital lig., 79, 82
    intermeniscal lig., 179
    interosseous lig., 26
    intersesamoidean lig., 36, 77
    interspinous lig., 416
    intertransverse lig., 416
    intervertebral disc, 416

lateral lig. of urinary bladder, 238
ligamentum arteriosum, 309
ligamentum venosum, 309
long plantar lig., 186
median lig. of urinary bladder, 238, 334
meniscal ligg., 177
meniscofemoral lig., 177
nuchal lig., 416, 418, 421
of accessory carpal bone, 73
of distal sesamoid bone
of ergot, 113, 547
of femoral head, 131, 169
of head of fibula
of manus of horse, 78, 80
of manus of ox, 84
of ungual cartilages, 78
olecranon lig., 69
orbital lig., 432
palmar lig.
    metacarpophalangeal jt., 77
    proximal interphalangeal jt., 81
palmar annular lig., 36
patellar ligg., 177
phalangosesamoidean lig., 85
posterior cruciate lig., 177
proper lig. of ovary, 363
proximal digital annular lig., 85
proximal interdigital lig., 82, 84
proximal sesamoidean lig., 64
pulmonary lig., 267
radial annular lig., 69
radioulnar lig., 69
round lig. of liver, 256, 369
round lig. of urinary bladder, 309
round lig. of uterus, 367
sacroiliac lig., 167
sacrosciatic lig., 167
sacrotuberous lig., 167
sesamoidean lig., 77, 82
supraspinous lig., 416
suspensory lig., 36, 64, 78
suspensory lig. of distal sesamoid bone, 82
suspensory lig. of ovary, 238
tibial collateral lig., 176, 186
tibiofibular ligg., 183
transverse acetabular lig., 169
transverse lig. of genual joint, 179
transverse humeral lig. (see retinaculum)
triangular ligg., 238
ventral longitudinal lig., 416
yellow lig., 418
Line block, 416
Line of diaphragmatic attachment, 267
Line of pleural reflection, 267
Linea alba, 231, 234
Lips, 440
Liver, 256
Lobe
    kidney, 325
    liver, 256
    lung, 273
    pancreas, 260
    prostate, 349
Lordosis, 410, 513
Low foot, 556
Lumbosacral plexus, 209
Lung, 271
    auscultation, 276
    lobectomy, 273
    radiographic patterns in, 276
Luxation (see individual joint)
Lymph node, 318, 319
Lymphadenitis (guinea pig), 518
Lymphatic system, 293, 315
Lymphatic vessels, 322
Lymphocenter, 318
Lymphomatosis, 486
Macaca sp., 524
Magda block, 416
Magnum, 485
Malleolus, 136, 137
Malleus, 465
Mammary gland, 542
Mammary suspensory apparatus, 544
Marburg virus, 525
Marek's disease, 486
Margo plicatus, 242
Marmoset, 524
Meatus
    acoustic, 465
    ethmoid, 442
    nasal, 442
Mediastinotomy, 271
Mediastinum, 267, 270
Meniscectomy, 181
Menisci (genual joint), 176, 181
Meriones unguiculatus, 518
Mesentery, 237
Mesepididymis, 349
Mesocolon, 237
Mesocricetus auratus, 512
Mesoductus deferens, 238, 349
Mesoduodenum, 237
Mesoileum, 237
Mesojejunum, 237
Mesometrium, 238
Mesorchium, 238, 347
Mesorectum, 237
Mesosalpinx, 238
Mesovarium, 238
Microtus spine, 507
Middle ear, 465
Monkey, 522
Morgolian gerbil, 518
Moult, 471
Mouse, 507

Mouth, 440
Mutilocular adipose tissue, 507, 511
Murmur (cardiac), 279
Mus musculus, 507
Muscle
    abductor cruris caudalis m., 155
    abductor digiti I (pollicis) longus m., 58
    accessory gluteal m.. 151
    adductor m., 157
    anconeus m., 51
    articularis coxae m., 164
    articularis genus m., 164
    articularis humeri m., 67
    ascending pectoral m., 42
    biceps brachii m., 51
    biceps femoris m., 153
    brachialis m., 51
    brachiocephalicus m., 42, 44
    brachioradialis m., 59
    bulbospongiousus m., 357
    caudiomedial antebrachial mm., 39, 59
    caudal mm. of brachium, 39, 51
    caudal mm. of crus, 161
    caudal mm. of hip, 152
    caudal mm. of thigh, 153
    caudal tibial m.. 163
    caudofemoralis m., 164
    cleidobrachialis m., 42
    cleidocephalicus m., 42
    cleidocervicalis m., 42
    cleidomastoideus m., 42
    cleidooccipitalis m., 42
    cleidotransversarius m., 43
    common digital extensor m., 58
    coracobrachialis m., 50
    cranial m. of brachium, 39, 51
    cranial m. of thigh, 158
    cranial tibial m., 158
    craniolateral mm. of crus, 158, 159
    craniolateral antebrachial m., 39, 55, 56
    cricoaryternoideus dorsalis m., 452
    cricothyroideus m., 452
    deep digital flexor m., 60, 163
    deep gluteal m., 152
    deep pectoral m., 42
    deltoideus m., 47
    descending pectoral m., 39
    epaxial mm., 403
    extensor carpi obliquus m., 58
    extensor carpi radialis m., 55
    extensor carpi ulnaris m., 58
    extensor digiti I et II m., 59
    extensor hallucis longus m., 161
    external abdominal oblique m., 231
    external intercostal m., 270
    external obturator m., 152
    extrinsic mm., 39, 40
    facial mm., 438
    flexor carpi radialis m., 59
    flexor carpi ulnaris m., 59
    gastrocnemius m., 161
    gemelli m., 153
    gluteobiceps m., 153
    gracilis m., 156
    hamstring mm., 153
    iliacus, 158
    iliocostalis m., 403
    iliopsoas m., 158
    infraspinatus m., 50
    internal abdominal oblique m., 231
    internal intercostal m., 270
    internal obturator m., 153
    interosseous m., 36, 64
    interspinalis m., 403
    intertransversarius m., 404
    intrinsic mm., 39, 52
    ischiocavernosus m., 357
    lateral digital extensor m., 58, 160
    lateral digital flexor m., 163
    lateral mm. of hip, 149
    lateral mm. of shoulder, 39, 47
    latissimus dorsi m., 47
    long digital extensor m., 158
    longissimus m., 403
    medial digital flexor m., 163
    medial mm. of shoulder, 39, 50
    medial mm. of thigh, 156
    middle gluteal m., 151
    multitidis m., 403
    mm. of abdominal wall, 231
    mm. of eye, 438
    mm. of head, 436
    mm. of larynx and hyoid apparatus, 439, 452
    mm. of manus, 39, 61
    mm. of mastication, 438
    mm. of pelvic limb, 149
    mm. of pes, 164
    mm. of pharynx and soft palate, 438
    mm. of thoracic limb, 39
    mm. of tongue, 438
    mm. of trunk (epaxial), 403
    omotransversarius m., 43
    pectineus m., 156
    pectoral mm., 41
    pectoralis thoracicus m., 479
    peroneus brevis m., 161
    peroneus longus m., 160
    peroneus tertius m., 169
    piriformis m., 152
    polpiteus m., 163
    pronator quadratus m., 61
    pronator teres m., 61
    quadratus femoris m., 153
    quadriceps femoris m., 157
    rectus abdominis m., 235
    rectus femoris m., 157

retractor penis m., 357
rhomboideus m., 46
rotator m., 403
sartorius m., 156
semimembranosus m., 155
semispinalis m., 503
semitendinosus m., 155
serratus ventralis m., 46
soleus m., 161
spinalis m., 403
stapedial m., 465
sternocephalicus m., 43, 44
sternomandibularis m., 43
sternomastoideus m., 43
sternoocipitalis, 43
subclavius m., 42
sublumbar mm., 149
subscapularis m., 50
superficial pectoral m., 39
superficial digital flexor m., 59, 161, 162
superficial gluteal m., 151
supinator m., 59
supracoracoideus m., 479
supraspinatus m., 47
tensor fasciae antebrachii m., 51
tensor fasciae latae m., 149
tensor tympani m., 465
teres major m., 50
teres minor m., 50
transverse pectoral m., 39
transversospinalis m., 403
transversus abdominis m., 231
trapezius m., 46
triceps brachii m., 51
triceps surae, 161
ulnaris lateralis m., 58
vastus intermedius m., 157
vastus lateralis m., 157
vastus medialis m., 157
Mycobacterium sp,. 525
Mycoplasma pulmonis, 511
Myofibrillar hypoplasia, 490
Myology
    pelvic limb, 149
    thoracic limb, 39
Myringotomy, 467
Nasal cavity, 442
Nasal conchae, 433, 442, 499
Nasal diverticulum, 442
Nasal plane, 537
Nasopharynx, 449
Navicular disease, 36, 121
Needle teeth, 492
Nephrectomy, 328, 330
Nephrotomy, 330
Nerve
    abducens n., 457
    accessory n., 457
    axillary n., 110
    branch to the coccygeal m., 218
    branch to the levator ani m., 218
    caudal clunial nn., 211, 223
    caudal cutaneous antebrachial n., 103
    caudal cutaneous sural n., 218, 228
    caudal gluteal n., 211
    caudal rectal nn., 218
    cervical spinal n., 101
    common digital nn., 111, 222
    common peroneal n., 218
    communicating branch, 112
    cornual n., 436, 454, 457
    cranial clunial nn., 223
    cranial gluteal n., 211
    cranial nn., 454, 457
    cutaneous antebrachial nn.
        caudal, 103, 120
        cranial, 111, 120
        lateral, 102, 120
        medial, 110, 120
    deep peroneal n., 218, 219
    dorsal branch of ulnar n., 112
    dorsal metatarsal nn., 223
    facial n., 457, 458
    femoral n., 210
    fibular n., 218
    genitofemoral n., 209
    glossopharyngeal n., 457
    hypoglossal n., 457
    iliohypogastric n., 209
    ilioinguinal n., 209
    inferior alveolar n., 455, 456
    infraorbital n., 454, 455
    ischiatic n., 211
    lateral cutaneous femoral n., 209, 223
    lateral cutaneous antebrachial n., 102
    lateral cutaneous brachial n., 111
    lateral cutaneous sural n., 223
    lateral thoracic n., 111
    long thoracic n., 111
    lumbar spinal n., 415, 417
    mandibular n., 457
    maxillary n., 454, 457
    median n., 103
    mental n., 456
    middle clunial nn., 223
    musculocutaneous n., 110
    obturator n., 210
    oculomotor n., 457
    of bovine manus, 113, 116
    of bovine pelvic limb, 217, 225
    of bovine pes, 222, 225
    of bovine thoracic limb, 106
    of canine pelvic limb, 213
    of canine thoracic limb, 108
    of digit of horse, 219, 221
    of digit of ox, 118, 225

of equine manus, 112, 114
of equine pelvic limb, 215, 219
of equine pes, 219, 220
of equine thoracic limb, 104
of pelvic limb, 209
of ruminant digit, 102, 118, 225
of thoracic limb, 101
olfactory n., 457
ophthalmic n., 457
optic n., 457
palmar branch of ulnar n., 112
palmar digital n., 111
palmar metacarpal nn., 113
palmar n., 112
pectoral n., 111
perineal n., 218
peroneal n., 218
phrenic n., 288
plantar digital n., 220
plantar metatarsal n., 219
plantar nn., 219, 222
proper digital nn., 111
pudendal n., 218
radial n., 102
recurrent laryngeal n., 289, 452
sacral spinal n., 408
saphenous n., 210, 222
sciatic n., 211
spinal cord contribution, 101, 210
spinal nn.
    dorsal branch, 101
    ventral branch, 101
subscapular n., 111
superficial peroneal n., 218, 219
suprascapular n., 110, 111
sympathetic trunk, 289
thoracic spinal n., 417
thoracodorsal n., 111
tibial n., 218
trigeminal n., 457
trochlear n., 457
ulnar n., 103
vagus n., 289
vestibulocochlear n., 457
Nerve block, 121
  caudal cutaneous sural n., 229
  cornual n., 456
  diagnostic, 121
  dorsal branch of ulnar n., 123
  inferior alveolar n., 456
  infraorbital n., 454
  maxillary n., 454
  median n., 122
  mental n., 123
  musculocutaneous n., 456
  palmar n., 122
  palmar branch of ulnar n., 123
  palmar digital n., 121
  perineal n., 359
  peroneal n., 228, 229
  Peterson's, 456
  plantar n., 228, 229
  plantar digital n., 228
  pudendal n., 359
  radial n., 122, 123
  saphenous n., 228, 229
  surgical, 121
  tibial n., 229
  ulnar n., 122, 123
Neurology
  pelvic limb, 209
  thoracic limb, 101
New world monkey, 524
Nictitating membrane, 461, 464
Nomnia Anatomica Veterinaria, 1
Nonhuman primate, 555
Norway rat, 509
Nose, 442
Obturator paralysis, 200
Odontology, 379
Off level foot, 556
Old world monkey, 522
Omasum, 247
Omentopexy, 242
Omentum, 237
Omphalocele, 236
Onychectomy, 82
Onychomys sp., 507
Oophrectomy, 363
Open knees, 74
Optic disc, 460, 463
Oral cavity, 440
Oropharynx, 449
Oryctolagus cuniculus, 519
Os clitoridis, 375
Os penis, 354
Osselets, 81
Ossifying pachymeningitis, 414
Ostectomy of femoral head and neck, 176
Osteochondrosis, 67, 69, 189
Osteology
  pelvic limb, 125
  thoracic limb, 111
Osteotomy
  bullar, 436
  femoral, 182
  pelvic, 129
  symphyseal, 126
  tibial tuberosity, 182
  wedge, 130
Ostium
  ileal, 249
  urethral, 336
  uterine, 367
Otitis, 467
Otoscopy, 467

Ovariectomy, 363
Ovariohysterectomy, 376
Ovary, 363
Over-at-the-knee, 74
Overriding (in fractures), 131, 134
Over-the-top procedure, 179
Oviduct, 365, 485
Owl monkey, 524
Pad
    cutaneous, 547
    dental, 387
Paddle, 556
Palear, 537
Palpebrae, 461
Pan panisius, 524
Pan troglodytes, 524
Pancreas, 260
Pancreatectomy, 262
Panosteitis, 135
Papilla
    duodenal, 248
    lingual, 441
    ruminal, 246
Papio sp., 524
Paradigit, 30
Paramesonephric ducts, 345
Parnasal sinuses, 443
Paraoophoron, 367
Parapatellar fibrocartilage, 136
Parapatellar incision, 182
Paraphimosis, 358
Paravertebral lumbar anesthesia, 414
Parts of the body, 4
Pastern axis, 553, 554
Pasteurella multocida, 522
Patella, 135
Patellar lock mechanism, 194
Patent ductus arteriosus, 309
Patent foramen ovale, 285
Paw placing, 110
Pectineal tenotomy (myotenectomy), 157
Pedal osteitis, 33
Pelvic osteotomy, 126, 130
Pelvis
    radiography, 174
    species differentiation, 126, 128
Penicillin toxicity, 513, 515
Penis, 351
    blood supply, 357
    erectice tissue, 352
    glans penis, 354, 355
    innervation, 357
    muscles of, 357
Percussion
    heart, 280
    lung, 276
    omasum, 248
    rumen, 246

Pericardial cavity, 277
Pericardium, 277
Periople, 549
Periosteal stripping, 18
Periostitis, 30
Pertioneal cavity, 236
Peritoneum, 237, 237
Peritonitis, 258
Peromyscus sp., 507
Persistent frenulum, 358
Persistent right aortic arch, 314
Persistent truncus arteriosus, 286
Pharynx, 449
Pygostyle, 476
Phimosis, 351
Phrenicotomy, 289
Physeal stapling, 18
Physis, 17, 22
Pig, 489
Pigeon-toed, 556
Pig-tailed macaque, 524
Pin, 17
Pinion, 473, 479
Pinna, 465
Pinworm, 509
Pituitary gland, 504
Placenta, 369
Placentation, 370
Plane (of body), 2
    Platyrrhine, 524
Pleura, 267
Pleural cavity, 267
Plica transversae colli, 537
Pneumothorax, 276
Pneumovagina, 372
Paatsama's technique, 179
Point of maximal intensity, 280
Poll evil, 418
Polyarthritis, 490
Polydactyly, 490
Polythelia, 544
Popped knees, 73
Porphyrin, 512
Portal circulation
    hepatic, 307
    renal, 485
Portocaval shunt, 315
Post-legged, 189
Pregnancy diagnosis
    cow, 70
    mare, 371
    ultrasound, 371
Pregnancy ketosis (guinea pig), 518
Premature closure of physes, 23
Prepuce, 352
Primate, 522
Probe patency (of foramen ovale), 285
Process

    accessory, 408
    anconeal, 22
    articular, 404
    cartilaginous (of patella), 135
    caudate (of liver), 256
    ciliary, 460
    condyloid (-lar), 433
    cornual, 433
    coronoid, 22, 433
    frontal, 433, 476
    hemal, 410, 411
    jugular, 432
    mammillary, 408
    mastoid, 432
    palmar (of distal phalanx), 31, 32
    papillary (liver), 256
    spinous, 404
    styloid
        ulnar, 20, 22
        radial, 17
        medial, 22
        lateral, 22
    suprahamate, 11
    temporal, 433
    transverse, 404
    uncinate, 478
    ungual, 31, 32
    urethral, 354
    vaginal, 347
    zygomatic, 433
Proctodeum, 480
Prognathia, 401
Proliferative ileitis, 513
Pronation, 153
Prostate, 349
Proud cut horse, 341
Proventriculus, 243
Pseudopregnancy (hamster), 513
Pseudorumination, 522
Psoroptes cuniculi, 522
Pterylae, 471
Pubovesicular excavation, 240
Pulmonary stenosis, 279, 281, 284
Pulse, 157, 199
Pumiced foot, 556
Pygmy chimpanzee, 524
Pyramidal disease, 33
Quarter, 552
Quarter crack, 561
Quick, 548
Quittor, 31, 560
Rabbit, 519
Rachiology, 403
Radial paralysis, 102
Radiography
    carpus, 70
    heart, 281
    limbs (see individual bones and joints)
    lungs, 276
    pelvis, 126, 174
Ranula, 440
Rat, 509
Rattus norvegicus, 509
Reciprocal apparatus, 195
Rectal palpation, 370
Rectal prolapse, 509
Rectogenital excavation, 240
Rectovaginal fistula, 372
Rectrix, 471
Rectum, 255
Red tears, 512
Reflex
    corneal, 458
    palpebral, 458
    panniculus, 111
    placing, 110
    pupillary light, 458
Regions of the body, 7
Reingestion, 522
Remix, 471
Reproductive system
    female, 363
    male, 339, 340
Respiratory mycoplasmosis, 511
Retained fetal membranes, 372
Reticulum, 247
Retina, 460, 643
Retinaculum
    extensor, 164
    flexor, 73
    transverse humeral, 51, 68
Ringbone, 33
Roaring, 289, 452
Rodentia, 507
Rumen, 243, 244
Rumen fistula, 247
Rumenotomy, 246
Ruminal paracentesis, 246
Sacculations, 252, 253
Sacculus rotundus, 520
Sacrococcygeal dysgenesis, 413
Sacrum, 408, 409
Saddle thrombus, 305
Saimiri sciureus, 524
Salivary cyst, 440
Salivary gland, 439
Sanguinis sp., 524
Scale, 473
Scissor mouth, 401
Scoliosis, 410
Scrotal plug, 518
Scrotum, 343
Scurvy, 23
Seedy toe, 560
Self-sucking, 442
Semen collection, 358

Seminal vesicle, 351
Seven-year-hook, 400
Sex determination
    birds, 485
        rabbits, 523
        rodents, 530
Sex skin, 522
Sexual dimorphism, 508
Shear mouth, 401
Sheath
    of rectus abdominis, 235
    prepuce, 532
Shifting leg lameness, 135
Shoe boil, 54
Sialocele, 440
Sialodacryoadenitis, 512
Sickle-hocked, 189
Sidebone, 31, 82
Siderotic plaque, 262
Sinus
    conchal, 449
    conchofrontal, 444
    frontal, 443
    infection in, 444
    inguinal, 540
    interdigital, 540
    infraorbital, 540
    lacrimal, 449
    lactiferous, 544
    mammary gland, 544
    maxillary, 444
    palatine, 449
    paranasal, 443
    renal, 325
    repelling teeth through, 448
    sphenoid, 448
    sphenopalatine, 448
    teat, 544
    trephination of, 445, 446, 447, 448
Skull, 429
Slobbers, 522
Sloping foot, 526
Small colon, 254
Small intestine, 248
Smooth mouth, 401
Snood, 476
Snuffles, 522
Sole, 31, 552
Sow mouth, 401
Spastic paresis, 163, 189
Spavin, 188
Spay, 376
Spermatic cord, 347, 348
Spina bifida, 410
Spinal anesthesia, 414
Spine, 403
    ischiatic, 125
    of frog, 552
    of scapula, 11
    of vertebra, 404
Splaying of digits, 103
Splayleg, 490
Splay-footed, 560
Spleen, 262, 322
Splenectomy, 264, 300
Splints, 74
Spondylitis, 414
Spondylolisthesis, 413
Spondylosis (deformans), 413
Spraddleleg, 490
Spur, 476
Squirrel monkey, 524
Standing under, 556
Stapes, 465
Stay apparatus, 189
    pelvic limb, 192, 195
    thoracic limb, 192, 193
Stenosis (heart valves), 279
Step mouth, 401
Sternum, 478
Stomach, 240, 241
Streptomycin toxicity, 509, 513, 519
Stringhalt, 160
Stump-tailed macaque, 524
Submucosal myotomy, 243
Sulcus (see groove)
Supination, 153
Suprarenalectomy, 300
Supraspinous bursitis, 418
Surgical approach
    cubital joint
        lateral, 69
        transolecranon, 69
    femur
        lateral, 155
    genual joint, 182
    hip joint
        craniolateral, 173
        dorsal, 173
        Gorman, 131, 152
        transtrochanteric, 131, 152
        ventral, 173
    humeral joint
        cranial, 43, 50
        lateral, 47, 50, 199
    humerus, 17
        craniolateral, 43
        medial, 54
        transolecranon, 69
    thorax
        intercostal thoracotomy, 47
        midsternal thoracotomy, 42
Suspensory apparatus, 77
Sustentaculum tali, 137
Sweeny, 47, 110
Symphyseal osteotomy, 126

Symphysis
    ischiatic, 126
    mandibular, 433
    pelvic, 126
    pubic, 126
Synoviocentesis (see individual j.)
    carpal j., 74
    coxal j., 170
    cubital j., 69
    distal interphalageal j., 72
    genual j., 170
    humeral j., 50, 68
    metacarpophalangeal j., 72
    pelvic limb structure, 170
    podotrochlear bursa, 72
    proximal interphalangeal j., 72
    tarsal j., 170
    thoracic limb structures, 72
Synovitis, 61
Synsacrum, 478
Syrinx, 482
Tail biting, 504
Tail bleed, 306
Tamarin, 524
Tarsal sheath of deep digital flexor m., 163
Tassel, 537
Teaser bull, 359
Teat, 542
Teeth, 379
    arrangement, 379
    carnassial, 386
    cheek, 379
    composition, 379
    floating, 401
    needle, 386
    roots, 382
    sectorial, 386
    supernumerary, 386
    surfaces, 380
    wolf, 393
Tendinitis, 61
Tendon
    Achilles' tendon, 162
    bowed tendon, 61
    calcanean tendon, 141, 162, 163
    contracted tendon, 60, 61
    cunean tendon, 158
    extensor carpi radialis tendon (rupture), 55
    mineralization of, 479
    of infraspinatus m., 50
    patellar tendon, 158
    prepubic tendon, 169
    subpelvic tendon, 169
    symphyseal tendon, 169
    tendinitis, 61
    tendosynovitis, 61
    tenosynovitis (tenovaginitis), 61
Tendonotomy (calcanean), 162

Tendosynovitis (tendovaginitis), 61
Tenectomy
    cunean, 158
    of lateral digital extensor m., 160
    of pectineus m., 157
Tenia, 252, 254
Tenon's capsule, 458
Tenosynovitis, 61
Testis, 339, 342
    degeneration, 341
    descent, 347
    hypoplasia, 341
    neoplasia, 341
Tetralogy of Fallot, 285
Third eyelid, 461, 464
Thoracentesis, 271, 276
Thoracic cavity, 267
Thoracic duct, 289, 322
Thoracotomy, 42, 47, 270
Thorax, 267
Thorough-pin, 163
Thrush, 560
Thymectomy, 507
Thymus, 288, 322
Thyroid cartilage, 451
Tied in knees, 74
Toe, 552
Toe crack, 561
Toed-in, 556
Toed-out, 560
Tongue, 441
Tonsillectomy, 450
Tonsils, 318, 450
Torus pyloricus, 242, 494
Torus ungulae, 552
Total hip prosthesis, 174
Trachea, 271
    collapse of, 273
Tragus, 465
Transtrochanteric approach (femur), 131, 152
Trephination, 444, 448
Trochanter
    greater (major), 130, 131
    lesser (minor), 130
    third, 130
Trocarization
    cecum, 252
    rumen, 246
    stomach, 243
Tubal ligation, 367
Tuber
    calcanei, 137
    coxae, 125
    olecrani, 22
    sacrale. 167
    scapulae, 11
    spinal (of scapula), 11
Tubercle

    greater (major). 13, 14
    infraglenoid, 11
    intermediate, 14, 16
    intervenous, 277
    lesser (minor), 13, 14
    pubic, 126
    supraglenoid, 11, 13
    trochlear, 131
    urethral, 373
Tuberculosis, 525
Tuberosity
    deltoid, 113
    ischiatic, 125
    metacarpal, 126
    radial, 17
    supracondylar, 130
    tibial, 136
Turbinates, 433
Tusk, 386, 492
Tympanic membrane, 465, 466
Typhlectomy, 252
Udder, 524
Ultimobrachial body, 486
Ununited anconeal process, 21, 22, 69
Ununited coronoid process, 22, 69
Upward fixation of the patella, 158
Urachus, 332
Ureter, 331
    dislodgement during castration, 345
Urethra, 335
Urethral calculi, 337, 357
Urinary bladder, 332, 333
    cord bladder, 335
    paralytic bladder, 335
Urinary calculi, 334, 337, 357
Urinary system, 325
Urodeum, 485
Urography, 330
Urolithiasis, 334, 337, 357
Uropygial gland, 473
Uterine tube, 365
Uterus, 367
    prolapse, 369
    torsion, 369
Uterus masculinus, 345
Uvulectomy, 449
Vaginal process, 347
Vagina, 372
Vaginal tunic, 347
Valgus deformity, 74
Valve
    of foramen ovale, 278
    of heart, 277, 278
Varus deformity, 74
Vascular lacuna, 199
Vascular ring disease, 314
Vein
    accessory cephalic v., 96, 99
    azygos v., 307
    axillobrachial v., 99
    brachial v., 486
    brachiocephalic v., 454
    caudal mesenteric v., 307
    caudal vena cava, 307
    cephalic v., 96, 98
    common iliac v., 307
    cranial mesenteric v., 307
    cranial vena cava, 306, 454
    deep circumflex iliac v., 307
    external jugular v., 454
    gastroduodenal v., 307
    gonadal v., 307
    hemiazygos v., 307
    hepatic v., 307
    lateral saphenous v., 203
    linguofacial v., 454
    lumbar v., 307
    maxillary v., 454
    medial saphenous v., 203
    medial tarsometatarsal v., 484
    median cubital v., 96
    milk v., 305
    of thoracic limb, 96, 97
    of pelvic limb, 203
    of head and neck, 454
    omobrachial v., 99,
    phrenic v., 307
    phrenicoabdominal v., 307
    portal v., 307
    pulmonary v., 307
    renal v., 307
    saphenous v., 203
    second dorsal common digital v., 208
    splenic v., 307
    subclavian v., 454
    superficial abdominal v., 305
    superficial caudal epigastric v., 305
    umbilical v., 308
    wing v., 486
Venipuncture, 87, 486
    cephalic, 96
Venous occlusion, 284
Vent, 480
Ventral slot procedure, 425
Ventricle, 277, 278
Ventriculus, 480
Vertebra
    caudal, 410
    cervical, 404
    lumbar, 408
    sacral, 408
    thoracic, 406
    transitional, 413
Vertebral formula, 402
Vesicogenital excavation, 240
Vesico-ureteral reflex, 331

Vestibular bulb, 373
Vestibule, 373
Viborg's triangle, 449
Volvulus, 249
Vulva, 373
Wall (of hoof), 549, 551
Wattles, 476
Web, 473, 474
Wet-tail, 513

Whitten effect, 508
Whorlbone disease, 151
Windsucker, 372
Wing lock, 471
Wing (locomotion), 560
Wishbone, 478
Wobbler, 413
Zygomatic arch, 429